MERENESS' ESSENTIALS OF PSYCHIATRIC NURSING

MERENESS'

Essentials of psychiatric nursing

CECELIA MONAT TAYLOR, R.N., M.A.

Associate Professor of Nursing,
Syracuse University,
Syracuse, New York

ELEVENTH EDITION

Illustrated

THE C. V. MOSBY COMPANY

ST. LOUIS • TORONTO • LONDON 1982

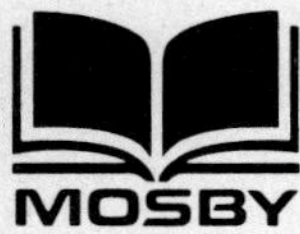

A TRADITION OF PUBLISHING EXCELLENCE

Editor: Alison Miller
Assistant editor: Susan R. Epstein
Manuscript editor: Elizabeth O'Brien
Design: Diane Beasley, Nancy Steinmeyer
Production: Barbara Merritt

ELEVENTH EDITION

Printed in the United States of America

The C.V. Mosby Company
11830 Westline Industrial Drive, St. Louis, Missouri 63141

Library of Congress Cataloging in Publication Data

Mereness, Dorothy.
Mereness' Essentials of psychiatric nursing.

Bibliography: p.
Includes index.
1. Psychiatric nursing. I. Taylor, Cecelia Monat.
II. Title. III. Title: Essentials of psychiatric nursing.
[DNLM: 1. Psychiatric nursing. WY 160 M559]
RC440.M38 1981 610.73'68 81-14186
ISBN 0-8016-4890-4 AACR2

C/VH/VH 9 8 7 6 5 4 3 2 03/B/316

To the
Deans and Directors
of Schools of Nursing

who have worked tirelessly for the advancement of nursing education,
thereby making a major contribution to the improvement
of nursing care of all persons

Foreword

1940-1982: The evolution of a textbook

This text has played an important role in my life throughout my entire professional career. It was first published by The C.V. Mosby Company in the spring of 1940 and carried the title *Psychiatry for Nurses*. The major author was Dr. Louis J. Karnosh, Professor of Nervous Diseases at the medical school of Western Reserve University (now Case Western Reserve University) and Clinical Director of the Psychiatric Division of Cleveland City Hospital (now Cleveland Metropolitan General Hospital). Miss Edith Gage, Director of Nursing at the Psychiatric Division of City Hospital was the nurse co-author.

This book was one of the earliest psychiatric texts for nurses. It became available just as I began a student experience in psychiatric nursing at City Hospital. Dr. Karnosh, who was interested in improving the nursing care of the mentally ill, always gave a series of lectures to each group of student nurses. He was a fascinating speaker who was a favorite of students. I was intrigued by the lectures, the new textbook, and the psychiatric nursing experience. Unfortunately, Dr. Karnosh was shot at his home and severely wounded by a distraught individual 2 weeks after the course began. He was able to give only two lectures to my student group. After 6 months he was able to return to work, but this was long after my experience at City Hospital had been concluded.

I was distressed because I had missed so many of Dr. Karnosh's lectures. Thus it was arranged at the University Hospital in Cleveland that I could be free on the day of his lectures to travel across the city by public transportation to hear the entire series. My classmates commented that I all but stood up and cheered during those lectures.

Edith Gage died about a year after the first edition of *Psychiatry for Nurses* had become available. Her position was filled by the instructor of psychiatric nursing. This created a vacancy about 6 months after I had completed the nursing curriculum at Western Reserve University. Dr. Karnosh suggested that I fill this vacancy. Although I had been a teacher before becoming a student nurse, and held a baccalaureate degree from a teachers' college, I knew nothing about teaching psychiatric nursing. The opportunity of working with Dr. Karnosh and learning more about psychiatric nursing overpowered my better judgment and I accepted the position in November 1941. Within a month the United States declared war on Japan. I was declared an essential worker and frozen in my position. This began a 4-year stint of teaching an ever-growing student body without an assistant or vacations.

Because of the epidemic of mental illness that the experience with the Armed Forces precipitated among American youth, and because so few nurses at that time had had any experience in psychiatric nursing, our students were a precious commodity. Many of them were made head nurses and supervisors of psychiatric units as soon as they were inducted into the U.S. Nurse Corps.

It was not until the third edition of *Psychiatry for Nurses,* which appeared in 1949, that I was involved in a revision of the text. My name was included in the flyleaf as the collaborator. In that edition I was allowed to add only a few comments concerning nursing care at the end of each chapter. Dr. Karnosh wrote in the preface of the third edition that psychiatric nursing had come into its own following World War II. This revision emphasized the shock therapies. A long chapter on syphilis of the central nervous system was included, and a new chapter on psychosomatic disorders was added.

The illustrations were pictures of actual patients, many of whom were unpleasant looking. Some purchasers of the text objected to these pictures. Since that time, a continuing effort has been made to identify meaningful illustrations for this text.

The fifth edition was published in 1958. My name appeared for the first time on the outside cover of the book. A chapter on psychopharmacology and a glossary were added.

The seventh edition appeared in 1966. My name was given the position as major author with Dr. Karnosh becoming the collaborator. The name of the text was changed to *Essentials of Psychiatric Nursing,* and the book was enlarged. This edition emphasized self-understanding on the part of the nurse and the development of psychiatric nursing skills. In 1968 this edition was published in the Philippines.

In 1970 the eighth edition was published. It carried me as the only author. Chapters on children and adolescents, individuals with faulty intellectual development, and community psychiatry were added. Additional case histories were included in each chapter and discussed from the standpoint of the implications for nursing. Each chapter was concluded with a list of important concepts that the content of the chapter had covered. Finding appropriate illustrations continued to be a challenge. In the eighth edition pictures of nurses actively involved in patient activities were included.

The ninth edition, which appeared in 1974, introduced Cecelia Monat Taylor as the second author. Mrs. Taylor completed the master's curriculum in Psychiatric Mental Health Nursing, which I developed and directed at New York University from 1955 to 1965. She and I had similar beliefs about psychiatric nursing and we worked together harmoniously. Mrs. Taylor was actively involved in psychiatric nursing at Syracuse University at the time I had left the field to become the Dean of the School of Nursing at the University of Pennsylvania. In this edition the philosophy was revised, the entire content was reorganized, much of the book was rewritten, and all of it was updated. We attempted to emphasize the fact that a great deal of the treatment in psychiatry was being given outside an institution.

In the tenth edition, published in 1978, the word *patient* was discarded in favor of *client* or *individual.* Again the book was enlarged. Emphasis was placed on understanding the psychodynamics of observed behavior and the use of the nursing process.

In 1982 the eleventh edition of this text will not carry my name as one of the authors. This entire revision has been the work of Cecelia Monat Taylor. For the first time this book will be accompanied by a workbook, the author of which is Carol Lofstedt.

During the past 25 years I have spent many summers, weekends, and Christmas vacations searching for new, appropriate articles to be added to each chapter's bibliography, reading all of the competing texts, doing background reading in current journals, writing and rewriting chapters that were being revised or being added, trying to develop more appropriate illustrations, and desperately trying to meet the publisher's deadlines.

In a sense, the development of this text, which has been published continuously for 40 years and has proved to be the most durable in the field, is the story of the development of psychiatric nursing itself.

Dorothy A. Mereness
Philadelphia, Pennsylvania

Preface

Since the beginning of time, a measure of societal progress has been the passage of familial generations who have had to face the challenge of retaining the value of the past while simultaneously adapting to the uncertainties of the future. To the degree that societies have been successful in meeting this challenge, they have prospered.

Similarly, professions are characterized by the passage of generations. Many authorities believe that psychiatric nursing began as an identifiable and valued profession in the 1940s due in large part to the establishment of the National Institute of Mental Health and the subsequent provision of federal training funds designed to support the integration of mental health concepts throughout undergraduate nursing curricula and to prepare psychiatric nurse specialists at the graduate level.

Most of the leadership in psychiatric nursing has been assumed by nurses prepared through these funds. Now in the 1980s National Institute of Mental Health training funds have been severely curtailed, and coincidentally those who have provided such valuable leadership are at the age of retirement. The new generation of psychiatric nurse leaders, however, has been well prepared to fulfill the vision of the past and to create a viable potential for the future.

It is within this transitional period that the eleventh edition of this textbook is published. As such, it truly marks the end of one era and the beginning of the next in psychiatric nursing. While characterized by a sense of loss and sadness for what was, this period also holds the potential of great change that will benefit not only nursing, but most importantly, the society it serves. Every effort has been made to have this book reflect the value of the past, while simultaneously providing direction for shaping the future.

The title of this text has become *Mereness' Essentials of Psychiatric Nursing* so that the name of the author who so greatly influenced not only this book but also the practice of psychiatric nursing will be permanently associated with this book despite the fact that she has retired from its authorship. She and her wise guidance will be sorely missed by those of us who have been her students and colleagues, as well as by those untold numbers of other student nurses and faculty who have known her only through this book.

Another major change is the addition of a learning and activity guide, authored by Carol Lofstedt. This guide has been carefully designed to correlate closely with the textbook to provide students with opportunities to test their knowledge and to apply the theoretical material presented in the text to clinical situations. We firmly believe that the use of this guide will greatly enhance students' learning in a manner not possible within the constraints of a textbook.

As with any revision of a major textbook, this eleventh edition represents a reorganization and revision of the entire book with the student's educational needs and the current and anticipated future practice of psychiatric nursing used as criteria. I continue in the belief that all nurses should have sound theoretical and experiential preparation in the care of the emotionally ill. At the same time it is important to emphasize that students of nursing who are preparing for beginning professional practice should not be expected to become psychiatric nursing specialists. Instead, they should be encouraged to use knowledge learned during earlier learning experiences and in turn to apply skills gained during the psychiatric nursing experience to the care of all persons. As a result, this edition retains material on concepts basic to psychiatric nursing, which includes topics such as personality development and the process of communication, the understanding of which is integral to the effective practice of nursing in any setting and with any client.

The philosophical beliefs introduced in the ninth edition have been enlarged and included as Chapter 1, since it is becoming increasingly clear that the wide variation in treatment modalities and the complexities of human behavior necessitate a framework to guide and direct the nurse in her practice.

Previously anticipated changes in the mental health needs of the society and in the mental health delivery system have become a reality and are reflected in this edition. Totally new chapters include Chapter 5, which addresses the topic of anxiety and its defenses; Chapter 11, which discusses therapeutic interventions with families; Chapter 18, which focuses on intervening therapeutically with the aging person; Chapter 28, which discusses the impact of the law on the current practice of psychiatric nursing; and Chapter 29, which raises issues that I believe have great influence in shaping the future of psychiatric nursing.

Most of the other chapters were markedly revised or enlarged, as were the appendixes, which now include the DSM-III classifications, the ANA Standards of Psychiatric–Mental Health Nursing Practices, the ANA Code for Nurses, and the AHA Patient's Bill of Rights.

The plan of suggesting sources of additional information from easily obtained books and periodicals has been maintained. Thus foreign periodicals or relatively unknown ones have not been used. In addition, references of several years ago have been retained when they are classics or still contain much currently valid information.

An attempt has been made to delete evidence of sexism in the language of this text; however, this has not always been possible. Therefore, for expediency and clarity, the client is often referred to in the third person, masculine gender, and the nurse is often referred to in the third person, feminine gender. Pronouns in quoted material have not been changed.

Having been responsible for the first time for the entire revision of this text, I am profoundly aware of the fact that it would not have been possible without the wise guidance and support of numerous friends and colleagues. I am also well aware of the fact that this statement in one form or another appears in the prefaces of almost all texts. Never before, however, has this sentiment had the meaning it now holds for me. The reader should be aware that no amount of financial remuneration or professional recognition can begin to balance the tedium, isolation, and just plain hard work involved in such an endeavor. The question that can then be asked is why embark on such an activity? After much introspection I have concluded that for myself the answer can be found only in consideration of love given and love received. Harry Stack Sullivan has defined love as putting the needs of another above one's own needs. In that sense, love has been the story of this revision.

Those who have so generously given of their love are the following:

Linda Beeber, M.A., R.N., whose insightful analyses of the interpersonally therapeutic responsibility and potential of the psychiatric nurse in regard to somatic therapies contributed much to my understanding and thus to the chapter on somatic therapies;

Leslie Brower, M.S., R.N., who assumed the tedious task of reviewing every bibliographic citation for its relevance and accuracy and making appropriate revisions;

Kathleen Hoppe, M.S.N., R.N., who contributed not only knowledge but also wisdom to the chapter on legal issues;

Merial R. Fitzgerald, R.N., and Rose Anne Tietenberg, R.N., who so generously shared their unpublished studies on battered women and child abuse;

Colleen Trody, M.S., R.N., and Elizabeth Neely, M.S., R.N., who 2 days before Christmas enthusiastically took the time to share with me their insights about the knowledge and skill necessary for the therapeutic care of aging persons; and

Betty Hansel, the departmental secretary who was able to cheerfully and willingly type draft after draft of manuscript while still meeting her responsibilities to other faculty.

Finally, this list of acknowledgments would not be complete without citing the unconditional love given by my daughter, Corliss, whose behavior throughout this endeavor evidenced maturity beyond her years.

It is my hope that this text will make a meaningful contribution to the education of nursing students and that they in turn seize the opportunity to engage in sustained human contact with clients through which both are given the opportunity to grow.

Cecelia Monat Taylor

Contents

SECTION ONE

A profile of the psychiatric nurse

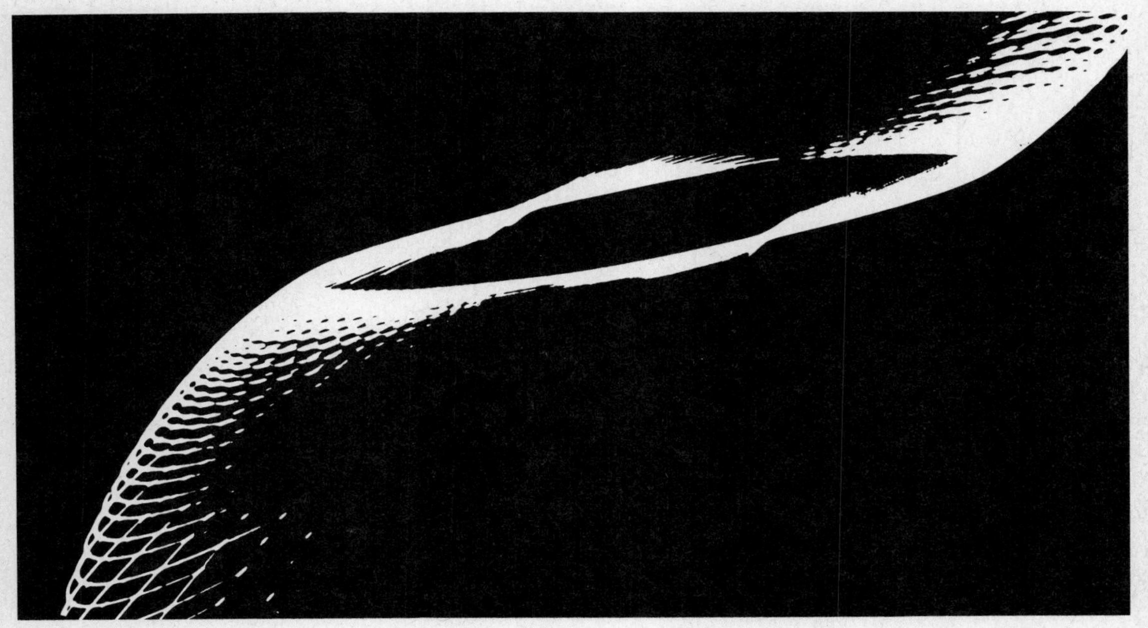

Section One focuses on the psychiatric nurse—her beliefs, her feelings, and her behavior. It is the first section of this text because of the belief that students who are beginning to study psychiatric nursing are most helped by a presentation of a broad conceptual framework designed to enable them to function in providing nursing care to the mentally ill.

Emphasis in this section is on the necessity for the psychiatric nurse to become aware of her beliefs, feelings, and behavior. Generally accepted beliefs, feelings, and role behaviors of psychiatric nurses are presented and discussed. However, since psychiatric nursing is as much an art as a science, students are encouraged to formulate their own beliefs, become aware of their own feelings, and develop their own approaches to the care of the mentally ill. This section is a useful one for the reader to review frequently as subsequent sections are studied.

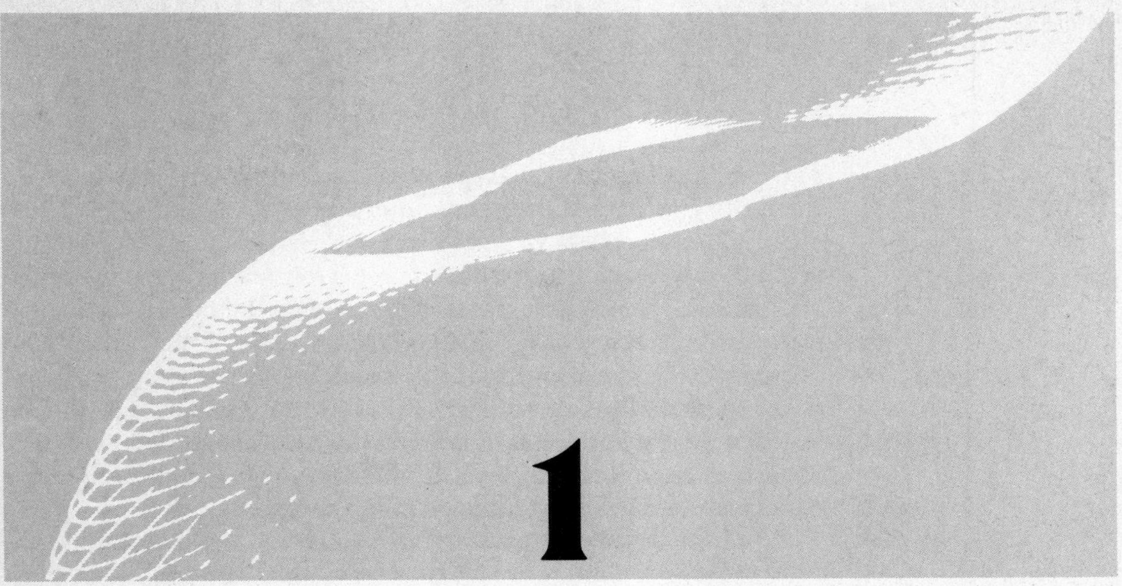

1

What a psychiatric nurse believes: a statement of philosophy

- Philosophical beliefs: their implication for psychiatric nursing
- What is psychiatric nursing?

It is well documented that the knowledge of human behavior and the ability to develop effective interpersonal relationships based on a sound theoretical framework are essential to all nursing practice and should be within the repertoire of all nurses. Psychiatric nursing, however, focuses primarily on the client's thoughts, feelings, and behavior. The psychiatric nurse is primarily concerned with those aspects of the lives of individuals that distinguish them as human beings. This is not to say that nurses who practice in other clinical settings are not concerned with the client's thoughts, feelings, and behavior, but rather that these concerns are not always their primary focus.

To practice psychiatric nursing effectively, the nurse must expand and deepen her knowledge of human behavior and her ability to develop interpersonal relationships beyond that which is necessary for the effective general practice of nursing. This is not to suggest that psychiatric nursing should become an area of specialization on the undergraduate level. Rather, the implication is that psychiatric nursing includes a knowledge base that is sufficiently unique to warrant its discrete study. This knowledge base should be made available to all beginning professional nurse practitioners so that the health needs of society can be met more effectively, since statistics reveal that mental illness is a major health problem in the United States. If nursing is to contribute to meeting the health needs of society, the mental health needs of people cannot be ignored.

The body of knowledge basic to psychiatric nursing practice is derived from both the behavioral sciences and nursing science. Because some of the theories may be incompatible, it is important that a text about psychiatric nursing make some introductory remarks reflecting the beliefs of the author about the nature of human beings and the nature of psychiatric nursing practice, on which the content of this text is predicated. This chapter is designed to achieve this goal by establishing a philosophical framework within which the remainder of the text should be viewed.

I suggest that the student read this chapter first. I hope that the student will find a need to refer continually back to it as the content in subsequent chapters is studied and that the student will reread this section as a summary of the entire text. I also hope that after having studied this text and having had concurrent clinical experiences the student will be motivated to identify and operationalize a philosophy of psychiatric nursing, whether it be in agreement with the beliefs stated in this chapter or not. The student's personal philosophy should serve as a guide in the use of the ever-increasing body of knowledge in the area of nursing care of the mentally ill.

PHILOSOPHICAL BELIEFS: THEIR IMPLICATION FOR PSYCHIATRIC NURSING

Human beings are viewed as complex systems of interrelated parts, the whole of which is greater than the sum of the parts. This view represents a *holistic perspective,* a stance that acknowledges the interdependence and interrelatedness of the parts to each other, to the person, and to the psychosocial environment.* Therefore alterations in any aspect of the system require responsive alterations in other aspects of the system. For example, the student is probably familiar with the fact that a person who is physically ill, for whatever reason and to whatever degree, has concomitant emotional reactions to this lack of physical well-being. Conversely, the student is also familiar with the physical side effects of emotional reactions, such as the stomach upsets, the lightheadedness, and the heart palpitations that accompany severe anxiety or fear. The view of human beings as complex, interrelated systems has relevance for psychiatric nursing. Although psychiatric nursing is concerned primarily with the individual's emotional state, one must never lose sight of the fact that the individual's emotions are only one aspect of the entire system and that the emotional state has a direct or indirect effect on the total physical well-being. It should be noted that mental illness does not provide immunity to physical illness and that mentally ill persons are as prone to the development of physical illness as are other members of the population. Therefore the psychiatric nurse needs to be constantly alert to the possibility of physical symptoms and must avoid the pitfall of assuming that all physical symptoms are simply manifestations of emotional stress.

The holistic view of human beings also provides direction for

*Flynn, Patricia Ann Randolph: Holistic health: the art and science of care, Bowie, Md., 1980, Robert J. Brady Co., p. 9.

viewing the individual as an integral part of his social system, simultaneously affecting that system and being affected by it. This view implies that an individual cannot be viewed accurately in isolation from his family, his community, and the reference groups to which he belongs. Novice psychiatric nurses have had the experience of assisting a mentally ill individual to achieve a more functional adaptation only to be surprised to observe that the behavior of another member of his family becomes increasingly maladaptive. This common phenomenon reflects the fact that the family operates as a holistic system—a unit—and change in one member requires a compensatory reaction on the part of the other members. This understanding is one of the bases of family therapy as a treatment modality. Although not all psychiatric nurses conduct family therapy, all psychiatric nurses can and should analyze the effect of the reciprocal relationship between the client and his family. In addition, the well-prepared psychiatric nurse has a broad-based knowledge of the norms and practices of the various subcultures and religions, enabling her to take these factors into account when assessing and intervening with clients who are members of such groups.

This text reflects the belief that each individual has a potential for growth, that is, a potential for developing increasingly satisfactory methods of adapting to his environment and to other people within that environment. This does not suggest that all individuals have equal potential for growth, but rather that each individual has a potential, no matter how small or great. This belief implies that the approach to the nursing care of a person cannot be determined solely by such factors as the duration of the illness, the degree of regression, or the extent of maladaptive behavioral patterns. Rather, the nurse must look on the nurse-client interaction as a new opportunity for the client to work toward fulfilling his potential for growth.

I endorse the belief that each individual, although sharing much in common with other persons, is unique and has inherent value. This belief is a product of the Judeo-Christian heritage of our society, is manifested in numerous ways through societal practices, and has many implications for the practice of psychiatric nursing. It guides the nurse in respecting the worth and dignity of persons at all times, without regard to the acceptability of their behavior. Thus the psychiatric nurse treats clients with respect, even though their behavior may be unacceptable. Inherent in this belief is the attitude that information about clients is treated with appropriate professional confidentiality and that client problems must not become topics for social chatter. This belief also implies that the treatment methods in which health professionals engage must not in themselves be dehumanizing, even though they may have desirable outcomes. In other words, because of the belief that all human beings have inherent worth and value, treatment modalities that are dehumanizing do not justify even desirable ends. The conviction that each individual is unique implies that the nurse has a responsibility to observe and listen carefully to each person as if he were the only one to whom care has ever been given. The nurse must not "tune him out," even though his story has been told 100 times before. Psychological experiments have demonstrated that each person's perceptions of and reactions to the same situation are always different, depending on many variables such as previous experience and present state of being.

In apparent contradiction to the belief that each individual is unique is the belief that all human beings are sufficiently similar that there is a basis, no matter how small, for understanding and communicating with one another. Harry Stack Sullivan, a renowned American psychiatrist, has said that we are all more human than otherwise. I ascribe to this belief of similarity among human beings and further believe that differences in feelings and behavior are more likely to be differences in quantity rather than in quality. For example, all persons have experienced anxiety, although most individuals have not been forced by anxiety to withdraw from reality as a means of coping. Almost everyone knows what it means to feel sad, or happy, or excited. Those who are mentally ill experience these same emotions, but to an exaggerated or diminished degree. This belief implies that nurses who work with the mentally ill must continuously strive to discover that area of similarity between the person and themselves which will serve as a means of establishing communication. Nurses cannot hide behind the belief that it is useless to try to help an individual because his background, experience, and behavior are different from anything with which they are familiar. This does not suggest that a common cultural or experiential background between a client and a nurse may not be helpful in establishing communication, but rather that nurses must continue to strive to communicate with clients even if their frame of reference is not immediately understood. Furthermore, in some situations when the nurse and the client share a great deal in common, the nurse may make the mistake of failing to recognize the client's uniqueness and of inappropriately attributing to him her own feelings and reactions.

I believe that all behavior has meaning. No behavior of an individual is accidental or occurs by chance. Rather, all behavior is purposeful and designed to meet a need or to communicate a message. This implies that the psychiatric nurse must develop skill in observing, interpreting, and responding when appropriate to all behaviors of the client, not just to those the client or the nurse deem meaningful.

Furthermore, I believe that behavior is a learned response based on the individual's perceptions of past events, especially those experiences he had during the influential years of infancy and childhood when the foundation of the personality is laid. Therefore I believe that an individual's present behavior represents the best possible adaptation he is capable of making at the time. It should be noted that all behavior was functional at the time it was learned. If, however, the interpersonal environment in which the behavior was learned and reinforced was unique or unhealthy, the behavior that was effective and adaptive in the original situation becomes ineffective and maladaptive when the person moves to a subsequent developmental stage or into the larger social system that operates in a more usual or healthy manner.

These convictions are central to the practice of psychiatric nursing, for they imply that it is possible for the client to unlearn old patterns of behavior and relearn new, more satisfactory patterns if provided with an environment that facilitates and supports this goal. They imply that the psychiatric nurse is less likely to judge clients' behavior and more likely to accept it. For example, adherence to these beliefs makes it inappropriate for the nurse to say that the client refuses to participate in group therapy; rather, the nurse is more likely to understand that at this time the client is not able to participate. In addition, these beliefs help to dispel the aura of hopelessness that often surrounds the care of the mentally ill. While it is important to be realistic about the changes any one individual can make, it is inappropriate to believe that a person's behavior cannot be changed or that his overall adaptation to life cannot become more adaptive.

Another belief within my philosophy that is central to the practice of psychiatric nursing is the understanding that an individual learns behavioral responses primarily in interaction with significant people in his environment. Human beings do not exist in a vacuum; their survival depends on interaction with other human beings. This concept is reflected in the frequently heard statement, "Man is a social animal." When one accepts this belief, it becomes clear that an individual cannot be expected to learn new patterns of behavior if he is not given an opportunity to interact with others who provide experiences that are more positive than those he has known previously. As the student will learn, many mentally ill persons have an unrealistic self-concept that often results in behavior that is not acceptable to others in the society or that is not adaptive.

When the individual seeks help from a treatment setting, he has little impetus to change if his characteristic behavior is met with the same negative, judgmental attitudes he has experienced from society. On the other hand, if in spite of his behavior the individual becomes involved with an interested, concerned nurse who values his worth and dignity, positive satisfactory behavioral responses are likely to be elicited. Much of the rest of the discussion in this text is based on this concept. This belief is particularly germane to the practice of psychiatric nursing because the nurse is the professional person who is most likely to spend the greatest amount of time with the client. Therefore the nurse has the unique opportunity of influencing the client's treatment experience in the direction of positive therapeutic results. It is the psychiatric nurse who has the greatest opportunity to provide the environment in which the client can unlearn old patterns of behavior that have proved to be unsatisfactory and learn new patterns of behavior that will be more satisfactory. I therefore believe that the psychiatric nurse's primary function is to provide corrective, emotional experiences for the client.

The beliefs just stated are fundamental to the following definition of psychiatric nursing.

WHAT IS PSYCHIATRIC NURSING?

Psychiatric nursing is the process whereby the nurse assists persons, as individuals or in groups, in developing a more positive self-concept, a more harmonious pattern of interpersonal relationships, and a more productive role in society. The achievement of these goals results in the establishment of patterns of behavior that are more satisfactory to others and more satisfying to the individual. Helping persons to accept themselves, to improve their relationships with other people, and to achieve their maximum development are the most fundamental goals in psychiatric nursing.

The therapeutic role of the psychiatric nurse cannot be described only in terms of routines and procedures, but it also must be discussed in terms of attitudes, feelings, relationships, and understandings. What the nurse brings as a person to the treatment situation is directly related to her therapeutic effectiveness.

It should be noted that this definition of psychiatric nursing does not refer to a specific clinical setting. Today the mental health needs of people are met through the activities of community organizations, including hospitals and mental health treatment centers. I hope that the content of this text will be useful in whatever setting the student provides nursing care for emotionally ill persons.

The remainder of this text is based on the beliefs stated in this introductory chapter and is devoted to presenting to the student that body of knowledge which I believe to be essential for all nurses when they work therapeutically with the mentally ill.

CONCLUDING STATEMENTS

1. Sound, effective interpersonal relationships are fundamental to the effective practice of nursing in all areas.

2. There is a body of knowledge specific to the care of the mentally ill with which all nurses should be familiar.
3. It is important for the student to develop an individual philosophy of psychiatric nursing that will provide future direction in the use of the constantly increasing body of knowledge in the field.
4. The author's philosophy includes the following beliefs:
   a. Human beings are complex systems of interrelated parts, the whole of which is greater than the sum of the parts. This view represents a *holistic perspective,* a stance that acknowledges the interdependence and interrelatedness of the parts to each other, to the person, and to the psychosocial environment.
   b. Each individual possesses a potential for personal emotional growth.
   c. Each individual is unique and has inherent value.
   d. Human beings are sufficiently similar in that there is always a basis for developing mutual understanding and communication.
   e. All behavior has meaning. It is designed to meet a need or to communicate a message.
   f. Behavior is a learned response based on the individual's perceptions of past events. An individual's present behavior represents the best possible adaptation the individual is capable of making at the time.
   g. Behavior is learned primarily as a result of the individual's interaction with significant persons in the environment.
5. With the stated philosophy as a basis, psychiatric nursing is defined as the process whereby the nurse assists persons in the achievement of a more positive self-concept, a more harmonious pattern of interpersonal relationships, and a more productive societal role. The achievement of these goals results in the establishment of patterns of behavior that are more satisfying to the individual and more satisfactory to others. The nurse may assist in achieving these goals by working with individuals or groups of individuals.

Suggested sources of additional information

CLASSICAL

Black, Sister Kathleen M.: An existential model for psychiatric nursing, Perspect. Psychiatr. Care **6:**178-184, July-Aug., 1968.

Schmieding, Norma Jean: Institutionalization: a conceptual approach, Perspect. Psychiatr. Care **6:**205-212, Sept.-Oct., 1968.

CONTEMPORARY

Brown, Martha, and Fowler, Grace: Psychodynamic nursing: a biosocial orientation, ed. 4, Philadelphia, 1972, W.B. Saunders Co.

Davis, A., and Aroskar, M.: Ethical dilemmas and nursing practice, New York, 1978, Appleton-Century-Crofts.

Fagin, Claire: Accountability, Nurs. Outlook **19:**249-251, 1971.

Flynn, Patricia Ann Randolph: Holistic health: the art and science of care, Bowie, Md., 1980, Robert J. Brady Co.

Gedan, Sharon: This I believe . . . about psychiatric nursing pracice, Nurs. Outlook **19:**534-536, 1971.

Rawnsley, Marilyn M.: Toward a conceptual base for affective nursing, Nurs. Outlook **28:**244-247, April, 1980.

Schwartz, Morris S., and Shockley, Emmy Lanning: The nurse and the mental patient, New York, 1956, John Wiley & Sons, Inc.

Ujhely, Gertrud B.: Am I my brother's keeper? Perspect. Psychiatr. Care **17:**204-211, Sept.-Oct., 1979.

OF PARTICULAR INTEREST

American Nurses' Association, Division on Psychiatric and Mental Health Nursing Practice: Standards of psychiatric–mental health nursing practice, Kansas City, Mo., 1973.

This is important reading for students of psychiatric nursing. The American Nurses' Association (ANA) describes each of the standards of psychiatric nursing, the rationale for each, and the assessment factors for each.

Peplau, H.: Interpersonal relations in nursing, New York, 1952, G.P. Putnam's Sons.

This classic book provides the reader with a description of psychiatric nursing. Included are discussions of the roles of psychiatric nursing, its functions, and its impact on various settings, all within an interpersonal conceptual framework.

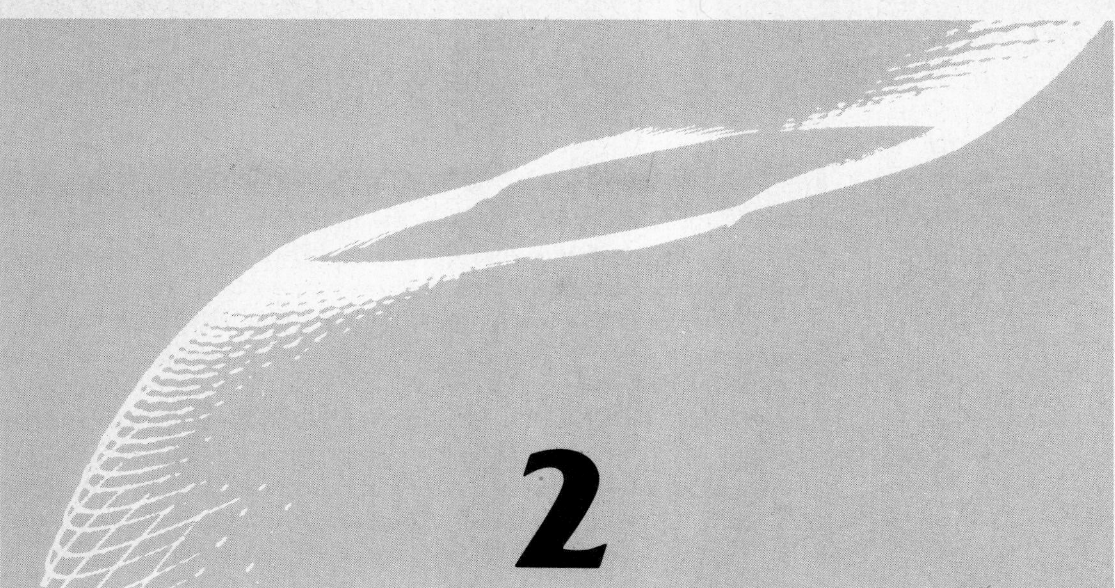

2

What some psychiatric nurses feel: the importance of self-awareness

---

- Recognizing and coping with personal reactions
- Emotional involvement versus an objective attitude

In many ways mentally ill persons are the most challenging group of individuals with whom the nurse has an opportunity to work. In a very real sense the relationship the nurse and the client develop can be one of the most important factors in the client's therapeutic experience. Whether the nurse can be a force for developing a truly therapeutic situation for the client depends on her ability to provide him with new and more positive experiences in living with other people. To accomplish this the nurse continuously strives to understand the client's behavior and the emotional needs expressed by that behavior. However, since it is the relationship between the nurse and the client that has the potential for becoming a therapeutic experience for the client, it is not sufficient for the nurse to understand only the client. In addition, she must develop self-awareness.

The effective psychiatric nurse constantly adjusts and readjusts her approaches, attitudes, and feelings. To do this the nurse gives much thought and consideration to her own behavior as it influences the behavior of others. In other words, the nurse needs to be prepared to make positive use of her own personality, the primary tool she has at her disposal, as she works therapeutically with clients. Many nurses successfully achieve the ability to make therapeutic use of their personality without actually recognizing it or being able to analyze how success was accomplished. However, psychiatric nurses cannot trust to luck in the hope of developing the self-awareness that is fundamental to being therapeutically effective. Although the effective practice of psychiatric nursing probably does not require unique personality attributes or attitudes, it does require an interest in developing a therapeutic approach to clients and a consistent, thoughtful effort directed toward developing awareness of self and others.

All psychiatric nurses will not be able to have professional help in understanding the reciprocal relationship that develops between themselves and clients and co-workers. However, it is possible for all nurses to develop an interest in learning to become aware of and to confront their own feelings and behavior. They can consider their own responses, and they can develop the habit of studying responses they evoke from others. Nurses can develop the practice of recognizing and acknowledging their feelings and examining them in group discussions with other professional people who are also striving to develop and improve awareness of self. Nurses can learn a great deal by studying their own behavior and the behavior of others and by asking themselves such questions as, "Why did I do what I did?" "What do I do that elicits the responses I get from others?" "How can I alter my behavior to achieve more desirable responses on the part of the other person?"

RECOGNIZING AND COPING WITH PERSONAL REACTIONS

Although one of the most effective tools available to the psychiatric nurse is the therapeutic use of her own personality, when the nurse is burdened with personal fears and anxieties, it is difficult for her to focus attention or interest on the client and his emotional problems. To overcome this difficulty it is necessary for the nurse to become aware of these fears and anxieties, to learn to identify their source, and to modify her reactions to them. Until this goal is achieved, it is unlikely that it will be possible for the nurse to achieve the knowledge, skills, and attitudes that will allow her to become a therapeutic influence.

Personal fears and anxieties related to working with the mentally ill usually disappear as knowledge and understanding develop. One of the most helpful ways to view such feelings objectively is to share them with other people who are likely to have had similar experiences. When fears are discussed with an empathic peer group under the guidance of a wise leader or teacher, one discovers that they are almost universally shared by others. This knowledge, plus the experience of examining these feelings objectively, makes them more easily understood and accepted. Furthermore, although helping mentally ill persons through the use of a therapeutic relationship is the nurse's primary goal in psychiatric nursing, nurses who are most successful in achieving this goal often find that they themselves grow in maturity and self-understanding as a result of the self-examination required by the relationship. This very fact is what is initially so frightening to the novice, but with perseverance and appropriate supervision the nurse frequently finds that therapeutic relationships with clients result in mutual self-growth.

Although every nurse will have individualized fears and anxieties, nurses who are beginning an experience in psychiatric nursing often share many of the same concerns. These include fear of bodily harm, fear of becoming mentally ill, fear of personal inadequacy, fear of loss of emotional control, fear of rejection by clients, and fear of harming clients emotionally. Each of these fears will be discussed separately in an effort to help the nurse recognize that these feelings are not unusual and that it is possible to cope with such reactions.

Fear of bodily harm

New situations are feared by most people. Some nurses fear the clinical practice of psychiatric nursing not only because it is a new experience but also because of many preconceived ideas about the behavior of mentally ill persons. Nurses may have heard discussions about unusual and frightening behavior of such individuals. These discussions often exaggerate the behavior that is being described and tend to arouse fear on the part of the listener.

The nurse with these feelings can cope more readily with the situation by acknowledging any concerns about personal safety, by facing the fact frankly, and by examining these fears to discover where they came from and what they involve. As has been suggested, it is usually helpful to discuss such attitudes in situations in which students and teacher can help each other in examining, understanding, and coping with these feelings. This method is particularly effective when the discussion focuses on a specific individual whose behavior is causing concern.

Much of the fear of mentally ill persons grows out of cultural attitudes and beliefs that are handed down from one generation to another. In spite of attempts to educate the public about mental illness, there are still many persons who believe that all mentally ill individuals are dangerous and require drastic measures to control their behavior. Nurses who are being introduced to a mental health setting will be surprised at the large number of clients whose behavior is socially acceptable. They will be surprised to find that many mentally ill persons seem content to be inactive. Instead of requiring controls, many clients require stimulation and need to be helped to develop an interest in the available activities.

The nurse will learn that the behavior of mentally ill persons differs only in degree from that of any group of people of similar age, culture, and socioeconomic background. As the nurse learns more about human behavior and mental illness she will realize that all behavior has meaning, that all behavior is in response to a human need, and that abnormal behavior differs from normal behavior in degree but not in kind.

Fear of becoming mentally ill

Not too many decades ago it was commonly believed by lay people that if a person worked with the mentally ill for too long a period, he too would become mentally ill. This belief had its origins in the lack of understanding of the causes of mental illness and in the observation that many who did work with the mentally ill were in fact emotionally disturbed themselves. This latter phenomenon was a result of the fact that the care of the mentally ill was seen as such an undesirable job that only socially deviant persons who could not find employment elsewhere were willing to work in the asylums.

The nurse of today brings into the mental health setting all the biases and prejudices of the society at large. When the nurse realizes that the behavior of most clients is not as bizarre as had been expected, another fear may be elicited—the fear that she has more problems than the clients appear to have. Consequently, some nurses initially believe that they require psychiatric treatment or hospitalization. Although this may be true in a very few instances, the nurse will learn that most persons enter a treatment situation because of an increasing inability to perform the usual activities of daily living in regard to both work and family life. In contrast, the nurse who is functioning despite the emotional problems she may have learns that the ability to function productively is an important criterion of mental health.

Beginning students of psychiatric nursing frequently experience anxiety about their state of mental health as they learn more about the dynamics underlying mental illness. This probably results from the fact that the student can more easily identify with the mentally ill person than with the physically ill person. All human beings have experienced emotional traumas, anxiety, guilt, anger, and other emotions, but not all have experienced appendicitis, myocardial infarcts, or other forms of major physical illnesses.

Once again, it is important for the nurse to remember that none of the feelings and few of the experiences of mentally ill persons are different in kind from those she has personally known. In fact, the sensitive, empathic nurse will learn to use her familiarity with the various emotions as a tool with which to better relate to the client.

Fear of personal inadequacy

Nurses who are beginning an experience in psychiatric nursing sometimes find they have a strong desire to be helpful but simultaneously feel they are not skillful enough to assume a significant role in the treatment of the mentally ill person. These feelings present nurses with an uncomfortable personal dilemma from which they may seek to escape by developing an attitude of indifference. To allow this attitude to develop would be unfortunate, because indifference is one of the reactions with which most mentally ill persons have already had far too much experience in their relations with family and friends.

At the beginning of the psychiatric experience the nurse may feel that she is functioning without tools, because she cannot rely on many of the nursing activities that were so helpful to her in caring for physically ill patients. In fact, she may feel more empathy for the physically ill than she does for the mentally ill in the belief that mental illness, unlike most physical illnesses, is under the control of the individual. This belief probably stems from attitudes about mental illness that were learned early in life and persist in spite of scientific information. Actually, the symptoms of mental illness usually exist because the individual has unconsciously selected them to assist himself in coping with unbearable emotional conflicts or unmet personal needs. Through the use of knowledge, personal warmth, and interpersonal skills the nurse can assist the client to solve a problem or meet a need. The nurse does not carry out her functions alone or without direction, but she may be the most significant person with whom the client has a relationship. Although initially the nurse may feel that her interpersonal skills are not developed to a level that would make her feel adequate in the situation, with guidance, practice, and persistent study of self, the early feelings of inadequacy will be replaced with a developing ability to help the mentally ill.

Fear of loss of emotional control

Mentally ill persons present an inexperienced nurse with a unique situation. These persons are rarely in need of bed rest and are usually physically well. They may be the same age as the nurse herself or her parents. In many mental health settings the clients wear their own clothing and present a superficial picture of being personally and socially competent. Thus the inexperienced nurse may unconsciously apply to the group of clients with whom she is becoming acquainted the same ready-made standards of behavior that she uses for other groups of strangers. Her expectations may include behaviors she has learned to associate with age-groups, sex roles, and familial roles. She may not be emotionally or intellectually prepared for a profane outburst from a motherly looking client who appeared to be perfectly calm when introduced earlier. The nurse may react to such an outburst with horror in the same way she would respond if her mother became profane. The sarcastic remarks of an attractive young male client are understandably difficult to accept. The young female nurse may react with the same angry feelings that she would have in a social setting. Situations such as these give rise to the nurse's fearing loss of emotional control. She fears loss of control in the client, since his behavior seems without cause and unencumbered by the usual social constraints. In addition, she fears that she will react to these behaviors in an equally spontaneous way, thereby threatening her own sense of emotional control. When the nurse has an opportunity to increase her self-awareness, develop some understanding and insight into the behavioral patterns of individuals, and develop some skill in helping the individuals, then these fears will subside.

The nurse will quickly develop the habit of seeking answers to questions such as the following: "Why does this person need to behave in this way?" "What was there in the situation that precipitated this behavior?" "Where can I find information about the dynamics of this behavior that will help me to understand this client?" "How can I be of more help to him?"

It is understandable and reasonable for a nurse to react with controlled anger to some kinds of client behavior. For instance, it is reasonable for the nurse to be angry if a client deliberately trips her. In such a situation the nurse would undoubtedly speak to that individual about the fact that tripping other people is dangerous. It would be reasonable for her to make it clear that she disapproves of such behavior. The thoughtful nurse would wonder what it is about her that precipitated such a hostile reaction on the part of the client. It would be important to discuss this incident with other workers who are acquainted with the client to discover whether he reacts similarly to all persons or if this reaction is unique and directed toward specific workers. Finally, it would be important for the nurse, in cooperation with other members of the professional staff, to make some decisions as to how to help this person express his hostile feelings in a more appropriate way.

It is helpful for nurses to remember that the reality of the situation is always a good basis on which to develop an approach to any behavioral problem. In dealing with the incident just discussed, the nurse would appropriately place the emphasis on the dangerous aspects of such behavior as it involves other people, rather than on her personal anger.

Nurses who work with the mentally ill are not expected to operate as automatons who do not respond with appropriate feelings. Actually, the nurse who is rigidly controlling her personal behavior and her emotional responses will probably find it difficult to develop a helping relationship with mentally ill persons. The mentally ill need nurses who understand their own emotional reactions and who can analyze situations, determine how their emotions contribute to the situation, and identify the part the client's feelings are contributing. Clients can accept and learn from the nurse who responds emotionally in a sincere, genuine, and appropriate way.

Many clients have difficulty separating their thoughts and feelings from their actions. That is to say, many mentally ill persons believe that to feel or think negatively about someone results in harm to the person at whom these feelings and thoughts are directed. If the nurse expresses to the client only positive feelings about his behavior even when his behavior does not warrant these feelings, she is indirectly supporting the belief that there is something dangerous about expressing negative feelings. Conversely, the client can learn in an experiential way from the nurse's behavior toward him that *he* can still be accepted and valued by her even if his *behavior* is unacceptable to her.

Fear of rejection

Health care workers want to be liked by their clients. A large part of the satisfaction a nurse derives from her work comes from client approval and gratitude. Physically ill patients are usually ready and willing to accept the nurse. They often bring readymade attitudes to the hospital that encourage the immediate development of a cooperative, friendly relationship. Such patients often help bridge the gap that sometimes exists between strangers so that a relationship is usually established without too much thought having been given to this aspect of the patient's care.

In contrast, mentally ill persons, even when they are seeking help, may be shy, suspicious, withdrawn, and preoccupied with their own thoughts and problems. They may view the nurse as a stranger and observe her cautiously from a distance. By actions or statements some individuals may demonstrate what appears to be an obvious dislike for the nurse. This situation is disturbing and confusing, especially to the nurse who has not had previous experience working with mentally ill individuals.

As the nurse develops an understanding of mental illness, her concern about rejection by clients will become less acute. She will realize that some clients remain aloof even when they want very much to become acquainted, because they fear that they will not be accepted by the nurse. A client who appears to be disturbed by the nurse's presence may be misidentifying her. For example, the client may believe that the nurse is the hated woman who lived across the street. A male client may show dislike for a female nurse because he has always had difficulty with his sister; he may be treating the nurse as he would like to treat his sister. The nurse will learn to understand that rejection on the part of the client may be one expression of the mental illness for which he is receiving treatment.

As the nurse learns to know clients as people, as she develops some understanding of their individual needs, and as she develops skill in offering professional help to these people, they will begin to accept her. The nurse cannot expect to thoroughly like all clients nor can she expect all clients to genuinely like her. However, it is realistic to expect to develop some understanding and acceptance of all clients.

Fear of injuring clients emotionally

Nurses sometimes believe that the slightest change in the environment of a mentally ill person will precipitate an untoward emotional response. Because of this attitude nurses may feel that such a person must be approached with great caution. It is not unusual for a nurse to believe that the mentally ill individual is so emotionally fragile that he can be traumatized by an inexpertly phrased statement. These beliefs may cause some nurses to avoid contact with clients because of a fear that they may actually harm them emotionally.

It is important to remember that emotionally ill persons are not defenseless and that they withstand the inappropriate approach of new workers remarkably well. It may be helpful to note that if clients were in fact defenseless, it would be a relatively easy matter to interact with them in a manner that would result in emotionally corrective experiences. Mentally ill persons, like all human beings, are usually able to sense the innate friendliness behind a nurse's approach even if it is not skillfully executed. They likewise are able to sense the negative feelings that sometimes underlie the expertly phrased or executed statements and actions of a few professional workers. The most significant qualities of the nurse's approach to any client are sincerity, warmth of feeling, and genuine caring.

Clients usually have an avenue of escape available to them when a professional worker is upsetting to them. Except in rare instances, they are free to physically remove themselves from the worker by walking away. Instead of avoiding clients because of the fear of harming them emotionally, the nurse can help by developing understanding and skill as quickly as possible. Developing skill for working therapeutically with mentally ill persons requires that the nurse initiate a relationship with clients early in her experience, reflect thoughtfully on the content of the experience, discuss the aspects of the developing relationship with a more skilled and experienced professional person, and return to the client prepared to proceed with more understanding and in a more helpful way.

EMOTIONAL INVOLVEMENT VERSUS AN OBJECTIVE ATTITUDE

"Maintain an objective attitude" has been the theme of teachers of nursing throughout the years. Although students of nursing have been told to maintain an objective attitude, teachers have not always defined the meaning of these words. Many nurses adopt an aloof, impersonal approach to all patients because they interpret objectivity to mean social and professional distance. When the nurse enters the psychiatric nursing aspect of the curriculum, an even greater emphasis may be placed on objectivity in nurse-client relationships. This emphasis grows out of the hope that students will avoid possible pitfalls in the area of interpersonal relations. It is hoped that students will avoid becoming so emotionally related to the client that problems are viewed through the eyes of the client instead of through the eyes of a professional person. It is hoped that the nurse will focus on the client's needs and not on her own needs. It is hoped that emotional maturity of the client will be encouraged by making sure that he is free to relate to others. The goals of psychiatric nursing might more realistically be achieved if students are helped to develop a mature professional relationship with clients. Instead of emphasizing objectivity, nurses could more profitably receive help in identifying the client's needs and the ways in which the client can be assisted to satisfy these needs in a mature way. Instead of emphasizing aloof detachment, the nurse can more profitably use help in becoming aware of her own reactions in relation to the client.

Today psychiatric nurses are encouraged to become emotionally involved with their clients. In fact, many authorities believe that without such involvement the nurse can be of little real therapeutic help. However, it is essential to understand the meaning of involvement. Involvement implies that the nurse is genuinely and sincerely interested in the client, that she gives of her time and of herself without expecting anything in return, and that she is warm and helpful in a way that meets the needs of the client instead of her own. Finally, the nurse who is emotionally involved professionally with a client can help him to develop meaningful relationships with other appropriate people.

CONCLUDING STATEMENTS

1. To be effective, the psychiatric nurse must develop a self-awareness as well as an understanding of the client, since it is the relationship between the nurse and the client that has the potential for becoming a therapeutic experience for the client.
2. The nurse's own personality is the primary tool she has at her disposal as she works therapeutically with clients.
3. Until the nurse is able to cope with personal fears and anxieties in relation to psychiatric nursing, it is unlikely that she can become a therapeutic influence.
4. Sharing fears and concerns about psychiatric nursing with a peer group under the guidance of a wise leader is helpful to the nurse in understanding and dealing with such feelings.
5. The behavior of mentally ill persons differs only in degree from that of any group of people of similar age, culture, and socioeconomic background.
6. The symptoms of mental illness usually exist because the person has unconsciously selected them as useful methods for relieving tensions derived from emotional problems.
7. Although the nurse does not work alone or without direction, she may be the most significant person with whom the client has a relationship during his treatment.
8. The reality of the situation is always a good basis on which to develop an approach to any behavioral problem.
9. Clients need nurses who understand their own emotional re-

actions and who can analyze the situation, determine how their emotions may contribute to the situation, and identify the contribution made by the client's feelings.

10. The nurse learns to understand that rejection of other people may be one expression of the mental illness from which the client suffers.
11. The nurse cannot expect to thoroughly like all clients, neither can she expect all clients to genuinely like her. She can expect to develop some understanding and acceptance of all clients.
12. The most significant part of the nurse's approach to any client is the sincerity, warmth of feeling, and genuine caring that are conveyed to the client.
13. Many authorities believe that psychiatric nurses can be of little real therapeutic help to mentally ill persons unless they become involved in a mature, emotional relationship with them. It is essential for the nurse to have a clear concept of the meaning and significance of a mature, emotional involvement.

Suggested sources of additional information

CLASSICAL

Brill, Norman Q.: The importance of understanding yourself, Am. J. Nurs. **57:**1325-1326, 1957.

Frances, Gloria M.: How do I feel about myself? Am. J. Nurs. **67:**1244-1245, 1967.

Goldsborough, Judith D.: On becoming nonjudgmental Am. J. Nurs. **70:**2340-2343, 1970.

Goldstein, Joan: Exploring attitudes that affect nursing care, Nurs. Outlook **16:**50-51, June, 1968.

Holmes, Marguerite J.: What's wrong with getting involved? Nurs. Outlook **8:**250-251, May, 1960.

Hyde, R.M., and Coggan, C.M.: When nurses have guilt feelings, Am. J. Nurs. **58:**233-236, 1958.

Jacobs, Linda M.: Beginning practitioner's adjustment to a psychiatric unit, Nurs. Outlook **18:**28-31, Oct., 1970.

Johnson, Betty Sue, and Miller, Lynne C.: The interpersonal reflex in psychiatric nursing, Nurs. Outlook **15:**60-63, May, 1967.

Lewis, Garland K., and Holmes, Marguerite J.: Meddling with emotions, Nurs. Outlook **9:**405-407, July, 1961.

Lewis, John A.: Reflections on self, Am. J. Nurs. **60:**828-830, 1960.

Peplau, Hildegard E.: Professional closeness—as a special kind of involvement with a patient, client, or family group, Nurs. Forum **8:**342-359, 1969.

Rogers, C.R.: On becoming a person, Boston, 1970, Houghton Mifflin Co.

Schwartz, Morris S., and Shockley, Emmy Lanning: The nurse and the mental patient, New York, 1956, John Wiley & Sons, Inc.

Stevens, Leonard F.: Understanding ourselves, Am. J. Nurs. **57**:1022-1023, 1957.

Tuteur, Werner: As you enter psychiatric nursing, Am. J. Nurs. **56**:72-74, 1956.

CONTEMPORARY

Aiken, L., and Aiken, J.L.: A systematic approach to the evaluation of interpersonal relationships, Am. J. Nurs. **73**:863-866, 1973.

Benfer, Beverly A.: Clinical supervision as a support system for the care-giver, Perspect. Psychiatr. Care **171**:13-17, Jan.-Feb., 1979.

Gunderson, Kathleen, et al.: How to control professional frustration, Am. J. Nurs. **77**:1180-1183, July, 1977.

Kalisch, Beatrice J.: An experiment in the development of empathy in nursing students, Nurs. Res. **20**:202-211, 1971.

Levinson, Richard: Sexism in medicine, Am. J. Nurs. **76**:426-431, 1976.

McGoran, Saralee: On developing empathy: teaching students self-awareness, Part 1, Am. J. Nurs. **78**:859-861, May, 1978.

Reich, Stephen, and Geller, Andrew: The self-image of nurses employed in a psychiatric hospital, Perspect. Psychiatr. Care **153**:126-128, 1977.

Roe, Anne, and Sherwood, Mary: Nursing in the seventies, New York, 1973, John Wiley & Sons, Inc.

Sinkler, Gail H.: Identity and role, Nurs. Outlook **18**:22-24, Oct., 1970.

Sobel, David: Love and pain, Am. J. Nurs. **72**:910-912, 1972.

Thomas, A., and Sillen, S.: Racism and psychiatry, ed. 2, Secaucus, N.J., 1974, Citadel Press.

Van Devort, Dolores Walters: Both hands clapping, Am. J. Nurs. **73**:999-1000, 1973.

OF PARTICULAR INTEREST

Albiez, Sr. A.: Reflecting on the development of a relationship, J. Psychiatr. Nurs., pp. 25-27, Nov.-Dec., 1970.

This article is especially relevant for the beginning student. The author describes her feelings during her first student psychiatric nursing experience.

Coad-Denton, A.: Therapeutic superficiality and intimacy. In Longo, D., and Williams, R., editors: Psychosocial nursing: assessment and intervention, New York, 1978, Appleton-Century-Crofts.

The differences between an intimate social relationship and an intimate therapeutic relationship are discussed by the author. Included are nursing interventions designed to promote therapeutic intimacy.

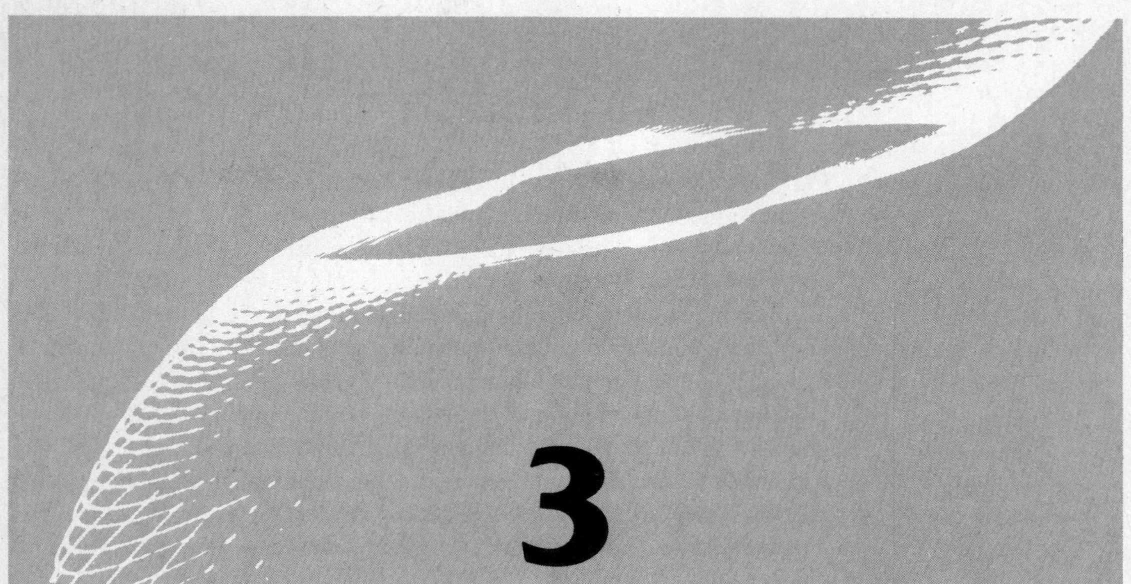

3

What all psychiatric nurses do: the nursing process

- Assessment of behavior
- Development of a plan for nursing intervention
- Principles of psychiatric nursing
- Nursing intervention through role utilization
- Evaluation of nursing care

All too often the same nurse who systematically plans, implements, and evaluates care for the physically ill individual relies on on-the-spot intuitive judgment in administering care to the mentally ill person. This practice is likely to result in therapeutic interactions that occur more by chance than by design, and as a result decrease the probability of the client's attaining a more satisfactory level of emotional well-being. Therefore it is important for the nurse to understand how the *nursing process* can be applied to the care of the mentally ill. Although the terms used to describe the nursing process vary, the process is always an adaptation of the problem-solving technique and involves the following steps of assessment, development of a plan, intervention, and evaluation.

ASSESSMENT OF BEHAVIOR

The first step in the nursing process is the assessment phase. The purpose of the assessment phase is to collect data about the client and to organize the data in a way that will be useful. It should be noted that the assessment of behavior concerns the present behavior of the client, not the events that have occurred in his past. The psychiatric nurse is the only health care professional who is primarily concerned with the current daily living activities of the client. The fact that the nurse's education has prepared her to assist the client to achieve a more satisfactory level of social performance, combined with her unique opportunity to observe and participate with him as he engages in these activities, provides the nurse with the singular opportunity to intervene in ways that could be very helpful to him.

Obviously, for the nurse to assess behavior she must have some knowledge of the client and have spent some time observing him. *Observation* is a frequently used term that refers to an active goal-directed process. Merely standing in the middle of a room looking is not observation. Rather, observation is characterized by the use of all appropriate senses—in addition to what I see in this room, what do I hear? what do I smell?—directed in such a way to collect specific information. The nurse should ask questions such as, "Am I observing this room to collect data about its decor or about the people in it?" "Am I interested in the people primarily as individuals or primarily as they interact with one another?" This implies, then, that observations are planned. Not meant to be implied, however, is that the nurse should not observe phenomena that she had not anticipated. In this regard it is important for the nurse to attend to her own intuitive feelings about a situation. Experience has shown that more often than not these intuitive feelings are manifestations of the nurse's unconscious perceptions that are based on reality. The observer needs to be alert to the client's facial expression, voice quality, neatness and appropriateness of dress and grooming, participation in activities, response to other clients and staff, and many other aspects of his behavior during the time he spends in the treatment setting, whether that be 1, 8, or 24 hours.

To validate the information gained from observations and to determine their significance, observations of the same or similar events need to be made repeatedly. For example, the nurse may observe that on one occasion a client who was unable to purchase his brand of cigarettes swore at the clerk and stalked out of the store. Many people occasionally feel this degree of frustration and sometimes act on it. If the client does not have a similar reaction in future situations, it is likely that this incident is relatively insignificant. On the other hand, if the nurse observes that on subsequent days the same client yells and walks away because he must wait for the elevator, and then later displays the same behavior because his meal contains food he does not like, the nurse would be correct in determining that she had identified a theme or pattern in this client's behavior that is likely to be most indicative of his problems. In some instances, however, behavior that is strikingly uncharacteristic of the client may be highly significant and should be recorded and communicated to other members of the professional team. As the nurse learns to understand more about the meaning of human behavior and learns to know the client as an individual, she will become more skillful in recognizing significant behavior.

In addition to the information the nurse gains from observing, she needs to collect further data about the client from all appropriate sources. Common sources of additional information are the client's chart, other health care workers, relevant texts and journal articles, and most importantly, the client himself. Much valuable observation is carried on simultaneously as the nurse interacts with the client in the role of a participant-observer.

The final step in the assessment phase of the nursing process is to sort and organize the data that have been collected according to themes. Themes are recurring patterns that may have different manifestations but that stem from the same source. For example, the nurse may observe that the client has an unkempt appearance, speaks deprecatingly of himself, and refuses to join in group activities that are new to him. Even though these behaviors superficially may seem to have no relationship, with a little study the nurse will learn that they all may be manifestations of a poor self-concept. The theme could then be stated as, "Presents himself as inadequate to the situation."

DEVELOPMENT OF A PLAN FOR NURSING INTERVENTION

The next step in the nursing process is the formulation of a nursing diagnosis. This step is the same as the formulation of a hypothesis in the problem-solving technique. The purpose of the nursing diagnosis is to provide direction for nursing intervention. The nursing diagnosis stems from a synthesis of all the available assessment data. It is often recommended that the nursing diagnosis be a statement that postulates the theme of the client's behavioral patterns with a potential explanation of this theme and its consequences. An example of a nursing diagnosis is, "Moderate anxiety, related to recent hysterectomy and marriage of youngest son, leading to inability to fulfill usual activities of daily living." This diagnosis, then, provides a fairly clear direction for the development of the plan for nursing intervention. It should be noted that many individuals may have more than one nursing diagnosis. As the nurse gains knowledge and experience she will learn that there is usually a high degree of interrelatedness among the various nursing diagnoses.

The plan for nursing intervention is derived from the nursing diagnoses and includes statements indicating what the nurse will do (the nursing goal), why (the rationale for the nursing goal), how the goal will be achieved (the nursing actions), and the anticipated results (the outcome criteria). Outcome criteria are

Table 1 *Example of a plan for nursing intervention*

Nursing diagnosis: *Moderate anxiety, related to recent hysterectomy and marriage of youngest son, leading to inability to fulfill usual activities of daily living.*

Nursing goal	Rationale	Nursing action	Outcome criteria
To convey a sense of worth	To help client develop a sense of worth that is not dependent on her ability to bear and raise children	Praise accomplishments, no matter how small When client verbally derogates self, disagree if appropriate without arguing	Increase in client's statements reflecting self-worth (e.g., "Yes, I did do that well.") Decrease in self-derogating remarks Well-groomed personal appearance, appropriately dressed

statements phrased in behavioral terms that enable the nurse to assess whether the goal has been achieved. See Table 1 for an example.

The plan for nursing intervention is highly individualized for each client. However, there are a number of principles of psychiatric nursing that should be reflected in the plan for intervention for all mentally ill persons.

PRINCIPLES OF PSYCHIATRIC NURSING

Principles are rules or laws that have proved to be applicable in most, if not all, situations. As such, the principles of psychiatric nursing provide general guidelines that should be used in the nursing care of all mentally ill persons, unless the assessment data indicate otherwise. The purpose of identifying principles is to allow the psychiatric nurse to give care to a client even though she might not yet know him well enough to formulate an individualized nursing care plan.

The basis of principles of psychiatric nursing is found in the beliefs the nurse has about the nature of human beings. At this point it may be helpful for the student to review Chapter 1 in which my beliefs are stated and from which the principles that follow are derived.

A major principle of psychiatric nursing is that *the nurse must view the client as a holistic being with a multiplicity of interrelated and interdependent needs.* This principle stems from a holistic perspective of human beings and directs that the psychiatric nurse must become skilled in understanding the interrelatedness of all the client's subsystems. As a result, the psychiatric nurse must develop effective interpersonal relationship skills while maintaining current knowledge and skill in the biophysiological realm. The necessity to do so is indicated by the numbers of individuals who become irreversibly ill or die from an undetected physical illness such as a brain tumor or coronary disease while receiving care for an emotional illness.

This principle is often cited as the rationale for employing a nurse whose educational background includes preparation in the biophysical, psychosocial realms, instead of a nursing assistant whose on-the-job training focuses only on the psychosocial realm.

A second principle of psychiatric nursing is that *the nurse can be most helpful to the client by focusing on his strengths and assets, not on his weaknesses and liabilities.* This principle is based on the belief that each individual has potential for growth. All clients have some strengths, no matter how few or insignificant they may seem. These strengths should be built on to encourage the emotional growth of the individual. For example, the client who dresses himself without undue difficulty can build on this behavior by being encouraged to choose clothing appropriate to the occasion and weather. As the client learns to make these choices, he may very well develop an increasing sense of autonomy, which in turn may carry over to other areas of his daily living. This example may seem overly simplistic, but it is given to illustrate how this principle can be used in frequently encountered situations.

When mental health care was limited to institutional care, an illness–pathological condition orientation was all pervasive. A client who was cooperative was all too often seen as being overly submissive; if the same client became assertive, he ran the risk of being labeled rebellious. The focus on illness and pathological condition not only tended to reinforce the condition and therefore stifle the client's growth, it also may have contributed to the development of illness. A positive outcome of the community mental health movement has been the necessity to focus on the healthy aspects of the client in an effort to enable him to maintain himself in the community and outside the institution. In many instances this orientation has been even more successful than had been originally anticipated. Some authorities believe this may be due to the fact that when an individual is helped to identify and accept his strengths, he is less threatened and therefore more open to exploring and altering his maladaptive behaviors. It should be noted, however, that a focus on the individual's strengths and growth potential does not mean that his weaknesses or pathological condition should not be taken into account when assessing his behavior. The lack of doing so and the subsequent misjudgments have accounted for many of the failures that have also accompanied the community mental health movement.

Most authorities agree that the most basic principle of psychiatric nursing is that *the nurse needs to accept the client as a human being who has value and worth, exactly as he is.* This principle stems from the belief that each individual is unique and has inherent value. Although the nurse needs to convey to the client a belief in his potential to change and grow, acceptance of him must not depend on his reaching these goals. That would be conditional acceptance and may convey, "I value you only because of what you could become." Most clients have a long history of being rejected in social relationships because their behavior did not measure up to usual societal expectations. Therefore such individuals enter treatment situations fully expecting the responses with which they are so familiar. If they do in fact receive these negative responses, they might just as well not have sought treatment, because they will be receiving very little constructive help. Since the nurse spends more time with the client than any other professional person, she has the greatest opportunity to convey a feeling of acceptance to him. Calling the client by his surname, such as Mr. Smith, until the client requests otherwise is an example of how acceptance can be conveyed.

Acceptance of individuals as human beings who have value and worth does not mean to imply that all behavior must be accepted or condoned as it is expressed. On the contrary, tolerance of all behavior, no matter how antisocial it may be, can convey to the client the idea that he is not important enough for the nurse to explore his behavior with him. Therefore another important principle of psychiatric nursing is that *the nurse must view the client's behavior as designed to meet a need or to communicate a message.* This principle is based on the belief that all behavior has meaning. The helpful nurse will make an effort to convey to the client her understanding of this fact and her willingness to help him meet the need or communicate the message in a socially acceptable way. Some clients have never been aware of the fact that there are socially acceptable means through which their needs can be met. When the nurse helps the client to evaluate the consequences of his present behavior and test new patterns of behavior, she will do a great deal in furthering his feeling of being a worthwhile human being. By treating the client's socially unacceptable behavior in this manner, the nurse communicates that she is not being punitive or judgmental, but is primarily concerned about the client's welfare.

A fifth principle of psychiatric nursing is that *the nurse has the potential for establishing a relationship with most, if not all, clients.* This principle is based on the belief that all human beings are sufficiently similar so that there is a basis, no matter how small, for understanding and communicating with one another. This principle does not mean, however, that any one nurse should or could have a relationship (as described in Chapter 9) with all clients. The student will learn that to effectively engage in a therapeutic relationship with a client is very time consuming and an emotionally and intellectually draining activity. Therefore such an intervention should be undertaken with clients who are most likely to benefit from the nurse's personality and style of interaction. However, the nurse can interact with every client in a helpful way if she continuously looks for areas of similarities between them to use as a basis for increasing her understanding of the client.

A sixth principle of psychiatric nursing follows directly from the one just discussed. This principle is that *the quality of the interaction in which the nurse engages with the client is a major determinant of the degree to which the client will be able to alter his behavior in the direction of more satisfying, satisfactory interpersonal relationships.* This principle stems from the belief that an individual learns behavioral responses primarily in interaction with significant people in his environment. In most settings the nurse has the opportunity of spending the greatest amount of time with the client. Hence she has the greatest potential for becoming a significant other to the client, and through therapeutic interaction, helping him to effect behavioral change. Rather than viewing this situation as a burden, the nurse can welcome it as an opportunity to provide the client with corrective emotional experiences through her interactions with him. The nurse who truly understands this principle will approach each interaction with the client in a concerned, thoughtful manner.

A final principle of psychiatric nursing is that *the nurse needs to view the client's behavior as the best possible adaptation he is capable of making at the time.* This principle stems from the belief that all behavior is a learned response based on the individual's perceptions of past events and that present maladaptive behavior represents an adaptation to previous unhealthy or unique situations. It then follows that if maladaptive behavior was learned, it can be unlearned and more adaptive behavior learned in response to healthier and more usual situations. This belief is one of the bases of the nurse-client relationship.

As the nurse interacts with clients, however, she soon learns that all mentally ill persons feel insecure and tend to cling to their behavior, regardless of how maladaptive it may be. This is because that which is known provides a modicum of security; the unknown (i.e., "What would happen if I changed my behavior?") is fraught with danger and elicits much anxiety. Therefore the client consistently tries to discredit the intentions of the nurse. It becomes important that the nurse not give the client reason to do so by behaving in an inconsistent manner.

If the client can experience consistency in the treatment environment and in the responses of the nurse with whom he relates, a great deal can be achieved in lowering his anxiety and increasing his feelings of emotional safety. These conditions in turn make the client more accessible to therapeutic interventions that are related to his attempts to alter his feelings and behavior. Therefore it is important that the routine of the treatment setting be explained to the client and that the nurse follow through on commitments and promises made to him.

A common problem in this regard is the frequently heard social response, "I'll see you later." To a mentally ill person, this response is likely to mean a very concrete promise. Consequently, he expects to see the nurse later when she in fact has no intention of seeking him out. When the nurse does not seek out the client, his ability to trust her and her word may be greatly diminished. Thus it becomes important for the nurse to say what she means and mean what she says.

Most mentally ill persons, especially those diagnosed as schizophrenics, have often experienced communications that conveyed a verbal message that was contradicted by a nonverbal message. For example, an 18-year-old boy asked his father for the use of the family car to take a girl friend to the movie. His father replied, "Sure, that's fine with me," but then angrily threw the car keys at the boy. To say the least, this situation was confusing and resulted in the boy not knowing how to respond. Obviously, it is important for the nurse to avoid such contradicatory messages when communicating with clients. It is far more helpful to the client if the nurse states frankly that she is irritated with his behavior, rather than conveying that attitude by nonverbal behavior while she discusses other matters. Even though it is difficult for the beginning psychiatric nurse to achieve this, it provides an opportunity for the nurse and the client to verbally explore their feelings about the situation rather than avoiding them. This concept is frequently referred to as congruence of behavior and is equally applicable in regard to positive feelings.

NURSING INTERVENTION THROUGH ROLE UTILIZATION

In the process of implementing the plan for nursing intervention in which principles of psychiatric nursing are employed, the nurse uses a variety of roles.

The psychiatric nurse's role shifts frequently as she strives to develop the environment into a therapeutic situation for the mentally ill. She fills the role of creator of a therapeutic environment when she provides opportunities for clients to experience acceptance in social relationships. Frequently she fills the role of socializing agent when she helps individuals or groups to plan and participate in parties. The nurse finds that she must assume the role of counselor when clients need someone to listen with understanding and empathy while they talk about troublesome problems. The nurse is sometimes a teacher, especially when she helps clients learn to function in more socially acceptable ways. Frequently she fills the role of mother surrogate when she gives emotional support and understanding or when she performs a nurturing activity such as feeding a client. Sometimes she functions in the more familiar role of nurse as she performs technical nursing duties such as administering medications or treatments. Some nurses who have advanced educational preparation function in the therapist role, meeting with individuals, families, or groups at specified times and engaging them in a process designed to assist them in making fundamental changes.

The nurse probably never functions in any single role at any given time; usually she fulfills all or several of these roles at once. For the sake of clarity, however, these roles will be discussed separately.

The nurse as creator of a therapeutic environment

One of the major therapeutic contributions the nurse can make is to develop a warm, accepting atmosphere. Although this atmosphere is related superficially to the physical equipment and decor of the environment, these attributes are no substitute for genuine human warmth, which springs solely from other human beings. If the situation is to be therapeutic for clients, it is essential that the nursing staff members who are in close daily contact with the clients be honest, sincere, friendly people who really care about others. If the nurse is able to establish a warm, accepting atmosphere, the way will have been prepared so that the contributions of the other members of the psychiatric treatment team can be of maximum effectiveness.

A feeling of security is an essential element in developing a therapeutic climate. When clients are provided with an emotionally secure climate, feelings of acceptance, friendliness, warmth, safety, and relaxation are present. Many emotionally ill people enter a treatment setting because they are fearful, anxiety-ridden, and insecure in their relationships with other people. A therapeutic climate should make it possible for such individuals to behave as they need to behave because of their illness, secure in the knowledge that they will not be rejected and that they do not need to fear retaliation.

Another essential element in creating a therapeutic climate is an attitude that anticipates positive change and growth. If the climate is to be therapeutic, everyone working with clients must project an attitude that encourages improvement and positive change in behavior.

The nurse as socializing agent

Another important role is that of socializing agent. In fulfilling this role the nurse helps clients participate successfully in group activities. Physical facilities in many mental health settings are ideal for organizing and directing group activities. In a residential setting, group activities are particularly needed during that period in the day which comes after the evening meal. Many scheduled activities stop before supper, and clients are frequently faced with long, unoccupied, dull evenings. The clever, imaginative nurse who cares for clients during the evening hours has a real opportunity to contribute to the mental health of these persons. Such a simple activity as an evening snack period can be the focus for group singing, group games, or group conversation. Activities organized by the clients themselves uncover and use hidden talent. In this way the group has an opportunity to recognize and encourage its own members and to contribute to developing the strengths of individuals. A dining room situation may lend itself to group activity. In such a situation the nurse has an opportunity to create a leisurely, happy experience from which a feeling of belonging can develop. Mealtime is too often viewed solely from the standpoint of nutrition. Sometimes clients are hurried so that the staff can get on to some other activity. Conversation is sometimes discouraged because it slows up eating. The nurse who supervises the dining room may stand about like a policeman and may view the task solely from the standpoint of getting the clients fed as efficiently and quickly as possible. When the nurse ascribes to these views, she misses a valuable opportunity to facilitate positive learning experiences for clients.

The nurse makes a contribution to improving the socialization skills of clients by encouraging and developing the healthy aspects of their personalities. Many mentally ill persons have used withdrawal because of their extreme sensitivity and anxiety in relation to other people. The treatment setting provides opportunities for these individuals to learn to achieve success in social situations by creating opportunities through which they develop feelings of security with other people. The skillful nurse uses recreational activities, the dining room situation, and even activities centering around housekeeping chores to help clients learn to participate successfully in common social situations.

The nurse as counselor

Empathic listening is another important aspect of psychiatric nursing. There is probably no more important task than listening to a client in a positive, dynamic, empathic way without at the same time giving advice, stating opinions, or making suggestions. This type of listening encourages the client to think through his problems and to arrive at a decision that is helpful to him. It helps the client to discharge anxiety and tension. It conveys to the client the realization that the nurse really cares.

Empathic listening demands a great deal from the nurse both in time and in emotional energy. It demands that she be skillful in reflecting the client's comments to him in such a manner that he will realize that she is interested in the discussion and wants to hear as much as he needs to tell. Some nurses may not understand the vital importance of this kind of listening and may feel that they should stop the client's outpouring of problems. Unfortunately this is easily done by a comment such as, "You can tell all that to your therapist tomorrow. He's the one who needs to know these things." The nurse may respond with the even less helpful comment, "Things will be better tomorrow. Just keep a stiff upper lip."

Sometimes clients pour out problems more freely to the nurse than to anyone else. However, the role of the psychiatrist is to deal primarily with the problems of the unconscious, whereas the nurse deals with reality-oriented concerns. Therefore the nurse seeks to assist the client to channel those problems that are the legitimate concern of the psychiatrist to him. The nurse and the psychiatrist need to work out together their mutually therapeutic roles with the client who actively seeks help from both of them.

The role of the nurse is to help the client with problems of reality that deal with the here and now. There are scores of times when clients discuss problems with the nurse that do deal with the areas that are her special concern, and it is in these situations that her role as a counselor is most frequently helpful.

Among the nurse's therapeutic responsibilities as a counselor is the giving of reassurance. Many situations in the life of a client require that someone give some reassurance. Sometimes the nurse may suggest that reassurance should more logically be provided by the psychiatrist, religious counselor, or social worker. The nurse needs to learn what services are available and how she can help to procure the assistance the client needs. However, more often than not it is up to the nurse to provide the needed reassurance. Such needs appear in every area of the client's life. There is the client who cannot sleep because he fears the treatment scheduled for the morning; the client who is upset because her husband did not visit as he had promised and she is now sure that he does not love her; the client who believes he is doomed forever because he has committed an unpardonable sin; and the client who is afraid of everything. The list is endless, and the needs for reassurance frequently appear at 11 PM or at 3 AM when no help may be readily available. It is for this reason that many day-care centers provide staff members who are available by phone during the entire 24-hour period. Often the staff members are nurses or trained aides whose prompt intervention can prevent the need for hospitalization.

Obviously no set of rules or suggestions will serve as a solution in each of these many situations. Probably the most effective reassurance for fearful, upset clients is a nursing staff that does not change frequently and whose members are consistently kind and accepting. Sitting beside a client may in itself be reassuring to him. This may help him feel that someone on whom he can depend is there, ready to help in whatever way possible. Listening is one of the better ways of offering reassurance. Although logical, reasonable answers are frequently not helpful, they may be reassuring for some clients. Effective reassurance is dependent on the situation, the nurse, her relationship with the client, and his personality. Obviously a suspicious client will require a different kind of help than will a depressed one.

Another aspect of the nurse's counseling role is in helping clients find acceptable outlets for anxiety. The client who is found sobbing hopelessly may be helped by a simple suggestion that she walk up and down the hallway with the nurse. Another client who is tense or excited may respond to the nurse's suggestion that she take a hot tub bath before going to bed. Some other ways in which the nurse may help clients find outlets for anxieties include assisting clients to participate in simple tasks, to become involved in some group activity, or to talk about their feelings.

The nurse as teacher

If purposeful therapeutic interventions can provide the individual with opportunities to learn to live more happily and more successfully with other people, they will make a significant contribution to the client's emotional growth. If the client is merely treated for the purpose of safeguarding his family, the community, or himself, and if he relies entirely on the judgment of professional personnel, it is questionable how worthwhile the experience can be. It is in helping the client to learn to cope in a more mature way with interpersonal relationships that the nurse has a role as a teacher.

Problems of behavior manifested by mentally ill persons are as varied as life itself and encompass every aspect of living. Some clients, like children, must learn many simple tasks involved in living. They need help in learning to dress appropriately for the occasion; to assume responsibility for tasks assigned; to care for physical needs so that they can be acceptable to others; to eat in socially prescribed ways; to accept a reasonably flexible schedule for eating, sleeping, and bathing; and to cope with many other aspects of group living.

The nurse may fill the role of teacher as she helps a client learn a new game, dance step, or song so he may participate more actively in recreation. She may actually take the role of dance partner or may participate in a game to help a shy, frightened client become integrated into a group. The nurse may participate in an activity requiring only two persons to help a hostile, suspicious client learn that some people can be trusted. She may continue to participate with this client over a period of time until she is able to help him move into some group activity without her supporting presence.

The psychiatric nurse in her role as a wise and understanding teacher helps clients learn to participate in more socially acceptable and satisfying living activities.

The nurse as mother surrogate

Traditionally in this culture the nurse has been a trusted person who performs personal services for sick people. Many of these services are similar to those a mother performs for children. Nurses who are permanently assigned to mental health settings almost invariably become mother surrogates for some of the clients with whom they are closely associated. The role of mother surrogate is part of the traditional role of the nurse, and, although it does not imply becoming the client's mother, it includes many mothering activities that may be required for some persons who are mentally ill. Although most mentally ill persons are able to bathe, dress, and feed themselves, there are a few who are too emotionally ill to carry out these simple tasks. For some of these persons the nurse may need to assume the traditional protective, supportive, mothering role when she gives physical care.

The nurse, like a wise mother, realizes that it is important for clients to assume responsibility for their own physical care as soon as possible. Thus she gives physical care to emotionally ill persons in an empathic and understanding way but looks for and seizes every opportunity to encourage them to assume responsibility for their own care as soon as possible. The wise nurse withdraws from the task of feeding or bathing a client just as rapidly as he is able to take over the responsibility for himself. In this way the nurse supports the client's increasing autonomy.

The psychiatric nurse not only carries out the mothering role in relation to the physical needs of clients, but she is also like a mother in relation to managing the house or treatment setting. It is she who develops many of the policies concerning the environment, which profoundly affect the lives of the clients. She is indirectly responsible for almost every aspect of the time the client spends in the treatment setting, from housekeeping to calling a physician if the client needs emergency medical care. The nurse sets the tone of the treatment situation, much as a mother sets the tone of the family.

One of the most therapeutic aspects of the nurse's traditional role as mother surrogate is in assisting individuals and groups of clients to set limits for their own behavior. This aspect of the nurse's role probably overlaps with the teacher role.

Clients who interact with each other over time may react toward each other as if they were members of the same family. These reactions are usually unconscious but are nonetheless real and may serve as a basis for much emotional and social unlearning and relearning. The nurse's role as mother surrogate offers her an opportunity to provide clients with healthy experiences in the area of emotional relationships. She may be able to supply the warm, accepting mothering relationship that some persons require to move toward more mature behavior. She may serve as the object of many of the angry, hostile feelings that some clients cannot admit or express toward their own mothers. With the help of the professional person who is directing the care of the client, the psychiatric nurse may be able through her mothering role to supply an emotional experience that may be significant in the client's total therapeutic regimen.

In summary, the role of the nurse as a mother surrogate is the most significant in providing experiences that may prove to be corrective of the client's earlier unsatisfactory interpersonal experiences.

The technical nursing role

The traditional role of the nurse includes those technical aspects involved in pouring and administering medications, carrying out medical and surgical treatments, and observing and recording client behavior. Unfortunately it is this aspect of nursing that many people identify as nursing care. The technical aspect of the nurse's role is of great value but is not always as therapeutic in the mental health setting as are some other roles that the nurse assumes or is cast in by clients and co-workers. Occasionally a mentally ill person can accept a nurse as a helpful counselor or teacher only after her ability to carry out the technical aspects of the role has been demonstrated. Therefore the nurse needs to be alert to the fact that such procedures as administering medications and taking vital signs provide her with an opportunity to enhance the therapeutic relationship with the client as well as to achieve the goals of the procedure.

One of the nurse's most significant responsibilities is the accurate and perceptive observation and recording of the client's behavior. In carrying out this function skillfully and meaningfully the nurse contributes to the understanding that all members of the psychiatric team bring to bear on the client's problems. Since nurses are the professional persons who are with clients during the entire treatment period, they have a unique opportunity to help other professional workers understand clients' needs through effective recording of samples of conversation, sleep patterns, interpersonal relationships, socialization activities, and descriptions of personal habits.

It is suggested that the client's behavior be described rather than labeled. Instead of recording that a client is hallucinating, it is more meaningful to record exactly what was observed. The following is an example of this type of recording: "Stood near the ventilator for 10 minutes with hand cupped around ear as if trying to hear better. Carried on an animated conversation. Although no other person was present, the client could be heard saying, 'How dare you call me those names! You are a liar!' "

Instead of recording that the client is disoriented and misidentifies people, it would be more meaningful to record the following: "Mr. J. greeted the nurse by saying, 'Good morning, Mary. Have you cooked breakfast yet?' In the afternoon he asked, 'When are we going to have breakfast?' Client believes that this nurse is his wife, and he is not able to differentiate between morning and afternoon."

By recording her observations in this manner, the nurse permits the reader of her recordings to make his own assessment of the meaning of the client's behavior.

The nurse as therapist

For a number of years some nurses who have had the benefit of an appropriate educational experience in psychiatric nursing have been developing the role of the nurse therapist. When the nurse functions in the role of the nurse therapist, the principles developed through the practice of psychotherapy are used.

Nursing therapy has developed differently in each situation, but basically it follows the same general guidelines.

The role of the nurse therapist is carefully explained to all levels of the professional staff and to all clients in the clinical situation. Every attempt is made to be sure that the role is understood before any therapeutic activity is initiated. The nurse works collaboratively with other mental health professionals in the situation and confers regularly with those responsible for developing the treatment plans for the clients with whom she is working. The nurse's work becomes a part of the total treatment plan for the client.

The nurse therapist strives in a professional capacity to help the individual with emotional problems that can benefit from her particular skills and knowledge. She works with clients who require help in improving their ability to cope with the daily problems of living. In contrast, the psychiatrist more frequently works with persons who require help in making fundamental changes in the area of psychopathology or ego psychology.

Early in the initial phase the nurse therapist establishes with the client the ground rules for the relationship. Thus the nature of the relationship and the responsibility of the nurse therapist and the client are discussed. The time, frequency, place for the sessions, and approximate total number of meetings to be held are established.

The relationship passes through the same three phases experienced in the other relationship therapies discussed in Chapter 9 of this text. Thus there is an initial phase of getting acquainted and testing one another, a second phase in which the work of the therapy is achieved, and a termination phase during which the emotional involvement in the relationship is decreased gradually. The length of each phase depends on the individuals involved, the problems presented by the client, and his reaction to termination.

It is essential for the nurse's professional development, as well as for the client's welfare, that she identify a skilled professional therapist to function on a regular basis as her preceptor or her supervisor while she is working in the role of a nurse therapist.

With this in mind, the nurse therapist should record each therapy session in such a way that it can be used to (1) review the dynamics of the relationship, (2) analyze the problems that have been presented, and (3) evaluate client progress against the established treatment goals.

Clinical example of role utilization

The following situation is an example of the way in which the nurse functions in a variety of roles that are sometimes carried out almost simultaneously.

> "Please take me back to the ward, Miss S., I feel sick." Tall, dark-haired, 17-year-old Sam G. had walked across the dance floor and was pleading with the nurse to be allowed to leave the regular Wednesday evening dance. The dance was part of the recreational program for clients. Both Sam and the nurse knew that clients were usually encouraged to remain at the dance until it was over. She also knew that Sam had not made such a request before, and intuitively she felt that something at the dance had been upsetting to him.
>
> Miss S. quietly made the necessary arrangements with the staff member in charge of the dance and took Sam back to the homelike unit. Then she took his pulse, temperature, and respirations to be certain that he was not physically ill. When she found that these physical signs were within the normal range, she suggested that he help her make some sandwiches. Together they went into the kitchen where they prepared a snack for the other clients who would soon be returning from the dance. Sam seemed happy to help. He and the nurse chatted and joked together. He spoke at length about his mother's illness and his family's financial problems, but he did not mention feeling ill.
>
> After finishing the sandwiches and cleaning the kitchen, they went together into the living room and sat down on the couch. "Do you think that my face is changing?" he asked. "I just looked in the bathroom mirror, and it seems to me that my nose is getting a lot longer."

The nurse looked carefully at his face and said, "It looks just the same to me. It seems to you that your nose is getting longer?"

Soon the other clients arrived from the dance. The unit was filled with the busy noise of 25 people discussing the dance and eating the evening snack. Sam took part in all this activity but sought the nurse several times to ask questions: "Do you think you ought to call my doctor?" "Will I be able to sleep tonight?" "You think that I am going to be all right, don't you?"

Each time Sam came to ask a question, the nurse took time to listen carefully to his questions and to answer truthfully and sincerely. She did call the doctor who was on duty that evening and told him about Sam's behavior. He agreed to come to see Sam. Because the doctor was not well acquainted with him, the nurse spent several minutes telling him briefly about Sam's family problems. She pointed out that he had been anxious and tense during the evening and had seemed to cling to her and to be asking for reassurance. The doctor talked with Sam. He felt that by allowing Sam to leave the dance, the nurse had been able to help him avoid an anxiety attack. The doctor told the nurse that her empathic listening and her efforts at reassuring Sam had been partially successful. The next day Sam's regular therapist was able to help him look more objectively at the problem that had been so upsetting to him. As a result of the nurse's intervention and the doctor's help, Sam was able to attend the dance the following week without experiencing undue anxiety.

This example is typical of situations that the psychiatric nurse frequently encounters. In her interaction with Sam the nurse used the technical nursing role by taking and evaluating his vital signs. She simultaneously engaged in the roles of mother surrogate and socializing agent when she worked with Sam to prepare and serve snacks for the other clients. The therapeutic effectiveness of this activity became apparent when Sam spoke about his family's problems and then became able to communicate his concern about his physical appearance. The nurse's response to this concern reflects the role of counselor, since she listened attentively and responded in a reassuring way. The nurse displayed an understanding of the necessity for professional collaboration by calling the physician and carefully sharing with him her assessment of the client. In summary, the nurse saw this clinical situation as an opportunity to use a variety of nursing roles, which proved to be very helpful to the client. Without an awareness of the therapeutic potential of these activities, the nurse might have

Table 2 *The nursing process*

Step	Purpose	Examples of nursing action
Assessment	To collect data	Observe present behavior of the client, using all the appropriate senses. Read client's chart and relevant texts and journals. Talk to client, his family, and other health workers.
	To validate data collected from observation	Make repeated observations; discuss perceptions with others. Read relevant texts and journals to confirm observations.
	To analyze data	Sort and organize data according to themes.
Development of a plan	To establish a nursing diagnosis	Synthesize all available assessment data. Postulate themes of the client's behavioral patterns with a potential explanation of the theme and its consequences.
	To plan for nursing intervention, using a nursing diagnosis as a basis	Individualize a plan for intervention and identify the nursing goal, rationale, nursing action, and outcome criteria. Use the principles of psychiatric nursing: 1. The nurse views the client as a holistic being with a multiplicity of interrelated and interdependent needs. 2. The nurse focuses on the client's strengths and assets, but does not ignore his weaknesses and liabilities. 3. The nurse accepts the client as a human being who has value and worth, exactly as he is. 4. The nurse views the client's behavior as designed to meet a need or to communicate a message. 5. The nurse has the potential for establishing a relationship with most, if not all, clients. 6. The quality of the interaction in which the nurse engages with the client is a major determinant of the degree to which the client will be able to alter his behavior in the direction of more satisfying, satisfactory interpersonal relationships. 7. The nurse views the client's behavior as the best possible possible adaptation he is capable of making at the time.
Intervention	To implement plan for nursing intervention	Function in a variety of roles while using principles of psychiatric nursing: 1. Creator of a therapeutic environment 2. Socializing agent 3. Counselor 4. Teacher 5. Mother surrogate 6. Technical role 7. Nurse therapist
Evaluation	To make planned, critical assessment of care	Review assessment data for accuracy and currency. Review nursing diagnoses for accuracy and currency.
	To revise or confirm plan of care	Review plan for nursing intervention. Compare client's response to intervention with outcome criteria.
	To make self-assessment	Evaluate own behavior. Revise or confirm plan for the nursing intervention based on overall evaluation.

insisted that Sam remain at the dance and thereby could have contributed to the exacerbation of an acute anxiety attack in the client.

EVALUATION OF NURSING CARE

The final phase of the nursing process is that of evaluation of nursing care. The steps of the nursing process previously cited have been described as if they were discrete entities, and the phase of evaluation is frequently seen as the last step in this process. In reality, however, all phases of the nursing process may occur simultaneously, and some form of evaluation must take place continuously. Therefore it is imperative that the nurse review the assessment of the client's behavior and the plan for nursing intervention, as well as the outcome of the nursing intervention. The outcome of the nursing care should be evaluated against the outcome criteria the nurse established as she planned for the care. As previously stated, outcome criteria need to be stated in behavioral terms and as specifically as possible.

The focus of evaluation should be on the adequacy of the steps of the nursing process, as well as on the changes in behavior that may or may not have been the result of the planned nursing intervention. Therefore the client's behavior and the nursing diagnosis need to be continuously reassessed and revised as indicated. Inherent in all aspects of evaluation is the necessity for the nurse to evaluate her own behavior and determine the degree to which it does or does not facilitate achievement of the goals of the plan for intervention. It should also be noted that evaluation frequently serves the purpose of identifying those aspects of care that are indeed helpful to the client and that therefore should be continued. See Table 2 for a summary outline of the nursing process as used in psychiatric nursing.

CONCLUDING STATEMENTS

1. The nursing process is an adaptation of the problem-solving technique. Thus the steps of the nursing process are assessment, development of a plan, intervention, and evaluation. The plan of nursing care is derived from the nursing diagnoses and is highly individualized for each client.

2. The purpose of the assessment phase is to collect data about the client and to organize the data in a way that will make it all useful:
   a. Observation of behavior is an active, planned, goal-directed process.
   b. Themes are recurring patterns that may have different manifestations but that stem from the same source.
3. The nursing diagnosis stems from a synthesis of all the available assessment data. The plan for nursing intervention is derived from the nursing diagnoses and is highly individualized for each client.
4. Basic principles of psychiatric nursing that should be reflected in the plan for intervention for all clients include the following:
   a. The nurse must view the client as a holistic being with a multiplicity of interrelated and interdependent needs.
   b. The nurse can be most helpful to the client by focusing on his strengths and assets, but does not ignore his weaknesses and liabilities.
   c. The nurse needs to accept the client as a human being who has value and worth, exactly as he is.
   d. The nurse must view the client's behavior as designed to meet a need or to communicate a message.
   e. The nurse has the potential for establishing a relationship with most, if not all, clients.
   f. The quality of the interaction in which the nurse engages with the client is a major determinant of the degree to which the client will be able to alter his behavior in the direction of more satisfying, satisfactory interpersonal relationships.
   g. The nurse needs to view the client's behavior as the best possible adaptation he is capable of making at the time.
5. During the intervention phase of the nursing process the nurse uses a variety of therapeutic roles, often simultaneously:
   a. In the role of creator of a therapeutic environment the nurse develops an accepting atmosphere.
   b. In the role of socializing agent the nurse can provide opportunities for clients to achieve greater success in social situ-

ations by helping them to develop feelings of security with other people.

c. In the role of counselor the nurse performs the critical task of listening to a client in a positive, dynamic, empathic way without at the same time giving advice, stating opinions, or making suggestions. The nurse is concerned with the client's reality problems that deal with the here and now.

d. The nurse has a role as a teacher in helping the client learn to deal in a more mature way with interpersonal relations and group living.

e. The nurse's role as a mother surrogate offers her an opportunity to provide clients with healthy experiences in the area of emotional relationships.

f. The technical aspects of the nurse's role are of great value but are not always as therapeutic in the psychiatric situation as some other roles the nurse assumes or is cast in by patients and co-workers. Technical procedures should be used as a means of enhancing the therapeutic relationship.

g. The potential of providing therapy through the nurse-client relationship is one of the most challenging roles being accepted by psychiatric nurses today.

6. The evaluation phase of the nursing process includes review of the assessment of the client's behavior, the plan for nursing intervention, and the outcome of the nursing intervention. The outcome of the nursing intervention should be evaluated against the outcome criteria, which the nurse established as she planned for the care.

Suggested sources of additional information

CLASSICAL

Gregg, Dorothy E.: The psychiatric nurse's role, Am. J. Nurs. **54**:848-851, 1954.

Gregg, Dorothy E.: The therapeutic roles of the nurse, Perspect. Psychiatr. Care **1**:18-28, Jan.-Feb., 1963.

Hays, Joyce Samhammer: The psychiatric nurse as a social therapist, Am. J. Nurs. **62**:64-67, June, 1962.

Holmes, Marguerite: The need to be recognized, Am. J. Nurs. **61**:86-87, Oct., 1961.

Hyde, Naida: Psychotherapy as mothering, Perspect. Psychiatr. Care **8**:73-78, March-April, 1970.

Meldman, M.J., McGowan, Marjorie, Higgins, Joan, and Schaller, Donna: Nurse psychotherapists in a private practice, Am. J. Nurs. **69:**2412-2415, 1969.

Morimoto, Francoise R.: The socializing role of psychiatric ward personnel, Am. J. Nurs. **54:**53-55, 1954.

Peplau, Hildegarde E.: Interpersonal relations in nursing, New York, 1952, G.P. Putnam's Sons.

Sabshin, Melvin: Nurse-doctor-patient relationships in psychiatry, Am. J. Nurs. **57:**188-192, 1957.

Schwartz, Morris S., and Shockley, Emmy Lanning: The nurse and the mental patient, New York, 1956, John Wiley & Sons, Inc.

CONTEMPORARY

Aiken, Linda, and Aiken, James L.: A systematic approach to the evaluation of interpersonal relationships, Am. J. Nurs. **73:**863-867, 1973.

Briggs, Paulette Fitzgerald: Specializing in psychiatry: therapeutic or custodial, Nurs. Outlook **22:**632-635, 1974.

Davis, Ellen D., and Pattison, E. Mansell: The psychiatric nurse's role identity, Am. J. Nurs. **79:**298-299, Feb., 1979.

Dethomaso, Marita Tribou: "Touch power" and the screen of loneliness, Perspect. Psychiatr. Care **9:**112-118, May-June, 1971.

Lathrop, Vallary G.: Aggression as a response, Perspect. Psychiatr. Care **16:**203-205, Sept.-Dec., 1978.

Lenarz, Dorothea M.: Care is the essence of practice, Am. J. Nurs. **71:**704-707, 1971.

Loomis, Maxine E.: Nursing management of acting-out behavior, Perspect. Psychiatr. Care **8:**168-173, July-Aug., 1970.

Robinson, Lisa: Psychiatric nursing as a human experience, Philadelphia, 1977, W.B. Saunders Co.

Roman, Linda, and Swietnicki, Colette: There's a man in my locker, Perspect. Psychiatr. Care **9:**59-73, March-April, 1971.

Snyder, Joyce C., and Wilson, Margo F.: Elements of a psychological assessment, Am. J. Nurs. **77:**235-239, 1977.

Travelbee, Joyce: Interpersonal aspects of nursing, ed. 2, Philadelphia, 1971, F.A. Davis Co.

OF PARTICULAR INTEREST

Hauser, M., and Feinberg, D.: Problem solving revisited, J. Psychiatr. Nurs., pp. 13-17, Oct., 1977.

Problem solving and creative thinking are combined in this article as a framework for addressing nursing problems in challenging situations.

Kalisch, B.: Strategies for developing nurse empathy, Nurs. Outlook **19:**714-718, 1971.

This article describes the author's experiment to develop empathy in nursing students. It is excellent for the purpose of defining the concept and discriminating between empathy and related concepts.

SECTION TWO

Concepts basic to psychiatric nursing

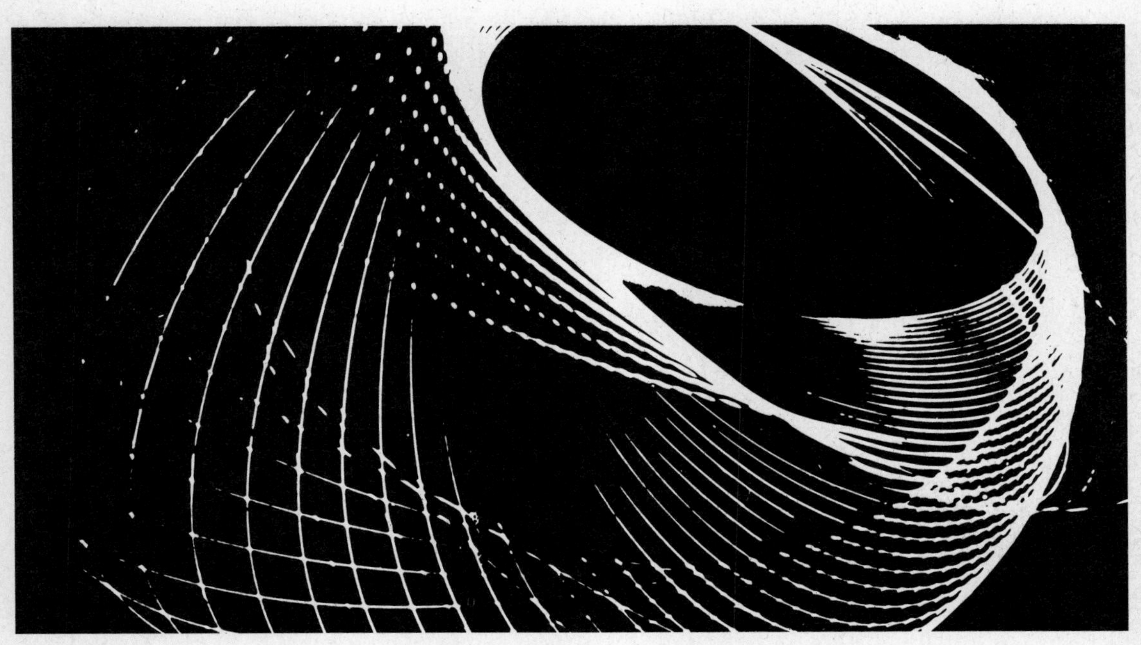

Section Two provides an in-depth discussion of personality development, anxiety and its defenses, and mental health and the cause and prevention of mental illness. An understanding of these topics is not only basic to psychiatric nursing, but also to all nursing practice, since they focus on the understanding of the dynamics underlying human behavior. Therefore the reader may find this section enlightening not only during the study of psychiatric nursing, but also throughout the entire student experience. As is also true of Section One, the understanding of subsequent sections of this text is predicated on knowledge of the material presented in this section.

These topics are presented early in the text because of the belief that one must understand the development and manifestations of mental health to adequately understand the development and manifestations of mental illness.

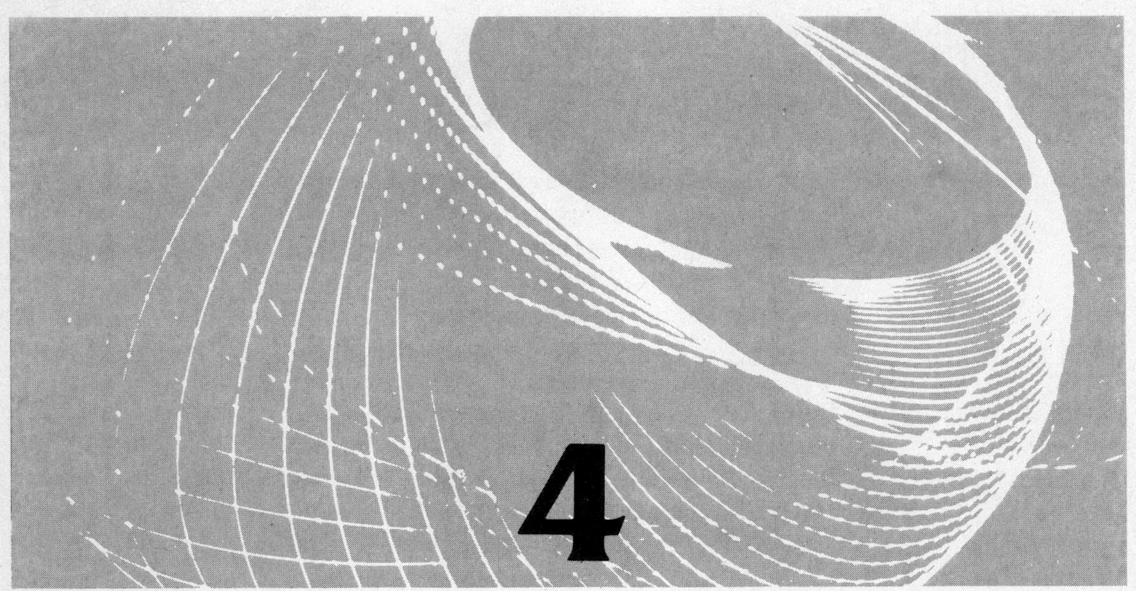

4 Personality: its structure and development

- Definition of personality
- Major theorists
- Basic concepts
- Development of the personality

Understanding human behavior and the many adjustment problems that arise in the lives of people depends to a large extent on understanding the process through which the personality develops. It is therefore important to recognize the relationship between the early experiences that human beings undergo and the development of the personality.

DEFINITION OF PERSONALITY

Before a discussion of personality development can become meaningful, it is essential to understand the definition of the term *personality* used by students of human behavior. Unfortunately this word has been used to convey many different meanings and ideas. In ordinary conversation it usually refers to the personal response that the individual evokes from others. It is not unusual for someone to comment that an individual has a pleasing personality or that a certain person has a poor personality. When used technically, the word personality refers to *the aggregate of the physical and mental qualities of the individual as these interact in characteristic fashion with his environment.* Thus it can be seen that personality is expressed through behavior. The characteristic combinations of behavior distinguish one individual from another and endow individuals with their own unique identity.

This definition of personality includes the individual's biological and intellectual endowment, the attributes he has acquired through experience, and his conscious and unconscious reactions and feelings. Personality development is a complex and dynamic process that is constantly evolving from what it was to something different, yet it always retains a certain identifiable consistency. It is important to remember that from birth to death personality is ever changing and ever developing. This fact makes it possible for individuals of all ages to profit from corrective experiences and to modify behavior in a positive direction. This is the rationale underlying all psychotherapeutic endeavors on the behalf of clients.

MAJOR THEORISTS

Much of the information we have today about the evolution of personality has been derived from psychological theories and not from scientific research. Actually, much of our current knowledge is based on theories proposed by Sigmund Freud who lived from 1856 to 1939. He did much of his important work in Vienna around the turn of the century and is given most of the credit for developing the foundational theories of personality development. It was Freud's writing that first stressed the crucial importance of early childhood experiences in the development of human personality and the relationship between some of the emotional problems in adult life and the negative influences that sometimes occur during the early years.

During and after Freud's pioneering work, many other theorists addressed themselves to the study of personality development to better understand human behavior. Investigators such as Erik Erikson and Harry Stack Sullivan have adapted, modified, and enlarged on Freud's basic theories; their work has resulted in theories that are seen as significantly different from those of Freud.

Erik Erikson was born in Frankfurt, Germany, in 1902 of Danish parents. His mother and father had separated before he was born, and when he was about 3 years old, his mother married a pediatrician who was a German Jew. With this mixed cultural heritage Erikson had difficulty establishing his own sense of identity. In fact, he made up the name Erik Erikson, which reflects the concept that the child (Erik) is the father (son of Erik) of the man (Erik Erikson). It is likely that his own personal quest for identity was a major factor in the development of his theory of personality development, referred to as the *Eight Ages of Man.* At age 25 Erikson left Germany to go to Vienna where he studied the new discipline of psychoanalysis. He immigrated to Boston, Massachusetts, in 1933, fleeing fascism, and has spent the remainder of his life in the United States.

Harry Stack Sullivan was born in Norwich, New York, in 1892 and died while on a trip to Paris, France, in 1949. Sullivan became a psychiatrist during the early years of Freud's profound influence on American psychiatry. However, unlike many of his colleagues, he studied only in the United States, working closely with a group of psychoanalysts and social psychologists who were pulling away from the classical psychoanalytical model established by Freud. Sullivan's theories postulate that the most critical factor in personality development is the individual's relationship with other significant people. His theories emphasize the nature and the quality of these relationships. This fact is best illustrated by his reference to the mothering one to distinguish between the roles of the biological mother and the person (male or female) who provides nurturing experiences for the infant. Although Sullivan viewed the relationship between the infant and the mothering one as foundational to personality development, he also placed great emphasis on the importance of relationships with significant others such as peers, spouse, and one's own children as the person progresses throughout life. Therefore Sullivan's theory is referred to as the *interpersonal theory of psychiatry.* In view of the fact that the nurse's role with mentally ill persons is almost totally focused on the relationship that is developed with them, Sullivan's theory seems to be particularly applicable to nursing practice.

Although some psychiatrists feel that it is important to adhere strictly and consistently to the tenets of one school of thought, psychiatric theories currently in use in the United States are becoming increasingly eclectic. That is, concepts from various schools of thought are being used in combination to develop a usable theory of personality development. The necessity of an eclectic approach is particularly apparent in nursing practice, since the role of the nurse in interaction with patients is probably more varied than in any other discipline. Consequently, the following discussion will outline the basic concepts of Freud, Erikson, and Sullivan with a subsequent discussion of each stage of personality development as described by these theorists. It is hoped that this approach will enable the student to compare and contrast these theories and use that which is applicable as she plans, implements, and evaluates nursing care.

BASIC CONCEPTS

Freudian concepts

Freud's theories are often referred to as *intrapsychic,* because they emphasize the internal emotional life of the individual as the most significant factor in the development of the personality. Even though Freud deviated widely from the accepted medical theories and practices of his day, his theories are largely based on a biological model. For example, Freud believed that each individual is born with a genetically determined amount of *libidinal energy,* a form of psychic energy that seeks pleasure in an attempt to avoid tension or pain. In this sense, libidinal energy is viewed as sexual energy. This energy cannot increase or decrease in amount but must be shared among the various parts of the personality. Freud developed his conception of the stages of personality development largely around the concept of libidinal energy, and delineated each stage of development according to the area of the body on which he believed the energy was focused. For example, the first stage of development is characterized by the libidinal energy being concentrated on the mouth. It is through the mouth that the infant expresses tension and pain, and through the mouth that pleasure is perceived. As the child matures physiologically, the libidinal energy shifts from the mouth to other parts of the body until adulthood when the libidinal energy is focused on the genital area, enabling the individual to establish a mature heterosexual relationship, which Freud saw as the hallmark of the normal development of personality. Therefore Freud delineated only five stages of personality development, seeing this process as being complete at adulthood with major personality alterations unlikely thereafter under usual circumstances. Because of the libidinal energy theory and its relationship to the development of the personality, Freud's theory of personality development is called the *psychosexual theory.*

Freud's topographical descriptions of the psyche are important for the student to understand, since these concepts are used almost universally in the United States and contribute much to understanding human behavior.

Levels of consciousness. One way in which Freud described the mind topographically was from the standpoint of levels of consciousness. These levels are referred to as the conscious, the preconscious or subconscious, and the unconscious parts of the mind.

The *conscious* part of the mind is aware of the here and now as it relates to the individual and his environment. It functions only when the individual is awake. The conscious mind is concerned with thoughts, feelings, and sensations. It directs the individual as he behaves in a rational, thoughtful way.

The *preconscious* or *subconscious* is that part of the mind in which ideas and reactions are stored and partially forgotten—it is not economical for human beings to burden the conscious mind with a multitude of facts that are infrequently used and currently not in demand. The preconscious also acts as a watchman, since it prevents certain unacceptable, disturbing unconscious memories from reaching the conscious mind. These two functions make the preconscious an extremely valuable device. Material relegated to this handy storehouse can usually be brought into conscious awareness if the individual concentrates on recall.

The *unconscious* is by far the largest part of the mind and is sometimes compared to the large hidden part of an iceberg that floats under the water. In this comparison the small part of the iceberg that appears above the water represents the conscious mind. The unconscious is the storehouse for all the memories, feelings, and responses experienced by the individual during his entire life. The unconscious is one of Freud's most important concepts. Freudian theorists believe that the human mind never actually forgets any experience but stores in the unconscious all knowledge, information, and feeling about all experiences. These memories cannot be recalled at will. The individual is rarely aware of the unconscious mind, except as it demonstrates its presence through such means as dreams, slips of the tongue, unexplained behavioral responses, jokes, and lapses of memory. Psychotic symptoms are expressions of unconscious thoughts or feelings. Material stored in the unconscious has a powerful influence on behavior because the accompanying feelings continue to act as motivating, dynamic forces. The individual is unaware of the ideas themselves, but he may continue to experience an emotional reaction as if the material were in the conscious mind. It is this theory that underlies the belief that all behavior has meaning. In other words, no behavior occurs by accident or chance; rather, all behavior is an expression of feelings or needs of which the individual frequently is not aware.

Structure of the personality. The second topographical description developed by Freud is frequently referred to as the structure of the personality. This structure includes the concepts of the id, the ego, and the superego.

The *id* is part of and derived from the unconscious. It is unlearned, primitive, selfish, and the source of all libidinal energy. It contains the instinctual drives, included in which are the drive for self-preservation, the drive to reproduce, and the drive for group association. The id is without a sense of right and wrong and ruthlessly insists on the immediate satisfaction of its impulses and desires.

When the new individual is born, he is said to be a bundle of id, seeking only to satisfy his needs and to find release for physiological tensions. By crying, the infant insists on receiving attention when tensions build up. He disregards all other factors in his environment as he demands that his needs be met.

During the individual's entire life the id persists in pushing the organism toward the achievement of its primitive, instinctual goals. It is described as operating on the basis of the *pleasure principle.* That is to say, the id presses for avoidance of pain at all costs and seeks to maintain pleasure. Pleasure in this sense refers to release of tension and the establishment of emotional and physiological equilibrium. Pain refers to tensions that are present when the infant is cold, hungry, frightened, or anxious. As the child matures, the concept of pain encompasses additional aspects of body equilibrium, including sexual tension, tensions that result from cultural pressures, and tension from physiological needs. Throughout the individual's entire life the id insists that the individual seek release of tension, regardless of the social outcome. It is the duty of other parts of the personality to censor the id and to keep it under control.

The development of the *ego* is a result of the individual's interaction with the environment. It is initiated when the infant recognizes the breast or the bottle as part of the environment rather than as part of his own body. The ego promotes the individual's satisfactory adjustment in relation to his environment. Its main function is to effect an acceptable compromise between the crude pleasure-seeking strivings of the id and the inhibitions of the superego. The means through which the ego achieves this goal is reality testing. The ego deals with the demands of reality as it strives to control and derive satisfaction from the environment. Thus as the individual matures, the ego becomes the rational, reasonable, conscious part of the personality and strives to integrate the total personality into a smoothly functioning, unified, coherent whole. In the mature adult it is the ego that represents the self to others and individualizes him from other human beings.

Chronologically, the *superego* develops last. Its development is partially a result of the socialization process that the child undergoes. The superego incorporates the taboos, prohibitions, ideals, and standards of the parents and the other significant adults with whom the child associates. It operates mostly at the unconscious level and at this level is an inhibitor of the id. The superego is blindly rigid, strictly moralistic, and as unrelenting and ruthless as the id. There are two aspects of the superego. One is called the *conscience*. The conscience is the part of the superego that punishes the individual through guilt and anxiety when his behavior deviates from the strict standards of the superego. The other aspect is called the *ego ideal*. The ego ideal rewards the individual through feelings of euphoria and well-being when his behavior emulates those standards believed by the superego to be desirable. It is important to understand that neither the punishing nor the rewarding functions of the superego are based on the reality of the situation. Rather, they are based on the individual's internalized standards of right and wrong, good and bad, which were learned at an early age and which are stored for the most part in the unconscious mind.

If the individual does not develop an ego that is strong enough to arbitrate effectively between the id and the superego, he will surely develop intrapersonal and interpersonal conflicts. When the id is not controlled effectively, the individual functions in antisocial, lawless ways because his primitive impulses are expressed freely. If the superego is so strong that the individual's life is dominated by its restrictions on behavior, he is likely to be inhibited, repressed, unhappy, and guilt-ridden. Thus a mature, effective, stable adult life is dependent on the development of an ego powerful enough both to deal with and to adequately test reality to mediate successfully between the demands of the id and the superego.

Eriksonian concepts

Erikson's theories build on and include Freudian concepts. However, their emphasis is not on Freud's intrapsychic theories, but rather on the ability of the ego to develop in a healthy, adaptive manner given a facilitative environment. Therefore Erikson's theories are variously referred to as neo-Freudian, ego psychology, and cultural. Erikson has also extended the stages of personality development to include the totality of the life span, introducing the very important idea that personality development does not cease at the achievement of adulthood. This belief helps to explain the fundamental changes in an individual's feelings and behavior that characteristically occur during his adult life.

A major contribution Erikson has made to the understanding of personality development is his identification of *developmental tasks* for each developmental period. These developmental tasks are age-specific achievements that are largely culturally determined. Achievement of each task increases the ego strength of the individual and enhances the probability of satisfactory achievement of subsequent tasks. Erikson sees the individual's ability to satisfactorily complete each developmental task as dependent not only on his genetic endowment and intrapsychic development, but also primarily on the quality of his interaction with the environment. It is important to understand that the developmental tasks identified by Erikson include both positive and negative outcomes. This means that the individual who has not satisfactorily achieved the developmental task for a specific stage of development will develop as a result, a nondesirable and less healthy attribute in its stead. The most obvious example is the developmental task of the first developmental period—basic trust versus basic mistrust. The infant who is not successful, for whatever reason, in developing a sense of basic trust will not be left with an ego structure that demonstrates a mere lack of trust. The alternative is the development of an even more negative characteristic—a sense of basic mistrust. The significance of this paradigm is illustrated simply by the difference between the feelings of "I'm not sure that I can trust you." and "I'm sure that I cannot trust you." Therefore to fully understand Erikson's theory of personality development, the student must understand the negative as well as the positive outcomes of each developmental period.

Sullivanian concepts

Sullivan's theories are firmly based on the belief that human beings are more basically different from, than similar to, all other animals. The uniqueness of human beings, according to Sullivan, lies in their interdependence; and it is as a result of their interactions with each other, not their physiological endowment, that the personality is developed. As previously stated, Sullivan's theories are referred to as *interpersonal,* because of their emphasis on human interaction. Sullivan believed that all human behavior is goal directed toward the fulfillment of two needs—the need for satisfaction and the need for security. The need for satisfaction represents the biological needs of the person for such things as air, food, and sex. The need for security represents the emotional needs of the individual for such feelings states as interpersonal intimacy, status, and self-esteem. When these needs are perceived, internal tension results, and the individual employs a variety of methods to meet the need and thereby reduce the tension. Sullivan called these methods *dynamisms,* and it is partially around the dynamisms characteristic of each age group that Sullivan based his theory of personality development. For example, during the first stage of development, the oral cavity is used almost exlusively by the infant as the method to meet his needs for satisfaction (by crying to be fed) and his needs for security (by crying to be held). Therefore the stage of infancy is characterized by the oral dynamism, and the oral cavity becomes important because it is the means through which the individual establishes interpersonal contact, which in turn is the means through which his needs are met and tension is reduced. In fact, the individual not only gets his needs met through interpersonal contact, but also through this contact he establishes the fact of his own existence. Sullivan believed that it is due to the response of significant adults to the individual when he was an infant and child that the individual's self-concept develops. Sullivan defined the self-concept as the result of the reflected appraisals of significant others.

The concept of anxiety is central to Sullivan's theory of personality development. He postulated that anxiety is a response to feelings of disapproval from a significant adult. It is important to understand that these feelings may or may not be based in reality, and that the adult whose disapproval is feared may be real or a symbolic representation. The development of the personality then consists of a series of interpersonally based learnings in which dynamisms are used as the individual attempts to gain approval and avoid the anxiety associated with disapproval.

DEVELOPMENT OF THE PERSONALITY

It has been said that the first 6 years in a child's life contribute the most to personality development. When one considers that these years provide the foundation for future patterns of behavior, this statement appears to be true. However, the student must understand the influence of all stages of development on the personality to accurately assess the behavior of the adults for whom she provides nursing care. The following is a description and discussion of each of the developmental stages according to the theories of Freud, Erikson, and Sullivan.

Infancy

The period of infancy roughly extends over the first year and a half of life. Freud referred to this period as the *oral stage,* because the child's libidinal energy is focused on his mouth and its functions to the exclusion of all other considerations. This singular focus on self is technically referred to as *primary narcissism,* which means self-love.

In the first months of life the infant is unable to differentiate between himself and his environment. He therefore feels that all that happens to him is caused by him. This feeling of being all powerful is termed *omnipotence.* The infant's awareness of himself is in terms of comfort or discomfort, and his total being is focused on fulfilling the demands of the id, which insists on relief from hunger and cold, which are perceived as a diffused tension. He seeks relief from this tension by using his mouth, lips, and tongue to cry, suck, and swallow. These activities provide him with the greatest pleasures, since they reduce discomfort. In the earliest months the infant is dependent on a nurturing adult to supply the nipple that meets his need for sucking and through which he obtains milk to swallow, appeasing the tension caused by hunger. Accidentally the infant soon finds his thumb and discovers that he can meet his own needs for sucking. Although sucking his own thumb provides pleasure, it is experienced as being different from sucking the nipple. Through this simple realization the infant begins the complex, lengthy process of differentiating himself from the environment. In this way the ego or the recognition of the self or the "me" begins to develop.

When weaning is initiated, the infant begins to receive fewer oral satisfactions from his environment. When the cup and solid food are substituted for the breast or bottle, the infant feels frustrated. With the adoption of more rigid schedules the infant is denied the complete attention of the mother. He may react to these frustrations orally in an aggressive, sometimes destructive way and may begin to bite and may seek symbolic oral gratification by sucking other objects.

Because food and love are given simultaneously during the oral period, oral needs become synonymous with protective love and security. These needs are universal and continue throughout life in one form or another. In adult life, release of tension through oral gratification is achieved through chewing gum, smoking, eating, and drinking. Freud believed that these activities are residuals of the oral stage of personality development.

Erikson's view of the oral stage is very similar to the Freudian view just described. Unlike Freud, however, Erikson emphasizes the significance of the mother-child relationship in the achievement of the developmental task of the oral stage—basic trust versus basic mistrust. Erikson theorizes that if the infant's great need for love and attention is met consistently and unconditionally by a giving, loving mother, he will learn to trust her. Since the infant cannot help but view his mother as representative of the world at large, this attitude of basic trust in her will strongly influence his perceptions of other people and the environment. Therefore a healthy resolution of the oral stage of personality development, according to Erikson, results in the development of a basic sense of trust in the mother, which serves as the basis for the development of future trusting relationships. On the other hand, if the infant's experiences with his mother are characterized by inconsistencies and anxiety, he will learn to mistrust her and subsequently generalize this attitude to the world at large. It does not take much imagination to appreciate the many great differences between the feelings and behaviors of adults who have achieved a sense of basic trust and those who have achieved a sense of basic mistrust.

Sullivan referred to the first year and a half of life as the stage of infancy, rather than the oral stage, because he believed that the oral cavity has significance only in that it is the vehicle through which the infant establishes interpersonal contact. Sullivan introduced several very important concepts regarding the first stage of development. He coined the term *mothering one* to reflect the belief that the most important person in the infant's life is the individual who consistently nurtures him, and that this person does not necessarily have to be the biological mother. In fact, whether the mothering one is the biological mother or not, Sullivan believed that this person and the infant have to establish an interpersonal relationship, wherein they become highly significant to each other. This relationship is unique to the stage of infancy and is characterized by the *empathic linkage,* a symbolic emotional umbilical cord that makes the infant and the nurturing adult highly sensitive to each other's feeling states. Other theorists refer to this process as bonding. It is through the empathic linkage that both positive feelings of love and acceptance and negative feelings of anxiety and rejection are conveyed. Sullivan also believed that the development of the self-concept begins in the stage of infancy and is closely related to the quality of the infant's feeding experiences. Since self-concept develops as the result of the reflected appraisals of significant others, if the infant frequently experiences satisfaction and security from the mothering one during the feeding process, he begins to see himself as being a worthwhile individual; that is, he will begin to develop a "good me" self-concept. Conversely, if the infant's experience with the mothering one is frequently fraught with tension and inconsistency, the foundation is laid for the development of a "bad me" self-concept, wherein the individual begins to see himself as being not worthwhile. If the infant is severely deprived during this stage, he will respond with massive amounts of anxiety that threaten his very life. To preserve his life the infant defends himself by disassociating the anxiety-generating experiences. As a result, he cannot develop a sense of self from reflected appraisals, so he develops a "not me" self-concept. This situation lays the foundation for the subsequent development of severe emotional problems.

All three theorists agreed that the successful resolution of the first stage of personality development greatly enhances the probability of a successful resolution of subsequent stages.

Early childhood

The period of early childhood is a phase of personality development that occurs roughly between the ages of 18 months and 3 years. Freud termed this period of time the *anal stage,* because the libidinal energy shifts from the oral cavity to the anus and the urethra.

In the early part of this period the child freely gratifies his love of self with the pleasurable sensations involved in evacuating the bladder and bowels naturally and without restriction. Although the mouth remains an important zone of pleasure, the child derives his greatest pleasure from the anus and the urethra during these early years.

Ego development continues in this period as the child continuously develops a better defined concept of self. Superego development is initiated as the mother begins to insist that the child accept certain restrictions and controls regarding toileting. It is at this point that the child experiences the first major frustration of his id drives. He is forced to come to terms with the reality of the situation. To retain the love of the mother the child must learn to postpone the immediate pleasure of urinating or evacuating until the appropriate time and to use the appropriate place. The necessity for making an adaptation to the wishes of the mother regarding toileting places the child and the mother in conflict. As the mother makes demands on the child in an attempt to force him to accept her standards in relation to toileting, the child develops ambivalent feelings toward her, that is, he simultaneously loves and hates her.

Freud believed that if great stress is placed on the child in relation to remaining clean during this period, he may grow up to be compulsively clean and meticulous. On the other hand, he may unconsciously deal with his anxiety by the use of reaction formation as a defense mechanism and become very untidy and unconcerned about cleanliness in his adult life. Other adult attitudes thought to be traceable to rigid toilet training include stubbornness, hoarding and collecting, excessive concern with bowel function, and sadistic or masochistic tendencies.

Erikson identifies autonomy versus shame and doubt as the developmental task of the anal stage. Of great significance, according to Erikson, is the mother's response to the child's interest in assuming control over himself by controlling his urine and feces. If she treats the child with respect as an individual who is separate from her, he will begin to develop a sense of autonomy, or self-sufficiency. On the other hand, if his efforts to do for himself are ridiculed or interfered with, he will develop a sense of shame and doubt in his capabilities.

Sullivan used the term *early childhood* to refer to this period of life. He acknowledged the shift in the child's interest from his mouth to his anus but emphasized the sense of power the child feels as he attempts to control himself and others, particularly the mothering one. This feeling of power often puts the child and the mothering one in conflict as the mothering one attempts to toilet train the child. The process and outcome of this power struggle are believed to serve as the prototypical experience for similar interpersonal conflicts in later life. Of equal importance during this stage of development is Sullivan's belief that the child sees his feces as an extension of himself, and therefore the mothering one's response to the child's pleasure in his feces is seen by the child as a reflection of her view of him. In that way the self-concept established in the stage of infancy is reinforced or altered.

Later childhood

The period of later childhood is a phase of development that includes the ages from 3 to 6. Freud called this period the *phallic stage.* This descriptive term refers to the fact that the focus of pleasurable sensations has shifted from the mouth and the excretory organs to the genitalia and that the child begins to identify with the parent of the same sex and unconsciously wishes to replace that parent in the family situation. Thus it is not uncommon to hear a girl in this age-group speak of "marrying Daddy" or a little boy say, "Go away, Daddy, I will take care of Mommy."

Between the ages of 3 and 6 years children begin to examine purposefully their own bodies and the bodies of their playmates. They discover that pleasurable sensations can be aroused from manipulation of the penis or the clitoris. They also become aware of the difference between the sexual structure of men and women and wonder about the girl's lack of an obvious sexual organ. Children of this age may conclude that the penis can be lost in some way, since some people whose bodies they have observed have apparently lost this organ. Anxiety about the loss of the sex organ may develop among children in this age-group. Fears may be expressed by a little boy concerning the loss of his penis through punishment or an accident. These fears are referred to as *castration fears.* Unfortunately some parents reinforce these fears by threatening to cut off the penis if the child is observed fondling it. A little girl notices that she has no penis and may conclude that she lost it or that it has been taken away. She naturally wants what she observes some other children possess. This attitude on the part of a little girl is called *penis envy.* It is sometimes basic to the problem of *sibling rivalry.*

It should be noted that some theorists believe that any evidence of castration anxiety or penis envy in children of this age is a result of cultural conditioning and not an inherent element in personality development. This view is particularly popular among feminists, and a serious student of human behavior would be wise to keep an open mind, observing for behavioral changes in children as cultural changes are adopted.

During this period the little boy who has always had a great deal of attention and love from his mother begins to feel very possessive toward her. He wants her for himself, and he resents the close tie that he feels exists between his mother and father. He develops competitive feelings toward his father and tries to become a rival with him for his mother's love. The father is such a large and formidable opponent that the little boy develops a good deal of resentment and fear of him. This situation is referred to as the *Oedipus complex*. It may precipitate castration fears, because the little boy may begin to fear that the father will punish him for his resentment toward him and his attempt to replace him in his mother's life. Eventually the little boy concludes that being like his father is a more effective way of achieving his mother's love and attention. Thus he begins to take on the masculine behavior of his father. This is referred to as *identification* (Fig. 4-1). In this way the little boy begins to learn the role of the male in the culture.

Similarly, during this period the little girl begins to identify

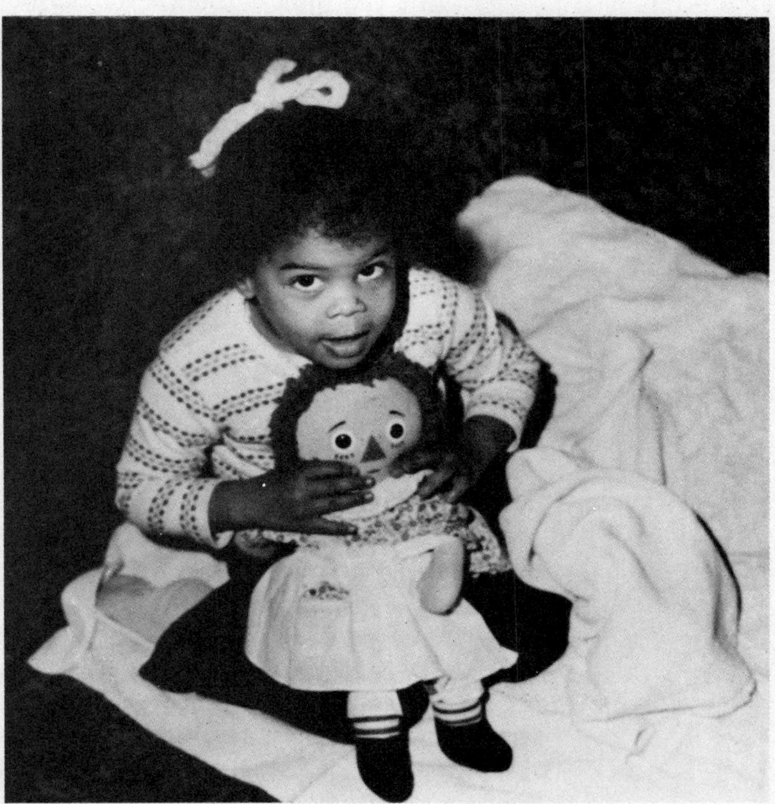

Fig. 4-1 *Role identification is the major developmental task to be initiated during the stage of later childhood.*

with the feminine role. The process through which the girl passes in identifying with the parent of the same sex is not as clearly understood as is the process for little boys. The girl feels that somehow her mother is responsible for the fact that she does not have a penis. She also notices that she does not have breasts as her mother does. She may blame her mother for not having provided her with a complete body and may display a good deal of hostility and antagonism toward her. The little girl turns to her father for love and affection and frequently competes openly with the mother for his attention. She begins to imitate her mother because she feels that in this way she may be able to please her father. This is a difficult period for the little girl who must keep her mother's love and approval because she is still dependent on her. It is essential that the child maintain a positive relationship with her mother if she is to accomplish the task of identifying with the feminine role.

The birth of a baby in the family at this time presents both boys and girls of this age with a particularly difficult adjustment problem. The 3- to 6-year-old uses almost all of his energy in controlling his incestuous desires toward the parent of the opposite sex and his rage toward the parent of the same sex. The necessity to compete with a helpless infant for the attention of the parents often results in a great deal of overt sibling rivalry.

Superego development is also at its height at this time, since the issues involved are seen, in our society at least, as moralistic ones. Therefore unless this stage is successfully resolved, the potential exists for the child to develop long-lasting feelings of guilt because of his incestuous wishes for the parent of the opposite sex and his rage against the parent of the same sex.

Erikson identifies this stage of development as having the developmental outcomes of initiative versus guilt. He agrees with Freud that children of this age desire to exclusively possess the parent of the opposite sex. To achieve this goal the child makes the first move, that is, he takes the initiative. In a healthy family environment, the child inevitably fails to achieve his goal, but he learns a great deal about being assertive and is able to turn his failure into the process of learning how to become a spouse and parent in the future. If, on the other hand, the child experiences a great deal of punitiveness and withdrawal of basic approval, his feelings of guilt that are already present will be reinforced and remain in subsequent stages.

Sullivan designated this period of life as later childhood. Sullivan believed that the major significance of this stage of personality development is that the child becomes capable of giving up his personal and private language and substitutes language that has universal meaning. The importance of the acquisition of the tool of language cannot be overemphasized, since it allows the child to begin to check out his perceptions and feelings with others. The term that describes this process is *consensual validation*. The ability to consensually validate experiences with others is a major factor in enabling the child to develop relationships with peers in the neighborhood or in the nursery school.

Latency

The stage of personality development that occurs roughly between the ages of 6 and 12 was called *latency* by Freud. This term was chosen because Freud believed that the child's libidinal energy was not focused on any one area of the body as it had been in the previous three stages. He believed that this energy was lying dormant, and therefore nothing of psychosexual significance occurred during this stage. The relatively stable behavior and even-tempered nature of most children of this stage attest to the temporary intrapsychic equilibrium established by the id, ego, and superego.

Erikson recognizes the very important role that school experiences play in the personality development of the child during this period. Although he agrees with Freud that no specific area of the body is of particular interest to children during this stage, he believes that psychic energy is being actively used in pursuit of knowledge and skills. In other words, the child is purposefully involved in acquiring tools through which he can deal with his environment both in the present and in the future. According to Erikson, if the child is successful in this endeavor, he will have achieved the developmental task of industry. If the child is unsuccessful, he will feel inadequate and develop a sense of inferiority.

Sullivan saw this period of time as being very critical to the development of a healthy adult personality. He divided Freud's and Erikson's 6-year span into two periods: the *juvenile era,* lasting roughly from ages 6 to 10; and *preadolescence,* lasting roughly from ages 11 to 12, or the onset of puberty. During the juvenile era the child turns away from his parents as being the most significant people in his life and looks to peers of the same sex to fill the functions of providing him with a sense of security and companionship. This is the period of gang formation and fierce gang loyalties. The gang requires strict adherence to the rules of the group, and the child slavishly complies with them. During this period the child tries to find his place among his peers. In so doing he acquires two very important interpersonal tools: the ability to compete and the ability to compromise. As the child tests out these modes of behavior with his peers, their responses help him to learn to use both appropriately.

Another very important function of the peer group is the reinforcement or alteration of the self-concept. A child who enters this stage of development with a positive or "good me" self-concept is very likely to behave in a manner that elicits responses from his peers that confirm and reinforce his view of self. In instances when the child enters this period with a negative or "bad me" self-concept, positive reflected appraisals from his peer group can do much to alter his view of self. This fact indicates what a very significant role the peer group plays in the life of the child during this period.

During preadolescence the child maintains great interest in the group but simultaneously develops an intense love relationship with a particular person of the same sex who the child perceives to be very similar to himself. Sullivan called this special relationship a *chum relationship.* Up until this time the child's love has been self-centered, but in the chum relationship the child experiences for the first time the capacity to put the needs of someone else ahead of his own. Sullivan saw this experience as a necessary prerequisite to the establishment of a satisfactory heterosexual relationship in subsequent stages of development. The emotional intimacy that the chums experience also helps them to explore and clarify their feelings in a way that builds self-esteem.

Sullivan also stressed the importance of the school experience in the development of the child's personality. It is at school that children meet significant adults who greatly influence the development of their self-concepts. In this culture, success at school is rewarded with much approval, whereas lack of success often begins a series of defeats that carry over into adult life. The self-concept of children who do poorly in school may be irreparably damaged by the reactions of teachers, the significant adults in that important environment. On the other hand, understanding, helpful teachers may provide the child with a positive basis for self-evaluation and in some instances may constitute an opportunity for corrective interpersonal experiences with adults. Teachers are of tremendous importance in the lives of children and need to be aware of their potential for providing therapeutic experiences in their day-to-day contacts with children.

Puberty and adolescence

The stage of puberty and adolescence covers the years from age 12 to approximately age 18. Because all theorists agree that this stage of development is initiated by the active functioning of the sexual glands and because individuals mature physiologically at different rates, it is difficult to make a definite statement concerning the span of years included in adolescence.

Freud saw adolescence as the final stage of personality development characterized by a reactivation of libidinal energy and the focusing of this energy on the genital area. As such, he designated this period as the *genital stage.* Although Freud believed that this final stage lasted for the rest of the person's life, he emphasized that the intense work of this period was completed when the individual achieved a satisfactory heterosexual relationship with a mate and began the life cycle anew by establishing a family.

Adolescence may be the most problematic stage of personality development. As the adolescent matures physiologically he is faced with the necessity of handling powerful sexual urges that threaten to put the influence of the id out of balance with the influences of the ego and superego. Because of this imbalance of psychic forces, unresolved conflicts and unsolved problems of earlier developmental periods often reemerge at this time. This is particularly true of the Oedipal conflict because of the similarity of the sexual urges experienced at both stages. Therefore the adolescent is simultaneously drawn toward his parents and driven away from them. This ambivalence is manifested by much conflict between the adolescent and his parents as the adolescent vacillates between behaving in a dependent, immature, childlike way and in an independent, mature, adult manner.

Erikson builds on Freud's theory by elaborating on the conflictual nature of the parent-child relationship. Erikson sees the developmental task of adolescence as the development of a sense of identity versus role diffusion. It is during this time that the individual must emancipate himself from his parents, not only physically but also emotionally by establishing for himself his own sense of identity. He must answer the most fundamental questions of "Who am I?" and "What am I?" This requires many decisions regarding familial, occupational, and social roles. To be sure, the adolescent is strongly influenced by his family's norms and values as he struggles to make these decisions. However, if he is to successfully master this developmental stage, he must accept these norms and values as his own, or reject them and establish new guidelines for himself. In other words, the adolescent's primary task is to develop an ego that has integrated previous learnings and experiences so that he develops a sense of continuity and sameness in his life. Unsuccessful mastery of this stage results in a diffuse, fragmented sense of self, the most problematic aspect of which is often the shifting between an adult and a child orientation.

Sullivan designated the period between 12 and 17 or 18 years of age as early adolescence. As the person experiences sexual urges (termed *lust* by Sullivan), he turns from the chum relationship to the task of establishing a relationship with a peer of the opposite sex. The peer group remains an important aspect of the adolescent's life during this stage because it serves the important function of providing security and consensual validation of the adolescent's feelings and behaviors. The influence of the peer group in regulating the adolescent's behavior is very strong.

Successful resolution of the stage of adolescence is greatly impeded when the child is seen as unacceptable by his peer group, perhaps because of physical handicaps or major cultural differences. The consequence of this nonacceptance may be a prolonged clinging to parents or parent figures to feel a sense of security and belongingness. Another pitfall of this stage occurs when the adolescent's peer group is composed of individuals who are antisocial in nature and engage in delinquent behavior. Although the adolescent will avoid the anxiety of isolation by identifying with this group, it is also likely that he will develop behaviors that are antagonistic to the society at large and that will impede him in the successful achievement of subsequent developmental tasks.

Early adulthood

The period of early adulthood has its onset at the end of adolescence and continues until middle age. It is almost impossible to state a chronological age range for this period with any degree of accuracy, although many authorities state that it usually begins sometime in the person's twenties and is concluded in the late thirties or early forties. As the life span increases and the entry into the adult work world is delayed by the need for increasingly advanced education, it is obvious that the age ranges of the later developmental periods will have to be reevaluated.

As previously stated, Freud believed that the healthy young adult will have achieved psychosexual maturity. By this he meant that the individual will have integrated his libidinal drives in a manner that enables him to love a member of the opposite sex with whom he hopes to establish a home and nurture a family. At the same time the mature adult retains enough self-love to seek satisfaction for his own needs without being destructive to others. In addition, he is able to direct positive feelings toward other people in his environment, to work effectively, to achieve creatively, and to fully use the capacities with which he has been endowed without being hampered by crippling anxieties. The ability to achieve these mature capabilities depends to a large extent on the person's heredity and constitutional endowment. However, psychosexual development is powerfully influenced by the experiences that the person has during his early formative years.

Although Freud's theory of psychosexual development does

not preclude the potential influence of events on personality in the individual's adult life, Freud postulated that the early developmental stages were critical and that the final stage begins in the late teens and lasts until senility, with major personality development alterations being unlikely during this time under usual circumstances.

Erikson, on the other hand, sees the personality as continuing to develop dynamically throughout the remainder of the life span. During early adulthood Erikson sees the necessity for the individual to continue making decisions about significant aspects of life, such as choosing a mate with whom the individual can experience both physical and emotional intimacy. Erikson expresses this by stating that the task to be mastered during this period is the development of intimacy versus isolation. The ability to develop an intimate relationship with an adult of the opposite sex is highly dependent on satisfactory mastery of previous developmental tasks and leads to the establishment of a safe and congenial family environment in which children can be raised. Accepting the role of parent and the responsibility for nurturing, safeguarding, and rearing children is essential if the culture is to be perpetuated. Obviously the individual's ability to be successful in these activities is determined to a large extent by his experiences as a child within a family—hence the expression that the child is the father of the man. Erikson also emphasizes the significance of successfully building one's lifework during this stage. Children cannot be effectively nurtured unless the family has a reasonable degree of social and financial security. Thus acceptance of family responsibilities requires that the young adult be reasonably effective in performing some aspect of work.

If the developmental task of intimacy and its concomitant responsibilities are not achieved, the young adult is likely to develop a sense of emotional isolation having the sense that he "does not fit." Although the young adult who retreats into isolation often does so to avoid the emotional pain risked by the vulnerability associated with intimacy, he ironically discovers that the price of self-protection is not having his needs met, which increases the need to protect himself.

Sullivan referred to early adulthood as the stage of late adolescence. He believed that the major task of this period is the incorporation of intimacy (which developed during preadolescence with a chum) with lust (which became the mode of relating during early adolescence) so that these are not experienced in isolation from each other. Sullivan viewed this mode of relating as the hallmark of adult maturity, and therefore did not identify any subsequent stages of development.

Middle age

As previously stated, neither Freud nor Sullivan identified developmental dynamics beyond the achievement of adulthood. However, both these theorists implied that it may take the remainder of the individual's life for him to develop the maturity that theoretically should have been achieved by middle age. Erikson, however, continued to elaborate on developmental tasks specific to later life.

According to Erikson, the developmental task of middle age is the development of generativity versus stagnation. Erikson believed that as the emotionally healthy individual grows older it becomes increasingly important to him that he transmit his values to the next generation, thereby helping to ensure his own immortality through the perpetuation of his culture. Therefore it is not unusual to see the middle-aged adult become very involved in activities that are concerned with his community and the society at large. On the other hand, the individual who developed a sense of isolation during the previous period becomes increasingly self-absorbed and is often acutely aware of "marking time." This person gets little fulfillment from interpersonal relationships or work and has few if any meaningful goals. Hence Erikson's descriptive term, *stagnation.*

Current literature about the stage of middle age makes it clear that this period is one about which we still need to learn more. Several authorities believe that the middle-aged person, because of physiological alterations, aging parents, and increasing awareness of community and societal needs and grown children who lead lives independent of him, confronts his own mortality for the first time. It is believed that this confrontation results in much uneasiness about the status quo and a subsequent reevaluation of one's goals and purposes in life. Persons who have previously led relatively unexamined lives often find themselves in a state of crisis, which they may attempt to hide from others, since to them their concerns do not seem to be reality based. Societal manifestations of this middle-age turmoil are a marked increase in the divorce rate and major shifts in career patterns.* For example, the woman who has been relatively satisfied as a homemaker for the past 15 or 20 years feels as if she has been left out of the mainstream of life and suddenly develops a need to become involved in a career outside the home. Likewise, it is not uncommon for a husband and father at this stage of life to feel that the occupation in which he has been involved for the previous 20 years is unsatisfying, regardless of his monetary or social success.

It is understandable that this reaction on the part of either wife or husband, or both, causes much disequilibrium in the family system. As a result, it is believed, many middle-aged persons decide they have made a mistake, not only in choice of vocation, but also in marriage partner, geographical location, and hobbies. It is unfortunate that many decisions are made precipitously on the basis of these feelings and that these feelings are not recognized as being valid within the developmental context in which they occur.

Margaret Mead, world famous anthropologist, eloquently pointed out that the needs and requirements of marital partners, like those of their children, change as the relationship matures. Thus the maintenance of a happy and successful marriage relationship requires that the partners continuously seek to relate to each other as individuals whose needs are in a process of dynamic evolution.

Old age

The role of aged individuals who have retired from an active social and economic life is unique in this culture. Unfortunately the wisdom that they have accumulated through the years is not con-

*Sheehy, Gail: Passages—predictable crises of adult life, New York, 1976, E.P. Dutton & Co., Inc.

sidered to be of value as it is in some cultures. Aging persons find it necessary to adjust to a reduced income, waning physical strength, and deteriorating health. This may be an anxiety-producing experience, since it represents a loss of power and independence. Loneliness is another experience with which elderly people must cope. Frequently their friends and marital partners die, leaving them in the position of being socially isolated. Such lonely individuals who are no longer able to cope efficiently with their own physical requirements need to adjust to the establishment of living arrangements that are acceptable, while at the same time being faced with the need to accept a dependent role. Older persons need to establish social relationships with a group of interested, sympathetic peers. This need leads many older individuals to seek an affiliation with a "golden age" club or a similar organization.

The preceding statements about the stage of old age are pessimistic in tone because of the current nature of the society in which we live and the ways in which elderly people are viewed. It should be clear that the older person must inevitably make many adjustments to altered physiological, social, and financial states. If, however, his previous developmental tasks have been satisfactorily achieved, it is quite possible for him to make the necessary adjustments with grace, dignity, and a minimum of undue anxiety.

The major dynamic of the old-age period is the acceptance of the inevitability of death. To develop this acceptance the individual engages in a life review. If on the whole the aged person is able to feel satisfied with the uniqueness and achievements of his past life, Erikson believes the person will develop a sense of ego integrity, which in turn enables him to view death as the ultimate conclusion of life. If, on the other hand, the individual's life review finds him lacking, he will develop a sense of despair, because time is too short for him to undo and redo his life to achieve the sense of fulfillment he lacks.

As with middle age, old age is a period of life about which much more can be learned. Interest in and concern about this stage of development are increasing as the number of older persons in our society increases.

CONCLUDING STATEMENTS

1. Personality refers to the aggregate of physical and mental qualities of the individual as these interact in characteristic fashion with his environment.
2. All individuals progress through a lifelong dynamic sequence of stages of personality development.
3. Much of our current knowledge concerning personality development is based on the theories proposed by Sigmund Freud's theory of personality development, which is based on the shifting of libidinal energy to various areas of the body. Hence Freud's theory of personality development is called the psychosexual theory.
4. The levels of consciousness were described by Freud as the conscious, the preconscious, and the unconscious.
5. According to Freud, the structure of the personality includes the id, the ego, and the superego.
6. Erik Erikson builds on Freud's theories by identifying eight developmental stages that encompass the entire life span, referred to as the Eight Ages of Man.
7. Erikson's theory of personality development is variously referred to as neo-Freudian, ego psychology, or cultural.
8. Harry Stack Sullivan's theory of personality development emphasizes the uniqueness of human interdependence. Therefore his theories are referred to as interpersonal.
9. Sullivan theorized that personality development consists of a series of interpersonally based learnings in which dynamisms are used as the individual attempts to gain approval and avoid the anxiety associated with disapproval.
10. A theoretically eclectic approach to the understanding of personality development is particularly applicable to the practice of nursing.
11. Freud identified five stages of personality development: the oral stage, the anal stage, the phallic stage, the stage of latency, and the genital stage. These descriptive terms represent the area of the body on which the libidinal energy is focused.
12. Erikson identifies developmental tasks specific to eight stages of development. These are basic trust versus basic mistrust,

autonomy versus shame and doubt, initiative versus guilt, industry versus inferiority, identity versus role diffusion, intimacy versus isolation, generativity versus stagnation, and ego integrity versus despair.

13. Sullivan identified significant interpersonal learnings that take place during each of seven stages of development. During the stage of infancy, the self-concept is learned; during early childhood, the use of power; during later childhood, the use of language, which can be consensually validated; during the juvenile era, the ability to compete and to compromise; during preadolescence, the ability to experience intimacy; during early adolescence, the development of a heterosexual orientation; and during late adolescence, the integration of intimacy and lust in a heterosexual relationship.

Suggested sources of additional information

CLASSICAL

Berlien, Ivan C.: Growth as related to mental health, Am. J. Nurs. **56:**1142-1145, 1956.

Bowlby, John: Maternal care and mental health, Series No. 2, Geneva, 1952, World Health Organization.

Brill, A.A.: Freud's contribution to psychiatry, New York, 1944, W.W. Norton & Co., Inc.

Caplan, Gerald: Prevention of mental disorders in children, New York, 1961, Basic Books, Inc., Publishers.

Committee on Psychiatric Nursing, National League for Nursing Education: Psychological concepts of personality development, Am. J. Nurs. **50:**122-125, 182-184, 242-243, 1950.

English, O. Spurgeon, and Pearson, G.H.J.: Emotional problems of living; avoiding the neurotic pattern, ed. 3, New York, 1963, W.W. Norton & Co., Inc.

Erikson, Erik H.: Childhood and society, ed. 2, New York, 1964, W.W. Norton & Co., Inc.

Munroe, Ruth L.: Schools of psychoanalytic thought, New York, 1955, The Dryden Press, Inc.

Sullivan, Harry Stack: The interpersonal theory of psychiatry, New York, 1968, W.W. Norton & Co, Inc.

Thompson, Clare: The different schools of psychoanalysis, Am. J. Nurs. **57:**1304-1307, 1957.

CONTEMPORARY

Arnold, Helen M.: Snowwhite and the seven dwarfs: a symbolic account of human development, Perspect. Psychiatr. Care **117**(5):218-222, Sept.-Oct., 1979.

Bowlby, John: Attachment, New York, 1980, Basic Books, Inc., Publishers.

Bowlby, John: Separation, New York, 1980, Basic Books Inc., Publishers.

Cumming, Elaine, and Henry, William E.: Growing old; the process of disengagement, New York, 1979, Arno Press, Inc.

Dresen, Sheila E.: Staying well while growing old: autonomy, a continuing developmental task. V. Am. J. Nurs. **78**:1344-1346, Aug., 1978.

Ehmann, Virginia E.: Empathy: its origin, characteristics, and process, Perspect. Psychiatr. Care **9**:72-80, March-April, 1971.

Geller, Joseph: Developmental symbiosis, Perspect. Psychiatr. Care **13**:10-12, Jan.-March, 1975.

Gibney, Helen A.: Masturbation: an invitation for an interpersonal relationship, Perspect. Psychiatr. Care **10**:128-134, July-Sept., 1972.

Graves, Joy Dan: Psychoanalytic theory—a critique, Perspect. Psychiatr. Care **11**(3):114-120, 1973.

Lidz, Theodore: The person: his and her development throughout the life cycle, New York, 1976, Basic Books, Inc., Publishers.

May, Robert: Sex and fantasy: patterns of male and female development, New York, 1980, W.W. Norton & Co., Inc.

Rouslin, Sheila: Developmental aggression and its consequences, Perspect. Psychiatr. Care **13**:170-175, Oct.-Dec., 1975.

Woods, Nancy Fugate: Human sexuality in health and illness, ed. 2, St. Louis, 1979, The C.V. Mosby Co.

OF PARTICULAR INTEREST

Erikson, Erik H.: Childhood and society, ed. 2, New York, 1964, W.W. Norton & Co., Inc.

This classic text presents the author's psychosocial theory of personality development in a sensitive, insightful manner.

Rogers, C.: On becoming a person, Boston, 1961, Houghton Mifflin Co.

Personal growth is discussed in this text both from the individual's point of view and as it affects the therapeutic process.

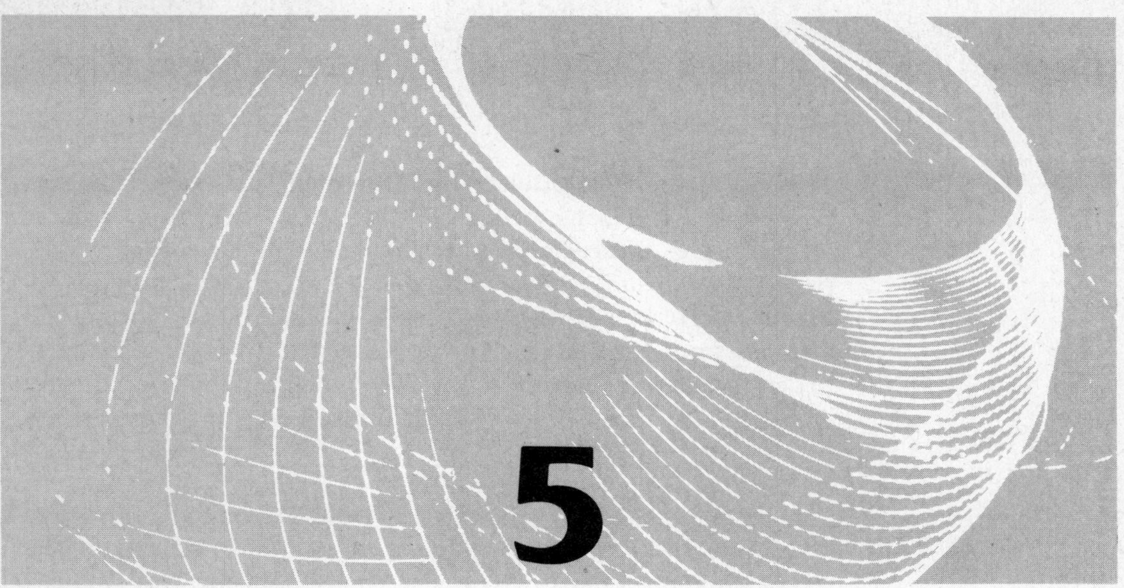

5

Anxiety: its development and defenses

- Definition and characteristics of anxiety
- Origin of anxiety
- Defense mechanisms of personality

Anxiety is the most universal of all human emotions. It is experienced by all persons throughout the entire life span. Despite its all-pervasive nature, however, anxiety cannot be observed directly. Rather, its presence can only be inferred from behavior. Since anxiety is a basic factor in the development and manifestation of human behavior, it is necessary for the psychiatric nurse to acquire an in-depth understanding of its origin, characteristics, and the usual means by which individuals deal with it.

DEFINITION AND CHARACTERISTICS OF ANXIETY

Anxiety is defined as a vague sense of impending doom, an apprehension or sense of dread, which seemingly has no basis in reality. Lay persons refer to anxiety as "being nervous."

Anxiety, unlike any other emotion, is always perceived as being negative. In contrast to anxiety, emotions that are usually considered to be painful sometimes bring pleasure. For example, most people do not enjoy being angry. On occasion, however, it is satisfying to experience anger when one feels it is justified and shares it in common with others. Another characteristic of anxiety is its extreme communicability. Almost like a living organism, anxiety is transferred with amazing rapidity from one individual to another, often out of a level of awareness.

When the individual experiences anxiety, he cannot distinguish it from fear, a feeling state that occurs in response to a specific identifiable environmental threat. Because anxiety cannot be distinguished from fear, the physiological response is the same in that the autonomic nervous system is activated and the body becomes ready for "flight or fight." Since an identifiable environmental threat is not present, the individual cannot discharge the tension of anxiety by fleeing or fighting and consequently may experience such symptoms as a pounding heart and a dry mouth, the perception of which serves to increase anxiety. Furthermore, when an individual becomes aware of being anxious, he often frantically searches for a reason to explain this feeling in the hope of abolishing it. Rarely is he successful, and his explanation often describes the result of his anxiety, not its cause. For example, a young woman who believes she is anxious because of the responsibilities she must assume in the care of her young infant may really be experiencing a conflict between a desire to be dependent and the need to be independent, which in turn creates anxiety, making her increasingly less able to care for the infant. Therefore her explanation of her anxiety is not its cause but rather its manifestation.

Anxiety occurs in degrees. Although it is never seen as desirable, mild anxiety serves the function of motivating the person and making him more physically and mentally alert. When the level of anxiety is extremely high, the individual may be incapable of action or may react with unusual behavior or what appears to be irrational behavior. This irrational behavior is referred to as a panic state.

ORIGIN OF ANXIETY

Most authorities believe that anxiety occurs most often as a result of a threat to biological integrity, an unconscious symbolic conflict, or a threat to the self-concept.

Freud believed that anxiety results from the emergence of id impulses that are unacceptable to the superego. In other words, the ego detects a real or potential conflict between the id and the superego, which results in anxiety, thereby alerting the ego to the necessity for intervention. He believed that all persons experience anxiety initially during the birth process when the respiratory and cardiovascular systems must undergo rapid, extensive changes to support extrauterine life. He also viewed the birth process as the prototypical separation. These two factors—the threat to life and separation—are associatively linked to each other and to the experience of anxiety. In subsequent developmental stages, he theorized that unconscious conflicts are perceived as life threatening, are associated with separation, and result in anxiety.

Sullivan viewed anxiety as always occurring in an interpersonal context. That is, anxiety is generated when the individual anticipates or actually receives cues that signal disapproval from one or more significant others. This presents an individual with an approach-avoidance dilemma in that there is a desire to approach or please the other person because he is seen as being significant, but to do so incurs the risk of disapproval of self—a threat to the very existence of the individual as he knows himself. According to Sullivan, the human being first experiences anxiety as an infant when either his need for satisfaction, which is physiologically based, or his need for security, which is interpersonally based, is not met by the mothering one. The student will remember that Sullivan's theory of personality development also emphasized the empathic linkage between infant and mothering one through which anxiety is readily communicated. The empathic linkage makes the infant and mothering one uncommonly sensitive to discomfort in each other. The infant, because of his inability to solve problems, has no alternative but to believe that the mothering one's anxiety, which is communicated to him via the empathic linkage, is caused by him, even though the source of this discomfort may be external to him. This phenomenon, which all adults have experienced, by definition, during their infancy, is the basis for Sullivan's belief that anxiety is interpersonally based.

Children brought up by parents or other significant adults who punish them severely for minor indiscretions or who consistently disapprove of their behavior no matter how hard they try to please may develop persistent severe anxiety that becomes a lifelong problem. Corrective experiences to counteract such a long-standing problem require consistent long-term in-depth treatment.

Some authorities distinguish between normal anxiety and neurotic anxiety. *Normal anxiety* consists of the feelings of tension, nervousness, and apprehension that accompany a realistic situation. Thus the feelings of fear and tension a bridegroom experiences before his wedding are called normal anxiety and arise out of what he feels may be a threat to his identity as an adequate male.

Anxiety that is aroused by the individual's own unacceptable thoughts, feelings, wishes, or desires and that would cause the loss of approval or love from significant individuals or groups is sometimes termed *neurotic anxiety*. Individuals who develop overwhelming sexual thoughts and desires that are unacceptable to the social group frequently respond with behavior described as panic.

DEFENSE MECHANISMS OF PERSONALITY

When the individual unconsciously experiences a basic conflict between id impulses and the demands of the superego or perceives a serious threat to his biological integrity or sees his self-concept threatened, he experiences a degree of anxiety that cannot be tolerated for long. This uncomfortable situation is reflected in the individual's behavior. Some method of developing a compromise or otherwise relieving the tension and anxiety is essential. The human being usually is able to relieve the conflict by using a certain form of adaptation, that is, *defense mechanisms.* These methods of thinking and acting are actually patterns of behavior initiated during one of the earlier phases of personality development. They are further developed and elaborated as the individual grows and struggles with problems. Even during their early development, they are used to protect the individual from threatening aspects of his environment or from his own feelings of tension and anxiety, which are unacceptable and upsetting to him. Thus the use of these defense mechanisms is a matter of resorting to earlier patterns of behavior that have already proved helpful in relieving tension and anxiety. Many of these methods of thinking are wholly unconscious, whereas others are partially conscious and partially unconscious.

All persons use defense mechanisms to a certain degree to relieve intrapsychic tension. Under abnormal stress the use of the mental mechanisms may become a very prominent characteristic of behavior and may be so bizarre and unusual as to suggest that the individual is mentally ill.

In a sense, mental mechanisms are a means of protecting the individual from situations he perceives as dangerous. In this regard they serve a very important function by helping the person to maintain biological integrity and self-esteem.

A mention should be made of *coping mechanisms.* A coping mechanism, unlike a defense mechanism, is based on a conscious acknowledgment that a problem exists. As a result, the individual engages in reality-oriented problem-solving activities designed to reduce the tension. It is for this reason that coping mechanisms are considered to be more healthy adaptations than defense mechanisms. For example, when a student unexpectedly fails an examination, he would be using the defense mechanism of projection if he believes that the reason he failed is because the teacher is inadequate. While this would reduce his anxiety, it would not be helpful in enabling him to pass the course. On the other hand, if this student were able to acknowledge his failure to himself, he would then be able to engage in the coping mechanism of going to the instructor for help. By understanding his errors, his anxiety is reduced and he is able to learn what is necessary to pass the course.

The following is a discussion of commonly used defense mechanisms identified by Freud. These are called ego defenses, because they use psychic energy derived from the ego and serve to protect it from anxiety. It should not be forgotten that a defense mechanism may originate in more than one stage of personality development, or it may originate in one stage and be reinforced in others. Defense mechanisms are not clear-cut and almost never appear as isolated phenomena.

Compensation. Compensation is a pattern of adjustive behavior by which tension or anxiety is relieved as the individual makes up for a personal lack or a feeling of inadequacy by emphasizing some personal or social attribute that overshadows the weakness and gains social approval.

The origins of this device can be seen in the young infant who substitutes his thumb or a toy for the nipple or the bottle to relieve tension and make up for some of the pleasurable sensations of sucking that may be lacking in sufficient quantity.

Obviously compensation is far more complicated in adults than in infants and is usually prompted by feelings of guilt or inferiority. It may explain much of the behavior observed in adults who work zealously to promote philanthropic enterprises. Compensation may be operating in the behavior of a man who is very small in physical stature but who is extremely successful in the business world through his aggressive practices. It may also be one of the mechanisms operating when a young person who is paralyzed as a result of a car accident is able to achieve many honors for outstanding scholarship in college.

Displacement or substitution. Displacement or substitution refers to the discharge of emotions, feelings, or ideas on a subject entirely different from the one to which the feelings rightly belong. This is usually a safety operation, with the feelings being discharged away from the actual source of the emotion because it is not considered safe to express them directly. Displacement may be used by a teacher who is angry with an immediate supervisor and does not show these feelings in his presence but reacts with unreasonable anger when a pupil accidentally breaks a windowpane on that same day. The teacher may be displacing the angry feelings by expressing them toward the student rather than toward the supervisor. Actually the teacher has unconsciously substituted the student for the supervisor and has displaced the feelings accordingly.

Denial. Denial is the process whereby the individual truly does not recognize the existence of an event or feeling. Denial is a commonly used defense in severe emotional illnesses such as schizophrenia. It is often seen as a reaction of the healthy individual when he is unexpectedly confronted by a disasterous situation. For example, the wife of a policeman who has just been killed in the line of duty may calmly respond to the informant, "You must have made a mistake! I just had breakfast with him no more than 2 hours ago. I'm getting ready to shop now, so you'll have to excuse me."

It is important to understand that the mechanism of denial operates on a totally unconscious basis in response to the sudden onset of massive amounts of anxiety. Denial should not be confused with lying, which is a conscious effort to avoid responsibility in a situation.

Fixation. Fixation refers to the point in the individual's development at which certain aspects of the emotional development cease to advance. For reasons that are usually obscure, further development seems to be blocked. This blocking appears to arise from the inability of the individual to solve problems that occurred during the specific phase of development at which progress ceased. Thus the individual is unable to achieve the developmental tasks of that phase, and since it is not possible to entirely bypass a stage, he is always handicapped in proceeding to the stages that follow. Individuals who have not experienced the love and security required in the oral stage of development may spend the remainder of their lives pursuing this pattern of behavior. Many adults are said to be fixated at the oral-dependent level of development. They seek to find ways of meeting this need. Since food and liquid intake are so closely allied to love and security in the unconscious emotional life, some fixated individuals may imbibe huge quantities of alcohol or compulsively overeat.

Suppression. Suppression is the conscious and intentional dismissal to the preconscious mind of impulses, feelings, and thoughts that are unpleasant or unacceptable to the individual. Suppressed material is easily recalled and is thus available to the conscious mind.

Sublimation. Sublimation is a mechanism by which the energy involved in primitive impulses and cravings is redirected into socially constructive and acceptable channels. This is one of the chief mechanisms operating when a child learns to redirect the pleasurable sensations involved in expelling excrement at will into the more socially acceptable patterns of toilet training.

Sublimation is one of the more positive mechanisms of adjustment and is at least partially responsible for much of the artistic and cultural achievement of civilized people. It is operating when a woman redirects her sexual drives, which might be expected to result in a home and children, into a successful career as a nursery school teacher. It is probably operating when a young man who has lost his lover turns to writing poetry about love.

Reaction formation. Reaction formation occurs when an individual expresses an attitude or act that is directly opposite to his unconscious feelings or wishes. Thus the individual is denying, in a sense of the word, his true feelings or desires. People who are extremely friendly, overly polite, and very socially correct frequently have unconscious feelings of anger and hatred toward many people. These true feelings may be evident in slips of the tongue or in their biting humor.

Reaction formation sometimes develops out of rigid toilet-training experiences. One evidence of reaction formation may be observed in adults who are untidy about their homes and their personal hygiene but whose mothers required meticulous conformity to rules of cleanliness and tidiness.

Identification. Identification is a much used and extremely useful mechanism, since it plays a large part in the development of a child's personality and in the process of acculturation. Through the process of identification the individual takes on desirable attributes found in the personalities of people in his environment for whom he has admiration and affection. He integrates these personality attributes into his own ego. Thus the little boy takes on masculine attributes that he admires in his father. The student integrates into his personality makeup the attributes he admires in his professor. Another form of identification is observed when an individual develops an unreasoning sympathy for a criminal because of an unconscious sense of guilt.

Introjection. The mechanism of introjection is closely related to identification, and the two are difficult to distinguish. Introjection rests on the psychoanalytical concept of oral receptivity and refers to the fantasied swallowing or incorporation of a loved or hated object or person into the individual's own ego structure. Introjection is operating when the child develops the superego by incorporating the ideals and standards of the parents. When introjection is operating in adults, it suggests that the entire personality of a second person has been incorporated and has replaced the original personality. A psychotic patient who claimed to be Moses wore a beard, let his hair grow long, talked in biblical phrases, and acted as Moses might have acted. What he believed to be the personality of Moses had been incorporated by the patient, and he had given up his own personality. In contrast, identification is a mechanism by means of which an individual's ego is added to, not replaced. Introjection may operate in a less constructive way than identification, especially when it is observed in adults. For instance, a depressed person may unconsciously feel that he has incorporated another person within himself. He may attempt to commit suicide to kill the introjected person whom he unconsciously hates.

Undoing. Undoing is a mechanism wherein the individual engages in certain behaviors as a means of symbolically canceling out unconscious thoughts or feelings that are unacceptable and therefore associated with anxiety. Although the individual is aware of his behavior, he is not aware of its purpose, and it often seems irrational even to him. Undoing is seen as the basis of compulsive behavior. Undoing behavior is frequently highly repetitive, since it does not achieve its aim of actually canceling out the anxiety-producing thought or feeling.

Isolation. Isolation is a phenomenon when the feeling is detached from the event in the individual's memory, enabling the person to recall the event without its attendant anxiety. This mechanism is evident in situations when an individual relays a harrowing experience without any evidence of fear.

Rationalization. Rationalization is a mental mechanism that is almost universally employed. It is an attempt to make one's behavior appear to be the result of logical thinking rather than the result of unconscious desires or cravings. It is used when the individual has a sense of guilt about something he does or believes or when he is uncertain about his behavior. It is a face-saving device that may or may not deal with the actual truth. Rationalization should not be confused with falsehoods or alibis, since the latter are conscious avoidance maneuvers. Rationalization is almost totally unconscious, and although it is used to put the individual in the best possible light, it does not have the deliberate aspect of other conscious avoidance maneuvers.

The person who does not want to keep an appointment because to do so would create anxiety and says that the appointment slipped his mind is not telling a falsehood, but rather is using rationalization as a defense mechanism. Although rationalization relieves anxiety temporarily, it is not an effective mechanism of adjustment because it assists the individual to avoid facing the reality factors in the situation.

Repression. Repression is a widely used and completely unconscious mechanism. Painful experiences, unacceptable thoughts and impulses, and disagreeable memories are forcibly dismissed from consciousness. The psychic energy with which they were invested becomes an active free-floating source of anxiety in the unconscious mind. Many painful experiences are repressed during early childhood and become unconscious sources of emotional conflict in later life. Selfish, hostile feelings and sexual impulses are frequently repressed. Such repression always causes internal conflict. This repressed material may find escape through conversion into physical defects, into obsessions, and into morbid anxiety that arises without apparent reason.

Regression. Regression occurs when an individual is faced with a conflict or problem that cannot be solved by using the adjustment mechanisms with which he customarily solves problems. In such a situation he may resort to behavior that was successful at an earlier stage in his development but which he had presumably outgrown. Thus regression is a return to patterns of earlier immature behavior. Any retreat into a state of dependency on others to avoid facing acute problems can be called a regressive trait. "Crying on someone's shoulder" is symbolic of the infant's seeking comfort on the maternal bosom. Although some seeking for a dependency relationship is a benign form of regression, this dynamism may become the main element in the development of a serious psychosis.

Projection. Projection is a frequently used unconscious mechanism that relieves tension and anxiety by transferring the responsibility for unacceptable ideas, impulses, wishes, or thoughts to another person. The mechanism is used when the individual cannot accept the responsibility for his own hostile, aggressive thoughts. Although all people use this mechanism to some extent, it is not a healthy method of adaptation and is more frequently used by mentally ill persons than by more healthy individuals. It is operative in such psychotic symptoms as delusions and hallucinations. In the latter, the individual hears voices saying things about him that he unconsciously fears are true. The paranoid person may project his own inner hate of others by saying that a group of people is plotting to kill him. Less pathological use of projection is evident when a worker blames the boss for his difficulties on the job or when a student blames the teacher for his failure on the final examination. Paranoid persons frequently project their feelings of sexual inadequacy on others. Thus a common delusion concerns the unfaithful spouse when the actual lack of fidelity is in the mind of the accuser.

Symbolization and condensation. A symbol is an idea or object used by the conscious mind in lieu of the actual idea or object.

Instinctual desires may appear through symbols, the meanings of which are not exactly clear to the conscious mind. These symbols are the language of the unconscious. Such symbols appear in dreams or in fantasies and may emerge through various rituals or obsessive behavior.

Symbols may become further merged by condensation to represent a wide range of emotionally painful ideas that thus become lumped together so as to lose their painful significance. When they rise to the conscious level, they take the form of an apparently incoherent jumble of words, the real meaning of which is hidden in the unconscious. Such condensations of thinking are frequently noted in the apparently irrational language of the schizophrenic individual. However, these condensations have meaning and significance for him.

Conversion. Conversion refers to the expression of emotional conflicts through a physical symptom for which there is no demonstrable organic basis. When disagreeable experiences and unacceptable desires are repressed into the unconscious, they may reappear as a physical symptom without the individual's being aware of any connection between the two phenomena. Thus a child who is torn by a conflict arising out of chronic friction between her parents, both of whom she loves, may find herself suddenly blind. This symptom literally relieves her of the necessity of looking on such incompatibility. A young girl who fears that she must account for her misbehavior may suddenly develop a paralysis of her vocal cords. Conversion is not always expressed in such a direct and easily recognized manner. Frequently it is difficult to determine just what conflicts in the repressed unconscious produce a certain physical symptom. The symptom always serves to distract attention from the individual's real problems. This mechanism is entirely unconscious and is not used by mature, well-adjusted individuals.

• • •

Sullivan also identified protective measures against anxiety, which he called security operations. These include apathy, which is extreme indifference; somnolent detachment, which is falling asleep during anxiety-producing experiences; selective inattention, which is similar to Freud's mechanism of denial; and preoccupation, which is a consuming interest in a person, thought, or event to the exclusion of the anxiety-producing reality.

CONCLUDING STATEMENTS

1. Anxiety is the most universal of all emotions. It cannot be observed directly, but must be inferred from behavior.
2. Anxiety is defined as a vague sense of impending doom, an apprehension, or a sense of dread.
3. Anxiety has the following characteristics:
   a. It is always perceived as a negative feeling.
   b. It is extremely communicable.
   c. It cannot be distinguished from fear by the individual experiencing it.
   d. It occurs in degrees.
4. Anxiety occurs most often as a result of a threat to biological integrity, an unconscious symbolic conflict, or a threat to the self-concept.
5. Freud believed that anxiety results from the emergence of id impulses that are unacceptable to the superego.
6. Sullivan viewed anxiety as occurring when the individual anticipates or actually receives cues that signal disapproval from one or more significant others.
7. Defense mechanisms were identified by Freud. They use psychic energy derived from the ego and serve to protect the ego from anxiety.
8. All people use defense mechanisms to a certain degree to relieve intrapsychic tension and anxiety, but if these mechanisms become a prominent characteristic of behavior or are bizarre and unusual, the individual may be mentally ill.
9. Most defense mechanisms are initiated early during the development of the personality. They are not clear-cut and almost never appear as isolated phenomena.
10. Sullivan also identified protective measures against anxiety, which he called security operations.

Suggested sources of additional information

CLASSICAL

Freud, Anna: The ego and mechanisms of defense, New York, 1967, International Universities Press.

Horvath, Kathy: Incorporation: what is the nurse's role? Am. J. Nurs. **72:**1096-1100, 1972.

Nehren, Jeanette, and Gilliam, Naomi R.: Separation anxiety, Am. J. Nurs. **65:**109-112, Jan., 1965.

Peterson, Margaret H.: Understanding defense mechanisms, Am. J. Nurs. **72:**1651-1674, 1972.

CONTEMPORARY

Kerr, Norine: Anxiety: theoretical considerations, Perspect. Psychiatr. Care **16**(1):36-40, Jan.-Feb., 1978.

King, Joan M.: Denial, Am. J. Nurs. **66:**1010-1013, May, 1966.

Laughlin, H.: The ego and its defenses, New York, 1979, Jason Aronson Press.

Lidz, Theodore: The person; his and her development throughout the life cycle, New York, 1976, Basic Books, Inc., Publishers.

Snyder, Joyce C., and Wilson, Margo F.: Elements of a psychological assessment, Am. J. Nurs. **77:**253-239, Feb., 1977.

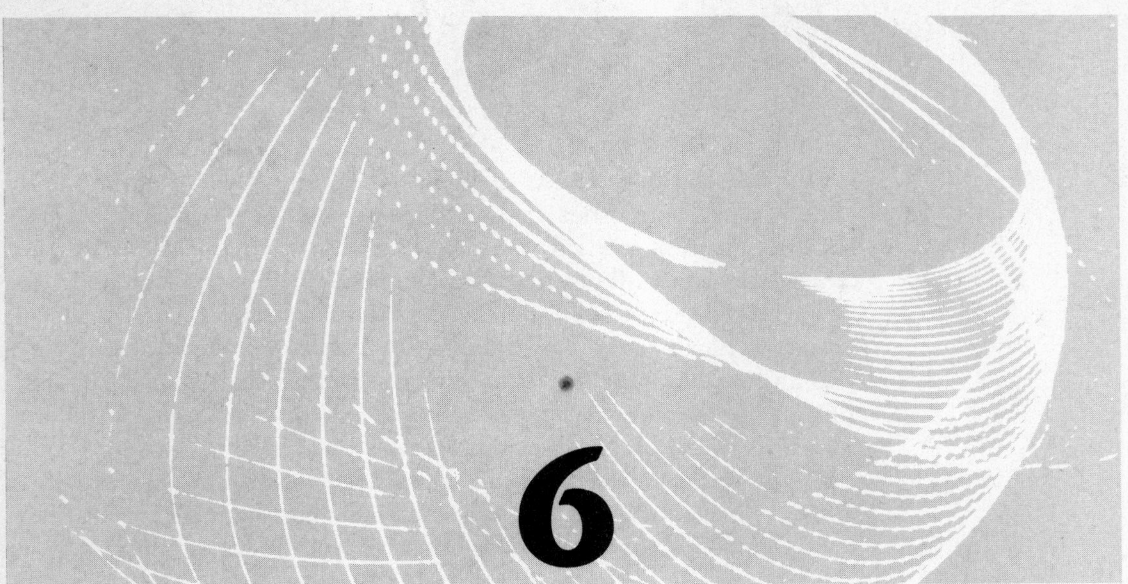

6

Mental health and the cause and prevention of mental illness

- Personality attributes of the mentally healthy individual
- Factors that may contribute to mental illness
- Prevention of mental illness

On few topics is there so little exact information available as there is on mental health and the cause and prevention of mental illness. Completely satisfactory definitions of mental health and mental illness still remain undeveloped. To a large extent these concepts are culturally determined and are defined differently in various parts of the world. Behavior that might be characterized as abnormal or mentally sick in one culture may be accepted and encouraged in another. For example, men who sit most of the day staring at the sun might be considered mentally ill in the United States, but in India they are considered to be holy and are provided for through the benevolence of the community.

Mental illness is a complex problem. It is thought to be a unique response involving an individual's personality as it interacts with his environment at a time when he is particularly vulnerable to stress. Early repetitive, negative interpersonal relationships within the famly situation apparently influence the future emotional health of an individual in many unfortunate ways. One of these ways is the lack of development of coping mechanisms that are adequate to meet the usual maturational and situational stressors of the society in which the individual lives. Human beings who have experienced severe interpersonal stresses in early life are apparently more vulnerable to stress during adolescence, middle age, and old age than are individuals who have developed a basic sense of trust and security during their very early experiences with other people.

PERSONALITY ATTRIBUTES OF THE MENTALLY HEALTHY INDIVIDUAL

Although it is impossible to provide the reader with a definition of mental health that would be universally acceptable to all authorities in all cultures, it is possible to discuss the attributes usually identified as being present in the personality structures of those who appear to have successfully mastered their environments. The ability to cope with the recurrent stresses of living and to achieve a relatively effective adjustment is referred to as mental maturity by many authorities, emotional maturity by others, and mental health by some.

Mental health is closely related to physical health because the human being is a unified, integrated whole. The dichotomy of body and mind has persisted much too long among some groups because the cause and effect relationship between the two is not always demonstrable in specific medical terms.

Currently, different medical standards exist for evaluating mental health and physical health. Those applied to mental health are stated in terms of personality attributes, adjustment to stress, interpersonal capacities, and the ability to cope with reality. Evaluations in these terms are of necessity complex and imprecise. In contrast, much of the evaluation of physical health can be done in terms of precise measurement in such areas as weight, blood pressure, biochemical content of the blood, and urinalysis.

Few people can be said to have achieved complete mental health or emotional maturity. Thus it is probably more helpful to evaluate the individual in terms of relative strengths or limitations in relation to the social norms and values existing in the community in which the individual lives. Because mentally ill people demonstrate some strengths as well as some limitations, it can be seen that the line of demarcation between mental health and mental illness is sometimes difficult to describe and is sharply defined in only a limited number of individuals. It also becomes clear that one can speak accurately of working with the healthy aspects of the personality.

Margaret Mead wrote that mental health is actually determined by a set of ratios involving the emotional, social, and psychological strengths with which an individual is fortified, the events he has experienced throughout life, the pressures he is currently undergoing, and the expectations society has established for him. Thus a young lawyer who loses his wife and two children in an automobile accident will be able to maintain emotional equilibrium and continue to carry on his law practice and his personal life after a reasonable period of grieving if the ratios stated above are favorable. His ability to carry on will depend on the strengths within his personality, the supports his family and friends provide, the number of crises he has experienced in the past, and the expectations of significant people in his life. If he has had other traumatic personal losses in the past, if his family and friends are not able to be with him or do not provide him with emotional support, if he is disappointed by not receiving the political appointment he was promised shortly before his wife was killed, and if he perceives that significant people in his life subtly believe that his burdens are overwhelming and he will not be able to carry on, he may unconsciously seek refuge in mental illness.

Mental health is always relative. It is relative to time, place, and situation. It has been demonstrated that the ability of individuals to maintain emotional equilibrium in the face of a devastating situation is different, depending on whether the problem is being faced alone or as a member of a group. Group membership is emotionally supportive and is usually a positive factor. This fact has been exemplified by the prisoners who were returned to the United States at the end of the Vietnam War. Although many of them had suffered tremendous deprivation for several years and had often undergone torture, most of these men were in much better mental health than psychiatrists had anticipated. A more recent example of the same phenomenon is the 52 Americans held hostage in Iran for 444 days. The explanation for these unexpected outcomes was the group relationship that was maintained throughout both ordeals. Individually these persons felt they were not alone in their misery. Their membership in the group was reassuring and supportive. In addition, as a group they were actively engaged in trying to do something about the situation, although this activity often had to be in the form of organized passive resistance.*

Most authorities agree that one of the major attributes of the mentally healthy or emotionally mature individual is the capacity to love and to be loved in return. This capacity is usually thought to embrace the ability to establish a satisfying heterosexual love relationship and the ability to carry through this relationship to its usual eventual conclusion of marriage and the establishment of a safe home environment for the nurturing of children. It follows that the establishment of a home and the nurturing of children require the capacity to effectively cope with a work situation.

The ability to love and be loved also includes the many appro-

---

*Mead, Margaret: Mental health in our changing culture, Ment. Hyg. **56:**6, 1972.

priate levels of love shared by the individual with parents, siblings, friends, and other individuals with whom he is involved. It is described by some authorities such as Marie Jahoda as adequacy in interpersonal relations.

The individual's level of self-acceptance and the way he perceives reality are usually mentioned as two other capacities significant in the development of emotional maturity. These capacities involve how effectively the individual has learned to accept his own limitations and abilities. In other words, the capacity to live comfortably with oneself is considered to be an important attribute. The way the individual perceives the world around him is equally important, since he copes with it in terms of his perceptions. Thus if the individual's view of the environment leads him to perceive it as a dangerous, hostile, threatening world, he will probably display attacking, suspicious, cautious behavior. On the other hand, if the individual perceives the world as a friendly, interesting, rewarding place in which to live, his method of coping with reality will be more acceptable, at least in this culture. Self-acceptance and the individual's perception of reality greatly influence another capacity, environmental mastery, which is almost always mentioned by authorities when writing about the emotionally mature, mentally healthy individual. Environmental mastery suggests that the individual is highly motivated and has made an investment in living that has necessitated the high-level development of his inherent abilities.

In addition, the mentally healthy or emotionally mature individual will have developed the capacity for independent thinking and action. This capacity is described by some as efficiency in problem solving and by others as autonomy or self-determination.

A final capacity usually included in such a discussion is the ability of the individual to effect a balance or synthesis of all psychological functions and personal attributes, which provides a unifying, integrated outlook on life and a sense of direction to the individual in relation to his role in it.

Thus it can be seen that mental health or emotional maturity is a highly individual attribute, that it cannot be defined in terms of the absence of disease, that it cannot be understood in terms of isolated symptoms, and that it is intimately related to the norms of the society in which the individual finds himself.

FACTORS THAT MAY CONTRIBUTE TO MENTAL ILLNESS

It is impossible to be definitive about the causes of a behavioral response that may be diagnosed as mental illness or to be specific about how this illness might have been prevented. The individual must be studied as a totality, as he is engaged with varying degrees of success in adjusting to his environment and as his environment affects him. No single set of facts can be considered separately when seeking the causes of mental illness. All the facts must be studied together if the behavior of any individual is to be understood. The only reasonable approach to the study of the cause of mental illness is a consideration of an individual's total life experience, with emphasis on genetic, physiological, intrapersonal, interpersonal, and cultural factors, each of which may have contributed to the problem. The following discussion presents some of the cues concerning the possible role of each of these factors in producing mental illness.

Genetic factors

Current knowledge concerning human heredity has not developed to a state in which definitive statements can be made about the influence of heredity on the development of mental illness. About the turn of the century it was a generally accepted belief that mental illness was inherited and that the tendency to develop certain psychotic reactions was transmitted with regularity from one generation to another. These ideas seemed to be given validity when it was observed that manic-depressive and schizophrenic syndromes did frequently appear in more than one generation of the same family. Today it is thought that the tendency to develop similar psychotic reactions among members of the same family may be a response to the environmental factors within the family rather than a result of heredity. It is reasonable to believe that children learn to behave in unusual ways when they are reared by parents who habitually respond in unusual ways to other people, to social situations, to work responsibilities, and to parenthood.

The question of the influence of heredity versus environment became a hotly discussed issue before Freudian theories became widely accepted in this country. People who were interested in the issue took sides, and two groups holding opposing views developed. For a time it appeared that the environmentalists had won the controversy. Today most well-read people take the rational view that both environmental and genetic factors significantly influence the way in which the individual reacts to life experiences.

More recently, the work of a famous geneticist, Dr. Franz Kallmann, focused the attention of scientists once more on the question of the role of genetic factors in the development of mental illness. His studies of identical twins with widely different environments were carried on for many years. He reported convincing evidence that may eventually lead to a greater understanding of the role of genetic factors in mental illness. Dr. Kallmann found in his study that if one twin developed schizophrenia, the other became ill with schizophrenia in 86% of the cases, even though these children were not reared in the same families and were not subjected to the same environmental influences. In the same study he found that if one twin developed manic-depressive psychosis, the other twin developed the same illness in 96% of the cases.

As scientific knowledge about human behavior evolves, scientists recognize the urgent need for more research and study of human genetics as it relates to the causation of mental illness. Disregarding the question of the genetic aspects of the cause of mental illness, the biological heredity of the individual is of great significance because body type, sex, intelligence, temperament, and energy endowment are largely determined by the combination of the genes that are contributed by each parent. These personal qualities that influence the new individual's life adjustment in specific ways are determined by his genetic endowment. In a sense the individual also inherits the family milieu into which he is born and the cultural forces with which he will be required to deal. These factors surely influence an individual's total response to life and play a large part in his ability to maintain an emotional equilibrium throughout life.

Organic factors

A large number of patients suffer from symptoms of mental illness in conjunction with a physical illness, but because of the temporary character of most of these mental reactions they are not recognized as being psychiatric conditions. It is interesting to note that the same organic problem may produce a wide variety of mental reactions in different persons. This suggests that personality plays an important role in behavioral response even when brain tissue is involved.

Traumatic brain damage is one of the common organic problems to which the human organism reacts with abnormal mental symptoms. Such an injury may result in a variety of mental symptoms, depending on the location and severity of the injury and the age and personality of the individual. The aftereffects of brain injury are frequently serious because of a progressive intellectual and emotional degeneration that may occur and the possibility that this degeneration may be accompanied by convulsive seizures.

Brain tumor is an organic condition that may be accompanied by a variety of mental and physical symptoms. The symptoms are dependent on the location of the tumor, its size, and, to some extent, on the type of tumor. Surgery is frequently helpful but may result in the same sequelae that follow brain injury.

Before the advent of the antibiotics, late syphilis, technically known as syphilitic meningoencephalitis, accounted for approximately 10% of all admissions to psychiatric hospitals. Although syphilis may be congenitally acquired, it is usually contracted after the age of puberty. Many more men than women were affected by this disease. Today it is rare for a patient to develop syphilitic meningoencephalitis, although the incidence of syphilis and other venereal diseases is again on the increase. The mental symptoms said to characterize syphilitic meningoencephalitis are depression, expansiveness, and agitation. However, the symptoms vary a great deal depending on the personality of the individual involved.

Delirium resulting from toxins in the blood or from a high blood level of certain drugs is a temporary condition that requires consideration and treatment of both the mental and physical symptoms. Bromides, barbituric acid derivatives, sulfa drugs, morphine, cocaine, marijuana, thiocyanates, and lead are examples of agents that produce such problems. In the last 20 years there has been an increase in the number of patients treated for personality disturbances resulting from the use of the amphetamines and the hallucinogenic agent D-lysergic acid diethylamide (LSD).

Withdrawal from a heavy and consistent intake of alcohol over a short period of time without adequate food intake can produce an acute condition called delirium tremens. A prolonged, excessive alcoholic intake can produce a chronic irreversible dementia that is accompanied by a gradual personality deterioration.

Most authorities agree that the excessive intake of alcohol is not the essential problem but rather that alcoholism is a symptom of a personality problem or an attempt to cope with an existing mental disorder.

Cortisone and adrenocorticotropic hormone (ACTH) may produce psychotic reactions in selected individuals. The symptoms usually disappear when the drugs are withdrawn. Thyroid and pituitary diseases may result in overactivity, emotional lability, anxiety, and overt fear or confusion and depression. These symptoms usually disappear when the physical condition is corrected.

Encephalitis, or inflammation of the brain, may cause specific abnormalities and may lead to psychic and physical disorders, depending on the organism that caused the condition, the age and personality of the individual, and the treatment provided. The acute form of encephalitis is characterized by lethargy, delirium, confusion, and stupor. In its chronic form it is recognized clinically as paralysis agitans and is characterized by shaking palsy associated with increasing irritability, insomnia, and neurotic behavior.

There are increasing numbers of researchers who are engaged in studies that point to a neurochemical correlate of mental illness, especially the schizophrenic and manic-depressive psychoses. Some hypotheses are (1) schizophrenics produce more or fewer corticoids than do normal individuals, (2) schizophrenia might result from faulty transmethylation of catecholamines, yielding a mescaline-like compound found more frequently in the urine of schizophrenic subjects than in the urine of normal persons, and (3) a disturbance in catecholamine metabolism is a major factor in manic-depressive psychosis. Although these and other research findings have promise in enlarging our understanding of factors that contribute to mental illness, it is unlikely that a singular, definitive causative factor will be identified in the near future. This pessimism is warranted because of the methodological problems encountered when studying human subjects and the large number of diverse behaviors that are labeled as indicative of mental illness in our society. Nevertheless, research in this area should continue to receive both cooperation and financial support.

Psychogenic factors

Psychogenic factors are involved with the individual's subjective and emotional feelings about himself. These include feelings of self-esteem, security, well-being, personal value, guilt, and inferiority. When an individual must cope with situations that increase negative feelings about himself, his anxiety level rises. Extremely high anxiety levels are unbearable and force the anxious person to seek defenses against these uncomfortable feelings. He may call on a variety of unconscious mechanisms with which he is able to defend himself against feelings of guilt, inadequacy, and insecurity. Specifically, one of these defenses may be projection or an unconscious blaming of others. Thus an individual may relieve guilt feelings about a sexual transgression by blaming his partner and claiming that it was not his fault but the fault of the woman whose behavior was seductive. A student may unconsciously defend himself against feelings of inadequacy by rationalizing and stating that although he failed a college entrance examination, he can play football better than anyone on his team. These are simple examples of normal defense mechanisms used to help an individual maintain an emotional equilibrium and relieve anxiety when intrapersonal feelings are involved.

If intrapersonal feelings continue to cause increased anxiety, it may become necessary for the individual to use more elaborate defense mechanisms. As time goes on, the elaborate defenses may prove inadequate and he may begin to use bizarre ways of defending himself. When this kind of defense becomes necessary, the individual is said to be mentally ill. Some situations that produce intrapersonal conflicts that may require more adjustment than the individual is capable of achieving include serious financial problems, loss of a deeply loved friend or relative, a broken marriage, loss of a job, failure to receive an important promotion, or disappointment in the integrity of a trusted friend. The foregoing conditions are often referred to as precipitating factors because the individual seems to give up his usual defenses and substitutes psychotic behavior at the time the serious intrapersonal conflict develops.

Age-related factors

There are some periods in life when the individual is more vulnerable emotionally than others. During these critical periods psychotic episodes are likely to occur more frequently than during other times throughout the life cycle. At these times individual defenses may not be adequate to deal successfully with the stresses that are presenting themselves.

These critical periods occur during the development of adolescence, middle age, and old age. They are stressful periods from both physiological and psychological standpoints.

During adolescence the young person is attempting to integrate rapid physical growth and genital maturity into the personality pattern. The individual is struggling to sever close family ties while at the same time seeking to be loved and accepted both at home and by the peer group. The adolescent's desperate need to belong to his age-group causes him to be influenced greatly by the social standards of his peers. Many of life's most significant decisions such as the choice of employment and of a lifetime marital partner are made during this period. Consequently these stresses cause some adolescents to suffer from a state of psychological confusion, and some actually become mentally ill. Young people seem to be most vulnerable between the ages of 17 and 25. During these years some adolescents or young adults develop a psychosis known as schizophrenia.

Four times as many women as men become mentally ill during late middle age. This critical period occurs during the late forties for women and during the late fifties for men. It is a critical period in life for several reasons, one of which is the declining activity of the reproductive function, which many men and women consider to be the factor that determines their masculine or feminine identity. Equally as important in the causation of mental illness during this period is the recognition that if the most cherished lifetime goals have not been achieved, there is little chance that they will be. Many married women with successful, busy husbands and children who are almost grown suddenly begin to feel that their life's work has been completed and that they are no longer useful or needed. This period is often perceived as the midpoint of life. If the future is viewed as being entirely downhill, a midlife depression can result.

After the age of 60, emotional disorders increase. This is an extremely critical period in the lives of many individuals because of the feelings of insecurity brought on by the changes in life-style caused by retirement, the threat of financial dependency resulting from the loss of income, and the fear of the loss of physical competence. Unfortunately degenerative conditions of the brain and nervous system do occur frequently after the age of 60, rendering some older individuals totally incapable of functioning independently.

Interpersonal factors

Interpersonal factors refer to the relationships that individuals develop with significant persons in their environment. Actually, the development of positive feelings is dependent to a great extent on the kind of interpersonal relations developed between the individual and the significant people in his environment during his very early life (Fig. 6-1). Adult feelings of security, well-being, personal value, and self-esteem originate and are powerfully influenced by the relationship that was developed with the mothering persons in the very earliest weeks and months of the individual's life. The feeding experiences are especially important in the development of an individual's attitude toward self and others. Likewise, experiences with other significant persons during childhood influence his attitudes toward himself and others, especially in relation to developing unconscious guilt feelings about

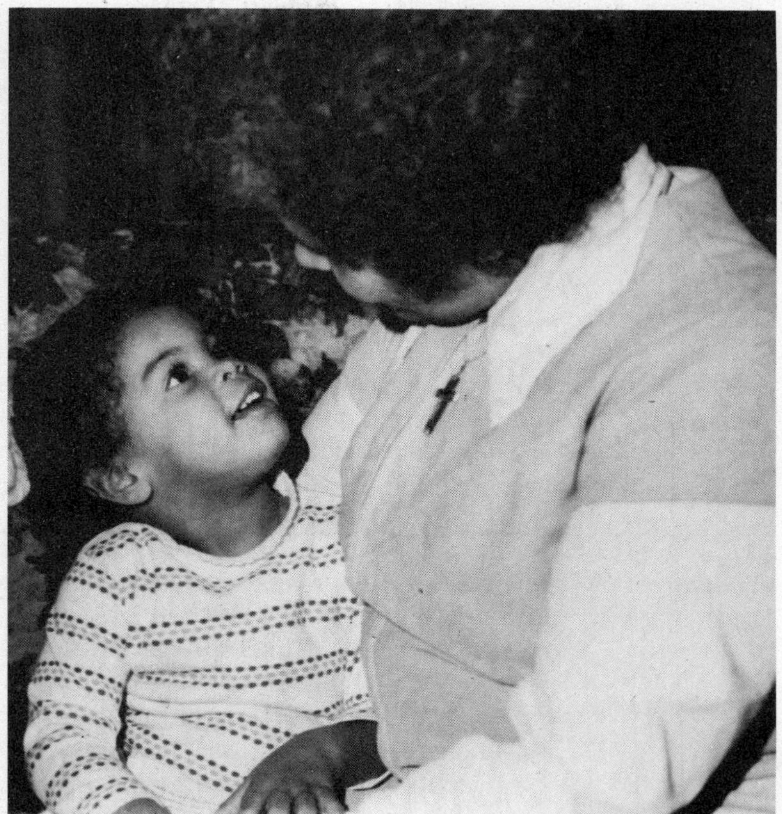

Fig. 6-1 *A trusting relationship with a significant person provides a basis for future mental health.*

sexual expression. It is possible to relate most of the anxiety-producing situations in an individual's adult life to some faulty relationships that existed with significant adults, particularly the mothering one, during his early life.

The early family relationships, especially with mother and father, influence the individual's ability to cope with the problems of adult life. When faulty relationships in some aspect of the individual's early life have never been corrected, he may not be able to adjust successfully to all the pressures of adult life. These faulty relationships that may influence the individual's future adjustment are referred to as *predisposing factors*. This suggests that they are dormant in the individual's unconscious life and may cause difficulty in the future, provided that a certain amount of intrapsychic stress occurs at a time when the individual is more vulnerable than usual.

A young man may be able to complete college, accept a responsible position, and carry on what appears to be a well-adjusted life until he becomes engaged to be married. The stress of assuming this additional financial and social responsibility added to the self-doubt that may develop concerning his ability to assume the masculine role in a marriage relationship may produce more anxiety than he is able to tolerate. At such a time his unconscious need for defense against anxiety may become so great that he may resort to unusual or bizarre ways of behaving.

Cultural factors

The culture into which an individual is born superimposes on him many values and ideas with which he must deal for the remainder of his life. It presents the individual with many conflicts between bodily drives and acceptable ways of directing these drives. For example, young people are physically ready for marriage long before our culture sanctions marriage.

The culture in the United States imposes on each person many ways of behaving simply because of one's sex. Sexual values are given to colors, furniture, occupations, hobbies, and almost everything else in life.

In the past, the roles of men and women have been clearly defined, but within the last 25 years these have been changing rapidly. The effect that sex-related role blurring or role changes will have on the mental health of future generations is yet to be determined. Some authorities believe that the effect will be to increase the incidence of mental illness, because children will find it difficult to identify with appropriate sex roles that are based on distinct functions for each sex. Conversely, other experts believe that the incidence of mental illness will decrease, since children will be encouraged by the society to engage in functions most suitable to them as persons, regardless of their gender. As with any other major cultural change, it will require several generations of alterations in child-rearing practices before definitive answers can be given to these questions.

Minority groups face problems superimposed on them by the culture. Members of a group that is different because of race or religion may face many situations that cause them as individuals to feel unsure, inadequate, and unwanted and to fear for the loss of personal security.

High cultural values have been placed on marriage, and a certain amount of disapproval is meted out to individuals who fail to marry after they have reached early adulthood. Single people eventually become members of a minority group and suffer some of the same discriminations with which minority groups must cope.

These examples should be sufficient to suggest that cultural conflict can lead to adjustment problems that may result in such a high level of anxiety that the individual is forced to use abnormal defenses.

PREVENTION OF MENTAL ILLNESS

Interpersonal factors

From the preceding discussion the reader has undoubtedly concluded that much of the emphasis on the prevention of mental illness should fall within the area of family relationships. There are few, if any, facts on which to base definitive comments concerning prevention of mental illness. Until there is a clear definition of mental illness, it will be difficult to know exactly what preventive measures are required. However, there are some clues that suggest that a child needs to be provided with emotional warmth, support, and security to provide for the emotional and social growth of his personality. Much adult behavior is determined by responses that the child experiences from significant adults in the early months of life. It appears at this point in our understanding of human behavior that stable, secure, loving family life, especially during the earliest years, is essential to the development of attitudes about self and others that will make it possible for individuals to adjust to the pressures of adult life and live in a satisfying and productive way. It is the responsibility of the home and the school, both of which deal with children during their early and formative years, to help children develop the capacity to live mentally healthy adult lives and to provide corrective experiences for children who have had negative relationships with individuals whose parenting behaviors were inadequate.

Biochemical factors

Since 1956 there has been widespread use of antipsychotic drugs, but not until recently has there been a drug that was said to prevent the recurrence of a cyclic manic-depressive reaction. Lithium carbonate has become increasingly prominent as a drug that prevents the recurrence of this condition when the recommended serum lithium level is established and maintained. Apparently the drug is effective for many individuals when they are able to tolerate it. This supports the belief that biochemical deficiencies ultimately may be identified as causing some forms of mental illness. If this proves to be the case, chemical substitutes could be taken throughout life, thereby preventing the onset of mental illness.

Cultural factors

Many authorities believe that prevention of mental illness will not be achieved on a widespread scale until efforts are directed at improving the quality of life for all persons in our society. These authorities conclude that many of our social problems such as poor housing, racial, religious, and sexual discrimination, and unavailability of quality health care to all are major elements in the cause of mental illness. Therefore these persons support broad social reform programs designed to alter the basis of these social ills. Although great strides have been made over the past few decades in alleviating some of these social problems, effective and economical means of eliminating them are yet to be determined.

CONCLUDING STATEMENTS

1. Mental health or emotional maturity is thought to be the ability to cope successfully with recurrent stresses of living and the achievement of a relatively effective adjustment to life.
2. Since few people can be said to have achieved complete men-

tal or emotional maturity, it is more helpful to evaluate the individual's relative strengths or limitations in terms of social norms and values.

3. Mental health or emotional maturity is evaluated in terms of personality capacities that involve interpersonal relations, self-acceptance, perceptions of reality, environmental mastery, self-determination, and resistance to stress.
4. Mental health and mental illness are culturally determined concepts and are defined somewhat differently in various parts of the world.
5. Mental health is always relative and is determined by a set of ratios involving the emotional, social, and psychological strengths with which an individual is fortified, the events he has experienced throughout life, the pressures he is currently undergoing, and the expectations society has established for him.
6. Mental illness is a complex problem that is thought to be a unique response involving an individual's personality as it interacts with his environment at a time when he is particularly vulnerable to stress.
7. The only reasonable approach to the cause of mental illness is the study of an individual's total life experience with consideration of genetic, physiological, intrapersonal, interpersonal, and cultural factors.
8. Current knowledge concerning human heredity has not developed to a level at which definitive statements can be made about the influence of heredity on the development of mental illness.
9. The tendency to develop similar psychotic reactions among members of the same family may be a response to the environmental factors within the family rather than a result of heredity.
10. Scientists recognize the urgent need for more research and study of human genetics as it relates to the cause of mental illness.
11. The biological heredity of the individual is of great significance, because body type, sex, intelligence, temperament, and energy endowment are genetically determined.

12. In a sense, the individual also inherits his family milieu and the cultural forces to which he must adjust throughout life.
13. There are some periods in life when the individual is more vulnerable emotionally than at others. These critical periods are adolescence, middle age, and old age.
14. The same organic problem may produce a wide variety of mental reactions in different persons, which suggests that personality plays an important role even in individual responses to involvement of brain tissue.
15. Current research indicates that alterations in a person's neurochemistry may be a contributing factor in the development of the schizophrenic and manic-depressive psychoses.
16. Some of the situations that may produce psychogenic conflicts include serious financial problems, loss of a dearly loved friend or relative, a broken marriage, loss of a job, failure to receive an important promotion, or disappointment in the integrity of a trusted friend.
17. Interpersonal factors refer to the relationships that an individual develops with significant persons in his environment and that exert a powerful influence on his mental health.
18. A stable, secure, loving family life assists individuals to develop attitudes about self and others that make it possible to adjust to the pressures of adulthood and to live a satisfying and productive life.
19. Lithium carbonate prevents recurrences of manic-depressive episodes when a recommended serum level is established and maintained.
20. Eradication of major social problems such as poor housing and discrimination may be a major factor in preventing mental illness on a widespread scale.

Suggested sources of additional information

CLASSICAL

Caplan, Gerald: Principles of preventive psychiatry, New York, 1964, Basic Books, Inc., Publishers.

Galdston, Iago: The American family in crisis, Ment. Hyg. **42:**229-236, 1958.

Hollingshead, August B., and Redlich, Frederick C.: Social class and mental illness, New York, 1958, John Wiley & Sons, Inc.

Jackson, Don D., editor: The etiology of schizophrenia, New York, 1960, Basic Books, Inc., Publishers.

Kallmann, Franz J.: Heredity in health and mental disorder, New York, 1953, W.W. Norton & Co., Inc.

Mead, Margaret: Mental health in our changing culture, Ment. Hyg. **56:**6-8, 1972.

Myers, Jerome K., and Bean, Lee L.: Family and class dynamics in mental illness, New York, 1964, John Wiley & Sons, Inc.

Norris, Catherine N.: Psychiatric crises: practical considerations, Perspect. Psychiatr. Care **5:**20-28, Jan.-Feb., 1967.

Opler, Marvin K., editor: Culture and mental health, New York, 1959, Macmillan Publishing Co., Inc.

Robischon, Paulette: The challenge of crisis theory for nursing, Nurs. Outlook **15:**28-32, July, 1967.

CONTEMPORARY

Aguilera, Donna C., and Messick, Janice M.: Crisis intervention: theory and methodology, ed. 3, St. Louis, 1978, The C.V. Mosby Co.

Burton, Arthur: Operational theories of personality, New York, 1974, Brunner/Mazel, Inc.

Chesler, Phyliss: Women and madness, Garden City, N.Y., 1973, Arno Press, Inc.

DeCourcy, Peter, and DeCourcy, Judith: A silent tragedy: child abuse in the community, Port Washington, N.Y., 1973, Alfred Publishing Co.

DeYoung, Carol D.: Nursing's contribution in family crisis treatment, Nurs. Outlook **16:**60-62, Feb., 1968.

Jaco, E. Gartley: Patients, physicians, and illness: a sourcebook in behavioral science and health, ed. 2, New York, 1972, The Free Press.

Jahoda, Marie: Current concepts of positive mental health, New York, 1979, Arno Press, Inc. (Edited by Gerald Grob.)

Kallman, Franz J.: Expanding goals of genetics in psychiatry, New York, 1962, Grune & Stratton, Inc.

Kolb, Lawrence C.: Modern clinical psychiatry, ed., Philadelphia, 1977, W.B. Saunders Co.

Landsberg, Gerald: The state of prevention in mental health, Perspect. Psychiatr. Care **15**(1):15-17, 1977.

May, Rollo: Power and innocence: a search for the sources of violence, New York, 1972, W.W. Norton & Co., Inc.

Myers, Jerome K., and Bean, L.L.: A decade later: a follow-up of social class and mental illness; in collaboration with Max P. Pepper, New York, 1968, John Wiley & Sons, Inc.

Plunkett, Richard J., and Gordon, John E.: Epidemiology and mental illness, New York, 1979, Arno Press, Inc.

Rosenthal, David: The genetics of schizophrenia. In Arieti, Silvano, and Brody, Eugene B., editors: American handbook of psychiatry, ed. 2, vol. 3, New York, 1974, Basic Books, Inc., Publishers, pp. 588-600.

Singer, Ann: Mothering practices and heroin addiction, Am. J. Nurs. **74:**77-82, 1974.

Wedge, Bryant: Changing perception of mental health, Ment. Hyg. **48:**22-31, 1974.

OF PARTICULAR INTEREST

Jahoda, Marie: Current concepts of positive mental health, New York, 1979, Arno Press, Inc. (Edited by Gerald Grob.)

This text is a classic presentation defining positive mental health and describing criteria of positive mental health.

Rosenhan, D.L.: On being sane in insane places, Science **179:**250-258, 1973.

This article provokes consideration of the definition of mental illness through description of an experiment testing mental hospitals' responses to psychiatrically "sane" people.

SECTION THREE

Interpersonally based therapeutic interventions

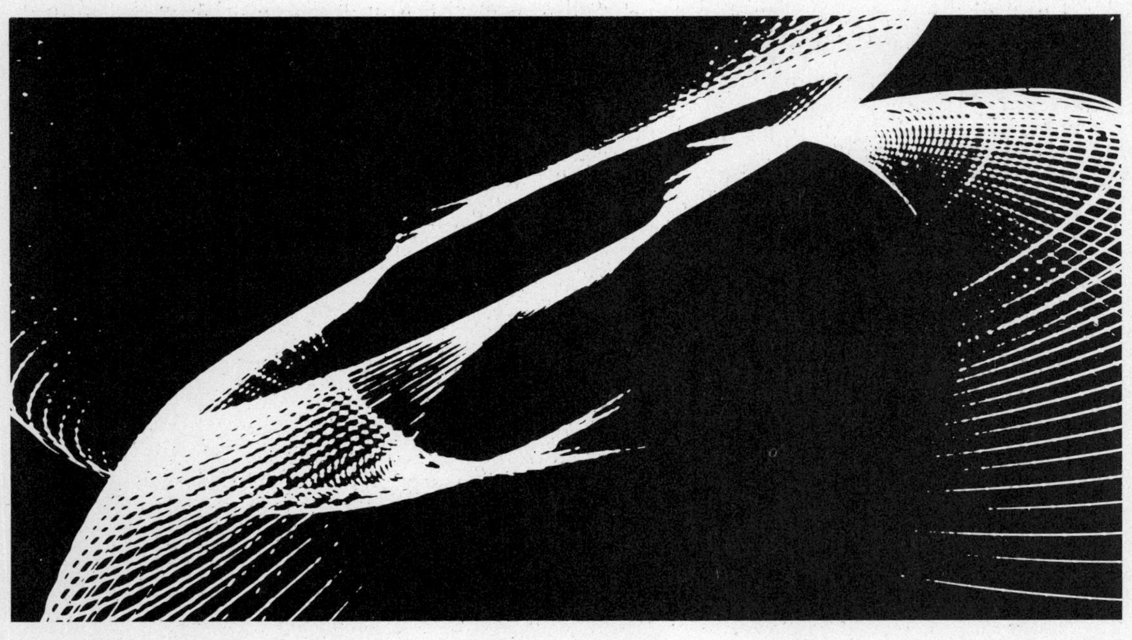

Section Three focuses on interpersonally based therapeutic interventions with individuals, groups, and families. Prior to the discussion of these modalities, the reader is introduced to the study of communication as a basis for therapeutic interventions and intervention in a crisis state. As with the previous two sections in this text, much of the material in Section Three is applicable to all nursing situations including situations in which the client is emotionally healthy. This section is presented early in the text because it describes processes that are applicable in intervening with clients regardless of the nature of their maladaptation.

Many nurses who work in psychiatric settings do not function as individual, group, or family therapists. However, the understanding of these treatment modalities is essential if the nurse is to effectively intervene with clients who are engaged in these treatments with another nurse.

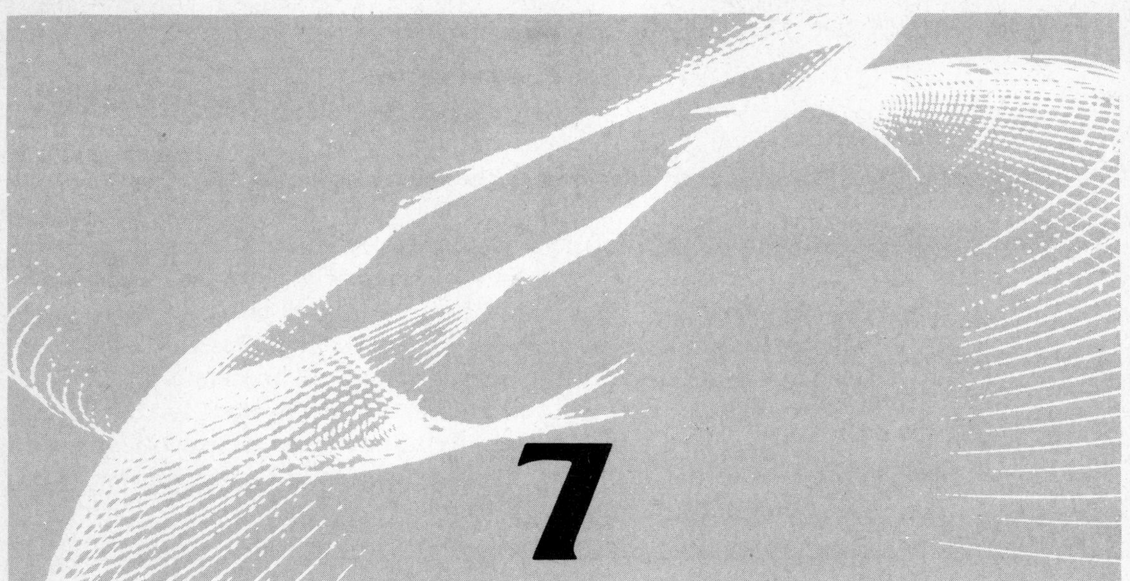

7

Communication as a basis for therapeutic interventions

- Modes of communication
- Developing effective modes of communication
- Using effective communication in the care of the mentally ill
- Special problems in communicating with the mentally ill
- Recording clients' conversations

Communication refers to the reciprocal exchange of information, ideas, beliefs, feelings, and attitudes between two persons or among a group of persons. Communication is considered to be effective when it accurately and clearly conveys the intended messages. The communication process is basic to all nursing practice and, when effective, greatly contributes to the development of all therapeutic relationships. An understanding of the principles of effective communication is essential for the psychiatric nurse, because her ability to intervene therapeutically with mentally ill persons is highly related to the effectiveness of her communication skills.

MODES OF COMMUNICATION

Everyone is familiar with communication through the written word. When written material is read, the reciprocal aspects of communication are limited to the reader's ability to understand and react to the ideas and concepts that the authors are attempting to convey. If the reader does not receive the intended message, effective communication has not been achieved.

Another mode of communication with which everyone is familiar is the spoken word. If persons who are speaking together understand the same language, a major reciprocal element is present as they exchange, question, challenge, clarify, and enlarge on statements.

A mode of communication of which people are not always aware is nonverbal communication, which is closely related to verbal communication and is usually an integral part of it. Nonverbal communication refers to the messages sent and received through such means as facial expression, voice quality, physical posture, and gestures. Thus a person's behavior conveys a great deal to the astute observer. Nonverbal communication is often referred to as *body language.* Because nonverbal communication, or body language, is always present, it has been said that a person cannot *not* communicate.

Inner feelings are expressed by the manner in which an individual conducts himself in even such simple activities as walking down the hall, opening and closing doors, reclining in an easy chair, speaking to other people, and asking questions. The nonverbal aspects of communication sometimes convey general attitudes, feelings, and reactions more clearly and more accurately than do spoken words. An understanding of the implications of nonverbal communication is important for all nurses, especially psychiatric nurses. Not only is it important for therapeutic reasons that the nurse be aware of the client's nonverbal behavior, she must also be aware of her own nonverbal behavior. Mentally ill persons are more aware of the nurse and her verbal and nonverbal behavior than many nurses realize. The nurse who works rapidly, walks down the hall briskly, closes doors emphatically, and answers questions sharply is likely to be seen as an angry person who is unapproachable. The nurse who smiles, speaks in a warm, friendly manner, and approaches her work calmly conveys an acceptance that may prompt the client to turn to her for help.

Another mode of communication, which is rarely recognized on a conscious level, is *metacommunication*. Metacommunication refers to the role expectation individuals have of each other in the context in which verbal and nonverbal communication take place. These role expectations strongly influence the nature of the verbal and nonverbal communication. For example, when a salesperson says to a customer, "May I help you?" it is understood by both individuals that she is asking whether she can be of assistance in helping the customer to make a purchase. On the other hand, when in a treatment setting the nurse asks the same question of a client, it is understood by both that she is asking if there is something she might do, such as listening or helping the client with activities basic to his needs. Metacommunication and nonverbal communication are present in all situations in which there are two or more persons, although verbal communication may be absent at times.

Communication is most effective when the three previously mentioned modes of communication—verbal, nonverbal, and metacommunication—are congruent. Imagine the reaction of the previously mentioned salesperson if the customer responded by saying, "Yes, you can help me. My child is ill and I am very worried about her." In this situation the customer's reply indicates that she is responding to only the verbal communication of the salesperson and is ignoring the metacommunication. Therefore the customer's reply illustrates incongruency between her verbal communication and her metacommunication, which is likely to result in an increase in the anxiety levels of both persons involved.

DEVELOPING EFFECTIVE MODES OF COMMUNICATION

The process of communication is not unique to human beings. Other species of animals communicate with each other. Only humans, however, have the ability to engage in the complex interaction evidenced by the use of language. In fact, the ability to engage effectively in this activity is seen by many as an essential characteristic of being human. Effective communication is a major means through which people express many of their needs and subsequently have them met, thereby experiencing satisfying, satisfactory relationships with others.

Developing modes of communication that are effective within the family, the culture, and the society in which one lives is an exceedingly complex learning process that begins at birth and comprises a large part of subsequent developmental stages. Although some of this learning takes place in a formal way through such societal agencies as the school, the foundation of the communication process is laid within the family long before the child is ready to attend school. In this respect the family acts as the representative of the society at large.

Much of the teaching and learning about communication within the family structure is achieved indirectly. For example, the child learns certain words by hearing them used in the home and without anyone actually teaching him to associate the word with the object. This is illustrated by the 4-year-old child of two college professors who was asked by his nursery school teacher to identify pictures of objects. His classmates identified one as a *suitcase* or *bag,* but he identified the same object as an *attaché case.* Furthermore, he was unable to identify the object called *apron* by the rest of his classmates. The strong academic influence and lack of domestic interest in this child's home were clearly demonstrated by the nature of his vocabulary.

In the same way the meaning of nonverbal communication is

learned. In some cultures a loud tone of voice signifies anger. In other cultures the opposite is true—that is, silence signifies anger, whereas loud, animated talking is indicative of nothing more than enthusiasm. To survive, children must learn to attach meaning to both the verbal and nonverbal communications of their family members, since they are highly dependent on these persons for having their needs met. It is a comment on the great intellectual potential of human beings to note how quickly the child does learn the meaning of highly complex messages.

It is not sufficient, however, for the child merely to learn the meaning of the messages he receives. He must also learn ways of responding that are acceptable within the family structure, and this is no simple task. Witness, for example, the child who lives within a family in which the verbal response to situations that are frustrating or anger-producing is to swear. Not infrequently the first time the child repeats a swear word in response to his anger or frustration, he is told by the adults that he is using a bad word that is forbidden and if he continues to use it, he will be punished.

Despite the complexity of learning the communication process, the majority of children are capable of doing so in a relatively short period of time and quickly become able to adapt that which they have learned in the home to the demands of the larger society. The previously mentioned 4-year-old quickly learned what an apron was and how it was used and that an attaché case is only one type of bag. In some instances, however, this adaptability is not possible or becomes possible only after much difficulty. The difficult adaptation to the communication in a different culture can be observed when adults travel rapidly between countries by jet airplane. Many travel agencies make available to their customers brochures describing the customs and frequently used words of the countries to be visited to lessen the communication shock experienced by the traveler.

The preceding examples illustrate communication problems that are normal from the standpoint of mental health. There are instances, however, when the learning of the communication process is fraught with overtones of emotional abnormality, which may produce a pattern of communication that is dysfunctional within either the family itself or society at large. *For our purposes, we can consider any communication to be dysfunctional if it does not accurately and clearly convey the message intended.* All persons occasionally experience dysfunctional communication. However, when this becomes a pattern (the rule rather than the exception), it frequently is a manifestation of mental illness and, in addition, is a factor in perpetuating the illness.

USING EFFECTIVE COMMUNICATION IN THE CARE OF THE MENTALLY ILL

Mentally ill individuals need the opportunity to communicate with others who are sincerely interested in their problems and who care about them as people. It is important for the nurse to learn to communicate in such a way that her conversation will become a part of the total therapeutic environment. The ability to communicate therapeutically with clients requires that the nurse have an attitude of acceptance and genuine interest in them.

A climate of mutual trust and respect must be developed before mentally ill persons can feel safe enough to communicate with a nurse. This is not an easy climate to establish; it requires time, patience, knowledge, and skill. However, the nurse is rewarded for her efforts by the knowledge that when a client is helped to converse effectively with a professional person, an emotionally supportive experience often results.

Initiating a conversation

When the nurse joins the professional staff of a treatment facility, she and the clients are strangers to one another. They must become acquainted before therapeutic communication can take place. Most clients approach the nurse cautiously at first, as they approach other strangers. Some shy individuals may not approach the nurse at all. A few of the more aggressive ones may insist on monopolizing her total attention. The wise nurse will use some of the same skills in building a relationship with a mentally ill person that she has used successfully to build relationships with other strangers.

If the nurse has not already been introduced to the clients, she will begin by introducing herself. It will be helpful if she explains her status at the same time. This can be done by saying, "I am Miss Jones, a student nurse, and I will be here for 4 weeks." Or she might say, "I am Miss Smith, a graduate nurse, and I have come to work here for a while." If the nurse cannot recall the name of a person to whom she has introduced herself, she might say, "Will you please help me learn your name? I am sorry that I do not know it." With this invitation most persons will introduce themselves. Thus the nurse will begin the necessary task of learning the names, faces, and personalities of the client population with whom she will be working.

After the nurse and the clients have been introduced, it is appropriate for the nurse to initiate a conversation. A conversation is one of the most common of the shared activities in which people engage. It is the logical beginning for any relationship. Just as the nurse initiates conversational topics with other strangers, she may find it helpful with clients to introduce a neutral conversational topic appropriate for the time and place. If the time of year is right, baseball may be an appropriate topic. If the client seems interested in baseball, the nurse may choose to initiate a conversation with a question about a recent game. For example, she may begin by saying, "I did not have a chance to follow the game yesterday. What was the final score?" Other neutral topics that may be used include the headlines in the newspaper, the weather, or an approaching event. If the nurse notices that one person is holding a newspaper, she may begin a conversation by inquiring, "What interesting happenings are in the headlines today?"

Having introduced a topic, the sensitive nurse will wait for a response and will not feel compelled to avoid silences by immediately adding her own comments or opinions. After ample opportunity has been given for a response, it is suggested that she introduce a second conversational idea that logically follows the first.

Clients often ask new nurses personal questions such as, "Are you married?" or "What nursing school are you from?" or "Where do you live?" The natural curiosity of clients about the personal life of the professional staff is understandable. However, if the conversation is allowed to be focused on the personal life of the nurse, it quickly loses its original goal—to achieve communication that is therapeutic for the client. If the nurse wishes to do so, it would seem logical for her to respond to factual questions such as, "Are you married?" with a simple "Yes" or "No." If further personal questions directed at the nurse continue, she might say in a friendly way, "Why do you ask?" or comment, "I wonder if we could not find a more relevant topic than my personal life to discuss." Personal questions directed to the nurse alert her to the need for focusing future conversation more carefully. It may suggest that the specific individual in question hopes to direct attention away from his own problems.

Developing effective verbal communication

To be effective, the nurse's verbal communication must be guided by goals. The nurse's therapeutic potential will be greatly increased if a conscious effort is made to establish a goal for each interaction before initiating a conversation. The identified purpose for the interaction will provide a guide as to the appropriate approach and attitude to be used, the approximate length of the conversation, and the manner in which it will be terminated.

Certainly the nurse should avoid approaching anyone with a barrage of words. In their desire to communicate effectively, nurses sometimes resort to asking a series of questions. Unfortunately this is too often the type of conversation that is reported when nurses are asked to tell about a recent conversation with a client. "How are you today?" is one of the usual questions with which many nurses begin a conversation. Such an opening sentence usually does little to develop a conversation.

Frequently the nurse interacts with the client for the purpose of giving or getting specific information. Although the attitude toward the client should be friendly, the nurse should initiate the conversation by explaining the purpose of the questions she will ask. In this instance it is appropriate that the questions be more direct than those usually employed. Such a conversation would be brief and terminated with a polite expression of thanks.

Direct questions may be perceived by a mentally ill person as threatening to personal security. "Why did you come to the hospital?" or "How do you feel about your job?" may touch on sensitive feelings. Thus direct questions are usually helpful only when specific information must be obtained or when the person is confused. When a client is responding to intrapsychic stimulation, it may be necessary to use direct questions to communicate with him.

A second goal for initiating an interaction may be to establish a beginning rapport that can serve as a basis for developing a meaningful future relationship. With such a goal, attention would be focused on the client in a friendly, relaxed way to convey a willingness to listen. In such a situation, emphasis is on getting acquainted and establishing a feeling of mutual trust.

If the purpose of the interaction is to encourage the person to express his thoughts and feelings, a nondirective approach would undoubtedly achieve the most positive results. In such a situation the client would be encouraged to initiate the conversation. Responding to his comments by reflecting his thoughts back to him might be helpful in encouraging him to continue expressing his feelings without introducing new or unrelated ideas. For example, if the client speaks of his unhappy home life, the nurse might respond by saying, "It sounds to me as if you are saying that your home life is unhappy." In addition, this type of response gives the client an opportunity to either accept or reject the nurse's impression of his communication.

A general rule to follow when talking with clients is to encourage them to take the conversational lead. Although the nurse may initiate communication and may keep the conversation alive, the conversation must focus on the interests and concerns of the client if it is to be of value.

Some nurses attempt to communicate with clients by doing most of the talking while the client sits or stands passively nearby. If the client responds at all in a situation like this, it is usually to give a one-word answer. When the nurse communicates in such a way, her comments usually fall into the category of giving advice or persuading the client to do something that someone believes will benefit him. Neither advice nor persuasion is of much help if the goal is to assist the client to become a self-directing adult. Giving advice suggests that one person is attempting to impose his values and personal choices on a second person who is not capable of making such choices. The giver of advice often begins the conversation by saying, "If I were you." The nurse is not the client and cannot know the choices that are best for him to make in most situations. She does not know all the past experiences that influence his present thinking and feeling and therefore is not qualified to make suggestions about his many problems and concerns. Advice may result in a temporary and positive response because it may relieve the client from the responsibility of making an immediate decision. In the long run it is likely to encourage the client to remain dependent on some other person for decisions.

Furthermore, giving advice is not always a safe practice. If the advice is accepted and the situation remains unimproved or worsens, the giver of the advice is likely to be blamed. Instead of offering advice, it is more helpful to explore mutually the positive and negative aspects of the possible decisions that are available. Ultimately the goal of the professional person is to help the client identify the decision he can feel most comfortable about making.

Nurses make many comments that they hope will give reassurance but actually fall short of this goal. Even though the nurse intends to be helpful, it is rarely helpful to make comments such as the following: "Don't worry," "Your doctor says this medicine will help you," "There are a great many people who are worse off than you are," and "Don't cry, you don't want people to see you crying." Such comments are meaningless and are likely to convince the client that the nurse is not able to understand his problems. The client's reassurance is never achieved by use of meaningless clichés. Instead, reassurance is more likely to be achieved by the nurse's spending time with the client and by listening to his expressions of feelings as long as he seems to need to talk. It is reassuring to the client if the nurse considers the problem thoughtfully and asks intelligent, reality-oriented questions about the situation. It is reassuring to the client when the nurse accepts his tears without comment or assures him that crying is a reasonable thing to do under the circumstances, provided, of course, the circumstances do warrant such expression. It is reassuring to the client when the nurse listens to his personal problems without showing surprise or disapproval when he talks about past social behavior that is unusual or below the standards that the nurse has set for herself. It is reassuring when the nurse agrees that the client has a problem and works with him in trying to think through solutions to it. It is reassuring when the nurse reflects back to the client the tone of the feeling she hears him expressing. For example, for the nurse to say, "It sounds to me as if you are really upset," conveys to the client that his feeling as well as the content of what he is saying is being understood. Once again, it should be noted that by a statement such as this the nurse is not imposing a feeling on the client, but rather expressing and owning her own response. It may be reassuring to the client if the nurse sits with him even when he does not feel like talking, thereby conveying a genuine interest in his problem and acceptance of him.

Persuasion suggests that some pressure is being placed on the client to accept a prescribed course of action. This, like advice, is not a practice likely to enhance movement toward more self-reliance.

Suggestion is an aspect of communication that may be helpful to some individuals. Much can be done to stimulate interest in activities and to help individuals alter social attitudes by using skillfully phrased suggestions. For instance, encouraging a client to participate in the activities offered by the occupational therapist may be accomplished by telling him about the activities available and by using suggestions such as, "You might enjoy the finger-painting class." At another time a second comment about this activity might be, "Everybody seems to have an interesting time when he goes to occupational therapy; I think you might too." The client who has refused to wash his hair for several weeks may do so if several people with whom he is acquainted comment about his attractive appearance when his hair was clean a few weeks before. One suggestion is usually not sufficient to alter an attitude or help a person accept a new idea. Suggestion must be used frequently and skillfully by persons whose opinion the client respects.

Developing effective nonverbal communication

One of the first steps the nurse can take in developing effective nonverbal communication is to examine her own feelings toward clients and, if possible, to focus her activities on those for whom she has genuine feelings of interest and acceptance. If the nurse attempts to work closely with clients about whom she has many negative feelings, she will surely communicate these feelings nonverbally. The nurse needs to recognize the importance of her personal feelings in developing a reciprocal relationship with a client. It is also essential to recognize the role of nonverbal communication and to understand that it is impossible for every nurse to work therapeutically with every mentally ill person. Equipped with this knowledge and understanding, the nurse can feel comfortable in admitting that she is not the appropriate person to be assigned to work closely with a specific individual with whom she has not been able to establish a positive relationship.

After examining her own feelings toward clients, there are a number of specific steps that the nurse can take to engage in effective nonverbal communication. One of the most important of these steps is to sit near a client when talking to him. Some nurses hesitate to sit beside clients even when they are trying to converse with them. This hesitancy probably comes from experience in previous nursing situations in which the nurse was expected to be constantly busy carrying out physical comfort measures or therapeutic treatment procedures.

When the nurse stands during a conversation she conveys the idea that she is in a hurry, that she expects the conversation to be a short one, and that she is prepared to remain for only a few minutes. In such a hurried atmosphere no one can expect a client to feel that there is interest or time enough for him to talk about anything important. Conversely, when sitting near or beside a mentally ill person, it is important not to sit in such a way that the person feels trapped or in danger of attack. Astute observation of the client's nonverbal behavior will quickly reveal if the nurse is sitting in a position that produces the best climate for conversation. Examples of behaviors likely to indicate that the client feels uncomfortable are the movement of his body or chair away from the nurse, his focusing his eyes elsewhere, and physical signs of anxiety such as restlessness and agitation. The nurse should not hesitate to alter her position if this seems appropriate from her observations of the client's behavior. When the nurse conveys her sincere interest in the client through her position and through the warmth of her voice and facial expression, the first step has been taken toward the establishment of a therapeutic nurse-client relationship.

Another important step the nurse can take in developing effective nonverbal communication is to develop her listening skills. Listening implies silence, but it does not imply passivity. The listener can and should be an active, alert, and interested participant, even though she may make very few verbal contributions. The nurse gives evidence of interest by being genuinely interested in the client and in what he is saying. This interest cannot be feigned. Evidence of genuine, sincere interest is shown by the expression on the listener's face, by the way the listener looks at the speaker, and by the verbal encouragement that is given to the speaker. Nodding the head to suggest that one understands or agrees is one way of giving encouragement. Comments such as, "I can understand that" or "That must have been difficult for you" or "I see, go on" are encouraging when said at an appropriate time with a friendly, interested tone. If the listener cannot follow the logic of the speaker or the sequence of the related incidents, it is best to ask the speaker to review that part of the story again. The nurse might say, "Could you explain that last statement again for me? I do not believe I understood it clearly." Or she might say, "I'm sorry, I didn't understand what you said a minute ago. Could you go over that last point again?" If the nurse fails to ask for clarification when it is needed, the client will soon discover that she has lost the sequence and meaning of the conversation and is trying to act as if she understands when she does not. This is one way of losing the client's confidence.

Effectively concluding a conversation

The conclusion of a conversation is as important as is the initiation of a conversation. The conclusion of a conversation will often set the tone for subsequent conversations between the nurse and the client. When the nurse needs to leave, she should break off the conversation in such a way that it can be resumed at another time. Thus she might say, "I have been interested in what you have been telling me, and I hope we can continue this discussion later on." Of course, such a statement must be true. If she has promised to talk with the client at another time, she must find a time for taking up the conversation again. She might begin by saying, "I have been thinking about our conversation of yesterday. I have some free time right now and I am wondering if we could talk some more about the last point that you were making." The nurse would use this statement only if there were a last point she wished to explore. If such a statement were not apropos, she would choose one appropriate for the conversation.

SPECIAL PROBLEMS IN COMMUNICATING WITH THE MENTALLY ILL

The need for congruent communication is great when one is attempting to relate therapeutically with mentally ill persons. They have had much previous experience in interaction with significant others who have communicated incongruent messages, particularly in regard to verbal and nonverbal modes of communication wherein the nonverbal message simultaneously contradicts the verbal message. The consequence of this communication is that the receiver must make a decision about which message he will respond to, with the awareness that, whichever choice he makes, he will be incorrect. When this type of communication is usual rather than exceptional, it may result in the receiver becoming unable to respond at all, that is, his behavior becomes immobilized. Some theorists believe that this pattern of communication is characteristic of dysfunctional families in which one or more members become schizophrenic as an adaptation to this form of disturbed communication. The technical term for this type of disturbed interaction is *double bind communication.*

Although it is currently believed that family therapy is the treatment of choice in such situations, in many instances it is not practical or feasible for this treatment modality to be employed. Therefore the nurse, as the professional person spending the most time with the client in the treatment setting, is the individual who has the greatest opportunity to create an environment in which the client can experience congruent communication. She can assist the client experientially to learn modes of adaptation that are more reality oriented and therefore more useful than his previous adaptation of retreating from reality into a psychotic reaction.

For the nurse to express congruent messages she must be aware of herself and her own feelings. This concept was discussed in Chapter 2. A helpful suggestion is for the nurse to make clear to the client what she is feeling, that is, to bring into verbal communication her nonverbal messages rather than letting the receiver guess their meaning. An example of this might be the nurse who says after being purposely tripped, "The feeling your behavior evokes in me is irritation." It is important to note that this statement conveys a very different message than if the nurse were to say, "You irritate me." In the former statement the nurse is expressing and owning her own feelings and not rejecting the client, whereas in the latter statement it may sound as if she is blaming and rejecting the client, which will be very likely to cut off further communication.

On the other hand, since nonverbal aspects of communication usually convey the intended message most clearly, mentally ill persons, like all others, usually sense the sincerity and kindness of the staff accurately. Thus it has been observed that a worker who is gruff and outspoken with clients may be respected and loved by them because he communicates nonverbally a basic attitude of kindness and a sincere interest in their welfare. A nurse who has adopted an unusually saccharine approach may be deeply resented by clients because she conveys nonverbally a feeling of rejection.

Many mentally ill persons struggle with the problem of not being able to trust other people. One of the ways a nurse can help such a person is to demonstrate that she can be trusted. If a client can begin to trust one person, it is possible that trust can eventually be extended to other people. When trying to help a client learn to trust her, the nurse sometimes finds herself in a dilemma. A client with whom the nurse is establishing a relationship may confide information that places her in an untenable position. On the one hand, she wishes to respect his confidences, while at the same time she hopes to carry out her responsibilities as a member of the professional staff. The following situation precipitated such a dilemma.

A client confided that he was planning to leave the city during the next weekend, ostensibly to visit his family. He told the nurse that he had stolen enough money from his friends to purchase a train ticket to a distant city where he was unknown and where he hoped to make a fresh start. The client cautioned the nurse not to tell anyone about these plans until after he had gone. The nurse had reason to be concerned about the client's safety, and now was in conflict about keeping the confidences, while still fulfilling her role as a member of the professional staff. She was understandably distressed about the situation.

Unfortunately the nurse failed to remind the client that she was a member of the professional staff and therefore had a responsibility to report his plan to the treatment team. A reasonable guide to follow is that the nurse has a responsibility to tell the client's therapist and the nurse in charge if the client tells her of plans that are dangerous to him or others or that interfere with the treatment plan. When the client begins to confide information to the nurse that should be shared with other members of the professional staff, she has a responsibility to remind him that she must report the conversation to the appropriate people. The nurse might ask the client, "Are you sure that you want to tell me this? You know it will be necessary for me to share this with the treatment team."

When a client confides his feelings about an emotion-laden situation to the nurse, she may be presented with another problem. If the information and feelings about which the client has told her should be handled in the therapeutic session, but for various reasons the client has not been able to share this information with his therapist, the nurse should suggest that she is not the appropriate person with whom this particular information should be shared.

When the nurse has established a relationship with the client that makes it possible for him to express his anxiety to her, she has a responsibility to listen with acceptance and understanding. In addition, she is obligated to encourage the client to share his feelings with his therapist. It is also suggested that the nurse ask the therapist for an opportunity to discuss the client and his problems.

RECORDING CLIENTS' CONVERSATIONS

The professional and nonprofessional staff in a mental health setting need to communicate continuously with each other. An effective communication system is one way of improving consistency of health care and of avoiding many errors that occur when information about the needs and behavior of clients is not shared. Talking together about clients and their behavior and needs is probably the best method to improve staff communication. The written records that are made by the professional staff are another important way of communicating with one another. Recording done by nurses should give an accurate account of the client's behavior, since the nursing staff has the opportunity of being with the client most continually. The most meaningful source of recorded material is the client's verbal and nonverbal communication. The nurse's record should quote and describe the client as accurately as possible and should be written in a reasonably short time after the conversation has taken place. The nurse's personal impressions and reactions should be avoided, except in situations in which the client's mood or attitude is being described. Psychiatric labels should be avoided because they contribute little information to the reader. Not only do these labels have stereotypical meanings, they may also convey different messages to different readers.

The nurse's record should emphasize the client's conversation and behavior and should be written simply, accurately, and straightforwardly. The reader should be free to make his own judgments concerning the meaning of the behavior about which the nurse has written.

CONCLUDING STATEMENTS

1. Communication refers to the reciprocal exchange of information, ideas, beliefs, feelings, and attitudes between two persons or among a group of persons.

2. An understanding of the principles of effective communication is essential for the psychiatric nurse because her ability to intervene therapeutically with mentally ill persons is highly related to the effectiveness of her communication skills.
3. Verbal communication, nonverbal communication, and metacommunication are three modes of communication. Nonverbal communication and metacommunication are present in all situations in which two or more persons are interacting; verbal communication may be absent at times.
4. Communication is most effective when the three modes of communication are congruent.
5. Communication is considered to be dysfunctional if it does not accurately and clearly convey the message intended.
6. The nurse works toward creating a climate in which the client can feel safe enough to converse with her freely.
7. Nonverbal communication often conveys general attitudes, feelings, and reactions more clearly and more accurately than do spoken words.
8. The nurse needs to examine her own feelings toward clients because she communicates these feelings nonverbally.
9. The therapeutic potential of the nurse's verbal interaction with the client will be greatly increased if it is guided by goals established before the conversation is initiated.
10. Conversation that is focused on the personal life of the nurse loses its real goal of achieving conversation that is therapeutic for the client.
11. Neither advice nor persuasion is helpful when the therapeutic goal is to help the client become a self-directing adult.
12. Reassurance can be helpful to clients if the method used is appropriate for the client and his problem, but statements that represent meaningless clichés are rarely reassuring.
13. Skillfully phrased suggestions are useful in altering social attitudes, in changing ideas, and in stimulating interest in therapeutic activities.
14. Direct questions are rarely helpful in stimulating conversation and may give the effect of probing into the client's personal life.

15. Clients should be encouraged to take the conversational lead.
16. Clients must be helped to understand that the nurse has a responsibility to share confidences with the treatment team when they confide behavior that may be dangerous to themselves or others or may interfere with the treatment goals.
17. The nurse's written records of conversations with clients should be accurate and should be written to avoid psychiatric terminology, labels, or personal impressions.

Suggested sources of additional information

CLASSICAL

Davis, Anne J.: The skills of communication, Am. J. Nurs. **63:**66-70, Jan., 1963.

Ehmann, Virginia E.: Empathy: its origin, characteristics, and process, Perspect. Psychiatr. Care **9:**72-80, March-April, 1971.

Gerber, Claudia B., and Snyder, Deanne, F.: Language and thought, Perspect. Psychiatr. Care **8:**230-233, 237, 1970.

Goldin, Phyllis, and Russell, Barbara: Therapeutic communication, Am. J. Nurs. **69:**1928-1930, 1969.

Goldsborough, Judith D.: On becoming nonjudgmental, Am. J. Nurs. **70:**2340-2343, 1970.

Hewitt, Helon E., and Pesznecker, Betty L.: Blocks to communicating with patients, Am. J. Nurs. **64:**101-103, July, 1964.

Lewis, Garland K.: Communication; a factor in meeting emotional crises, Nurs. Outlook **13:**36-39, Aug., 1965.

Lewis, Garland K.: Nurse-patient communication, Dubuque, Iowa, 1978, William C. Brown Co., Publishers.

Peplau, Hildegard E.: Talking with patients, Am. J. Nurs. **60:**964-966, 1960.

Peplau, Hildegard E.: Interpersonal techniques; the crux of psychiatric nursing, Am. J. Nurs. **62:**50-54, June, 1962.

Robinson, Alice M.: Communicating with schizophrenic patients, Am. J. Nurs. **60:**1120-1123, 1960.

Schwartz, Morris S., and Shockley, Emmy Lanning: The nurse and the mental patient, New York, 1956, John Wiley & Sons, Inc.

Travelbee, Joyce: What do we mean by rapport? Am. J. Nurs. **63:**70-72, Feb., 1963.

CONTEMPORARY

Amacher, Nancy Jean: Touch is a way of caring, Am. J. Nurs. **73:**852-855, 1973.

Bolzoni, N.J., and Geach, Barbara: Premature reassurance: a distancing maneuver, Nurs. Outlook **23:**49-51, 1975.

Burgess, Ann Wolbert, and Lazare, Aaron: Interviewing techniques. In Psychiatric nursing in the hospital and the community, ed. 2, Englewood Cliffs, N.J., 1976, Prentice-Hall, Inc., pp. 155-174.

Burkett, Alice D.: A way to communicate, Am. J. Nurs. **74:** 2185-2187, 1974.

Dethomaso, Marita Tribou: "Touch power" and the screen of loneliness, Perspect. Psychiatr. Care **9:**133-118, May-June, 1971.

Field, William E.: Watch your message, Am. J. Nurs. **72:**1278-1280, 1972.

Gruber, Louis N.: The no-demand, third person interview of the non-verbal patient, Perspect. Psychiatr. Care **15**(1):38-39, 1977.

Haggerty, Virginia C.: Listening, Nurs. Forum **10**(4):382-387, 1971.

Kalisch, Beatrice J.: What is empathy? Am. J. Nurs. **73:**1548-1552, 1973.

Lipkin, Gladys B., and Cohen, Roberta G.: The uses of the interview. In Effective approaches to patients' behavior, New York, 1980, Springer Publishing Co., Inc.

Underwood., Patricia R.: Communication through role playing, Am. J. Nurs. **71:**1184-1186, 1971.

Veninga, Robert: Communications: a patient's eye view, Am. J. Nurs. **73:**320-322, 1973.

Yoder, Susan A.: Alienation as a way of life, Perspect. Psychiatr. Care **15**(2):66-71, 1977.

OF PARTICULAR INTEREST

Reusch, J., and Bateson, G.: Communication: the social matrix of psychiatry, New York, 1968, W.W. Norton & Co., Inc.

These renowned authors discuss basic communication theory as it relates to psychiatric theory. It is highly recommended for the beginning student.

Snyder, J.C., and Wilson, M.F.: Elements of a psychological assessment, Am. J. Nurs. **77:**235, 1977.

In a concise, carefully organized format the authors present a model for psychological evaluation. Throughout is an emphasis on self-understanding and communication between nurse and client.

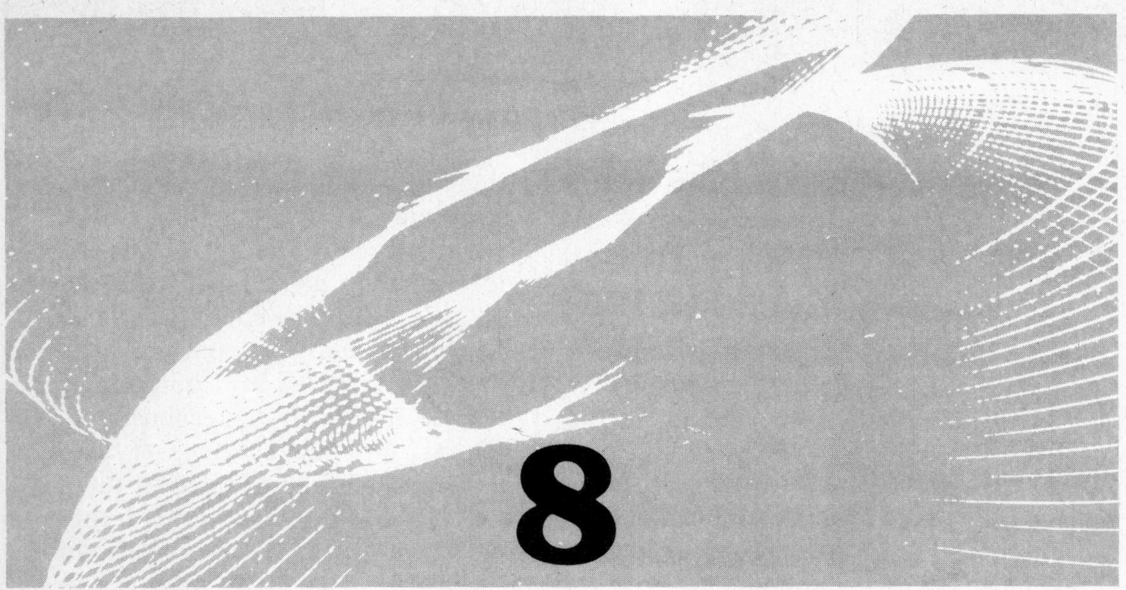

8

Intervention in a crisis state

- Definition of crisis
- Types of crises
- Characteristics of a crisis state
- Phases of a crisis state
- Techniques of crisis intervention

Crisis intervention continues to be a subject of interest to all health professionals. It is a technique that is successfully used by persons with a variety of backgrounds to aid individuals and families in understanding and effectively coping with the intense emotions that characterize a crisis. Once the client is able to deal with his emotions, he often is able to make appropriate decisions regarding behavior, which may be required for resolution of the problems that surround the crisis. Although the responsibility for crisis intervention does not fall into the province of any one health care discipline, a discussion of it is included in this text, since nurses are often in the position to engage in this technique or to counsel other health care workers in its use. Furthermore, psychiatric nurses are expected to have particular expertise in the understanding and management of emotional problems and are often looked to by their colleagues as consultants in crisis states.

DEFINITION OF CRISIS

The term *crisis* is often used by lay persons to describe a situation or a feeling state. It is not unusual to hear an individual say about an event, "It was a crisis." If in fact the event referred to was a turning point in a situation, the use of the term is correct according to the dictionary definition of the word. When referring to a feeling state, persons often report that they are in a crisis when they are very upset. Almost always this is an incorrect use of the word according to its technical definition.

Mental health authorities define a crisis as *a state of disequilibrium resulting from the interaction of an event with the individual's or family's coping mechanisms, which are inadequate to meet the demands of the situation, combined with the individual's or family's perception of the meaning of the event.* Therefore a crisis refers to an interactional process among these three variables that is reflected in the feeling state of the individual or family. Although anxiety usually underlies the feeling state, the individual may feel depression, anger, fear, or any other of a wide range of emotions. However, it is not the emotion that is unique to a crisis, nor is it the event. Rather, it is the meaning of the event to the individual or family and their inability to cope with it that produces the crisis. Therefore not every person who is anxious, depressed, angry, or fearful is in a crisis, nor does a traumatic event necessarily produce a crisis in those whom it affects.

Health professionals are greatly interested in crisis intervention because of a number of factors. First, more people are voluntarily seeking mental health care for problems that are not necessarily indicative of long-standing maladaption. In the past, because of the social stigma associated with mental illness, mental health counsel was sought only if the person was severely disturbed and exhibiting bizarre symptoms such as hallucinations or delusions. Although there is still more stigma associated with mental illness than with physical illness, society is gradually becoming more accepting of the value of mental health treatment; so a larger number of people voluntarily seek help for less severe problems. These problems are often individual or familial crises.

Second, as professionals have gained more experience in dealing with persons in a crisis, they have realized that former unresolved crises often emerge to consciousness in conjunction with the present crisis. Therefore intervention can be directed toward both the present and past situations, providing a unique opportunity to help the client resolve long-standing problems in a relatively short period of time.

Finally, crisis intervention is of great interest to mental health professionals because it provides a specific opportunity to prevent mental illness and to promote mental health. Prevention of mental illness is achieved by providing the client with assistance in using already established coping mechanisms that he has successfully used in the past or by assisting him in developing new defenses that are healthy adaptations to the situation. If this can be achieved, the necessity for the client to resort to pathological defense mechanisms, even mental illness, can be avoided.

Promotion of mental health through crisis intervention has been documented by researchers who have engaged in follow-up studies of individuals and families who have experienced crises. It has been demonstrated that there are three possible outcomes of a crisis state: (1) the client may reintegrate at a lower or less healthy level of functioning than the one prior to the crisis, (2) the client may reintegrate at the same level of functioning as previously, probably as a result of completely repressing the crisis situation and its attendant emotions, or (3) the client may reintegrate at a higher, healthier level of functioning than the level prior to the crisis experience. This last possible outcome was a startling realization at the time it was first described, since the goal had always been prevention of mental illness. The idea that people could actually grow and benefit from an emotionally traumatic experience opened up vast potential for increasing the level of mental health in a large population. In fact, some authorities see a crisis as a catalyst that disturbs old habits, evokes new responses, and becomes a major factor in charting new developments. Therefore the challenge that a crisis provokes may bring forth new coping mechanisms that serve to strengthen the individual's adaptive capacity and thereby, in general, to raise his level of mental health.*

Research studies have further documented that, although any one of the three outcomes can occur with or without skilled intervention, resolution of the crisis resulting in a lower level of functioning or the same level of functioning is more likely to occur without intervention, and resolution of the crisis resulting in a higher level of functioning is more likely to occur with intervention. Subsequently, to promote mental health as well as to prevent mental illness, an increasing number of communities have established crisis intervention centers. These centers may take the form of mental health emergency rooms, suicide prevention clinics, family guidance clinics, or telephone crisis services. Whatever the name, these centers are always staffed by personnel skilled in crisis intervention.

TYPES OF CRISES

There are two types of events that may precipitate a crisis state: developmental and situational. It should be understood, however, that very few events inevitably produce a crisis state in all persons. If the reader reviews the definition of crisis, it will be clear that the nature of the event is only one factor in the production

*Rapaport, Lydia: The state of crisis: some theoretical considerations. In Pared, Howard J., editor: Crisis intervention: selected readings, New York; 1965, Family Service Association of America.

of a crisis. In addition to the event, the other two necessary factors are the personalized meaning of the event to the individual and family, and the nature and extent of their coping mechanisms. These must interact in such a way as to produce a state of disequilibrium. For example, a hysterectomy may be well received by a 50-year-old unmarried career woman who sublimates her maternal needs through the children of friends and relatives and whose emotional energy is directed toward her profession. Another 50-year-old woman experiencing the same surgical procedure may be plunged into a state of crisis, since her identity unconsciously has been formed around her role as mother and homemaker, and the hysterectomy marks the end of her childbearing years, thus threatening her sense of self. To take this example one step further, the same career woman may enter a state of disequilibrium or crisis if she loses her job or retires, whereas the homemaker might respond to a loss of her outside job with an inner sense of relief.

Nevertheless, two types of events have been described that are likely to precipitate a crisis state in many individuals and families. The first event is the *transition period between developmental stages.*

Developmental crises are well documented. The reader will remember that each stage of development has its own developmental task, the achievement of which requires the individual to emphasize certain behaviors and to minimize others. Consequently, the family as a unit is called on to adjust and adapt to the changes experienced by each of its members. Although these changes in individuals are most pronounced during infancy and early childhood, they occur throughout the entire life cycle. Therefore any family unit is likely to have members who represent at least two different developmental stages. Many families have members who may be experiencing one of five or six different developmental stages, each stage having its own needs and manifestations. When this is the case, it is common to find family disequilibrium occurring because behaviors that meet the needs of one or more of its members may be in direct opposition to the needs of other members. An increasingly common example of such a situation is the phenomenon of adult children who return to the home of their parents to live after having been away for a few years. The reason this phenomenon is occurring more often is related in part to problems in the society at large. A scarcity of jobs and economic inflation make it difficult if not impossible for some young adults to become economically independent. Nevertheless, the young adult is developmentally ready to work on establishing his independence but is in a position of dependence on his parents. On the other hand, his parents are developmentally ready to address their generativity needs by engaging in civic-type activities, not by nurturing a family. It does not take much imagination to appreciate the nature and extent of the family disequilibrium that may result from this situation.

Developmental crises are characterized by their predictability. For example, behavioral scientists know that a young married couple will have new demands placed on them when their first child is born. No matter how eagerly they may anticipate this event, many young parents react with depression and frustration when the dependency needs of the infant cause them to alter their previous spontaneous life-style. During midlife this couple may go through an anxiety-laden period when they question the value of the direction they have taken in their marriage, family, and work. Finally, the same couple might become depressed and frustrated once again when they find that their long-anticipated freedom from responsibility for childrearing is limited by the financial and physical limitations of old age. Although the transition from one developmental stage to another is always fraught with a certain degree of increased individual and familial tension, these transitional periods can be prevented from becoming crises through the use of anticipatory guidance.

Anticipatory guidance is primarily an educative process that helps prepare the individual and family for behavioral changes that are likely to occur in the near future. This process has been greatly aided by the proliferation of information about behavior during each developmental stage, which is now available in newspapers, magazines, and paperback books. Therefore many families successfully engage in their own anticipatory guidance without requiring the assistance of health care professionals.

Public health nurses are in a unique position to provide anticipatory guidance. As they visit families in their homes, they have the opportunity to assess the entire family situation, even though they might be present to give care to only one member. For example, the nurse might counsel the mother of a 2-year-old in regard to the meaning of his negativistic behavior while visiting the home to administer a parenteral diuretic to the grandmother. The opportunities for anticipatory guidance by nurses are not limited to home visits. The nurse is in a position to assess the family dynamics when a member is hospitalized for a physical illness and visitors seek out the nurse to covertly ask advice about their problems rather than those of the patient. The astute nurse will recognize these clues and respond in a helpful way.

The second type of event that may combine with other factors to produce a state of crisis is called *situational.* By definition, most situational crises cannot be as accurately predicted as can developmental crises. Situational events that can precipitate a state of crisis include such major catastrophes as the unexpected death of a family member due to accident, the loss of a home through fire or flood, and sudden widespread economic depression as occurred in the 1930s. The event does not have to be as catastrophic as these, however, to precipitate a state of crisis. Any event, no matter how minor or even how desirable it may superficially appear, may combine with the individual's or family's perception of it to produce a situation that is felt to be *hazardous* to the equilibrium of the system. If the event is perceived as hazardous, and the individual or family does not have adequate coping mechanisms available to ward off such a threat, a state of crisis will ensue. Although most people would understand why a family might enter into a state of crisis after their home was burned in a fire that killed their infant daughter, few lay people would understand why a family might enter a state of crisis after the father receives a major promotion to the position for which he has been striving for many years. In this example the promotion might represent a threat to a satisfying life-style, a change in social class and social group, and increased responsibility for all family members. Therefore, although the family would undoubtedly gain many things they desire and have worked for, to do so they must give up the familiarity of the life they have known, and they may not have immediately available the coping mechanisms necessary to make a smooth adjustment.

Whether the type of event that precipitated the crisis is developmental or situational, the characteristics of the crisis state remain essentially the same.

CHARACTERISTICS OF A CRISIS STATE

A crisis state is not seen as an illness, but rather as an upset in the steady state of the system. The behaviors engaged in by those experiencing the crisis sequentially express feelings of being overwhelmed and an inability to cope, followed by attempts to cope, which may or may not be successful. Massive amounts of *free-floating anxiety* underlie these behaviors. The anxiety may be perceived as such, or it may take the form of depression or anger at various points in the crisis state. Since great amounts of anxiety cannot be sustained by the human being without serious damage to the personality organization, the individual consciously and unconsciously actively seeks to reorganize his personality in such a way that he rids himself of this unbearable emotion. Therefore *a state of crisis is self-limiting,* usually from 4 to 6 weeks in length. It is almost always resolved in this time frame, although not always in the healthiest way. If new, more adequate coping mechanisms are not developed within this time period, the individual is likely to repress the events and emotions surrounding the crisis to avoid further personality disorganization, which would result from prolonged maintenance of a high level of anxiety. Thus a pseudoresolution to the state of crisis is achieved.

As previously discussed, a crisis state seems to be a response to an event, whether developmental or situational, that is perceived as hazardous. Consequently, a crisis state is highly individualized, and an event that may precipitate a crisis in one individual or family may not necessarily have the same effect on another individual or family. Hazardous events are further categorized into three groups: (1) those that represent a *threat* to fundamental instinctual needs or to the person's sense of integrity, (2) those that represent a real or perceived *loss,* and (3) those that represent a *challenge.*

Another characteristic of the crisis state is that *it rarely affects an individual without also affecting those significant others who comprise the individual's social support system.* In most instances, this system is the family group. Therefore it is usually inappropriate to view an individual as being in a state of crisis without also taking into consideration the fact that it is highly likely that the family is also in a state of crisis. This point has numerous implications for intervention. Obviously any resolution to the crisis achieved by an individual in isolation from his previously established social system may be short-lived if it is not workable within the system as a whole.

Because of the mobility of the population in this country and the subsequent demise of the large, extended family, many persons have developed support systems that are not limited to, and in fact may not include, family members. Therefore it is important to recognize that friends and neighbors may serve as significant others to an individual even though these persons may not be relatives in the traditional sense. This social pattern is increasingly seen in older persons whose spouses have died and whose married children live at a great distance. In all instances, the individual being counseled should be the one who defines his significant social system, not the mental health worker who may be misled into making assumptions based on traditional societal patterns.

PHASES OF A CRISIS STATE

Whether it be an individual or a family that is in a state of crisis, the crisis seems to run through a series of definable, although overlapping, phases.

The initial phase is that of *denial,* which usually lasts for a period of hours. Denial is a defense mechanism that the mind unconsciously employs to protect itself from the sudden assault of intense anxiety. Denial is evident in the sitution where a 55-year-old executive calmly returns to his usual business activities after being informed by the corporate president that he has been fired. In most mentally healthy persons, the reality of the situation quickly becomes apparent and leads into the next phase of crisis, which is characterized by increased tension.

During the phase of *increased tension,* the persons involved make valiant efforts to continue their activities of daily living but do so while attempting to cope with ever-increasing amounts of anxiety. During this phase, therefore, the individual or family remains functional, although those who know them can easily see indications of increased tension in the form of hyperactivity or psychomotor retardation. A common example of this phase is seen in persons who are successfully making funeral arrangements for a loved one who has just died unexpectedly. The phase of increased tension is followed by disorganization.

During the phase of *disorganization,* those in a crisis seem to "fall apart." They can no longer continue with activities of daily living, become obsessively preoccupied with the event, and may remember earlier events they thought they had forgotten and that, unbeknownst to them, have a symbolic link to the current situation. It is during this phase that the person in a state of crisis is consciously flooded by a great deal of anxiety and fears that he may be "losing his mind." The fact that he is in a state of crisis may or may not be apparent to him. If it is not, as is often the case, it is usual for the person to become highly anxious about his anxiety, thereby compounding the problem. Therefore it is during this phase that most persons seek professional help, if this has not been done previously.

The next phase of a crisis is characterized by *attempts to reorganize.* With or without assistance, the individual or family attempts to bring previously used coping mechanisms to bear on the current situation. At this point the mechanisms used are likely to be short-range in nature and directed specifically at the immediate problem. For example, the homemaker who has not been able to mobilize sufficient energy to do the dishes for the last 3 days may wheel the portable television into the kitchen in an attempt to divert her mind sufficiently to get through the increasingly large stack of dirty dishes. The mechanism the woman in this example is using is suppression. If attempts at reorganization are successful at this point, they tend to build on one another and lead to general reorganization, the ultimate goal of crisis resolution. The affected persons gradually resume their normal activities of daily living, becoming anxious or depressed only when specific stimuli are present to remind them of the crisis situation. The attempt at reorganization lasts for weeks, if successful.

A phase characterized by an *attempt to escape the problem* occurs within a matter of days if initial attempts to reorganize are unsuccessful. Without appropriate intervention, it is during this phase that blaming commonly occurs. The persons involved tend to "escape the problem" by projecting responsibility for its existence onto other people, societal institutions, or a supernatural phenomenon such as God or fate. Blaming behaviors, at the very least, create increased tension in a system already overwhelmed by stress, and at worst lead to actions that ultimately compound rather than relieve the problem. For example, the husband who blames his wife's lack of supervision for their son's juvenile delinquency may initiate divorce proceedings only to find himself totally alone and still highly anxious a year later when the divorce becomes final. A couple who blames the rigid narrow-mindedness of the community in which they live for their failure to be accepted into the local country club may decide to move to a distant state only to find that they have left behind their primary support system in the form of co-workers. A highly religious person in this phase of crisis may officially leave his church as a means of publicly rejecting the God whom he blames for his problems. In so doing, he may also cut himself off from the human social system whose support he has used in the past and could benefit from now.

Regardless of whether the persons involved in the crisis resort to blaming behaviors or whether they attempt to escape the problem by consciously pretending it does not exist (as opposed to denial, which is an unconscious defense mechanism), this phase rarely results in a successful resolution to the crisis.

After failing at attempts to escape the problem, the individual or family moves into the phase of *local reorganization.* This phase has characteristics similar to the phase, attempts to reorganize, previously described.

After the local reorganization phase, the final phase of *general reorganization* occurs. It may take up to a year before new patterns of behavior are sufficiently well integrated into the individual's personality organization or the family's interactional structure and communication system to withstand additional stress on the system. However, the acute phase of the crisis is usually over within the 6-week time period, as previously mentioned.

Unsuccessful resolution of a crisis state occurs when, during any phase, the individual or family adopts pathological means of adaptation, which serves to obscure and compound the crisis. This is most likely to occur when the ego strength of the individual is already weakened or when the family has been using dysfunctional adaptations prior to the crisis. The outlook is particularly dim when skilled intervention is not sought or available and the persons involved resume functioning on a level lower than the one at which they had previously been functioning.

Pseudoresolution occurs when the crisis is repressed and the

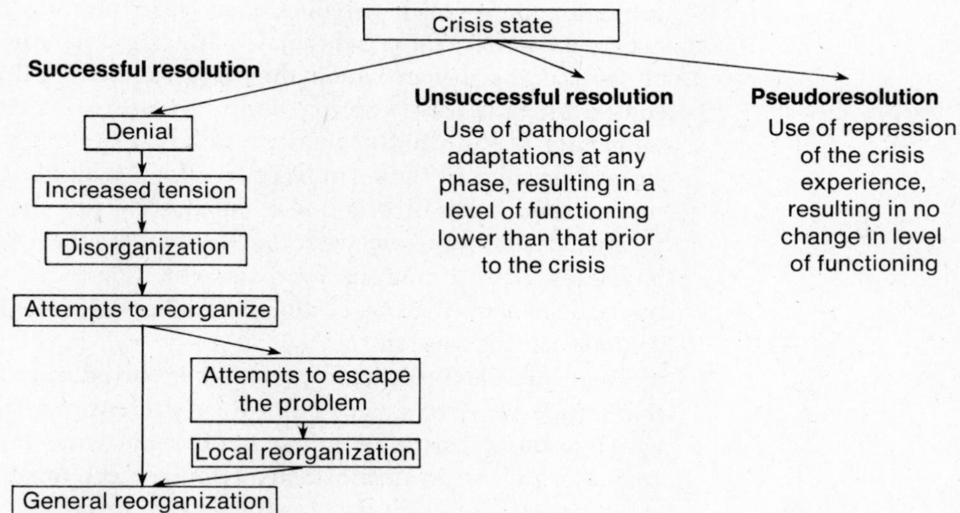

Fig. 8-1 *Processes leading to resolution of a crisis state. Successful resolution of a crisis state follows a series of phases before culminating in the ultimate goal of general reorganization. The initial four phases are experienced by all persons. Some persons may then move directly from attempts to reorganize to general reorganization. Others may need to take a temporary detour and attempt to escape the problem. When this attempt fails, they proceed to local reorganization, eventually reaching the goal of general reorganization. Successful resolution results in functioning at a level higher than that prior to the crisis.*

individual or family have learned nothing from the experience, returning to their former level of functioning. Although all may appear well, these people have missed a valuable opportunity to increase their repertoire of adaptive responses. Furthermore, future crises are likely to be compounded by the reemergence of the conflicts surrounding the previously unresolved repressed one. See Fig. 8-1 for a schematic representation of the processes leading to successful, unsuccessful, or pseudoresolution of a crisis state.

TECHNIQUES OF CRISIS INTERVENTION

The goal of crisis intervention is to assist the individual to seek new and useful adaptive mechanisms within the context of his social support system. By so doing, the mental health worker aids the involved persons to reorganize their individual personalities and their social system on a higher level of functioning than that which they had previously experienced. If this goal is achieved, these persons are better able to deal successfully with future developmental and situational events that inevitably will occur within their lifetimes.

It is important to note that many people who are in a state of crisis are not aware of this fact. They may come to, or telephone, a crisis intervention center with vague, diffuse complaints such as, "I can't sleep," "I'm afraid I'm losing my mind," or "I'm afraid that something dreadful is going to happen." On the other hand, friends or relatives may bring a person for treatment, stating that he is "not behaving like himself."

The initial step in intervention is to take the time to thoroughly assess the situation. Direct questions are appropriate, since the individual or family is likely to be in the phase of disorganization during which it is very difficult for them to focus their thoughts and feelings. In addition to collecting identifying data, it is important to ask specifically who else is involved in the problem. Rosenbaum and Beebe* describe this step as the identification of the protagonists.

---

*Rosenbaum, C. Peter, and Beebe, John E., III: Psychiatric treatment, New York, 1975, McGraw-Hill Book Co.

The next step is to define the event. It is not unusual for the persons involved to initially state that nothing unusual has occurred. If they respond in this way, it is not because they are lying, but rather because they are truly unaware of the significance of the event in their lives. To elicit this information, it is helpful to ask the person to review in detail what has occurred in his life over the past 2 weeks. If this account indicates nothing unusual, even with specific questioning, the interviewer asks the clients to go back 1 week further. Rarely is it necessary to go back further than 4 weeks. In the course of the narrative, the precipitating event will probably become clear to the interviewer and sometimes to the client as well. If the client is still unaware of the significant hazardous event, the interviewer can repeat back the situation the client has identified from the narrative and suggest that many people would find this situation troublesome. This intervention almost always elicits a surprised emotional response on the part of the client. The following is an example:

> Mrs. Curry received a regularly scheduled monthly visit from the public health nurse. Instead of finding her in the kitchen cleaning up after breakfast as was usually the case, the nurse found Mrs. Curry sitting on the living room couch, still in her nightgown and robe, crying and wringing her hands. The nurse sat down next to her and asked what was wrong. Mrs. Curry replied, "I don't know. I don't know. I just feel awful—as if something horrible is happening to me. Please help me." The nurse then asked if something unusual had happened since her last visit. Mrs. Curry replied, "No, nothing except I am going crazy." The nurse asked Mrs. Curry to tell her what the days had been like for her starting with 2 weeks ago. Although Mrs. Curry protested mildly at having to go through the last 2 weeks in such detail, she complied with gentle questioning from the nurse. The nurse was not surprised to hear that Mrs. Curry's mother-in-law had moved into the home 6 days ago. After 1 or 2 days of settling-in activities, the mother-in-law requested to cook the meals "for her son" so that she would feel useful. Mrs. Curry stated that she felt resentful about turning over the meal preparation to her husband's mother but in turn felt guilty about her reaction, since she would now have more free time. As a result, she dismissed her feelings as "unreasonable," agreed to her mother-in-law's request, and made arrangements to go clothes shopping with a friend late the following afternoon. When the following afternoon arrived, Mrs. Curry could not meet her friend because she was immobilized by anxiety, the source of which was unknown to her. Since that time she had been relatively sleepless

and decreasingly involved in the household activities. The above narrative was related by Mrs. Curry in a matter-of-fact way and with no particular emotion until the nurse said, "Many people find that when a new member of the family moves in, there is a major adjustment to make. I wonder if that's what could be troubling you?" At that point, Mrs. Curry began to sob but stopped wringing her hands.

Once the protagonists and the event have been identified, the involved persons are helped to develop a plan for coping with the crisis situation. To be effective in this step, the mental health worker needs to explore with the clients the resources that are available and known to them as well as to suggest resources available in the community about which they might not know. Most mentally healthy people have numerous interpersonal, social, and community resources available to them but may need help to identify the appropriate ones to use and to accept aid from. For clients to benefit from this step they need to be encouraged to make as many arrangements for help as possible by themselves. However, the wise mental health worker realizes that high levels of anxiety often interfere with cognitive comprehension and retention of information, so information is best written out. For example, if it is decided that the clients could benefit from a talk with a representative of a social service agency, the name and telephone number of the agency and a suggested day and time for the clients to call for an appointment should be clearly written out.

These steps in crisis intervention are designed to help the clients achieve a correct cognitive perception of the situation, which is enhanced by the worker's seeking the facts surrounding the situation and by her helping the clients to keep the problem in their consciousness.

Another vital aspect of crisis intervention is assisting the clients in managing their feelings. To achieve this goal, the clients need to develop an awareness of their feelings. Appropriate verbalization of them, assisted by the reflection of the mental health worker, leads to desensitization and mastery of the feelings that seem overwhelming. In helping clients deal with their feelings, it is important not to give them false reassurance, although it is helpful to tell them that they are likely to feel better in 1 or 2 months despite the fact that it may seem impossible at this point. As previously stated, it is also important not to encourage them to blame others. If the worker falls into this trap, the result is to support the clients' natural avoidance of looking at their own behavior, thereby decreasing their opportunities to develop more mature patterns of coping.

All these steps are usually gone through in the initial contact with the persons in a crisis. Obviously such an interview may take longer than the traditional 50-minute therapy hour. Since the best results in crisis situations seem to be achieved through intensive but short-term intervention, it is advisable to spend as much time as is necessary, as often as is necessary, with the clients without engendering unwarranted dependency. At the end of the first visit the mental health worker will make a specific appointment to see the clients again, preferably in a few days but no longer than a week later. In the meantime the clients should know how they can contact the worker and should be encouraged to do so if they feel it is necessary. Often the knowledge that help is readily available is sufficient to enable the clients to manage without a telephone call until the next appointment.

During subsequent contacts the clients are assisted to go through the same steps all over again. In addition, the plan that was made in the previous session needs to be evaluated in terms of its effectiveness. If it seems to be working, it should be reinforced by supporting the clients' efforts at implementation. If the plan is not working or if new factors have altered the situation, the plan needs to be revised accordingly, but always with the mutual agreement of those involved.

In summary, crisis intervention is designed to help essentially healthy persons who are in a state of disequilibrium to help themselves. This goal is facilitated by assisting them to achieve correct cognitive perception of the situation and to gain effective management of their emotions. Successful resolution of crisis situations results in the clients' developing a larger repertoire of adaptive mechanisms, which in turn enables them to function on a level higher than the level on which they were functioning prior to the crisis state. In this way, effective crisis intervention prevents mental illness and promotes mental health.

CONCLUDING STATEMENTS

1. Crisis is defined by mental health authorities as *a state of disequilibrium resulting from the interaction of an event with the individual's or family's coping mechanisms, which are inadequate to meet the demands of the situation, combined with the individual's or family's perception of the meaning of the event.*
2. Interest in crisis intervention is great because more people are seeking mental health care, because of the relization that formerly unresolved crises emerge and can be treated in conjunction with the present crisis, and because crisis intervention provides a specific opportunity to promote mental health and prevent mental illness.
3. There are three possible outcomes of a crisis state: (a) the client may reintegrate at a lower or less healthy level of functioning, (b) the client may reintegrate at the same level of functioning as previously, or (c) the client may reintegrate at a higher, healthier level of functioning. This last possible outcome has great potential for increasing the level of mental health in a large population and is most likely to occur with intervention.
4. Events that are likely to precipitate crises are developmental or situational.
5. Developmental crises can be prevented through the use of anticipatory guidance, which is primarily an educative process that helps prepare the individual and family for behavioral changes that are likely to occur in the near future.
6. A crisis state is not seen as an illness, but rather as an upset in the steady state of the system, which is characterized by massive amounts of free-floating anxiety.
7. A state of crisis is self-limiting, usually from 4 to 6 weeks in length.
8. A crisis state seems to be a response to an event that is perceived as hazardous. Hazardous events may represent a threat, a loss, or a challenge.
9. A crisis state rarely affects an individual without also affecting those significant others who comprise the individual's social support system.
10. Successful resolution of a crisis state follows a series of

phases before culminating in the ultimate goal of general reorganization. The initial four phases of denial, increased tension, disorganization, and attempts to reorganize are experienced by all persons. Some persons may then move directly to general reorganization. Others may need to take a temporary detour and attempt to escape the problem. When this attempt fails, they proceed to local reorganization, eventually reaching the goal of general reorganization.

11. Unsuccessful resolution of a crisis state occurs when pathological adaptations are used at any phase of the crisis state. The result of unsuccessful resolution is when the person is functioning at a level lower than that prior to the crisis.
12. Pseudoresolution of a crisis state occurs when the crisis experience is repressed and leads to no change in the level of functioning.
13. The goal of crisis intervention is to assist the individual to seek new and useful adaptive mechanisms within the context of his social support system.
14. The initial step in intervention is to thoroughly assess the situation, identifying the protagonists and the event.
15. Once the protagonists and the event have been identified, a plan for coping with the crisis situation is developed. To be effective, this plan must include awareness of available resources.
16. It is important to help the client to achieve a correct cognitive perception of the situation and to assist him in managing his feelings.
17. When engaging in crisis intervention, the mental health worker is well advised to spend as much time as is necessary, as often as is necessary, with the clients without engendering unwarranted dependency.
18. The plan for coping with the crisis situation should be continuously evaluated as to its effectiveness and relevance.
19. Successful resolution of crisis situations results in the clients' developing a larger repertoire of adaptive mechanisms, which in turn enables them to function on a level higher than the level on which they were functioning prior to the crisis state.

Suggested sources of additional information

CLASSICAL

Coles, Robert: Children of crisis (all volumes), Boston, 1967, 1970, Little, Brown & Co.

DeYoung, Carol D.: Nursing's contribution in family crisis treatment, Nurs. Outlook **16:**60-62, Feb., 1968.

Joint Commission on Mental Health of Children: Crisis in child mental health: challenge for the 1970's, New York, 1970, Harper & Row, Publishers.

Norris, Catherine N.: Psychiatric crises: practical considerations, Perspect. Psychiatr. Care **5:**20-28, Jan.-Feb., 1967.

Parad, Howard J., editor: Crisis intervention: selected readings, New York, 1965, Family Service Association of America.

CONTEMPORARY

Aguilera, Donna C., and Messick, Janice M.: Crisis intervention: theory and methodology, ed. 3, St. Louis, 1978, The C.V. Mosby Co.

Berliner, Beverly S.: Nursing a patient in crisis, Am. J. Nurs. **70:**2154-2157, 1970.

Burgess, Ann Wolbert, and Holmstrom, Lynda Lytle: The rape victim in the emergency ward, Am. J. Nurs. **73:**1741-1745, 1973.

Carter, A.B.: Rural emergency psychiatric services, Am. J. Nurs. **73:**868-869, 1973.

Chesler, Phyllis: With child, New York, 1980, Harper & Row, Publishers.

DeYoung, Carol D.: Nursing's contribution in family crisis treatment, Nurs. Outlook **16:**60-62, Feb., 1968.

Donner, Gail J.: Parenthood as a crisis, Perspect. Psychiatr. Care **10:**84-87, April-June, 1972.

Eisler, Richard M., and Hersen, Michel: Behavioral techniques in family-oriented crisis intervention, Arch. Gen. Psychiatry **28:**111-116, 1973.

Flomenhaft, Kalman, and Langsley, Donald G.: After crisis, Ment. Hyg. **55:**473-477, 1971.

Grier, Anne M., and Aldrich, C. Knight: The growth of a crisis intervention unit under the direction of a clinical specialist in psychiatric nursing, Perspect. Psychiatr. Care **10:**73-83, April-June, 1972.

Grollman, Earl A.: When your loved one is dying, Boston, 1980, Beacon Press.

Hall, Joanne E., and Weaver, Barbara R., editors: Nursing of families in crisis, Philadelphia, 1974, J.B. Lippincott Co.

Hitchcock, Janice Marland: Crisis intervention—the pebble in the pool, Am. J. Nurs. **73:**1388-1390, 1973.

Hurwitz, Arlene: Child abuse: a program for intervention, Downstate Medical Center, College of Nursing, Brooklyn, N.Y., Nurs. Outlook **25:**575-577, Sept., 1977.

Irwin, Theodore: How to cope with crisis, Public Affairs Pamphlet No. 464, New York, 1971, Public Affairs Committee.

King, Joan M.: The initial interview: basis for assessment in crisis intervention, Perspect. Psychiatr. Care **9:**247-256, Nov.-Dec., 1971.

Kuenzi, Sandra Hicks, and Fenton, Mary V.: Crisis intervention in acute areas, Am. J. Nurs. **75:**830-834, 1975.

Lieb, Julian, Lipsitch, Ian I., and Slaby, Edmund Andrew: The crisis team, a handbook for the mental health professional, New York, 1973, Harper & Row, Publishers.

McGill, Michael E.: The 40 to 60 year old male, New York, 1980, Simon & Schuster, Inc.

Maloney, Elizabeth M.: The subjective and objective definition of crisis, Perspect. Psychiatr. Care **9:**257-267, Nov.-Dec., 1971.

Pisarcik, Gail, et al.: Psychiatric nurses in the emergency room, Am. J. Nurs. **79:**1264-1266, July, 1979.

Reese, Mary Ellen: Moving on, New York, 1980, Peter H. Wyden/Publisher.

Rueveni, Uri: Networking families in crisis, New York, 1979, Human Sciences Press.

Salerno, Elizabeth Meehan: A family in crisis, Am. J. Nurs. **73:**100-103, 1973.

Sheehy, Gail: Passages: predictable crises of adult life, New York, 1976, E.P. Dutton & Co., Inc.

Tatelbaum, Judy: The courage to grieve, New York, 1980, Lippincott and Crowell.

Tuckerman, Alan J.: Disaster and mental health intervention, Community Ment. Health J. **9:**151-157, Summer, 1973.

Wallace, Mary, and Morley, Wilbur: Teaching crisis intervention, Am. J. Nurs. **70:**1484-1487, 1970.

Williams, Florence: Intervention in maturational crises, Perspect. Psychiatr. Care **9:**240-246, Nov.-Dec., 1971.

Wise, Doreen James: Crisis intervention before cardiac surgery, Am. J. Nurs. **75:**1316-1318, 1975.

OF PARTICULAR INTEREST

Aguilera, Donna C., and Messick, Janice M.: Crisis intervention: theory and methodology, ed. 3, St. Louis, 1978, The C.V. Mosby Co.

This book is one of the most concise, comprehensive texts available in crisis intervention theory and practice. It is clearly organized and meaningful to the practitioner.

Mitchell, C.E.: Identifying the hazard: the key to crisis intervention, Am. J. Nurs. **77:**1194, 1977.

In this article the author underlines the importance of identifying a precipitant in the state of crisis. Included are assessment criteria and intervention strategies.

9

Intervention with individuals

- Common patterns of nontherapeutic interpersonal interventions
- Developing therapeutic interpersonal interventions
- Types of therapeutic interpersonal interventions
- Developmental phases involved in the therapeutic relationship
- Differentiating between social and therapeutic relationships

All interpersonally based therapeutic interventions take place within the context of human interaction. Although interventions that are therapeutic possess common elements, they are developed differently by each person, depending on the characteristics of the individuals involved. If an intervention is to become therapeutic, it is necessary to recognize the client as a unique, important human being who experiences hopes, fears, joys, and sorrows as do all other people. It is necessary to understand that the client has his own special set of problems and reactions to life. It is important for the nurse to interact with him so that she develops and reflects an understanding of his emotional responses and the probable meaning of his behavior. Through her sensitivity the nurse can develop a recognition of some of the client's emotional needs and an appreciation for some of the ways in which she can be helpful to him. In many instances the nurse will be most helpful to the client by interacting with him in a way that turns out to be different from the previous social interactions he has experienced. Many mentally ill persons have a long history of having failed at establishing and maintaining satisfying interpersonal relationships. To the degree that the nurse's interactions with the client reflect acceptance of him and consistency in response to him, they will be therapeutic by providing experiences that are corrective of earlier, less helpful interpersonal experiences.

The use the nurse makes of her own personality can be a great therapeutic influence in the experience of the client if she uses understanding and skill. It is the only tool that is uniquely hers and that she alone directs. The nurse may give dozens of daily medications and may assist with many somatic therapies, but these activities are medically directed. Aside from assisting the physician in carrying out therapeutic measures, the major way in which the nurse directly influences the care of the client is through the use she makes of herself as she deals with the client in face-to-face interactions.

COMMON PATTERNS OF NONTHERAPEUTIC INTERPERSONAL INTERVENTIONS

Some of the characteristic ways in which nurses intervene nontherapeutically with clients are discussed here in the hope of assisting readers to examine the quality of their own professional behavior. Frequently the nurse relates to the client as a manager.

The role of controller of the situation is an easy one for the nurse to adopt, since she has had some practice with this role in other settings. Young nurses may adopt an authoritarian attitude because they feel insecure and unfortunately have patterned their behavior after that of older nurses who have behaved in an authoritarian way.

It is important for the nurse to look objectively at her professional behavior with clients. If it has qualities of authoritarianism, she should ask herself why this is true. What secondary satisfactions are derived from this controlling attitude? Is this the best method of helping clients become more self-respecting and self-directing? Obviously the nurse who rigidly controls the client's environment will not be able to create a climate in which the client can achieve maximum personal, emotional, and social growth. Development of emotional maturity is achieved only through practice in making decisions and in directing one's own behavior.

Inexperienced nurses sometimes relate to clients of the opposite sex in a seductive way. This often appears to be the only approach that some nurses are able to make to clients of the opposite sex. Nurses who use this method of relating to mentally ill persons confuse their professional and social roles. They probably give little thought to the meaning their behavior has for the client. Such an approach suggests that the nurse is not fully aware of the client's emotional problems and does not realize that seductive behavior may add to already disturbing feelings with which the client is trying to cope. Nurses who use seductive behavior in relating to mentally ill persons should seek the guidance of a mature counselor. They may need help in finding more appropriate channels through which they can express their own emotional needs.

Many nurses give little thought to the characteristic way in which they relate to clients. Some prefer to view their work role as a series of tasks to be performed. Such a nurse is probably seen by clients as a person who is busily engaged in performing tasks as a means of avoiding contact with them. She may interact with clients only when she is involved in performing a specific technical nursing task. Such a nurse should ask herself why she finds it necessary to remain aloof from clients. An evaluation of her professional behavior may reveal fears or an attitude toward mentally ill persons that can be altered.

Some nurses interact with clients solely through socialization. This approach might be called the role of the social technician. A nurse who uses this approach may spend much time initiating social activities and encouraging clients to participate. She may focus all conversation with clients on social activities. This approach makes it possible for her to avoid involving herself with clients except superficially, and it discourages clients from sharing emotionally upsetting problems with her. Clients often do need help in participating in social activities, but this is only one of their many needs. A nurse's focusing only on the social needs of clients limits her effectiveness.

The quality of the interaction between the nurse and the client is closely related to the motivation that underlies the nurse's attitude toward nursing and her perception of her role as a nurse. It is important for the nurse to evaluate her interactions with clients. Because motivations are partially if not wholly unconscious, it is difficult to examine one's own motivations. Therefore the nurse will need guidance in evaluating her characteristic approaches to clients. It is suggested that this can be accomplished best through a series of conferences with an expert in psychiatric nursing, during which nurse-client interactions are discussed in depth. As a result of these discussions and of the increased knowledge and experience gained, the nurse can often develop other patterns of nursing interventions with clients that are more therapeutic.

DEVELOPING THERAPEUTIC INTERPERSONAL INTERVENTIONS

The foundation of all interpersonally based therapeutic interventions is *acceptance*. This is a commonly used word among nurses, although it is not universally understood or used by them. Other behaviors that are equally important in psychiatric nursing are those expressed by the adjectives *nonjudgmental* and *consistent*. All these concepts are basic in developing therapeutic interventions with any client. They are discussed here in the hope of helping the nurse to make effective use of them in caring for mentally ill persons.

Acceptance implies that the nurse treats the client as an important individual who has inherent worth and not as a diagnostic entity or a set of psychiatric symptoms. Actually, the use of diagnostic terms may encourage the nurse to adopt an impersonal attitude toward the client. The nurse implies that she is accepting the client by calling him by name and by recognizing that he has the same basic personal rights she herself possesses. Acceptance implies that the nurse tries to understand the meaning the client is conveying through his behavior. An accepting nurse recognizes that the client handles his behavior as well as he is able at a given time. She encourages the client to express his feelings to her, realizing that in this way he is able to relieve emotional tensions. She does not censor him for statements and feelings that may not be conventionally acceptable, realizing that his behavior is an expression of his illness. She recognizes that his comments may not be directed toward her personally.

The word *nonjudgmental* is usually used in conjunction with the word *attitude* and is closely related to the concept of acceptance. One cannot be achieved without the other. A nonjudgmental attitude is neither condemning nor approving. Through tone of voice and manner the nurse conveys to the client a helpful attitude without morally judging his behavior. A nonjudgmental attitude toward the behavior of a mentally ill person implies that the nurse recognizes that the behavior, like physical symptoms displayed by physically ill persons, is neither good or bad nor right or wrong, but rather an expression of emotional need. She realizes also that the client's behavior will change when his illness improves.

Acceptance of mentally ill persons and their behavior is often difficult to achieve, and almost everyone occasionally falls short of the ideal. The behavior of some mentally ill persons is offensive at times. This is true, for example, of the behavior of clients who are so confused that they soil themselves. It may be impossible for the nurse to avoid feeling repelled by the sight of a person grossly soiled, but it is possible for her to avoid making him feel that he is an offensive person. Joking in front of a client about his behavior or describing his shortcomings to others within his hearing is neither respecting nor accepting him.

Being *consistent* is another important aspect to be considered in developing therapeutic interventions. The consistent nurse maintains the same basic attitude toward the client so that he derives security from being able to predict her behavior. Not only should the client be able to expect the same positive attitudes and approaches from an individual nurse, but also the entire nursing staff should interact with consistency from the standpoint of basic attitudes and overall policies. Consistency helps lessen the client's anxiety by simplifying decision making and by avoiding uncertainties.

All mentally ill persons experience some loss of self-esteem and self-confidence. If an intervention is to be helpful to a client, it must assist him in reestablishing his self-confidence and restoring his self-esteem. This is a slow process that requires consistent work over a period of time. Recognizing the client as being an important human being, expressing genuine interest in him, spending time with him, conversing with him, and listening with understanding to his expressions of feeling are all ways of helping him feel worthwhile, important, and wanted. On the other hand, indifference, insincerity, and an impersonal attitude toward the client reinforce his sense of unimportance and further convince him of what he may believe—that he is lacking in value as a person.

Behavioral examples of verbal and nonverbal approaches that may be therapeutic are discussed in depth in Chapter 7 of this text. They are summarized here in Table 3 because of their applicability to all types of interpersonally based therapeutic interventions.

It is not possible for a nurse to intervene in a way that has the same therapeutic potential and the same meaning for each individual client. It is possible, however, for the nurse to learn to know the names and something of the needs of all clients with whom she comes in close contact. With many of these persons the nurse can expect to develop a positive working relationship. With a limited number she will be able to develop a mutual give-and-take that will have the potential of growing into a therapeutic relationship. It is with these individuals that she will be able to

Table 3 *Behavioral examples of therapeutic verbal and nonverbal approaches*

Verbal approach	Nonverbal approach
Use client's name when speaking to him.	Develop awareness of own feelings about client.
Allow client to take the conversational lead.	Convey interest and empathy.
Restate client's words for the purpose of validating the meaning.	Sit near client and give him undivided attention.
Reflect client's words and feelings when the conversation lags.	Look at client.
Ask questions for the purpose of clarifying.	Nod head appropriately.
Assist client to test reality, to think through his problems logically.	Remain with client when his feelings are acute.
Help client to plan activities to provide an outlet for his feelings.	
Withhold advice and personal opinions.	
Avoid words that connote judgment.	
Avoid a barrage of questions.	
Avoid monologues.	
Withhold false reassurance.	
Remain silent if a response seems unnecessary.	

carry on discussions that have therapeutic potential, because she will know them well and will have developed a genuine interest in them as people.

TYPES OF THERAPEUTIC INTERPERSONAL INTERVENTIONS

There are at least three types of one-to-one situations in which the psychiatric nurse is often involved. These situations are differentiated on the basis of the degree of nurse-client involvement and whether the goal of the intervention is immediate, short-range, or long-range. As the nurse engages in each of these situations with clients she variously assumes the roles of creator of a therapeutic environment, socializing agent, counselor, teacher, mother surrogate, and technical nurse. Therapeutic use of these roles is discussed at length in Chapter 3 of this text.

The first situation in which the nurse and client are likely to engage is one in which the nurse and the client do not know each other, and the client is in immediate, severe difficulty that requires the nurse to intervene. The nature of the difficulty can range from a life-threatening situation, such as a suicidal attempt, to the client's being overwhelmed by a particular emotion, such as grief, and expressing this behaviorally. Ideally the person who intervenes in such situations should be one who knows the client and understands the plan of treatment for him. This, however, is not always possible because of the necessity for immediate action or the unavailability of the appropriate staff member or because the client is new to the treatment setting. When such situations arise, the nurse must not avoid intervening merely because she does not know the client. Rather, she must bring to bear on the situation her knowledge of the dynamics of human behavior and her skill in psychiatric nursing. In these emergency situations the nurse will do well to employ the principles of psychiatric nursing and good common sense. The client has a right to be protected from harming himself, either physically or emotionally, and from harming others.

Needless to say, once the emergency situation is resolved, immediate efforts should be made to contact those mental health personnel who are involved with the client's treatment or to establish a long-range treatment plan and begin its implementation if one has not already been developed.

The second situation is one in which the nurse and client know each other but the nurse does not have major responsibility for this particular client's treatment. Unfortunately, some nurses believe that if they are not assigned to the care of a particular client, they have little or no responsibility to behave in a thoughtful, goal-directed manner when interacting with him. This is not the case, and, in fact, the value of the therapeutic interventions of other staff can be lessened by thoughtless, offhand behavior of a particular nurse. Although it is not possible for the nurse to have in-depth knowledge of all the clients in any treatment setting, it is possible and important for her to be aware of the treatment goals for all clients with whom she is likely to come in contact, no matter how superficially. With this awareness, the nurse's on-the-spot interactions with the client can be designed to support and enhance the treatment that is being implemented by other nurses and mental health personnel.

This situation is particularly common in psychiatric nursing, since, unlike many physically ill persons, emotionally ill persons usually have physical mobility and are not dependent on the nurse to approach them at the bedside. It is not uncommon for an emotionally ill person to seek out a nurse other than the one to whom he is assigned to validate statements made to him by his assigned nurse or to otherwise engage the two nurses in a power struggle. The client's motivation may or may not be conscious and may be a manifestation of the stage of the relationship in which the client and his nurse are engaged. In any event, the manner in which the nurse responds is frequently an important factor in enhancing or impeding the therapeutic endeavors of others. These on-the-spot, seemingly casual interactions should have as their goal support of the overall treatment of the client.

The third one-to-one situation in which the psychiatric nurse finds herself is one in which she seeks to develop a therapeutic relationship with a client in an effort to provide corrective interpersonal experiences. Because such a relationship requires an in-depth knowledge of the client and much time and energy on the part of the nurse, it is possible for the nurse to have only a few such relationships in progress at any point in time. An understanding of the porcess of these relationships will make clear that it is inappropriate to use the term *nurse-client relationship* to describe all interactions between the nurse and all clients with whom she comes in contact. This is not to say that all nurse-client interactions should not be therapeutic, but rather that in only a few will the nurse be intensely involved in an ongoing relationship with the client, which is designed to provide corrective interpersonal experiences. Since the nurse can be involved in only a few nurse-client relationships at any one time, it is important that she make the best use of her time, energy, and skills by devoting them to those clients whose nursing diagnosis indicates a potential for benefiting from this type of nursing intervention. Not all nurses work equally effectively with all clients, since the nurse's own personality is the major tool she has for intervention. Therefore, when the nursing care plan indicates that a nurse-client relationship is desirable, the nurse who develops such a relationship should be one whose self-awareness indicates that she would be likely to be effective with the particular client. Since both nurses and emotionally ill persons are more human than otherwise and have the same wide variety of personality structures, it is unlikely that there ever would be a client for whom a suitable nurse were not available.

DEVELOPMENTAL PHASES INVOLVED IN THE THERAPEUTIC RELATIONSHIP

Every therapeutic relationship that a nurse develops between herself and a client has an initial phase, referred to as the *orientation phase* or the *getting acquainted period.* It is during this phase that the nurse and client agree on a mutually acceptable contract that serves to establish the parameters of the relationship. The goals of this phase are the development of trust and the establishment of the nurse as a significant other to the client.

Although in some instances the client initiates the relationship, more frequently it is the nurse who first approaches the client. She does so by introducing herself by name and position and suggesting that she would like to work with him on his problems by meeting with him for a specific period of time and at a specified time and place. It is also important for the nurse to ask the client how he would like to be addressed. Most clients respond positively to this approach, ironically because the nurse is not yet an important part of their life and the idea of developing a relationship with her is not threatening. Once the time and place of their conversations is agreed on, it is imperative that the nurse adhere strictly to this schedule. The nurse should also suggest a duration for each conversation, for example, 45 minutes. This period of time must be adhered to, despite the fact that the client may at various times attempt to entice the nurse to stay longer with him by bringing up highly charged emotional issues 5 minutes prior to the end of the session. The nurse can handle this by acknowledging that the issues at hand sound important and by suggesting that the client reintroduce them at the beginning of their next meeting. This approach is therapeutic because it illustrates that the nurse will follow through on what she had promised—in this instance, sessions of a 45-minute length—and therefore can be trusted to do what she says. It is important to understand that clients sometimes unconsciously introduce highly significant issues shortly before the end of planned sessions as a means of letting the nurse know what is disturbing them without running the risk of having to discuss these issues at length, since they know that the session will soon be over. If the nurse succumbs to the temptation to continue the discussion beyond the agreed time, the client will learn that he has to be more guarded with her in the future.

Some clients, rather than attempting to lengthen the sessions, try to shorten them by overt means such as walking away or covert means such as falling asleep. The nurse can effectively deal with such situations by remembering that this period of time is set aside solely for interaction with this client and by stating this to him. If the client then still walks away or falls asleep, the nurse should remain in the designated meeting place for the remainder of the decided time. This behavior of the nurse also indicates to the client that she can be trusted to do what she has promised, despite his behavior.

As the nurse becomes more meaningful to the client, his behavior toward her often appears increasingly negative. He may not appear for the scheduled sessions or his language may become profane or he may resist talking about himself and state a preference to discuss the nurse's personal life. At this point many nurses become discouraged and disappointed, since the earlier sessions had seemed to run smoothly. If the nurse does not view this change in the client's behavior as a test to determine just how much he can rely on her to be accepting and nonjudgmental of him, the nurse might feel that it would not be wise to continue the relationship. To act on this feeling would be a mistake, since the client's increase in testing behavior most frequently indicates that the nurse is becoming a significant other to the client and therefore he must test her reliability before finally allowing himself to trust her. Therefore, rather than discontinuing the relationship, the nurse must respond to the client's behavior with meticulous consistency. If she continues to do so, the client will soon have a decreased need to test her, and the first phase of the relationship will be over.

The second phase in a therapeutic relationship between a nurse and a client is called the *maintenance* or *working phase.* The characteristics of this phase are highly individualized to the nature of the client's problems. Because each individual is unique and because the working phase of a relationship is so highly individualized to the particular client and nurse, few specific parameters can be given to guide the progress of this phase. An exception, however, is the necessity for limit setting, which often arises during this phase.

Limit setting is required when the client is threatening physical harm to himself or others, when he is destroying property or threatening to do so, and when his verbal hostility is upsetting and causing other clients or personnel to become tense and upset. If the client who requires limit setting is willing to discuss his behavior, it may be sufficient for the nurse to point out that he is causing a dangerous and disturbing situation and to request that he stop. For some persons such a request will be sufficient. However, others will require a more direct approach. In such an instance the nurse must speak firmly and explain that unless his disturbing behavior stops, he will have to be segregated from the group and placed in a room alone or will be given a medication that will assist him to gain control of his behavior.

If the nurse initiates and enforces limit setting in an empathic and nonpunitive manner, the client will often feel a sense of relief because another person has assumed the responsibility for identifying and enforcing the boundaries of his behavior. Rather than damaging the relationship, limit setting often serves to further convince the client that the nurse cares about him as a worthwhile individual.

In summary, the maintenance or working phase of the nurse-client relationship is the time when the work of the relationship is carried on, and unless both the nurse and the client are actively involved in working to identify and solve the client's problems, the relationship cannot be maintained. In maintaining a therapeutic relationship with a client, the nurse will undoubtedly encourage him to express his concerns, fears, hopes, and problems. Sometimes she will be able to achieve this by asking leading questions that will be direct and specific. The nurse needs to recognize when she is able to handle the client's expressed concerns and, when it is necessary, to seek help from other members of the clinical team who are better prepared to cope with the specific problem. Therefore it is important for the nurse to understand how she and the other members of the clinical team share responsibility for the client's therapy.

The third phase of the therapeutic relationship is referred to as the *termination* or *concluding phase.* It is unrealistic to expect a relationship to continue indefinitely. This fact should be considered and included in the plan from the outset.

When the nurse learns that it will be necessary for her to leave the client, she should discuss this fact with him as soon as possible. If the nurse knows at the outset that the relationship will be terminated at a specific time, the plans for the work of the nurse and the client should always include this fact. Terminating a relationship can be a traumatic experience for both the nurse and the client because they may have shared much that is personal and important. At such a time many clients express the feeling that the nurse is forsaking them. The loss of a trusted nurse is an especially difficult problem for a client who has been unable to trust other people. It is not unusual for clients to act out their frustration at the news of the impending loss of a trusted nurse.

In view of the possible traumatic difficulties that the departure of the nurse presents to the client, the nurse must seek to understand the client's sense of loss and to help him express his feelings and cope with them. The goal of this phase of the relationship is to help the client to review what he has learned through the process of the relationship and to transfer these learnings to his interactions with other persons.

Although the client with whom the nurse has established an ongoing therapeutic relationship will require special help in accepting her departure, the entire group of clients with whom the nurse has been working will respond in a variety of ways to her expected loss. Ideally, clients in a psychiatric setting should experience a relatively constant professional staff with whom they can establish meaningful relationships and work out emotional problems. Clients, like all people, will react to an anticipated loss in a variety of ways, depending on the characteristic way in which they respond, their unique emotional needs, and the relationship they have developed with the departing staff member. Some clients may become depressed and unconsciously believe that they have been personally responsible for the loss of the nurse. Other clients may not be able to accept the loss of this valued person and may repress the knowledge. They may report that no one told them that she was leaving. Other clients may respond with anger and may insist that the administrator take steps to see that the nurse does not leave.

When the nursing staff members are prepared for a variety of responses on the part of clients, they can understand, accept, and cope with the behavior. This means that they will need to spend time talking with and listening to clients. They will need to make themselves more available than usual to deal with the clients' many feelings about the situation and to reassure clients that they are not being abandoned. Sometimes it is helpful to encourage the clients to channel their feelings into some constructive activity. One way of helping to redirect clients' concerns is to help them organize and carry out a party to honor the departing nurse.

It is unfortunate when clients are not given an opportunity to express their feelings about such a situation or helped to handle their feelings. When this happens, as it does when a valued staff member simply disappears without any explanation, the feelings are not avoided but appear in many unusual behavioral reactions. A group of clients who have suffered such an unexplained loss may suddenly rebel against the entire nursing staff, or the physician may find that many old symptoms that clients were handling effectively have been reactivated.

When it is not the nurse but the client who is ready to leave the therapeutic situation, the nurse needs to be especially alert to the feelings of loss that she may have. If she does not allow herself to recognize these feelings, she might express them indirectly by showing undue concern for the client's future welfare, by encouraging him to stay for a few more sessions, or by otherwise encouraging his dependence on her. If the termination phase is not handled skillfully by encouraging the client to assume the independence he is ready for, the nurse can negate the value of the work that has been done in the preceding stages.

DIFFERENTIATING BETWEEN SOCIAL AND THERAPEUTIC RELATIONSHIPS

Sometimes it is difficult for nurses to differentiate between social and therapeutic relationships when dealing with mentally ill persons. The problem is even more complicated because mentally ill individuals usually are not physically ill and therefore are not bedridden. They frequently give the superficial impression of being socially and emotionally well. Nurses who have not developed an understanding of emotional illness may find it difficult to accept the fact that they are dealing with sick people. Thus their role confusion is understandable.

In a social relationship the needs of both the involved individuals are considered. The needs of both must be met in a satisfying way if the relationship is to continue. A social relationship usually develops spontaneously without a conscious plan. The goal of such a relationship is usually shared by the participants and is frequently limited to personal pleasure. The participants in a social relationship share mutual concern regarding reciprocal approval. This may develop more or less satisfactorily without conscious awareness of the emotional significance of the relationship.

In contrast, the therapeutic relationship focuses on the personal and emotional needs of the client. Such a relationship is therapeutically oriented and is planned after consideration has been given to the needs of the client and the therapeutic ability of the nurse. There is always a therapeutic goal toward which the nurse. There is always a therapeutic goal toward which the nurse is working, but it is not always shared with the client. When the nurse has accepted this role, she must strive to be consciously aware of the developing relationship and its meaning. She should seek help in reflecting objectively on the meaning of the interaction between herself and the client so that she will be prepared to guide the client in developing more mature behavior. In a therapeutic relationship the nurse does not necessarily seek the client's approval. She reevaluates the situation constantly so that she can distinguish between the client's actual needs and his demands.

When it is time for the relationship to be terminated, the nurse releases the patient emotionally and strives to help him move forward to more appropriate relationships.

Following are examples of the development of both a social and a therapeutic relationship between a nurse and a client.

A young student of nursing, Miss S., was assigned to a unit where she was to receive an initial experience in psychiatric nursing. The unit was populated by young men and women in their late teens or early twenties. The living quarters for the two groups were divided by a large living room. The clients gathered in the living room for group meetings, social activities, and conversations. Clients came and went freely in this unlocked unit. Some of the clients were employed during the day and returned to the hospital in the evening. Other clients were continuing their schoolwork in a nearby high school.

Miss S. participated enthusiastically in the social activities of the group. She frequently sought permission to participate in some of the activities planned for the evening hours. Permission was granted because it was the only possible way for her to become acquainted with several of the clients. When it was learned that Miss S. did not know how to dance, some of the young men volunteered to teach her. She learned quickly and was particularly successful in dancing with one young man, Jim L. They were approximately the same age and had a few friends in common, since they had grown up in the same general area in the city. The student nurse began to focus a good deal of attention on Jim. At client parties she insisted that he dance with her most of the time. Because Jim was popular with the female clients, they became annoyed with the student nurse and complained about her to the physician in charge. When Miss S. was asked to stop attending ward parties, she arranged to meet Jim in the afternoon away from the hospital. She began writing Jim daily notes that were delivered by fellow students.

When the instructor became aware of this problem, she asked Miss S. to come to her office for a talk. Miss S. discussed the situation freely. She said that she enjoyed having the opportunity to associate with Jim and could see no reason why questions were being raised. She admitted that she planned to drop the relationship as soon as the psychiatric nursing experience was completed. Miss S. said her friendship with Jim was an interesting interlude for both of them while it lasted. She was surprised to learn that Jim had requested a transfer from the unlocked unit to a unit where he would not be allowed so many privileges. She did not realize that Jim was desperately afraid of falling in love with a girl and that her relationship with him had reactivated many of his old fears and self-doubts.

In this situation the nursing student focused on her own social needs and on what she believed were Jim's social needs. Her stated goal for the relationship was immediate personal pleasure. Miss S. had given little thought to the meaning this relationship had for Jim or what effect her behavior would have on her professional role with other patients. She did not seek guidance in evaluating the relationship. As a result of Miss S.'s failure to differentiate between a social and a professional relationship, her experience with Jim was not helpful to him or satisfying for her.

On this same unit another nurse was able to develop an effective therapeutic relationship. Miss L., a young graduate nurse, came to work on the unit shortly after Miss S. left.

> Miss L. became interested in Bill A., a young man approximately the same age as Jim. He was painfully shy and avoided social contact with other people. He did not know how to dance and felt so inadequate that his only role in social situations was that of an observer. He did not take advantage of the privileges available to clients housed in this unlocked unit. He was intellectually capable but had quit high school because of his shyness and fear of people.
>
> Miss L. was sorry that Bill had not completed high school; as a result of discussions with the clinical team, it was decided that her goal would be to help him free himself of his fear of people to the extent that he would be able to return to school. She realized that this was a long-term goal and that it would be necessary for Bill to take many small steps forward before he could make such a move. She began her work immediately by sitting beside him for a few minutes each day. Getting acquainted with him was difficult because he was always deeply involved in reading. At first he was almost rude when she asked if she might sit down for a few minutes to talk. After many days Bill seemed to look forward to their daily chats. Finally she noticed that he closed the book when she approached.
>
> After several weeks Miss L. suggested that they take a walk together to the occupational therapy department to see what was going on there. He reluctantly accompanied her. On their tour of this department she talked about the many interesting available activities. She discovered that Bill had once done oil painting but feared criticism so much that he destroyed each painting before it was completed. Making use of this knowledge, Miss L. was able to obtain some oil painting equipment so that Bill could paint in a single room away from inquisitive people. Miss L. stopped to see his work daily and discovered that he had a great deal of talent. Other nurses came to praise his work. Finally he was able to

transfer his work to the occupational therapy department and eventually gave his consent to have several of his paintings hung in the lobby of the hospital.

One evening Miss L. gently encouraged Bill to accompany her to one of the social affairs given by the clients. During the first party he began to learn to dance. With encouragement and praise he learned to dance well and attended most of the social activities planned by the clients. He began dancing with other nurses, and finally he felt sure enough of himself to ask young women clients to dance.

After Miss L. had known Bill for over a year, she suggested that they go for a walk together outside the hospital. As usual he was reluctant to comply, but with encouragement he accompanied her. Several months after his first venture outside with Miss L., Bill began going out regularly with other clients to attend movies and football games and to visit art galleries. After working closely with Bill for 2 years, Miss L. suggested that they visit the high school near the hospital. As usual, Bill needed much encouragement, but he finally made the visit with her. Eventually he was able to enroll as a student and completed his high school work.

CONCLUDING STATEMENTS

1. If an interpersonally based intervention is to become therapeutic, it is necessary for the nurse to recognize the client as a unique, important human being who, like all persons, experiences hopes, fears, joys, and sorrows and has his own special set of problems and reactions to life.
2. To the degree that the nurse's interactions with the client reflect acceptance of him and consistency in response to him, they will be therapeutic by providing him with encounters that are corrective of earlier, less helpful interpersonal experiences.
3. The use the nurse makes of her personality is the key to her success in face-to-face interactions with clients.
4. The quality of interaction between the nurse and the client is closely related to the motivation that underlies the nurse's attitude toward nursing and her perception of her role as a nurse.
5. The foundation of all interpersonally based therapeutic interventions is acceptance, which implies that the nurse treats the client as an important person who has inherent worth

and not as a diagnostic entity or a set of psychiatric symptoms.

6. The nurse who maintains a nonjudgmental attitude realizes that the unusual behavior of the mentally ill person is neither good or bad nor right or wrong but an expression of emotional need.
7. If the nurse maintains consistency in her approach toward the client, she helps to lessen his anxiety by minimizing his uncertainty about her and the necessity for him to make decisions.
8. If intervening with a client is to be therapeutic for him, it must assist him in reestablishing his self-confidence and restoring his self-esteem.
9. There are at least three types of one-to-one situations in which the psychiatric nurse is usually involved. These situations are differentiated on the basis of the degree of nurse-client involvement and whether the goal of the intervention is immediate, short-range, or long-range.
10. One of the types of one-to-one interactions is called a nurse-clent relationship, which has three developmental phases: the orientation or getting-acquainted phase, the maintenance or working phase, and the termination or concluding phase.
11. A therapeutic relationship focuses on the personal and emotional needs of the client, whereas in a social relationship the needs of both the involved individuals are considered.

Suggested sources of additional information

CLASSICAL

Bressler, Bernard, and Vause, Mary Ella: The psychotherapeutic nurse, Am. J. Nurs. **62:** 87-90, May, 1962.

Burkhardt, Marti: Response to anxiety, Am. J. Nurs. **69:** 2153-2154, 1969.

Connolly, Mary Grace: What acceptance means to patients, Am. J. Nurs. **60:** 1754-1757, 1960.

Hale, Shirley L., and Richardson, Julia H.: Terminating the nurse-patient relationship, Am. J. Nurs. **63:**116-119, Sept., 1963.

Hays, Joyce Samhammer: Focusing on feelings, Nurs. Outlook **10:**332-333, May, 1962.

Kachelski, M. Audrey: The nurse-patient relationship, Am. J. Nurs. **61:**76-79, May, 1961.

Rogers, Carl R.: A counseling approach to human problems, Am. J. Nurs. **56:**994-997, 1956.

Schwartz, Morris S., and Shockley, Emmy Lanning: The nurse and the mental patient, New York, 1956, John Wiley & Sons, Inc.

Speroff, B.J.: Empathy is important in nursing. Nurs. Outlook **4:** 326-328, June, 1956.

Tudor, Gwen E.: A sociopsychiatric nursing approach to intervention in a problem of mutual withdrawal on a mental hospital ward, Perspect. Psychiatr. Care **8:**11-35, Jan.-Feb., 1970.

CONTEMPORARY

Arnold, Helen M.: Four A's: a guide to one-to-one relationships, Am. J. Nurs. **76:**941-943, 1976.

Bayer, Mary: Saying goodbye through graffiti: it all began when we were about to discharge Hilda, Am. J. Nurs. **80:**271, Feb., 1980.

Bishop, Barbara R.: The psychiatric nurse as a therapist—not a baby sitter, Perspect. Psychiatr. Care **10:**41-43, Jan.-March, 1972.

Burgess, Ann Wolbert, and Lazare, Aaron: Techniques in the therapeutic process. In Psychiatric nursing in the hospital and the community, ed. 2, Englewood Cliffs, N.J., 1976, Prentice-Hall, Inc., pp. 108-128.

Caudle, Patricia: Found: one person, Am. J. Nurs. **73:**310-313, 1973.

Cloud, Elizabeth D.: The plateau in therapist-patient relationships, Perspect. Psychiatr. Care **6:**112-121, July-Sept., 1972.

Delgado, Melvin: Therapy Latino style: implications for psychiatric care, Perspect. Psychiatr. Care **17**(3): 107-113, May-June, 1979.

Dillon, Kathryn M.: A patient-structured relationship, Perspect. Psychiatr. Care **9:**167-172, July-Aug., 1971.

Eisenman, Elaine P.: Primary care in a mental health facility, Nurs. Outlook **24:**640-645, 1976.

Feather, Roberta, and Bissell, Brenda: Clinical supervision vs. psychotherapy: the psychiatric mental health supervisory process, Perspect. Psychiatr. Care **17**(6):266-272, Nov.-Dec., 1979.

Gruber, Louis N.: The no-demand, third person interview of the non-verbal patient, **15:**38-39, 1977.

Kerr, Norine J.: Discussion of "common errors in communication made by students in psychiatric nursing," Perspect. Psychiatr. Care **16:**184-187, July-Aug., 1978.

Lego, Suzanne M.: The one-to-one nurse-patient relationship, Perspect. Psychiatr. Care **18**(2):67-89, March-April, 1980.

Loesch, Larry C., and Loesch, Nancy A.: What do you say after you say mm-mm? Am. J. Nurs. **75:**807-809, 1975.

Mitchell, Ann C.: Barriers to therapeutic communication with black clients, Nurs. Outlook **26:**109-112, Feb., 1978.

Ruffin, Janice E.: The relevence of racism to the goals of psychotherapy, Perspect. Psychiatr. Care **14:**160-164, 1976.

Sayre, Joan: Common errors in communication made by students in psychiatric nursing, Perspect. Psychiatr. Care **16:**175-183, July-Aug., 1978.

Sene, Barbara S.: Termination in the student-patient relationship, Perspect. Psychiatr. Care **7:**39-45, Jan., 1969.

Stokes, Gertrude A., and Fitzpatrick, Patricia: Teaching students psychotherapy, Am. J. Nurs. **77:**249-253, 1977.

Thomas, Mary D., Baker, Joan M., and Estes, Nada J.: Anger: a tool for developing self-awareness, Am. J. Nrs. **70:**2586-2590, 1970.

Vidoni, Clotilde: The development of intense positive counter transference in the therapist toward a patient, Am. J. Nrs. **75:**407-409, 1975.

White, Cheryl L.: Nurse counselling with a depressed patient, Am. J. Nurs. **78:**436-439, March, 1978.

Will, G.E.T.: A sociopsychiatric nursing approach to intervention in a problem of mutual withdrawal on a mental hospital ward, Perspect. Psychiatr. Care **8:**11, 1970.

Zahourek, Rothlyn P., and Crawford, Carole M.: Forced termination of psychotherapy, Perspect. Psychiatr. Care **16:**193-199, July-Aug., 1978.

OF PARTICULAR INTEREST

Boettcher, E.: Nurse-client collaboration: dynamic equilibrium in the nursing care system, J. Psychiatr. Nurs. **16:**7, Dec., 1978.

Nurse-client collaboration as it parallels nursing process is the focus of this article. The clinical example used is helpful in planning care, implementing plans, and evaluating outcome.

Lego, Suzanne M.: The one-to-one nurse-patient relationship, Perspect. Psychiatr. Care **18**(2): 67-89, March-April, 1980.

In one of the most comprehensive articles of its kind the author discusses the history of the one-to-one therapeutic relationship in psychiatric nursing. She brings together factors such as published research, literature patterns, and related trends that have influenced the emergence of this therapeutic mode.

10

Intervention with groups

- Characteristics of groups
- Use of groups in the care of the mentally ill
- Nurses as group therapists
- Group therapy
- Socialization groups: a remotivation technique
- Selection of a therapeutic group
- Growth and self-actualization groups

Human beings spend the vast majority of their time in group situations. They live, work, play, learn, and worship in groups. Group association is such a prominent part of everyone's life because human beings are inherently social and because in complex, technological societies individuals are interdependent and must rely on each other for services. Therefore the nature of our humanness and the nature of the society in which we live dictate the necessity for a social structure organized around groups.

The individual's first experience with groups occurs in infancy when he is incorporated into his family—a specialized type of natural group. The second major group situation most people experience is school. In fact, significant group associations continue throughout the entire life span. Despite the pervasiveness of groups in our society, however, few persons give any thought to the nature and function of groups.

A group is not a mere collection of individuals. Rather, a group is an identifiable system composed of three or more individuals who engage in certain tasks to achieve a common goal. Furthermore, to be a group the members must relate to each other, usually around the tasks and goals of the group. The individuals who ride the elevator in a skyscraper office building to get to their offices may share the common goal of getting to work, but they rarely relate to each other about this goal. Therefore they would not be considered a group. If, on the other hand, the elevator stalled between floors and its occupants expressed their fears to each other, offered each other emotional support, made plans to get themselves out of their predicament, or otherwise began relating to each other, they would quickly become a group in the technical sense of the word.

As identifiable systems, groups share certain characteristics regardless of their differences in size, task, or goal. Since nursing care is often rendered in group situations, it is important for the nurse to develop an understanding of these characteristics.

CHARACTERISTICS OF GROUPS

Groups can be composed of as few as 3 or as many as 20 members. The upper limit of membership size is determined by the number of individuals who can easily relate to each other at the same time. In most group situations, it is not possible for more than 20 people to meet this criterion, and even then difficulty is encountered. When a group is larger than the number of individuals who can comfortably relate to one another simultaneously, *subgroups* are formed. For example, the 100-member senior class at the local high school cannot possibly function as a total group, but is likely to be an aggregate of subgroups. Groups that are very small (3 or 4 members) also are not likely to be the most effective, since there may be insufficient membership to fulfill all the roles necessary for the achievement of the group's goal.

All groups have goals. These may be multiple or single. Multiple goals may have equivalent importance, or they may be prioritized according to their value. Group members may or may not be equally aware of and supportive of the goals of the group. However, the group's effectiveness is strongly related to the degree to which the members are aware of and supportive of the goals. When the goals have been achieved, the group either disbands or determines new goals. Natural groups, such as families, tend to remain as groups by redefining their goals. Groups that have been formed around a single goal tend to disband after achievement of that goal. An example of such a group is the aforementioned senior high school class. The graduating seniors commonly feel a strong group association and promise to maintain contact with each other after graduation, but because the group has achieved its goal and disbands, the group members rarely follow through on their promise.

A group is a system and, as such, functions in a manner designed to maintain its equilibrium. Therefore the behavior of any one member affects and is affected by all other group members and must be seen as reflective of group behavior. Learning to view group behavior from a holistic perspective, rather than as a summation of individual interactions, is a difficult task for most students. A commonly used example that may be helpful in this regard is that of a symphony orchestra. If the listener attends to only the music played by each individual, he will have a distorted impression of what the finished piece sounds like, because each musician contributes only a part of what is necessary to the completed piece. However, when the listener attends to the contributions of all the musicians put together, a synchronized, harmonious piece is heard. This example not only illustrates the concept that the whole is different from and greater than the sum of its parts, but it also implies that each part is necessary and of great value. In a group, individuals have great value, but the result of their interactions is a product that can be best appreciated only when viewed from a group perspective.

The interactional behavior of the group's members has a great deal to do with the group's ability to achieve its goal. The term used to designate the behavior of group members is *role.* A role is the characteristic behavioral pattern employed by a group member and is determined by the personality of the individual and the needs of the group. At any point in time the group has a need to address the tasks necessary to achieve its goal, while simultaneously maintaining its life. Addressing the task is achieved through roles that have a content orientation, and group maintenance is achieved through roles that have a process orientation.

The content of a group is the overt verbal exchange, while the process is the underlying meaning the content has to the group, not to the individual. For example, Mr. Jones might say, "I'm not sure how to proceed." If Mr. Jones is viewed as an individual rather than as a group member, the content of his statement could lead one to believe that he feels insecure, a somewhat negative assessment. If this same content is viewed within the context of a group, it would be more appropriate to interpret the process as a need of the group for orientation and Mr. Jones as fulfilling the role of orienter. This interpretation not only conveys a positive tone, but is more accurate than the individually based one.

The roles assumed by group members relate to either the content or to the process of the group. Task- or content-oriented roles as suggested by Robert Bales* include coordinator, orienter, recorder, observer and commentator, opinion seeker or giver, elaborater, information seeker or giver, and initiator. Roles related to

---

*Bales, Robert: Interaction process analysis: a method for the study of small groups, Reading, Mass., 1950, Addison-Wesley Publishing Co., Inc.

group maintenance or a process orientation include energizer, encourager, dominator, aggressor, compromiser, blocker, harmonizer, and rejecter.

These lists of roles are not intended to be reflective of all the possible roles a group member could assume. However, they do represent the most commonly seen behaviors of group members, and they also illustrate the reciprocal nature of content and process interactions (e.g., information seeker or giver, encourager or blocker).

Since human beings have numerous experiences in many groups, by the time they reach adulthood most have developed a large repertoire of group behaviors. Therefore any one individual may assume different roles in different groups and different roles at different times in the same group, dependent in part on the needs of the group. Consequently, it is impossible to predict with complete assurance the role any individual will assume in a group. Furthermore, since the behavior of any group member affects and is affected by all other group members, it is not unusual for an individual to behave in a group in a way that is quite different from the way he behaves when relating to only one other individual.

To function effectively, groups develop rules or *norms* that govern their operation. Some norms may be externally imposed, but the norms that have the most meaning are those that have emerged from within the group. For example, group members are much more likely not to smoke if that norm was established by themselves rather than by the superintendent of the building in which they meet. Norms are sometimes fully known to all members and therefore can be explicitly stated. Other norms are not consciously formulated by the group, but rather have evolved as a result of the group's experience. Whether the group norms are explicit or implicit, their purpose is to influence the behavior of the group. Since implicit norms cannot be overtly conveyed, individuals who join an established group may be in a precarious position because they may unknowingly violate an implicit norm and receive a negative, nonverbal reaction from the others. The violation of implicit group norms is the basis of many social faux pas. The power of implicit norms is attested to by the excruciating embarrassment experienced by the person who has committed a faux pas, even when the reality of his error does not warrant such a reaction.

Another characteristic of groups is that each group has a unique identity, while at the same time sharing much in common with all other groups. The student will recognize this characteristic as also being true of individuals. The uniqueness of each group is based on the specific interactional combination of its size, its goals and the tasks designed to achieve its goals, the roles its members characteristically assume, and the norms the members establish to govern its operation. On the other hand, all groups share enough in common that an individual is able to apply that which he has learned in previous group associations to new group experiences. When a group is first formed, its members tend to behave in the ways they found to be successful in previous groups. As the group develops its own unique characteristics its members modify their behavior to a greater or lesser degree to adapt to the group's uniqueness, thereby further enlarging their repertoire of group behaviors.

The unique identity of a group is often recognized by both its members and nonmembers. The reader is familiar with the "in-group, out-group" phenomenon where two superficially identical groups are valued very differently by their members. The group term for the value placed on a group by both its members and nonmembers is *attractiveness*. An in-group is seen as being attractive, an out-group unattractive. The degree of attractiveness a group has is determined to a large extent by its unique identity, and the mere altering of a few members, goals, or norms does not succeed in altering the group's identity or resultant attractiveness.

Finally, all groups, just like individuals, go through predictable developmental phases. However, the time at which the group moves from one phase to another is not as uniform as it is with individual development. Rather, the speed of group development is determined by a number of factors unique to the group, such as the anticipated duration of the group's life, the developmental strengths and weaknesses of its members, the importance the group places on its goal, the relevance of its norms to its goals, and the group's attractiveness. In addition, groups may skip developmental phases for a variety of reasons. All groups, however, must go through a beginning and ending phase. These and the intermediate phases of group development are described in conjunction with the discussion of group therapy in this chapter.

USE OF GROUPS IN THE CARE OF THE MENTALLY ILL

During World War II many members of the civilian population as well as large numbers of Armed Forces personnel required psychiatric help. It became obvious that the traditional treatment methods used at that time could not provide the help required by the large population of mentally ill individuals. To make maximum use of psychiatrically trained personnel, a plan was initiated through which individuals were encouraged to talk out their problems in groups. Thus the concept of *group therapy* was born. As psychiatrists worked with this method and developed an effective technique that could be taught to others, it became obvious that not only was group therapy a more efficient means by which relatively few personnel could treat a large number of persons, but more importantly that this mode of therapy had effects that could not be achieved through individual, one-to-one therapy. Some theorists believe the one reason for this positive effect is that groups tend to simulate the familial situation, wherein the leaders are seen in the role of parent figures and group members are seen as siblings. Therefore it becomes possible for persons who have had difficulty in their early family relationships to work through experientially many problems as a result of their interaction with other group members. Group members may also find support and reassurance in the realization that others have problems that are similar to theirs.

As more experience has been gained with group methods, it has been recognized that group therapy has unlimited therapeutic possibilities in the treatment plan for a wide variety of individuals. It is now the treatment of choice for many persons and is frequently used in conjunction with individual therapy.

NURSES AS GROUP THERAPISTS

As more is learned about the group approach to emotional problems, there appears to be a place for a variety of groups having a wide range of therapeutic goals and led by people with varied backgrounds and preparation. For a number of years psychiatric nurses have been actively involved in providing leadership for groups in many different treatment situations. Some have chosen to function as the only therapist in the group. In such situations the nurse has usually had the benefit of leadership preparation before undertaking this role. However, a few nurses without previous experience or preparation have accepted the leadership role and have learned as the group worked together. In such situations it is wise for the nurse to seek supervisory guidance from a group psychotherapist in the treatment situation. Many nurses have functioned as co-therapists with a member of another discipline or with another nurse. Acting as a co-therapist is probably an ideal learning situation and provides an opportunity for the co-therapists to reconstruct and evaluate the group discussion after each session has been concluded. The practice of reconstructing and evaluating each group session is highly desirable, even for experienced group psychotherapists. As with the members, the group situation is likely to elicit feelings in the leader that unconsciously stem from her experiences in previous groups such as her family. Through discussion of the dynamics of each group session with an objective, skilled supervisor, the nurse is likely to avoid the pitfalls resulting from nonobjectivity.

The remainder of this chapter is devoted to a discussion of those types of groups in which the nurse is most likely to have a leadership role. For information on other types of therapeutic groups the reader is referred to Chapter 23 of this text.

GROUP THERAPY

Considerations in establishing a therapy group

Group psychotherapists differ in their approach when establishing a therapeutic group. Questions involving the size of the membership, the frequency of meetings, and the characteristics of the participants must be decided. As might be expected, authorities answer these questions according to their personal treatment philosophies.

Some group psychotherapists insist on a balanced group, which means that only individuals of the same age, sex, and diagnostic category should be included. Others do not believe that a balanced group is necessary or even conducive to the best possible group interaction. Another consideration is whether to include persons with different levels of intelligence or verbal skills. Since group therapy depends on effective communication skills, this may be an important consideration.

Certainly a decision must be made as to how large the group will be. Most authorities agree that a group should not be larger than 10, but many group leaders prefer a group no larger than six. They also agree that the membership of a group should be stable.

A definite place in which to hold the group meeting must be identified. It should be quite, comfortable, and private. The frequency and time of meeting must be decided as well as the date when group meetings will begin and end. When these decisions have been made and the group has come together for the first time, these norms should be shared with the members so that they will understand the nature of the contract they have with each other and with the group leader.

Some group leaders prefer to talk with potential group members before the actual group meetings begin. In this way each individual is acquainted with the nature of the sessions prior to the first meeting.

Characteristics of group therapy

The therapeutic group, like other groups, has a specific goal. It differs from a social group because its goal is to assist individuals to alter their behavioral patterns and to develop new and more effective ways of dealing with the stresses of daily living. To achieve this goal, individuals meet together regularly for a stated period of time to express their ideas, feelings, and concerns; to examine their current ways of behaving; and to develop new patterns of behavior.

The group leader works to develop among the group members a sense of trust in her as an individual and as a group leader. She avoids being critical or judgmental of the behavior of individual members of the group and relies on group action to control unacceptable behavior. The group leader strives to convey to the group members her acceptance of them as individuals and her respect for them as people. She avoids exerting undue control over the group or being the authority in the situation.

For a group to have maximum therapeutic effect, it is essential that members learn to know and trust not only the leader but also each other. Therefore this becomes an important goal, the achievement of which is facilitated by the leader when she refers questions back to the group, encourages participation from all members, and shows acceptance and respect for each individual. By engaging in these behaviors, the nurse leader acts as a role model for the members. The inexperienced group leader will be surprised at how quickly the group members learn to act toward each other in the manner suggested by her behavior.

Group development

Every group, like every individual, progresses through several developmental phases. The first developmental phase of a group is the *preaffiliation* or *getting acquainted phase.* During this time, group members behave toward each other as strangers and are obviously distrustful of each other and of the leader. Their expectations of the group activity are, of necessity, determined by experiences they have had in other groups. Although members are likely to be overtly polite to each other, their behavior also indicates an approach-avoidance dilemma. That is, most members are eager to become involved with each other but simultaneously fear the risks that such involvement may entail. It is during this stage that the leader is most effective when she provides structure, protects members from embarrassment by not allowing them to prematurely reveal highly personal information, and gently invites trust.

The second developmental period is the *phase of experiencing intragroup conflict* and is characterized by power and control issues. Unavoidably, conflict will emerge during this time, since the members are in the process of establishing their positions in the group relative to the positions of other members and the leader. Often group members look to the leader for sanction or condemnation of another member. If the leader falls into this trap, she is likely to find the group critical of her because of her decision. In this instance it is always wise to deflect the question about a member's behavior back to the group by a comment such as, "I wonder what the rest of you think about Mr. Jones's question? "It is during this second phase of group development that the group attempts to formalize relationships through the establishment of explicit norms. These attempts should be supported as long as they do not infringe on the rights or safety of one or more members. Throughout the group process the leader has the responsibility to protect the safety of the individuals and property, but the necessity for doing so becomes greatest during this second phase of group development. It is during the second phase that the group sessions may seem nonproductive in that the members alternate competitive, aggressive behavior with apathetic withdrawal. Interrelated with this phenomenon is the great danger of membership dropout.

If the leader can help the group safely navigate through this phase, characteristics of the third phase will emerge. This is called the *working phase* or the *phase of intimacy and differentiation.* During this phase the work of the group is achieved. It is a period of relatively high communication in which members appropriately share personal feelings and concerns about emotional problems.

It is during the working phase of the group that the members' sense of belonging, or group cohesiveness, is at its highest. When a group is cohesive, its members tend to feel emotionally close to one another, and individuals respond well to advice offered by other members. Consequently, during this period there is an opportunity for emotional reeducation and relearning. The members discover through the reactions of the other group members that there are many different reactions to their feelings and behavior. They come to realize how universal their problems are and that they are not as unique in their difficulties as they may have believed.

The last developmental phase is precipitated by the approaching time for the group to conclude its meetings. Thus it is the *termination phase* and may require a number of meetings to work through the feelings of the individuals involved. The goal of the termination phase is to help the group members integrate that which they have learned about themselves and the behavioral changes they have made so that these can be used in the future. If the termination phase is not handled skillfully, not only will this goal not be achieved, but the group members may leave the group feeling that the only thing to be gained by group association is more emotional pain. During this period the members relive previous periods when they experienced personal loss of someone very close to them. They may express feelings of being abandoned, rejected, or forsaken. The expression of these feelings provides an excellent opportunity to help the individual members of the group deal with these feelings and work through them.

Four phases of group development have been described. It should be noted, however, that these phases overlap one another and that only the first and the last phases are seen in all groups. Groups that meet for only a few sessions or groups whose members have a great deal of difficulty in trusting others are not likely to be able to move through the phase of experiencing intragroup conflict and the working phase. Consequently, the termination phase will not be as meaningful and therefore not as difficult as when the group has traveled successfully through all developmental phases.

Role of the leader

The group leader is the key to a successful group therapy experience. The leader needs to be aware of her own behavior and its effect on others. The effectiveness of the getting acquainted phase for the group is largely dependent on the way in which the leader orients the members to the group process, to each other, and to herself. The phase of experiencing intragroup conflict can be successfully resolved if the group leader is able to be supportive to the members and successfully establishes a feeling of acceptance and respect for all. As the group moves into the working phase, it is the leader who is able to involve the less verbal members by redirecting questions to them or by asking them how a situation seems to them. The leader sometimes provides essential factual information that is important in the resolution of an issue that has arisen. On occasion the leader may be useful in helping a member learn exactly what others think about his behavior or his responses. The leader assists members in exploring situations they bring to the group from the outside and helps them to think through and test out more appropriate ways of responding.

As the group develops, the leader will be confronted with a variety of specific problems in group interaction that will necessitate her intervention. Problems such as silence, monopolizing behavior, tardiness, and acting out on the part of members are common and require the skill of the leader if the group session is to be effective. It is beyond the scope of this text to discuss these problems and possible appropriate interventions, but the student should be aware that there are a number of excellent references available that will provide specific direction. It should be noted, however, that the most effective group leader is one who is able to vary her style of intervention based on her assessment of the needs of the group.

Skillful termination of a group requires first and foremost that the leader recognize her own feelings of loss. By recognizing her own feelings she is less likely to act them out by doing such things as "forgetting" the final meeting, acting punitively to members who express a sense of loss, or promising members that she will continue to contact them when this is not possible or desirable. The skillful group leader will understand that the anger at her and other members that is commonly expressed during this phase is a reflection of the severity of the loss the members are experiencing. She will not respond to anger with anger, but will help the group members to acknowledge their sadness about the disbanding of the group.

Finally, the skillful group leader will help the group members to identify what they have gained through their association. By conceptualizing these gains, the members will be able to take away someting concrete that helps to offset the emotional loss.

Many group therapists believe that it is most beneficial to the group if leadership is shared by two therapists, that is, if there are two staff members who act as co-therapists. In this situation one therapist is able to concentrate on the content being expressed while the other therapist focuses primarily on the group process. Although the co-therapists may change their function from one group session to another, it is believed that those co-leaders who are experienced and comfortable with each other can view the group more comprehensively and therefore provide the group with helpful direction in regard to both content and process.

SOCIALIZATION GROUPS: A REMOTIVATION TECHNIQUE

Psychiatric hospitals are frequently heavily populated with mentally ill persons who appear to have lost interest in reality, to have lost a sense of personal value, and who seem to be unaware of the other persons with whom they come in daily contact. Group interaction is one the most successsul ways of stimulating these people to rekindle their interest in their surroundings.

The nurse may be the only professional worker who is available or interested in developing some form of group experience that will encourage these individuals to begin to communicate with each other and with the staff. The primary goal of these group activities is to facilitate socialization and is most easily achieved by means of focusing on a task. If several persons come together as a group and carry on an activity for a few sessions, the initial attempt has been successful.

The focus of the group activity depends almost entirely on the individuals who are to be included as members. Their age, educational backgrounds, and physical health will greatly influence the choice of activities that can be suggested.

Some individuals might be interested in a current events discussion group. Others who evidence no interest in reading the newspaper or listening to the television news reports would not be interested in such a group activity. Some might be interested in forming a poetry reading group, whereas others would abhor such an activity. Some might enjoy sewing or knitting while they visit toegether; others would frown on this suggestion.

In view of this wide variation in personal abilities and taste, the first rule to follow in initiating any recreational or motivational activity is to be well acquainted with the individuals who will form the group membership. The nurse will find that it is wise to encourage the members to participate in selecting the focus for the group meetings. The wise group leader will formulate some tentative plans for the first meeting, but these need to be flexible and easily changed in case there are suggestions from the members.

The nurse leader will find that at first many persons will be reluctant to participate. Some individuals may require more than one friendly invitation to attend. Some who have lost interest in reality carry on an active fantasy life. Any group activity must compete with these fantasies for the individual's attention and enjoyment. Thus it is wise to offer the group members refreshments during the initial group meetings. As the group becomes cohesive, the members' interest in the group activity may become great enough to overshadow the food as the major enjoyment of the meeting.

It is wise to vary the focus of the group activity from time to time to maintain the interest of the group members. As the members become acquainted with one another, they themselves will suggest changes in the focus or the format of the meeting.

The following are some concrete suggestions for planning an effective socialization group experience*:

1. Develop a flexible plan that provides for change and spontaneity.
2. Encourage all group members to participate in the planning.
3. Keep the plan practical and within achievable limits.
4. Initiate activities that are within the abilities of the group members to handle.
5. Provide something specific such as refreshments that will give each group member some tangible satisfaction.
6. Avoid monotony by varying the focus of the group activity.
7. Maintain a consistency in the feeling tone of each meeting so that the expectations of the group members will be fulfilled.

SELECTION OF A THERAPEUTIC GROUP

It is important to note that the type of group activity that is most appropriate for the mentally ill person depends on a number of

*Brown, Martha, and Fowler, Grace R.: Psychodynamic nursing—a biosocial orientation, ed. 4, Philadelphia, 1972, W.B. Saunders Co.

variables, including the degree of ego strength he possesses and his current insight into his problems. Therefore it is likely that a person whose contact with reality is tenuous would benefit most from a socialization group rather than from a more formal group psychotherapy sesson. As the client gains more ego strength, he may be introduced into a group whose primary goal is that of supportive therapy. As members progress in this type of group, the focus of the group may very well change to that of insight therapy. This is not to say that socialization groups do not have therapeutic effects, but rather that the degree of stress that the person is able to tolerate should be a major determining factor in the decision as to the type of group in which he will participate. Furthermore, this determination should be made jointly by the interdisciplinary health care team, which is able to view the client from a variety of perspectives.

GROWTH AND SELF-ACTUALIZATION GROUPS

Other types of groups such as sensitivity, encounter, and self-help groups are becoming increasingly common and well known in our society. The nature of these groups will not be discussed within this text, primarily because expert leaders or facilitators of these groups believe that their primary goal is not and should not be therapeutic in nature, but rather educative, in the sense of self-growth, self-actualization, and increased self-awareness. Therefore these types of groups are rarely, if ever, used with mentally ill persons, and the nurse is not likely to be involved with them in a professional capacity. Nevertheless, there is much available literature about these subjects that the student nurse may be interested in exploring.

CONCLUDING STATEMENTS

1. The nature of our humanness and the nature of the society in which we live dictate the necessity for a social structure organized around groups.
2. A group is an identifiable system composed of three or more individuals who engage in certain tasks to achieve a common goal. In addition, group members relate to each other, usually around the tasks and goals of the group.

3. The size of an effective group is one that is large enough to fulfill all the roles necessary for the achievement of the group's goals, while being small enough so that its members can comfortably relate to one another at the same time.
4. All groups have goals. In effective groups the members are aware of and support the group's goals.
5. Since a group is a system, group interactions need to be viewed from a holistic perspective, rather than as a summation of individual interactions.
6. *Role* is the term used to designate the behavior of group members. The role assumed by any group member is determined by his personality combined with the needs of the group.
7. At any point in time the group has a need to address the tasks necessary to achieve its goal, while simultaneously maintaining its life. Addressing the task is achieved through roles that have a content orientation, and group maintenance is achieved through roles that have a process orientation.
8. To function effectively, groups develop norms that govern their operation. Norms that have the most meaning are those that have emerged from within the group. Norms may be explicit or implicit.
9. Each group has a unique identity, while at the same time sharing much in common with all other groups. The group's uniqueness is based on the specific interactional combination of a number of factors, such as its size and its goals.
10. The group method of treating people in need of psychiatric help was originally developed to make maximum use of the available psychiatrically trained personnel.
11. As psychiatrists worked with the group method of treatment, it became obvious that group therapy had certain advantages over the traditional methods of individual therapy, and now it is recognized as having unlimited therapeutic possibilities.
12. There appears to be a place in the treatment plan for a variety of groups having a wide range of therapeutic goals and led by individuals with varied backgrounds and preparation.
13. For many years psychiatric nurses have been involved in providing group leadership for a variety of groups in many different treatment situations.

14. The therapeutic group has as its goal the alteration of the behavioral patterns of the group members through the development of new and more effective ways of coping with stressful situations.
15. Before the group meetings are initiated, decisions must be made about the size of the membership, the frequency of the meetings, the place and time of meetings, and the characteristics of the members.
16. Each group progresses through several developmental phases, including the getting acquainted phase, and phase of experiencing intragroup conflict, the working phase, and the termination phase.
17. Group interaction is one of the most successful ways of stimulating persons who have lost interest in their surroundings.
18. The type of group activity that is most appropriate for mentally ill persons should be determined after consideration of a number of variables. In addition, as each individual progresses in treatment, the type of group activity appropriate to meet his needs will change.

Suggested sources of additional information

CLASSICAL

Armstrong, Shirley W., and Rouslin, Sheila: Group psychotherapy in nursing practice, New York, 1963, Macmillan Publishing Co., Inc.

Baker, Joan M., and Estes, Nada J.: Anger in group therapy, Am. J. Nurs. **65:**96-100, July, 1965.

Bales, Robert: Interaction process analysis: a method for the study of small groups, Reading, Mass., 1950, Addison-Wesley Publishing Co., Inc.

Brown, Donald I.: Nurses participate in group therapy, Am. J. Nurs. **62:**68-69, Jan., 1962.

Bueker, Kathleen: Group therapy in a new setting, Am. J. Nurs. **57:**1581-1588, 1957.

Bueker, Kathleen, and Warrick, Annette: Can nurses be group therapists? Am. J. Nurs. **64:**114-116, May, 1964.

Fagin, Claire M.: Psychotherapeutic nursing, Am. J. Nurs. **67:**298-304, 1967.

Getty, Cathleen, and Shannon, Anna M.: Co-therapy as an egalitarian relationship, Am. J. Nurs. **69:**767-771, 1969.

Glover, B.H.: A new nurse therapist, Am. J. Nurs. **67:**1003-1005, 1967.

Hargreaves, Anne G.: The group culture and nursing practice, Am. J. Nurs. **67:**1840-1846, 1967.

Pullinger, Walter F.: Remotivation, Am. J. Nurs. **60:**682-685, 1960.

Sink, Susan Mary: Remotivation; toward reality for the aged, Nurs. Outlook **14:**26-28, Aug., 1966.

Von Mering, Otto, and King, Stanley H.: Remotivating the mental patient, New York, 1957, Russell Sage Foundation.

CONTEMPORARY

Benton, Denise W.: The significance of the absent member in milieu therapy, Perspect. Psychiatr. Care **18:**21-25, Jan.-Feb., 1980.

Donner, Gail J.: Parenthood as a crisis, Perspect. Psychiatr. Care **10:**84-87, April-June, 1972.

Fochtman, Grace A.: Therapeutic factors of the informal group, Am. J. Nurs. **75:**238, 1976.

Gauron, Eugene F., et al.: The orientation group in pre-therapy training, Perspect. Psychiatr. Care **15**(1):32-37, 1977.

Gerace, Laina, and Rosenberg Lisa: The use of art prints in group therapy with aftercare patients, Perspect. Psychiatr. Care **17:**83-86, March-April, 1979.

Hankins-McNary, Lulu: The use of humor in group therapy, Perspect. Psychiatr. Care **17:**228-231, Sept.-Oct., 1979.

Johnson-Soderberg, Sherry: The theory and practice of scapegoating, Perspect. Psychiatr. Care **15:**153-159, 1977.

Joyce, Carol: The religious as group therapists: attitudes and conflicts, Perspect. Psychiatr. Care **15**(3):112-117, 1977.

Kahn, Alice N.: Group education for the overweight, Am. J. Nurs. **78:**254, Feb., 1978.

Lancaster, Jeanette: Activity groups as therapy, Am. J. Nurs. **76:**947-949, 1976.

Loomis, Maxine E., and Dodenhoff, Judith T.: Working with informal patient groups, Am. J. Nurs. **70:**1939-1944, 1970.

Marram, Gwen D.: The group approach in nursing practice, ed. 2, St. Louis, 1978, The C.V. Mosby Co.

Mealy, Anne R.: Sculpting as a group technique for increasing awareness, Perspect. Psychiatr. Care **15**(3):118-121, 1977.

Rogers, Carl: On encounter groups, New York, 1970, Harper & Row, Publishers.

Rogers, Carl: Facilitating encounter groups, Am. J. Nurs. **71:**275-279, 1971.

Rogers, Joanna, and Grubb, Pearl: The V.A. psychiatric patient: re-socialization and community living, Perspect. Psychiatr. Care **17:**72-76, March-April, 1979.

Rouslin, Sheila: Relatedness in group psychotherapy, Perspect. Psychiatr. Care **11**(4):165-171, 1973.

Sager, Clifford J., and Kaplan, Helen S., editors: Progress in group and family therapy, New York, 1972, Brunner/Mazel, Inc.

Sanderson, Marilynn R., and Blackley, Judith J.: Problems displayed "in vitro"—a particular advantage of group therapy, Perspect. Psychiatr. Care **17:**176-186, July-Aug., 1979.

Shaw, Dale, et al.: Multiple impact therapy, Am. J. Nurs. **77:**246-248, 1977.

Ward, Judy Trowbridge: The sounds of silence: group psychotherapy with nonverbal patients, Perspect. Psychiatr. Care **12:**13-19, Jan.-March, 1974.

Yalom, Irvin D., and Terrazas, Florence: Group therapy for psychotic elderly patients, Am. J. Nurs. **68:**1690-1694, 1968.

Yalom, Irvin D.: The theory and practice of group psychotherapy, New York, 1975, Basic-Books, Inc., Publishers.

OF PARTICULAR INTEREST

Marram, Gwen D.: The group approach in nursing practice, ed. 2, St. Louis, 1978, The C.V. Mosby Co.

This text introduces the reader to group work through a review of various group concepts and applications. It is especially relevant for the student of psychiatric nursing.

Whitaker, D., and Lieberman, M.: Psychotherapy through the group process, Chicago, 1964, Aldine Publishing Co.

This book is one of the classics in group therapy literature. It is easily read, and the clinical examples assist the reader in application of the concepts.

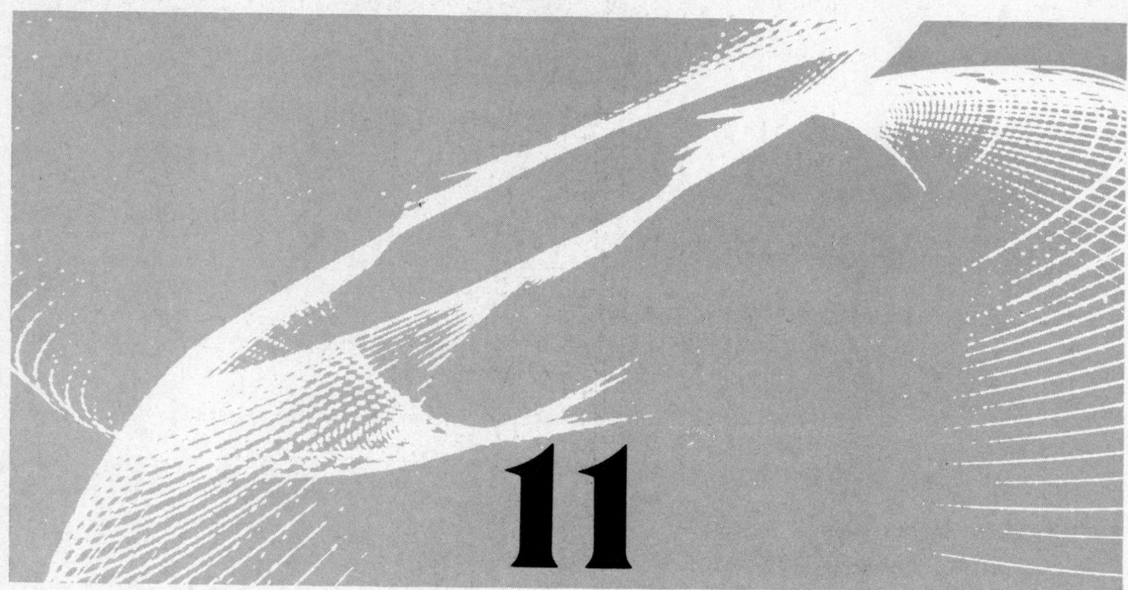

Intervention with families

- Family structure
- Definition of a family
- Functions of a family
- Developmental stages of the family
- The changing family
- The effective family
- The ineffective family
- The child-abusing family
- Family therapy
- Conjoint therapy

It is commonly asserted that the family is the most basic of all societal institutions. This assertion stems from two factors. The first of these factors is the universal tendency of human beings to organize themselves around the structure of the family. Second, it is believed that the experiences a child has as a family member have the most powerful influence on the kind of adult he will become. Therefore the society as a whole is very much affected by the family, both directly and indirectly, in both the present and future. Other societal institutions, such as the school and the church, are certainly fundamental to the society but are believed to be organizational structures that fulfill functions that historically have been delegated by the family. These societal institutions have developed in the belief that the collective society can fulfill certain functions more efficiently than can the singular family. However, the question of whether the society can fulfill these functions more effectively than the family is the subject of continuous debate, and dynamic fluctuations of functions between the family and other societal institutions can be observed over the course of generations.

The psychiatric nurse is often in a situation where she is dealing not just with an individual but also with a family. This contact may be direct and formalized, such as when engaged in family therapy, or direct but informal, such as when seeking information from or supplying information to family members. Some family theorists believe that even when the nurse is dealing only with an individual it is impossible for the interaction not to affect and be affected by that individual's family. Therefore interactions with an individual are seen as indirect interactions with that individual's family. This view stems from the belief that the family is a system, and consequently, the behavior of an individual is greatly influenced by his family, and in turn, any alterations in his behavior invariably affect his family. Whether one agrees with this view or not, it is hard to deny the fact that the effective psychiatric nurse needs to have an understanding of the family.

FAMILY STRUCTURE

In nonindustrial societies the family pattern most commonly observed is the *extended family,* where multiple generations live together and leave only for the purpose of joining another extended family through marriage. Prior to the industrial revolution, families in the United States often consisted of children, parents, and grandparents and perhaps one or more unmarried aunts or uncles. This pattern of family life provided the work force necessary for the productive management of the family business, usually the farm. When daughters married, they often left their family to join the family of their husband, while the sons' wives were incorporated into their family. This traditional family structure was also the mechanism whereby family resources, primarily land, were passed from generation to generation. The advantages of the extended family structure were multiple—physical and emotional resources were shared among a large group, and a broad division of labor was possible.

However, there were also many disadvantages. Families whose offspring were all female had to face the possibility of all the children leaving, thereby leaving the elderly parents in a very vulnerable economic and social position. Furthermore, although the prescribed roles of each family member provided stability and continuity, this prescription also thwarted individuality. The eldest boy was expected to continue the family business, leaving the younger brother, who might have been more interested and capable of so doing, the choice of either striking out on his own or working at the behest of his older sibling. The image we now have of the "good old days" as characterized by close-knit, warm, loving families is believed by most authorities to be a distortion of the reality of intense sibling rivalry and parental frustration.

The settlement of the Western frontier, which placed great value on rugged individualism, and the industrial revolution both contributed greatly to a dramatic change in the typical family structure. Individuals moved from settled rural areas to the unsettled West or to industrialized urban areas with the goal of making their own fortune. A pervasive belief in both instances was that more money could be earned with less labor. Initially that belief proved to be false as evidenced by the hardships of Western settlement and the horrors of the urban sweatshop. The mobility of American citizens along with waves of European immigrants combined to create cities where people lived in dense concentration. Population density and mobility mitigated against the perpetuation of the extended family, and the *nuclear family* structure became the norm.

The nuclear family is defined as a two-generational family where it is understood that the children will leave once they have achieved maturity. Therefore the nuclear family, as a family, is only a temporary arrangement. Although the nuclear family has the disadvantages of potential alienation from the family of origin and fewer emotional supports from within the family, it has the major advantage of facilitating upward social mobility because it tends not to predetermine the children's roles as inheritors of the family business.

DEFINITION OF A FAMILY

A family is traditionally defined as two or more people who are related by blood or by legal ties, such as marriage or adoption. However, a family also has the characteristic of identifying itself and being identified by others as such. Sharing a common surname is a manifestation of this characteristic, although it is not requisite to being a family, as evidenced by the increasing number of young women in our society who retain the surname of their family of origin after marriage. Another characteristic of a family is that it is a relatively permanent human affiliation. A family, therefore, has a history and a future.

In the complex, highly mobile, technological society in which we live, there are an increasing number of human groups that identify themselves as a family and that exist over a period of time, but whose members do not meet the traditional criteria of being related by blood or by legal ties. Therefore a more accurate and relevant definition of family may be one that reflects the functions of a family.

FUNCTIONS OF A FAMILY

A family is a specialized group that bands together in pursuit of the common goal of growth and development of its members. This goal is achieved through certain functions. While none of these functions are unique to the family, the combination of them is unique to this institution. The following is a list of functions considered by most authorities to belong to the family.

Regulation of sexual activity and reproduction. The family structure provides for socially sanctioned sexual activity between spouses, while at the same time enforcing the societal taboo against incest by defining parental and sibling relationships. Survival of the culture is ensured by systematizing reproduction within a context that is capable of providing for children who in turn become the vehicle for the transmission of cultural values and practices. Therefore a family conveys to its children its cultural heritage as a means of ensuring the culture's future.

Physical maintenance. The family structure provides a vehicle through which the physical needs of its members can be met. It provides an efficient means of organizing responsibility for meeting the needs of the individual for food, clothing, shelter, and health care. In this regard the family can be seen as an economic unit.

Protection. The family structure is designed to provide both literal and figurative protection of its members by providing a model for interacting with the society in a way that protects the family members from undesirable outside influences.

Education and socialization. Some authorities believe that the family's function of providing education and socialization is the most fundamental one in that it is through the family that children learn how to function in and relate to the world in which they live.

Recreation. Traditionally the family has been the structure in which the individual has engaged in leisure time activities that have served as a source of personal and group refreshment and renewal, leading to increased family cohesion. Unlike the last function of education and socialization, the function of recreation is seen as rapidly waning, with the advent of television and other passive or nonparticipant forms of recreation.

Status conferring. Another traditional function of the family that seems to be undergoing fundamental alteration is that of status conferring. Prior to the advent of industrialization in a democratic society with the emphasis placed on individualism, the individual was conferred social status by virtue of the family into which he was born. Although this is no longer strictly the case today, social status is still somewhat determined by the socioeconomic level of one's family of origin.

Affection giving. Only within the family can an individual be guaranteed unconditional acceptance by the mere fact of his relationship to that family. In all other societal interactions, the value placed on an individual is determined by such things as the quality or speed of his performance, his appearance, his social class, or his occupation. In functional families, acceptance is conveyed by a deep, enduring affection among the members.

• • •

A perusal of these family functions reveals that the family unit provides services that are essential to the survival and stability of the society, for example, by regulating sexual activity within the family society is protected from the consequences of wanton mating. Simultaneously, the family unit provides essential services to its members, such as physical maintenance and affection giving.

All functions of a family are not equally prominent at any given time. Each function is more specific to certain stages of family development than others and as such become developmental tasks of the family.

Family sociologist Evelyn Duvall* has outlined a series of developmental stages of the family. This concept is not without problems, but nevertheless provides a useful frame of reference from which many traditional families can be viewed.

DEVELOPMENTAL STAGES OF THE FAMILY

The first stage of family development is divided into two phases and is represented by the newly married couple who is childless. The initial phase begins at the time of marriage and consists of two persons (a dyad) who have made a major commitment to each other and therefore have the task of adjusting to living together as a married pair. This period of family life is fraught with great stress as the two persons negotiate to effect a union while at the same time attempting to maintain their individuality. In

*Duvall, Evelyn M.: Family development, Philadelphia, 1962, J. B. Lippincott Co.

other words, these two individuals are learning to assume the roles of husband and wife. The divorce rate during this stage is very high, probably due to the shattering of the romantic illusion fostered during the preceding courtship period. The second phase of this stage commences with the wife's pregnancy. The family goal during this phase is to adjust to the pregnancy, which often means a change in affective focus. Prior to pregnancy both the husband and wife are focused on each other, but during pregnancy the wife becomes increasingly self-absorbed as she emotionally prepares for the birth of the child. In addition, the husband may feel an increase in responsibility, especially if the couple decides that the wife should leave an income-producing job.

The second stage of family development begins when the first child is born and generally is believed to last until this eldest child enters school. The major change experienced by the husband and wife is the expansion of their roles to include those of father and mother. The family unit is reorganized around the needs of infants and preschool children, which often require dramatic shifts in priorities and activities.

The third stage of family development begins when the eldest child enters school and ends when this child becomes an adolescent. By definition, if there are younger siblings, the family unit needs to reorganize to fit into the expanding world of school-aged children, while still meeting the needs of the preschoolers. Through the school-aged child the family is often confronted for the first time with societal values that may be in conflict with the family values. The goal of this stage is for the family to protect the school-aged children from undesirable influences while still enabling them to fit into the larger social world.

The fourth stage of a family's development commences when the oldest child becomes an adolescent. The family goal during this very tumultuous time is to loosen family ties to permit greater freedom and heavier responsibility of the members. This task is not easy to achieve, since the children have a history of dependence on their parents and often overact to their newfound independence, resulting in an increase, rather than the desired decrease, in the control behaviors of the parents.

The fifth stage is referred to as the "launching" stage because it is during this time that the children are preparing to or are actually leaving home. This developmental task requires the reorganization of the family into an equalitarian unit, as opposed to the earlier superior and subordinate structure. At this time the family needs to be able to release its members. It superficially appears that parents would have the most difficulty with this task, but it often is equally difficult for children to assume adult responsibility and leave the family to start their own family.

The next stage is termed the *postparental family* and is characterized by the parents having to subsume their parental roles into their marital roles. In other words, the father and mother are left with no children to parent and find themselves with only each other to relate to. This stage is commonly referred to as the "empty nest syndrome" and is successfully navigated only if the parents are able to satisfactorily maintain their marital relationship during the childbearing and childrearing years. During this stage parents often become grandparents, an event that requires once again learning a new role. Although the grandparent role bears similarities with the parent role, it is fundamentally different because the ultimate responsibility for children rests with the parents, not the grandparents.

The last stage of family development is the period of retirement and postretirement years. During this time the couple prepares for the dissolution of the family by the death of one of the spouses. Couples who have satisfactorily achieved the earlier tasks and are able to view their families as satisfactory are able to thoughtfully prepare for this eventuality without undue anxiety.

THE CHANGING FAMILY

The structure, size, functions, and developmental stages of the family are undergoing many changes in today's society. For example, it is not uncommon for a family to consist of only one parent who is raising one or more children and fulfilling both roles of mother and father. Increasingly common are *blended* or *reconstituted families* that consist of a parent who had been previously married and has children. This parent is married to another parent who also has children from a previous marriage.

Such a couple may have children of their own, so that the family's task in this instance is to "blend" together three different sets of children into a functional family structure.

Finally, we are seeing an increase in the number of people who are joining together to form a family group based on mutual respect and common interests rather than for the purpose of procreation. These persons may or may not be related by blood or by law, but tend to reside in the same household. The household concept, or living under the same roof, has been the criterion used by the U.S. Census Bureau to define a family. With the multiplicity of family structures apparent in the society, this criterion may prove to be the most applicable. In any event, it is important for the nurse to extend her view of family beyond the traditional nuclear or extended family structure when dealing with individuals who do not live in these structures, if she is to accurately assess the individual's familial associations and dynamics. An example is the instance in which an adult woman was admitted to the hospital for surgery and was asked to supply the name of her next of kin. She responded by stating that her only blood relative lived at a great distance and was not involved in her day-to-day affairs, and that she preferred to have her housemate of 5 years listed as the person to be notified in an emergency. The admitting clerk replied that the person listed on the chart had to be related by blood or law. This situation reflects the legal and societal lag so often apparent in our society that put this woman in jeopardy by forcing her to either lie to get her needs met or to tell the truth but forego gratification of her needs—all at a time when she was already under the stress of ill health and impending surgery.

THE EFFECTIVE FAMILY*

The effective family is one that is able to facilitate the growth and development of its members while still maintaining cohesion as an identifiable system. This definition implies that the following patterns of behavior are characteristic of an effective family:

1. The family places the emotional, physical, and social needs

*Adapted from Sedwick, Rae: Family mental health, St. Louis, 1981, The C.V. Mosby Co., pp. 20-24.

of its members over other concerns, such as acquisition of possessions or status.
2. The family recognizes, values, and accommodates to differences among its members.
3. The family is sufficiently flexible so that changes stemming from within and outside the system can be accommodated without loss of family stability.
4. The family seeks and uses information from relevant outside sources, simultaneously maintaining its autonomy.
5. The family makes and carries out decisions, taking into account its goals and the age and experience of its members.

An effective family is not necessarily a family without problems. Rather, an effective family is one that has developed a structure and pattern of functioning that enables it to productively deal with its problems as they arise. Just as it is true of individuals, families must learn these processes, and many authorities believe that helping young families to develop effective patterns of functioning is the crux of mental health promotion.

Most young people receive no preparation for establishing an effective family. Therefore they unconsciously perpetuate the only patterns of familial functioning they know—the patterns they experienced in their families of origin. If fortuitously such learned patterns of behavior are conducive to effective family functioning, effective families will perpetuate. If, on the other hand, ineffective patterns are learned, the probability of perpetuating ineffective family patterns is greatly enhanced.

THE INEFFECTIVE FAMILY

Families that are unable to establish and maintain a structure and patterns of behavior conducive to effective functioning often show signs of continuous and irresolvable stress. Such stress may be manifested by the entire system as in instances where there is overt tension and hostility among members, or the stress may be focused on only one member who is covertly designated to assume and act out the family problems. In this instance the family member is often, although not always, a child. This phenomenon occurs because children are likely to be the most vulnerable, since they are so highly dependent on the family and their behavioral patterns are less firmly entrenched. Bed-wetting, learning difficulties, antisocial behaviors, and profound fears in a child are all seen to be symptoms of an ineffective family.

It is beyond the scope of this text to discuss the many types of family dysfunction. However, the following discussion of child abuse is presented as an example of one increasingly common and very serious form of ineffective family functioning.

THE CHILD-ABUSING FAMILY

The incidence of reported child abuse appears to be dramatically increasing. In one metropolitan area of New York State the incidence has increased almost 50% between 1978 and 1980. However, accurate statistics are difficult to obtain because the phenomenon is poorly defined. Child abusers often go to extraordinary lengths to conceal their actions, and friends, relatives, and health care workers are hesitant to "get involved." Nevertheless, it is known that the neglect or abuse of children occurs often enough to be of major concern to the legal and health care professions.

The form that child abuse can take ranges from violent, physical attacks that result in severe injury, to passive neglect that results in insidious malnutrition. Child abuse is not limited to physical maltreatment; it also includes emotional maltreatment such as continual yelling at and berating the child.

Children are the usual victims of family violence because they are relatively powerless and, until they reach adolescence, are certainly physically weaker than adults. The pattern of the powerless becoming victims of violence is seen not only in child abuse but also in wife battering and the tyrannization of the elderly in their homes and on the street.

The concept of powerlessness includes not only physical weakness but also social subordination. Children, women, and the elderly are all persons who traditionally have had less power in our society than has the young adult male. This situation is gradually changing. The values, needs, and rights of children, women, and the elderly are being recognized and becoming protected by law. These persons, therefore, are achieving a modicum of social power. Ironically some authorities believe that the very amelio-

Table 4 *Physical and behavioral indicators of child abuse and neglect**

Type of abuse/neglect	Physical indicators	Behavioral indicators
Physical abuse	Unexplained bruises and welts: —on face, lips, mouth —on torso, back, buttocks, thighs —in various stages of healing —clustered, forming regular patterns —reflecting shape of article used to inflict (electric cord, belt buckle) —on several different surface areas —regularly appear after absence, weekend, or vacation Unexplained burns: —cigar, cigarette burns, especially on soles, palms, back, or buttocks —immersion burns (socklike, glovelike, doughnut shaped on buttocks or genitalia) —patterned like electric burner, iron, etc. —rope burns on arms, legs, neck, or torso —infected burns, indicating delay in seeking treatment Unexplained fractures/dislocations: —to skull, nose, facial structure —in various stages of healing —multiple or spiral fractures Unexplained lacerations or abrasions: —to mouth, lips, gums, eyes —to external genitalia —in various stages of healing Bald patches on the scalp	Feels deserving of punishment Wary of adult contacts Apprehensive when other children cry Behavioral extremes: —aggressiveness —withdrawal Frightened of parents Afraid to go home Reports injury by parents Vacant or frozen stare Lies very still while surveying surroundings Will not cry when approached by examiner Responds to questions in monosyllables Inappropriate or precocious maturity Manipulative behavior to get attention Capable of only superficial relationships Indiscriminately seeks affection Poor self-concept
Physical neglect	Underweight, poor growth pattern, failure to thrive Consistent hunger, poor hygiene, inappropriate dress	Begging, stealing food Extended stays at school (early arrival and late departure) Rare attendance at school

*Heindl, Cathy, et al.: The nurse's role in the prevention and treatment of child abuse and neglect DHEW Publication No. (OHDS) 79-30202, Washington, D.C., 1979, U.S. Government Printing Office, p. 10.

Continued.

Table 4 *Physical and behavioral indicators of child abuse and neglect—cont'd*

Type of abuse/neglect	Physical indicators	Behavioral indicators
	Consistent lack of supervision, especially in dangerous activities or for long periods Wasting of subcutaneous tissue Unattended physical problems or medical needs Abandonment Abdominal distention Bald patches on the scalp	Constant fatigue, listlessness, or falling asleep in class Inappropriate seeking of affection Assuming adult responsibilities and concerns Alcohol or drug abuse Delinquency (e.g., thefts) States there is no caretaker
Sexual abuse	Difficulty in walking or sitting Torn, stained, or bloody underclothing Pain, swelling, or itching in genital area Pain on urination Bruises, bleeding, or lacerations in external genitalia, vaginal, or anal areas Vaginal/penile discharge Venereal disease, especially in preteens Poor sphincter tone Pregnancy	Unwilling to change for gym or participate in physical education class Withdrawal, fantasy, or infantile behavior Bizarre, sophisticated, or unusual sexual behavior or knowledge Poor peer relationships Delinquent or runaway Reports sexual assault by caretaker Change in performance in school
Emotional maltreatment	Speech disorders Lags in physical development Failure-to-thrive Hyperactive/disruptive behavior	Habit disorders (sucking, biting, rocking, etc.) Conduct/learning disorders (antisocial, destructive, etc.) Neurotic traits (sleep disorders, inhibition of play, unusual fearfulness) Psychoneurotic reactions (hysteria, obsession, compulsion, phobias, hypochondria) Behavior extremes: —compliant, passive —aggressive, demanding Overly adaptive behavior: —inappropriately adult —inappropriately infantile Developmental lags (mental, emotional) Attempted suicide

ration of this problem is contributing to its fulmination, a phenomenon that is not socially unusual. In other words, individuals who have no power and do not assert themselves are often not overtly abused. An example is the benevolent plantation owner who had a patronizingly paternal attitude toward his compliant slaves. Once the slaves began to assert themselves, however, much more systematic and spontaneous abuse occurred. Likewise, as children, women, and the elderly achieve more power they are more likely to constitute a threat and therefore be abused more often.

Table 4 lists physical and behavioral indicators of child abuse and neglect. It should be noted that the laws of most states require that health care personnel report to legal authorities situations in which child abuse or maltreatment is suspected; most state laws do not require proof before reporting child abuse or maltreatment. After a report is made the child protective agency is responsible for the actual determination of the situation.

Many health care workers, including nurses, are very hesitant to report incidents of suspected child abuse. Commonly expressed reservations include a fear of becoming involved in legal processes and a desire to protect the familial integrity. By not reporting suspected instances of child abuse, the health care worker is not only *not* protecting the family, but is indirectly contributing to the perpetuation of physical and emotionally dangerous family patterns.

Dynamics underlying child abuse

An understanding of the dynamics underlying child abuse includes societal, familial, and individual factors.

Societal factors. Dr. Harold Feldman, an expert on domestic violence at Cornell University, believes that family violence is a reflection of a society that endorses violence as a means of dealing with frustration and achieving goals. There has been a great deal of publicity regarding the amount of violence on television and in the movies. It is interesting to note that in our society a movie is more likely to be rated "X" if it portrays explicit sexual acts than if it depicts graphic details of a murder. More subtle forms of violence are socially sanctioned by the national preoccupation with such sports as football and boxing. In this way children learn that violent acts are socially acceptable outlets for anger and frustration.

Familial factors. It is a well-known fact that child abusers are people who have themselves been abused as children. Therefore there is a multigenerational pattern of child abuse. In addition, many authorities believe that the nuclear family structure contributes to the incidence of child abuse. In this family structure a small group of persons, the nuclear family, is often isolated from other sources of concerned support. Therefore an intensity of demands develops within the nuclear family, and there are few outlets to meet these needs. This leads to increased tension that may explode in the form of violence or neglect directed at the most powerless member of the family—the child.

Individual factors. Whether or not ineffective family functioning will manifest itself by child abuse is largely determined by the dynamics of the family members and how these interact with each other. The material on p. 217 lists behavioral indicators of abusive parents. These indicators, however, fail to reflect the very real human pain that many child-abusing parents experience. As previously stated, these individuals are most likely to have been abused children themselves. Therefore they have many unmet needs, are emotionally immature, and have limited control of their impulses. Many abusing parents, especially mothers, unconsciously look to their child as a vehicle through which their own needs can be met. When it becomes obvious that an infant or young child takes more than it can give, these parents may react with almost uncontrollable rage at once again being disappointed and deprived. In other words, these parents have many fundamental, unmet needs themselves that they look to their children to meet. When this need fulfillment is not forthcoming, they tend to react with violence, reflecting a primitive expression of frustration.

Why is it that one child in a family is consistently abused, while others develop unscathed? This question has no definitive answer, but some hypotheses can be stated. The abused child often has characteristics that set him apart from others in the family. These include birth order (youngest or oldest), physical char-

Behavioral indicators of abusive parents*

Parents of abused children may exhibit the following traits:

They are isolated from family supports such as friends, relatives, neighbors, and community groups; they consistently fail to keep appointments, discourage social contact, and never participate in school activities or events.

They seem to trust no one.

They themselves were abused or neglected as children.

They are reluctant to give information about the child's injuries or condition. When questioned, they are unable to explain or they offer farfetched or contradictory explanations.

They respond inappropriately to the seriousness of the child's condition either by overreacting, seeming hostile or antagonistic when questioned even casually, or by underreacting, showing little concern or awareness and seeming more preoccupied with their own problems than those of the child.

They refuse to consent to diagnostic studies.

They fail or delay to take the child for medical care, for routine checkups, for optometric or dental care, or for treatment of injury or illness. In taking an injured child for medical care, they may choose a different hospital or doctor each time.

They are overcritical of the child and seldom if ever discuss the child in positive terms.

They have unrealistic expectations of the child, expecting or demanding behavior that is beyond the child's years or ability.

They believe in the necessity of harsh punishment for children.

They seldom touch or look at the child; they ignore the child's crying or react with impatience.

They keep the child confined, perhaps in a crib or playpen, for overlong periods of time.

They seem to lack understanding of children's physical, emotional, and psychological needs.

They appear to be misusing alcohol or drugs.

They cannot be located.

They appear to lack control, or fear losing control.

They are of borderline intelligence, psychotic, or psychopathic. While such diagnoses are the responsibility of the psychiatrist, psychologist, or psychiatric social worker, even the lay observer can note whether the parent seems intellectually capable of childrearing, exhibits generally irrational behavior, or seems excessively cruel and sadistic.

---

*Child abuse and neglect: vol 1, an overview of the problem; vol. 2, the problem and its management, DHEW Publication, Washington, D.C., 1975, U.S. Government Printing Office.

acteristics (resembles paternal or maternal side of the family), particular skills or deficits, and identifiable personality characteristics (more or less intelligent, more or less assertive, likes solitary activities or activities involving others). In any event, the abused child seems to have particular significance not only to the parents but also to his siblings. The question arises as to why the abused child characteristically colludes with his family in concealing the events surrounding his injuries. Many social scientists believe the answer to this question lies in the fact that children so desperately need attention from significant adults that they are willing to submit to abuse if this appears to be the only way they can gain this attention. Family therapists postulate that the child knowingly assumes a role that is necessary for the survival of the family system. Regardless of why it occurs, it is well known that abused children block attempts to divulge the reality of the situation.

Role of the nurse

Because of the multifaceted dynamics operating in the ineffective family that abuses its children, treatment is very complex. Needless to say, the physical needs of the injured or neglected child must be met before attempts are made to alter the family's pattern of functioning. During the time the child is receiving treatment, the parents need a great deal of support and understanding. Health care personnel, including nurses, often have great difficulty avoiding the tendency to blame one or both parents. This attitude, which may be conveyed overtly or covertly, is counterproductive, since it reinforces the guilt and sense of worthlessness the parents already feel. It also reflects a lack of understanding that family units function as a system where each member contributes to the function or dysfunction of the unit.

The treatment of choice for the abusive family, as for all ineffective families, is family therapy. As psychiatric nurses become more educationally prepared, they increasingly become responsible for using this treatment modality.

FAMILY THERAPY

Family therapy as such is a relatively new treatment modality, although it has been unknowingly practiced in the past by the family physician and the public health nurse. These professional workers realized that the effectiveness of treatment of an individual was either enhanced or interfered with by the attitudes of his family. In addition, these professionals often became quasi-family members and were consulted and included during family crises. With the explosion of medical knowledge and the increase in medical specialization, the intimate knowledge of the family history and dynamics became unknown to the physician. Simultaneously, public health nurses assumed a greater number of technical functions that consumed a larger part of their role, giving them less time to act as family confidants. Until recently, it has seemed most expeditious of time and resources for the individual to be treated by professionals who were specialists. This approach has not only relegated the family to a position of second-class citizens but has deprived the individual of a valuable resource. Nowhere is this more dramatically illustrated than in the instance of emotional disorders.

Three of the earliest proponents of family therapy were Nathan W. Ackerman at Columbia University, Gerald Caplan at Harvard University, and Don Jackson at the University of California. Early in the 1950s these men wrote about the advantages of this method. The concept of family therapy is based on the belief that the family is a social system that has its own characteristic structure and pattern of communication. Although this structure and communication pattern are certainly related to the personalities of the family members, they cannot be explained by a mere summation of the traits of the individuals who comprise the family. In other words, the family as a unit is seen as a system, and the family members as components of that system who influence it and are in turn influenced by it. If one accepts this concept, it becomes inappropriate to refer to one member as being emotionally ill without looking at the family constellation, which, it is believed, has sanctioned the deviant behavior of one member and in turn is affected by it. In other words, the behavior of the "sick" member serves a function within the family. This belief is supported by two observations. First, it is not unusual for a person to be successfully treated for an emotional illness on an individual basis and for another member of the family to become ill, sometimes with very similar symptoms. This phenomenon suggests that the family structure and communication pattern, if they are to be maintained, require one member to be deviant. A second observation that supports the systems theory approach is the frequency with which family members bring one member for treatment with the statement that all is well within the family except for the stress-producing behavior of the one member. When that member is removed from the family, either through prolonged hospitalization or by geographical relocation, it is not uncommon for the family to enter into a state of acute disequilibrium that may manifest itself by such actions as divorce of the parents. This phenomenon is equally well documented in families in which a chronically physically ill person has died.

Lately there is a growing number of mental health professionals who believe that any attempt to treat individuals in isolation from their families is either futile or, if helpful to the individual, is at the expense of the equilibrium of his family system. Proponents of family therapy maintain that major strides in the promotion of mental health and the prevention and treatment of mental illness will occur only when the needs of the individual are considered within the context of the family system, which still remains as the fundamental social unit of our society. Although this may be seen as an extreme view, there is no doubt that family therapy is the treatment of choice when the identified client is a child or adolescent, and this treatment modality should be used in other situations when possible.

The goals of family therapy are to assist in resolving pathological conflicts and anxiety, to strengthen the individual member against destructive forces both within himself and within the family environment, to strengthen the family against critical upsets, and to influence the orientation of the family identity and values toward health. When therapy commences, the therapist assembles all family members, regardless of age, and pays as much attention to their behavior with each other as to the content of what they say. For example, the husband and wife may vehemently state how close they are to each other while at the same time sit as far as possible from each other. It is important for the therapist to avoid blaming one or the other member, and this pitfall will be avoided if the role of each member is seen in relation to the total family functioning. In one family therapy situation the identified client was a 20-year-old daughter who had made numerous suicidal attempts. This girl was hospitalized, and the entire family came to the hospital once a week for family therapy. The parents maintained that they had an unusually good relationship and could not understand why their daughter tormented them so with her life-threatening gestures. Several times during the course of therapy, their adolescent son took the risk of contradicting his parents by pointing out his observation that the parents' relationship was highly tension-laden, at which points the daughter would begin crying. This behavior on her part diverted the participants' attention to her, and successfully prevented the parents from having to face, much less talk about, their differences. The therapist interpreted this behavior not as being sick, but rather as the daughter's role in maintaining the family equilibrium.

It is the prerogative of the family to determine their own destiny, and often the major role of the therapist is to comment on the interactional process as it is observed. Bringing this process to a level of consciousness allows the family to evaluate its purpose and outcome. If the family desires a change, the therapist can be instrumental in modeling behaviors that can initiate such change.

Some family therapy sessions have been held in the home. As this trend develops, it appears likely that the role of family therapist will become increasingly identified with the prepared psychiatric nurse, since she is comfortable in the role of family visitor, is knowledgeable about family dynamics, and is becoming skillful in family therapy.

CONJOINT THERAPY

Conjoint therapy usually refers to therapy in which marriage partners engage in a therapeutic endeavor with a therapist (Fig. 11-1). The importance of this technique is supported not only by the well-being that can be attained by the marriage partners but also because these persons are seen by family theorists as the architects of the future family system. That is, treatment of the marital couple can have a profound effect on the promotion of mental health and prevention of mental illness of the growing family. Often it is found that couples who have marital conflict have incongruent expectations of each other, the most common being the expectation that each will have their dependency needs met by the other. When these expectations are simultaneously operationalized, both are disappointed. Frequently the mutual realization of these expectations moves the couple ahead to understand that both can have their needs met if they are willing to

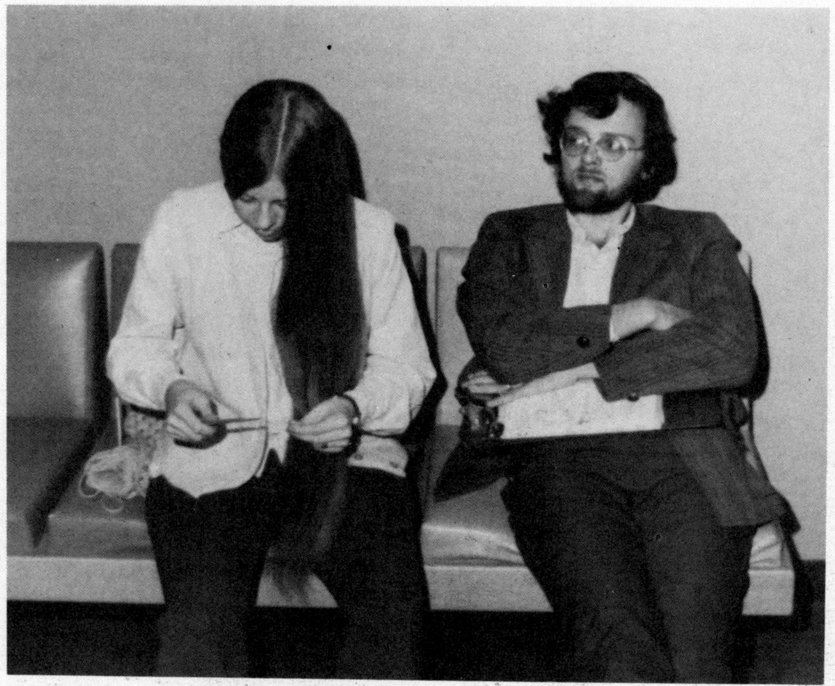

Fig. 11-1 *A couple awaits a conjoint therapy session.*

compromise. Several experts have written excellent texts about conjoint therapy, which the student is encouraged to read for additional information. Particularly recommended is *Conjoint Family Therapy* by Virginia Satir.

CONCLUDING STATEMENTS

1. The family is the most basic of all societal institutions, affecting and affected by the society.
2. Some family theorists believe that even when the nurse is dealing only with an individual, it is impossible for the interaction not to affect and be affected by that individual's family. This view stems from the belief that the family is a system.
3. The extended family is a type of family structure seen in non-

industrial societies and consisting of multiple generations living together.

4. The nuclear family is a type of family structure seen in industrialized societies and consisting of two generations.
5. A family is traditionally defined as two or more people who are related by blood or legal ties, although an increasing number of nonrelated groups are identifying themselves as a family.
6. The functions of the family include
   a. Regulation of sexual activity and reproduction
   b. Physical maintenance
   c. Protection
   d. Education and socialization
   e. Recreation
   f. Status conferring
   g. Affection giving
7. Traditional families progress through a series of developmental stages that are primarily related to role changes of its members.
8. The structure, size, functions, and developmental stages of the family are undergoing many changes in today's society. A common change is the blended or reconstituted family structure. It is important for the nurse to extend her view of the family beyond the traditional nuclear or extended family structure when dealing with individuals who do not live in these structures.
9. The effective family is one that is able to facilitate the growth and development of its members while still maintaining cohesion as an identifiable system. This goal is achieved by patterns of behavior characteristic of effective families.
10. Most young people receive no preparation for establishing an effective family and therefore perpetuate the behavioral patterns they learned in their families of origin.
11. Ineffective families show signs of continuous and irresolvable stress manifested by either the entire system or by one of its members.
12. The child-abusing family is an increasingly common type of ineffective family.

13. Child abuse ranges from violent, physical attacks to passive neglect. Maltreatment may be physical or emotional.
14. Children are the usual victims of family violence because they are relatively powerless, a concept that implies not only physical weakness, but also social subordination.
15. The laws of most states require that health care personnel report to legal authorities situations in which child abuse or maltreatment is suspected.
16. The dynamics underlying child abuse include societal, familial, and individual factors.
17. Child-abusing parents need a great deal of support and understanding that many health care workers find difficult to give.
18. Family therapy is the treatment of choice for child-abusing families as well as for all other ineffective families.
19. Family therapy is based on the belief that the behavior of any one family member affects and is affected by the entire family system. The family members are treated as a unit with the goal of assisting them to strengthen their identity so as to be better able to cope with both internal and external stressors.
20. Conjoint therapy usually involves only marital partners who are helped to become aware of their expectations of each other and of their marital relationship.

Suggested sources of additional information

CLASSICAL

Bulbuylan, Ann Agavni: The psychiatric nurse as family therapist, Perspect. Psychiatr. Care **7**:58-68, March-April, 1969.

Galdston, Iago: The American family in crisis, Ment. Hyg. **42**:229-236, 1958.

Gerrish, Madalene J.: The family therapist is a nurse, Am. J. Nurs. **68**:320-323, 1968.

Getty, Cathleen, and Shannon, Anna M.: Nurses as co-therapists in a family-therapy setting, Perspect. Psychiatr. Care **5**:36-48, Jan.-Feb., 1967.

Hitchens, Emily Wurster: Denial: an identified theme in marital relationships of sex offenders, Perspect. Psychiatr. Care **10**:153-159, Oct.-Nov., 1972.

Minuchin, S.: Families and family therapy, Cambridge, Mass., 1974, Harvard University Press.

Rohde, Ildaura Murillo: The nurse as a family therapist, Nurs. Outlook **16**:49-52, May, 1968.

Sager, Clifford J., and Kaplan, Helen S., editors: Progress in group and family therapy, New York, 1972, Brunner/Mazel, Inc.

Satir, Virginia: Conjoint family therapy, ed. 2, Palo Alto, Calif., 1967, Science and Behavior Books, Inc.

Smith, Lois Elaine, and Mills, Bernadine L.: Intervention techniques and unhealthy family patterns, Perspect. Psychiatr. Care **7:**112-119, May-June, 1969.

CONTEMPORARY

Auerbach, Stevanne: Confronting the childcare crisis, Boston, 1980, Beacon Press.

Barash, Dorothy A.: Cynamics of the pathological family system, Perspect. Psychiatr. Care **17**(1):17-24, Jan.-Feb., 1979.

Battered women: issues of public policy, Washington, D.C., 1978, U.S. Commission on Civil Rights.

Beavers, W. Robert: Psychotherapy and growth: a family systems perspective, New York, 1970, Brunner/Mazel, Inc.

Bowlby, John: Loss, New York, 1980, Basic Books, Inc., Publishers.

Braxton, Earl T.: Structuring the black family for survival and growth, Perspect. Psychiatr. Care **14**(4):165-173, 1976.

Bumagin, Victoria E., and Hirn, Kathryn F.: Aging is a family affair, New York, 1980, Lippincott and Crowell.

Carter, Elizabeth A., and Orfanidis, Monica M.: The family life cycle: a framework for family therapy, New York, 1980, Halsted Press.

Child abuse and neglect: vol. 1, an overview of the problem, DHEW Publication, Washington, D.C., 1975, U.S. Government Printing Office.

Child abuse and neglect: vol. 2, the problem and its management, DHEW Publication, Washington, D.C., 1975, U.S. Government Printing Office.

DeYoung, Carol D.: Nursing's contribution in family crisis treatment, Nurs. Outlook **16:**60-62, Feb., 1968.

DiAngi, Paulette: Barriers to the black and white therapeutic relationship, Perspect. Psychiatr. Care **14**(4):180-183, 1976.

Erickson, G.D., and Hogan, T.P., editors: Family therapy: introduction to theory and technique, Monterey, Calif., 1972, Brooks/Cole Publishing Co.

Fleming, Jennifer Baker: Stopping wife abuse, Garden City, N.Y., 1979, Anchor Press.

Fontana, Vincent J., and Esther Rovison: A multidisciplinary approach to the treatment of child abuse, Pediatrics **57**(5):760-764, May, 1979.

Geiser, Robert L.: The sexual abuse of children, Boston, 1980, Beacon Press.

Haller, Linda Lacey: Family systems theory in psychiatric intervention, Am. J. Nurs. **74:**462-463, 1974.

Heindl, Cathy, et al.: The nurse's role in the prevention and treatment of child abuse and neglect, DHEW Publication No. (OHDS) 79-30202, Washington, D.C., 1979, U.S. Government Printing Office.

Hofling, Charles K., and Lewis, Jerry M., editors: The family: evaluation and treatment, New York, 1980, Brunner/Mazel, Inc.

Kantor, David, and Lehr, William: Inside the family, New York, 1980, Harper & Row, Publishers.

Kaseman, Charlotte M.: The single parent family, Perspect. Psychiatr. Care **11:**113-118, July-Sept., 1974.

Leaman, Karen: Ambulatory nursing: recognizing and helping the abused child, Nursing (Horsham) **9**(2):64-67, Feb., 1979.

Lewis, Jerry, et al.: No single thread: psychological health in family systems, New York, 1980, Brunner/Mazel, Inc.

List, Julie Autumn: The day the loving stopped, New York, 1980, Seaview Books.

McDermott, John F.: Raising Cain—and Abel, too, New York, 1980, Peter H. Wyden/Publisher.

McKeel, Nancy L.: Child abuse can be prevented, Am. J. Nurs. **78:**1478-1482, Sept., 1978.

Martin, Del: Battered wives, New York, 1976, Pocket Books.

May, Rollo: Power and innocence: a search for the sources of violence, New York, 1972, W.W. Norton & Co., Inc.

Miller, Alice: Prisoners of childhood, New York, 1980, Basic Books, Inc., Publishers.

Miller, Jean: Cognitive dissonance in modifying families' perceptions, Am. J. Nurs. **74:**1468-1470, 1974.

Moore, Judith Ann, and Wallen, Andrea: The intake decision—individual psychotherapy or family therapy? In Kneisl, Carol Ren, and Wilson, Holly Skodol, editors: Current perspectives is psychiatric nursing: issues and trends, vol. 2, St. Louis, 1978, The C.V. Mosby Co.

Napier, Augustus Y., and Whitaker, Carl: The family crucible, New York, 1980, Harper & Row, Publishers.

Padberg, Joan: Bargaining to improve communications in conjoint family therapy, Perspect. Psychiatr. Care **75**:68-75, April-June, 1975.

Pincus, Lily, and Dare, Christopher: Secrets in the family, New York, 1980, Harper & Row, Publishers.

Rapoport, Robert and Rhona, and Bumstead, Janice, editors: Working couples, New York, 1980, Harper & Row, Publishers.

Reuveni, Uri: Networking families in crisis, New York, 1979, Human Sciences Press.

Scharer, Kathleen M.: Rescue fantasies: professional impediments in working with abused families, Am. J. Nurs. **78:**1483-1444, Sept., 1978.

Sedgwick, Rae: Family mental health: theory and practice, St. Louis, 1980, The C.V. Mosby Co.

Shaw, Dale, et al.: Multiple impact therapy: University of Texas Medical Branch in Galveston, Am. J. Nurs. **77:**246-248, Feb., 1977.

Smoyak, Shirley, editor: The psychiatric nurse as a family therapist, New York, 1975, John Wiley & Sons, Inc.

Taylor, John: The hyperactive child and the family: the complete what-to-do handbook, New York, 1980, Everest House.

Walker, Lenore: The battered woman, New York, 1980, Harper & Row, Publishers.

Wallerstein, Judith S., and Kelly, Joan Berlin: Surviving the breakup, New York, 1980, Basic Books, Inc., Publishers.

Weiss, Robert S.: Going it alone, New York, 1980, Basic Bokks, Inc., Publishers.

Weiss, Robert S.: Marital separation, New York, 1980, Basic Books, Inc., Publishers.

Wilkinson, Marcia B.: Power and the identified patient, Perspect. Psychiatr. Care **17**(6):248-253, Nov-Dec., 1979.

Willison, Marilyn: Diary of a divorced mother, New York, 1980, Peter H. Wyden/Publisher.

OF PARTICULAR INTEREST

Minuchin, S.: Families and family therapy, Cambridge, Mass., 1974, Harvard University Press.
Structural family therapy is described in this important text. Theory is highlighted throughout by relevant clinical examples.

Smoyak, S.: Family therapy. In Psychiatric nursing 1946 to 1974: a report on the state of the art, New York, 1975, American Journal of Nursing Co.
This extensive literature review outlines the role of the nurse in family therapies as it has developed historically.

SECTION FOUR

Therapeutic interventions with individuals whose behavior has become maladaptive

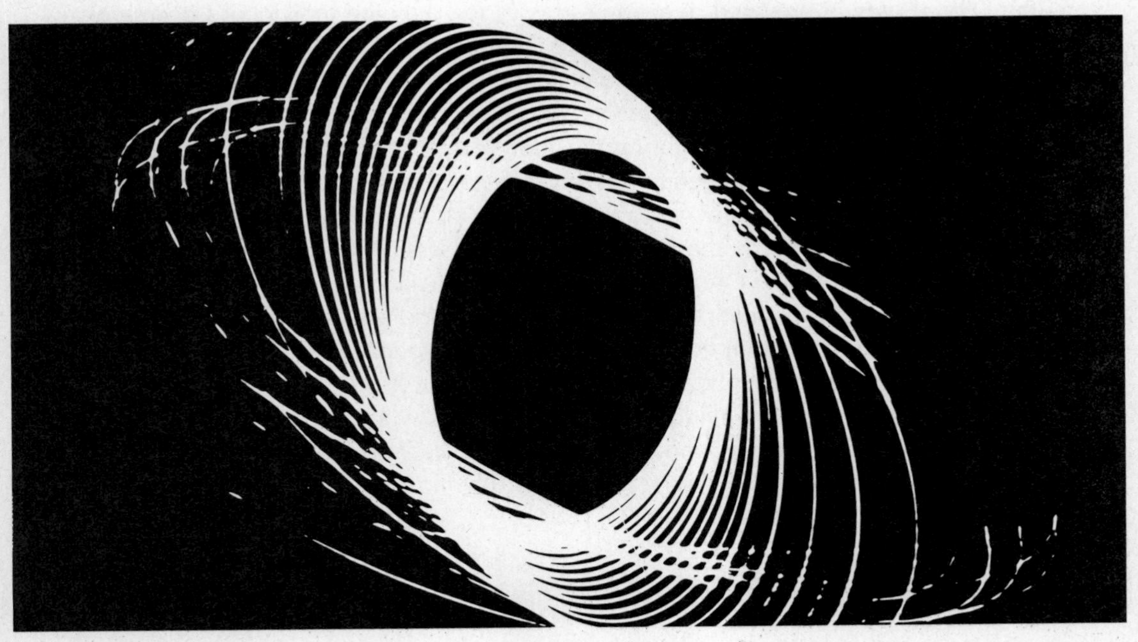

Section Four focuses on the nursing care of individuals who are suffering from the major forms of functional mental illnesses. As such, this section focuses on the practice of psychiatric nursing. The material is designed to be useful regardless of the setting in which the nurse and the client interact.

Particularly germane to this section is the latest revision of the American Psychiatric Association's Diagnostic and Statistical Manual of Mental Disorders (DSM-III), an outline of which is found in Appendix A of this text. This manual is the tool used by physicians to diagnose mental illness. This multiaxial evaluation is an attempt to assess individuals in a more comprehensive manner than was possible by use of the DSM-II, which provided direction for assessing only the individual's degree of mental health. While Axes I and II of the DSM-III still address this factor, Axis III provides for inclusion of physical disorders and conditions. Axis IV, an assessment of the severity of psychosocial stressors, and Axis V, an assessment of the highest level of adaptive functioning during the past year, complete this comprehensive evaluation. Although the American Psychiatric Association (APA) should be commended for its movement toward a holistic view of individuals, many psychiatric nurses have grave concern about the inclusion of assessments of psychosocial stressors and levels of adaptive functioning under the official diagnostic tool of psychiatrists. The basis of this concern is the belief that these assessments historically as well as currently fall within the province of nursing practice, not medical practice. Nurses are educationally and experientially prepared to assess the quality of the adaptive functioning of individuals and families; nurses are in the best position to collect, synthesize, analyze, and interpret data from assessing a social system. It is important, therefore, that nurses reaffirm their role in these areas.

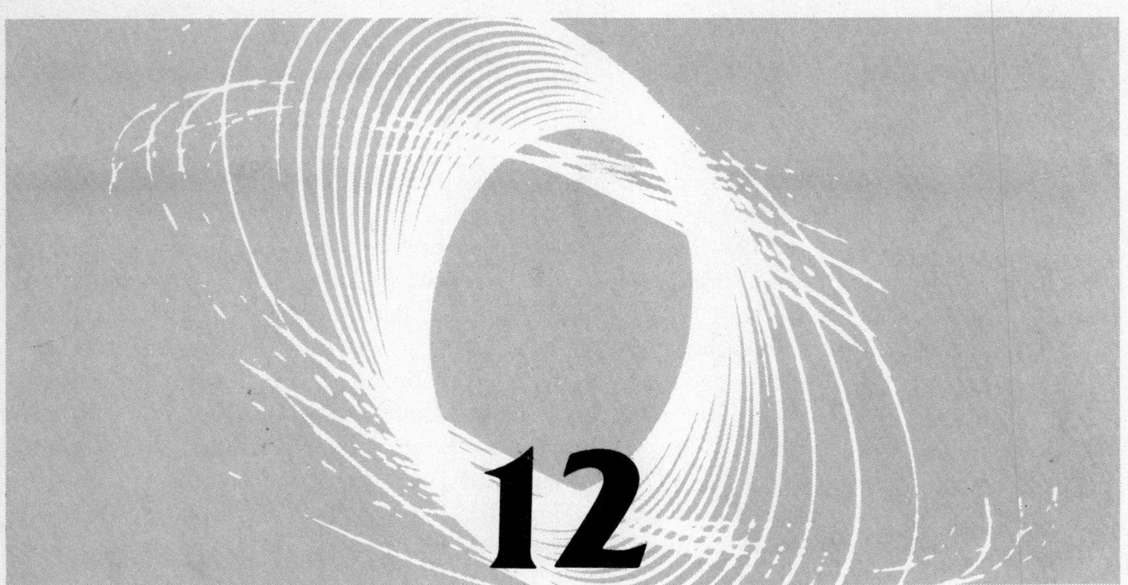

12

Behavioral patterns that reflect maladaptive thought processes

- Schizophrenic disorders
- Causative factors of schizophrenia
- Prognosis for individuals suffering from schizophrenia
- Nursing care of individuals suffering from schizophrenia

The ability of an individual to subjectively and behaviorally deal with the demands of living in a highly complex society presupposes that he is able to perceive reality accurately. An individual is able to perceive reality accurately only if he is experiencing a minimum level of anxiety and if he is able to consensually validate his perceptions with others whom he trusts. In mentally healthy people the process of consensual validation is learned early in life as a result of the development of trusting relationships with significant others. When an individual's level of anxiety is high, he perceives reality in a highly personalized way that cannot be consensually validated with others. If a high anxiety level and subsequent personalized perception of reality occur often early in life, they interfere with the development of basic trust. In cyclical fashion they also interfere with the accurate perception of reality even when anxiety is not heightened. Thus a pattern of reality distortion becomes established.

When an individual is functioning on the basis of a grossly distorted perception of reality, he is said to be *psychotic*. Psychotic behavior is primarily characterized by social deviance, when the individual behaves in a way that is outside the range of socially acceptable behavior. Therefore the designation of somebody being psychotic occurs as a result of society making a judgment about an individual's behavior as opposed to the individual making this determination himself. This is not to say that the psychotic individual does not feel distress; he may in fact be aware of being highly anxious, frightened, confused, or otherwise emotionally uncomfortable. He is very unlikely, however, to understand the significance of these feelings as representing an illness or disorder and therefore may not readily seek help.

When an individual's distorted perceptions of reality result from and contribute to maladaptive thought processes, that individual may be suffering from *schizophrenia*.

SCHIZOPHRENIC DISORDERS

Schizophrenia is one of the most serious illnesses that any individual can experience. Unfortunately, the majority of hospitalized mentally ill patients in the United States are afflicted with this baffling condition. It is believed to be a severe functional psychosis, which is defined as an extreme form of mental illness, having as its basis no demonstrable organic disease or intellectual deficit. Schizophrenia appears as a distorted reaction of an individual who lacks the capacities and feelings required for effectively handling the daily challenges of reality. There is either a total lack of normal feeling tone or a distortion of the emotions. An individual with schizophrenia frequently has a tendency to withdraw into a world of his own subjective construction, which is manifested behaviorally by an increasing inability to develop and maintain satisfactory interpersonal relationships. The individual frequently has great difficulty in identifying and communicating his feelings and thoughts to others, although he believes he has made many efforts to do so. Such an individual is frequently misunderstood by others, and it can be said that his communication patterns are dysfunctional.

To be diagnosed as schizophrenic, the individual must exhibit characteristic delusions, characteristic hallucinations, or other characteristic symptoms of thought impairment accompanied by blunted, flat, or inappropriate affect.

Delusions are false beliefs out of keeping with the individual's level of knowledge and his cultural group; the belief is maintained against logical argument and despite objective contradictory evidence. Delusions that are characteristic of schizophrenia include delusions about one's thoughts, feelings, and activities being controlled by some external force and delusions about one's thoughts being broadcast into the external world, inserted from the external world into one's mind, or removed from one's head by some external source. Religious and somatic delusions as well as delusions of grandiosity are also common.

Hallucinations are false sensory perceptions in the absence of an actual external stimulus. Although any of the five senses may be involved in a hallucinatory experience, auditory hallucinations are characteristic of schizophrenia.

Derailment (loosening of associations) is another characteristic symptom of schizophrenia and refers to a pattern of spontaneous speech in which the idea or trend of thought slips off of one track onto another that is completely unrelated. As a result, the person's speech may seem unintelligible to the listener even though individual words are understood.

The term *affect* refers to the feeling tone of the individual. The schizophrenic person characteristically exhibits a blunt or flat affect, in contrast to the healthy individual whose affect conveys a feeling that is indicative of his emotional state and is congruent with the content of what he is saying. In individuals with schizophrenic disorders one observes that the feeling tone conveyed by the individual does not enhance what he is saying. It is not unusual to spend a great deal of time talking with a schizophrenic person without learning what he is feeling, despite the fact that much of the conversation was his attempt to describe his feelings. It is also not unusual for the individual to convey a feeling tone that is inappropriate to the content of what he is saying; for example, he may laugh while stating how upset and sad he is because his mother just died.

Once the individual is diagnosed as schizophrenic, the individual's behavior is further categorized into types of schizophrenia. Psychiatrists have subclassified schizophrenia into five major types, depending on the predominant patterns of behavior displayed. These subclassifications are the disorganized (hebephrenic) type, the catatonic type, the paranoid type, the undifferentiated type, and the residual type. The *disorganized type* is characterized by severe personality disintegration, including hallucinations, inappropriate behavior (e.g., silly laughter), and regression. *Catatonic* behavior is characterized by an acute stupor associated with a sudden loss of animation and a tendency to remain motionless in a stereotyped position; this behavior may alternate with periods of excitement and explosive overactivity. The *paranoid type* is characterized by suspiciousness and ideas of persecution or grandeur called *paranoid delusions*. The *undifferentiated type* is characterized by the prominence of psychotic symptoms that fall into more than one subtype or that do not meet the criteria for any one subtype. The *residual type* is the schizophrenic diagnosis used for individuals who no longer exhibit overtly psychotic symptoms but do exhibit inappropriate behavior characteristic of schizophrenia.*

CAUSATIVE FACTORS OF SCHIZOPHRENIA

If one were to ask the schizophrenic person what caused his illness, he might respond by relating a particularly traumatic event that preceded the onset of his illness by days, weeks, or months. Although not all schizophrenic persons have such events in their lives, enough experience them to make it important to distinguish between a precipitating event and causation. Although there is much ongoing debate over the cause of schizophrenia, all authorities agree that the cause is likely to be a process of long standing, either physical or emotional or both. It is considered highly unlikely that a single event, either physical or emotional, no matter how catastrophic, would be sufficient to cause the drastic personality alteration seen in schizophrenia. The events reported by schizophrenic persons as the possible causes of their illness are usually viewed by authorities as precipitating factors. Lay persons express this concept when they refer to the "straw that broke the camel's back." The underlying physiological and psychological structure is so fragile that the traumatic event cannot be integrated within the context of reality, and the individual retreats into the illness to protect himself against total personality disintegration. It should be noted that many schizophrenic individuals are unable to identify a precipitating event; instead, the onset of the schizophrenic syndrome is usually insidious.

Although there is no conclusive scientific proof of the cause of schizophrenia, many authorities believe that it is related to factors that are inherent in highly complex cultures such as that of the United States. There are recent studies pointing to the influence of a genetic factor in schizophrenia, and some authorities believe that there is likely to be a certain biochemical composition that predisposes individuals to an inadequate adaptation to stress. Credence is given these theories by the number of schizo-

*Adapted from Morgan, James A., and Morgan, Mary D.: Manual of primary mental health care, Philadelphia, 1980, J.B. Lippincott Co.

phrenic individuals whose families report that, even as infants, these persons resisted attempts at cuddling, which set up a cyclically unsatisfying relationship between the infants and their parents. Whatever the cause, it is known that most individuals who develop behavioral patterns that can be classified as schizophrenic have experienced highly unsatisfactory family relationships in their early formative years. They are almost always products of family situations in which they could not develop warm, positive relationships with other significant members, particularly the mothering one. These individuals have not learned to trust others and have not developed a self-image enabling them to feel secure in their relations with others. This failure to develop an integrated ego and the necessary strength to resolve conflicts between the id and the superego presumably derives from early, persistent tension-laden parent-child relationships. Schizophrenic persons may not accept themselves as having real value or an identity that is uniquely their own. Frequently such individuals have not been able to identify with the parent of the same sex and may have a diffuse sexual identity and role. Such handicapped persons often direct their love energies toward themselves, since they are fearful of nonacceptance and rejection if they attempt to direct libidinal energies toward others. Because of extreme sensitivity, they often develop patterns of narcissism and introversion that eventually result in a life of activity and interest directed entirely toward satisfactions that focus on self.

Although there are many theories related to the causative, or etiological, factors underlying schizophrenia, the theory that seems to have the most relevance for nursing practice is the one that postulates that faulty interpersonal relationships in the early family relationship is a major contributory factor to the ultimate development of the illness. Several theorists, the foremost of whom is Gregory Bateson, have suggested that a particular type of dysfunctional communication is present in families in which there is a schizophrenic individual. This type of communication is called the *double-bind.* A double-bind communication is one that gives two contradictory messages at the same time, thereby forcing the receiver of the messages to make a choice between at least two feelings, thoughts, or behaviors that contradict each other. An example of this type of paradoxical communication occurs when the mothering one overtly and covertly conveys to her child that, to make her happy, he must love her most, while at the same time, he must love all in the family equally. Obviously the child cannot succeed in such a situation. If such patterns of communication become the rule rather than the exception, the child is likely to develop a high degree of anxiety that increasingly interferes with his ability to perceive reality accurately. It is hypothesized that the child adapts to his anxiety-laden environment by not responding to either aspect of the message, thereby avoiding overt or covert punishment and perhaps reducing anxiety to a manageable level. Although this adaptation serves a protective function, it does not enable the child to meet his needs and minimizes opportunities for the development of coping mechanisms that would be useful in other situations later in life.

It is important to understand that the initial adaptation of the child to his environment is functional in that it serves a protective purpose. Once learned, however, it becomes difficult if not impossible for the growing child to alter his response in other situations in which the communication is healthy. Therefore the response that was functional in the original situation becomes dysfunctional in other situations. Furthermore, the feedback given to this person is frequently negative, thereby establishing a vicious cycle that further increases the dysfunctional aspects of the communication. It is not uncommon for family members, teachers, and friends of a newly diagnosed schizophrenic person to give health personnel an account of an individual who had "always been a little different, shy, aloof," even though this may be the first time his behavior could be described as unusual enough to warrant medical attention.

The theory that faulty interpersonal relationships in early life are a major causative factor in the later development of schizophrenia has great relevance for nursing practice because it provides the nurse with the opportunity to provide the client with corrective experiences in which he can unlearn the previously learned dysfunctional patterns of relating and learn healthier patterns that are functional. It is often said that the most potent tool available to the psychiatric nurse is the therapeutic use of self, and it is through this use of self that the nurse provides experiences that have the potential to be corrective.

PROGNOSIS FOR INDIVIDUALS SUFFERING FROM SCHIZOPHRENIA

Schizophrenia is a disorder of the ego that causes the affected individual to have difficulty in perceiving himself in relation to others. This problem results in serious social maladjustment. As the individual matures, demands on his ability to integrate his activities with those of a group become greater, and thus his maladjustment becomes a progressively more serious handicap. The inability to cope with social pressures eventually results in a personality disorganization that is viewed by authorities as being extremely serious although not necessarily permanent. It is not coincidental that the initial acute onset of the illness often occurs during late adolescence or early adulthood when there are great societal pressures to make significant life decisions such as the choice of a career and mate.

Whether it will be possible to help such an afflicted individual to reestablish himself in his family and return to his work depends on several factors:

1. The character of the prepsychotic personality. The prepsychotic personality includes the effectiveness of the individual's adaptation before becoming mentally ill, the type of interests that were maintained, and the coping mechanisms that were used.
2. The nature of the onset of the illness. Did the illness develop insidiously over a long period of time as the result of progressively more unsatisfactory methods of coping with life's problems, or was the onset rapid and precipitated by a situation external to the life of the individual?
3. The timing and nature of the treatment. Was treatment sought early in the illness, and was treatment individualized and personalized?

An individual who has adapted reasonably well to the pressures of life before becoming ill will have a better chance of recovery, at least of returning to his prepsychotic level of effectiveness, than will someone who has never adapted effectively and therefore has limited ego strength. It is also obvious that someone whose illness has developed slowly and insidiously as a result of progressively worsening interpersonal relationships has a less optimistic future than does someone whose illness was precipitated only after experiencing great external stress.

Persons who receive psychiatric help very soon after the development of the illness and are given individualized, skilled, and highly personalized care have a good chance of making a social recovery. This is much less true of persons who receive psychiatric help after the illness has been full blown for a year or more.

Authorities suggest that expectations or recovery should be in terms of social recovery and not necessarily in terms of emotional recovery. Schizophrenic individuals who have been treated may maintain a marginal adjustment, still retaining an essential shallow affective response and shyness. They can be thought of as interpersonally fragile and may require professional help from time to time. Many schizophrenic individuals require a daily maintenance dose of one of the antipsychotic drugs.

Since the specific causes of schizophrenia are unknown, specific therapeutic measures have not yet been identified. In spite of all the therapeutic efforts currently being employed, about a third of the schizophrenic patients who receive professional help early make a fairly complete recovery, a third make a social recovery but require additional hospitalization from time to time, and a third require hospitalization for an indefinite period.

NURSING CARE OF INDIVIDUALS SUFFERING FROM SCHIZOPHRENIA

Nursing assessment

Since therapeutic intervention with the mentally ill, including the schizophrenic person, is increasingly taking place in a variety of settings and is no longer limited to hospital care, the following guidelines reflect nursing care necessary regardless of setting.

As stated in Chapter 3, to be of maximum help the nurse must assess the individual's behavior, develop a plan of care, and implement and evaluate the care. When assessing the behavior of an individual, it is important for the nurse to bear in mind that the classification of schizophrenia into five types is only of academic interest and has no practical significance from the nursing standpoint. It is valuable to recognize that the behavior of these persons is expressing a need and may fluctuate in an apparently unpredictable manner. It is necessary for the nurse to attempt to understand the needs of these persons rather than to focus on the diagnostic entities.

When making the initial assessment, it is important to determine whether the person has taken any psychotropic drugs and if so, the kind, dosage, and frequency. The purpose of these drugs is to alter emotional states biochemically, which brings about altered behavior. In addition, the drugs themselves may have side effects that are reflected behaviorally. It is important to differentiate between behavior induced by drugs and behavior reflecting the emotional state, since the subsequent intervention differs.

Chemotherapeutic agents are widely used in the treatment of emotional disorders and are not limited to the practice of psychiatry. Therefore, even if the person who is being assessed has not previously sought psychiatric help, it must not be assumed that he has not taken psychotropic drugs. For further discussion of the characteristics and effects of the major psychotropic drugs, see Chapter 22.

Behaviors that the nurse might commonly observe in the schizophrenic person are those that result from withdrawal (including hallucinations), feelings of suspiciousness, psychomotor retardation or overactivity, regression, social ineptitude, and unmet physical needs. Although each of these behaviors is discussed as a separate entity, it should be understood that they are all interrelated and stem from similar underlying dynamics. Therefore nursing care directed at altering one behavior will inevitably have an effect on others.

Withdrawal is characterized by retreating into a fantasy world of one's own design, termed *autism.* Autism is a form of thinking that does not take reality factors into account. The schizophrenic person creates a fantasy world of his own designed to fulfill needs and wishes that have not been met through the resources available in the world of reality. As such, this autistic world is unique to the person and is difficult for anyone else to understand. One can understand autistic thinking to some degree by recalling the daydreaming frequently engaged in by adolescents. The process is similar in that both autistic thinking and daydreaming are designed to meet unfulfilled needs. A major difference is that the daydreamer can easily call himself back to the world of reality, whereas the schizophrenic who is engaged in autistic thinking cannot.

It is not unusual to hear someone describe withdrawn behavior with phrases such as, "I feel there is an intangible wall between us" or "I just can't seem to get through to him." A withdrawn person frequently spends most of his time by himself, seemingly ignoring persons and situations around him. He may be mute and at best, speaks very little and in clipped, short phrases. Withdrawn behavior appears superficially similar to behavior resulting from depression. However, in a short time the observer will be able to distinguish between the two in that little or no feeling tone (affect) is perceived with the withdrawn person, whereas the depressed person conveys overwhelming feelings of sadness and hopelessness.

Hallucinations are common symptoms associated with withdrawn behavior. The individual experiencing hallucinations rarely offers this information spontaneously. Rather, he will be observed cocking his head to one side as if listening, staring into space as if watching something, and talking as if to someone, although no one is present.

Feelings of suspiciousness may be expressed very directly or quite indirectly. Some individuals refuse to eat because they are convinced that their food is poisoned in an attempt by others to kill them. This belief is an example of a delusion of persecution. Other persons may believe that those around them are talking about them and substantiate this belief by interpreting everyday events as referring to themselves (ideas of reference). More covertly, some persons may show evidence of suspiciousness by such subtle clues as darting their eyes around on entering a room or, in the case of women, carrying their purse with them at all times.

Obviously, all feelings of suspiciousness stem from and are accompanied by high levels of anxiety. In fact, developing feelings of suspiciousness is an unconscious means of reducing anxiety to a level that is manageable.

Psychomotor activity refers to the level of activity of the mind and the body. It is unusual for a schizophrenic individual to exhibit normal psychomotor activity, that is, both mental and physical activty that is congruent with the requirements of the situation. Rather, the person frequently exhibits retardation or overactivity in the psychomotor realm. An extreme example of psychomotor retardation is seen in persons who are diagnosed as being in a catatonic stupor. These persons move very slowly and can take hours to walk the distance of a city block or to eat a meal. Concomitantly, they speak very slowly, which reflects an extreme slowing down of mental processes. The term *retarded* as used in this context should not be confused with the same term when it is used to refer to an intellectual deficit of a person. As previously stated, schizophrenic individuals to not suffer from intellectual impairment, although this may appear to be the case because of their temporarily diminished ability to comprehend and respond to mental stimuli. Psychomotor overactivity is manifested by loud, rapid talking (pressure of speech) and frequent rapid gross motor movements that seem aimless. Despite the quantity of activity, fine motor movements are usually impaired. This person literally finds it impossible to sit still and frequently paces, swinging his arms and talking continuously.

Regression is behavior that is appropriate to an age level considerably below the chronological age of the individual. Therefore regression does not refer to a specific behavior but rather to a discrepancy between the observed behavior and that which one would expect to observe in a healthy individual of the same age and developmental stage.

The student may find it helpful to review Chapter 4 on personality development to gain a sound understanding of normalcy as a basis for determining deviancy from normal. This differentiation is a particular problem with schizophrenic persons who experience the initial acute onset of the illness during late adolescence or early adulthood. It will be remembered that this time of life is normally characterized by major fluctuations in behavior. Except for extreme cases, it becomes difficult to distinguish between the behavior resulting from conflicts experienced by the normal healthy adolescent and that which is a result of emotional disturbance in the adolescent who is also schizophrenic.

Behavior resulting from regression may include eating only when fed and being unable to dress oneself or carry out personal hygiene; in fact, the nurse is likely to observe disturbances in all activities of daily living.

Social ineptitude is a prominent feature of the behavior of schizophrenic individuals. Because of the dysfunctional nature of their early childhood experiences in interpersonal relationships, these persons have not learned many of the even rudimentary social skills healthy adults take for granted. Such common occurrences as meeting people for the first time can precipitate overwhelming anxiety in the schizophrenic individual and may lead to behavior that is highly inappropriate to the situation. It is not uncommon for schizophrenic persons to go to great lengths to avoid social situations and activities such as dating and team sports. Instead, they prefer to engage in solitary activities, which increase their social inexperience and result in a cycle of mutual withdrawal. Schizophrenic individuals frequently report that they have few if any friends; when the schizophrenic individual is encountered by the nurse in situations or settings where visitors or inquiries are to be expected, these two elements are in fact usually lacking.

Behaviors resulting from unmet physical needs may or may not be related to the emotional problems of the client. It cannot be overemphasized that emotional illness provides no immunity to physical illness. Therefore in the initial assessment it is imperative that the nurse determine the degree of general physical health of the client. Complaints by the individual of physical discomfort must be thoroughly investigated to determine whether they are related to physical abnormality or to the emotional state.

Because of the nature of the schizophrenic disorder, it is not uncommon to find a number of physical problems that stem from the dynamics of the emotional illness. Malnutrition is usual, either due to psychomotor retardation, suspiciousness, or generalized neglect of activities of daily living. Even though the client might not be able to tell the nurse his usual weight, the nurse can observe whether or not his clothing fits properly. If an individual has been taking psychotropic drugs for a period of time, especially the phenothiazines, he may be overweight, since these drugs have the effect of stimulating the appetite. Obesity should not be seen as evidence of a good nutritional state; many obese people are in fact malnourished because the foods that are high in caloric value frequently have limited nutritional value.

A lack of interest in physical cleanliness and personal appearance is often one of the first changes in behavior of schizophrenic persons. The schizophrenic person may be disheveled in appearance or may be dressed in a bizarre fashion.

The individual may be confused and therefore may not spontaneously report a physical condition of long standing such as diabetes or a hypothyroidism caused by thyroidectomy, either of which may require daily supplemental medication. The nurse should be alert to indications of these and other physical conditions by observing for such evidence as scars or injection marks.

Because of psychomotor retardation or overactivity, the person may have circulatory problems evidenced by peripheral edema or may be verging on a state of exhaustion.

Planning for nursing intervention

After assessing the behavior of the client and inferring his needs from these observations, the next step is to develop a plan of nursing care. To be effective this plan needs to be highly individualized. Therefore the suggestions that follow should be seen as general guidelines that should be used if they are appropriate to the needs of the client. All too often the individual is required to conform to the dictates of a set nursing care plan rather than one designed for him.

The problems of any schizophrenic person are essentially an exaggeration of the problems of his prepsychotic personality. Because he has usually been a shy, aloof, and emotionally sensitive individual, he has been unsuccessful in varying degrees in coping with the emotional aspects of the day-by-day problems of routine living. Because of this, he has attempted a solution by withdrawing from everyday problems and adapting through the use of more satisfying regressive, or infantile, behavior. To replace the world of reality, the individual often creates a fantasy world of his own that is devoid of certain emotional stresses. If such withdrawal into an unreal world continues, the person finds more and more relief in dealing with an environment derived from his autistic thinking. This reduces his interactions with others to the dependent and unpredictable behavior of a child. All nursing activities should therefore be related to a plan that is directed toward the prevention of regression and toward helping the client to accept and to remain in contact with reality. It seems logical that the nurse should strive to make reality as pleasant and as free of emotionally stressful situations as possible.

Underlying the withdrawal tendencies in schizophrenic persons is a consistent affective indifference or emotional impoverishment. This lack of appropriate feeling makes it difficult for the nurse to express warmth and demonstrate spontaneous interest in the schizophrenic person. It is helpful when the nurse understands that the schizophrenic individual feels lonely, isolated, and hungry for human contacts but is often incapable of inviting a friendly approach from another person. Only when the plan directs the nurse to approach the individual with an accepting attitude and with friendliness can she be a source of therapeutic help (Fig 12-1).

Schizophrenic behavior is invariably difficult to understand because it is unconsciously motivated and may have little logical relation to the immediate environmental situation. Frequently the client is out of contact with reality. This means that he is motivated by his thoughts and is not sure what is the real world and what is a result of his fantasies. Thus he may fuse or confuse his fantasy world with the world of reality. *Inappropriate* and *bizarre* may be accurate descriptive terms for much of his behavior, which is significant and meaningful only when considered from the standpoint of his emotional or instinctual needs. Although this behavior is often difficult to understand, it does have real meaning for the client, and if it is closely studied, the meaning often becomes obvious. One important aspect of the nursing care plan is to record what the nurse observes the client doing and saying.

Although most schizophrenic individuals show every outward manifestation of physical maturity, they are essentially struggling with many psychogenic conflicts that originated in child-

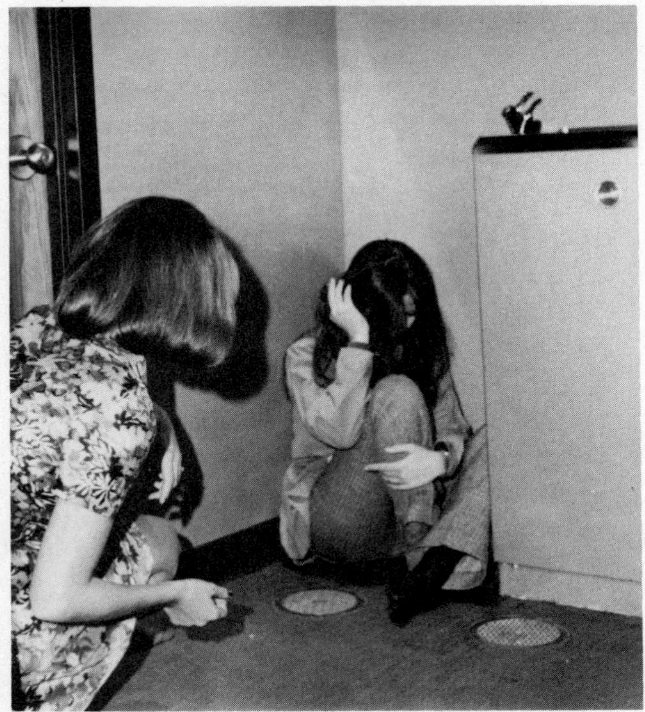

Fig. 12-1 *The withdrawn client requires individualized, concerned care.*

hood. Since their problems probably evolved at an early age from faulty emotional relationships between them and significant adults in their environment, corrective interpersonal experiences must be planned for and provided. Schizophrenic persons have often been deprived of a loving parent or have had a parent of the same sex who was so rigid and unloving that identification with this parent at the proper time was impossible. Such deprivation may have made it extremely difficult for the individual to trust or to give and receive love. Therefore it is highly desirable for the nurse to develop a relationship with the client in which she becomes a significant other. Specific information about the process of the nurse-client relationship is discussed in Chapter 9. The efficacy of using this approach with the mentally ill seems to be greatest in working with schizophrenic persons. The nurse-client relationship is a vehicle for providing a corrective emotional experience in which the client experiences, over a period of time, the unconditional positive regard of another person who communicates in a healthy functional way.

In group settings a corrective family situation can be simulated. Often a physician assumes the role of a kindly understanding father, a nurse that of a wise, accepting mother, and other clients that of siblings. If such a simulated family experience gives the client sufficient love and acceptance over a period of time, he can be helped to deal more realistically with his conflicts and can achieve some feeling of security. Calling the client Mr. Smith instead of John is a way of suggesting that he is expected to assume an adult role. Using a title that connotes respect, whatever it may be, is generally an incentive to more acceptable behavior and may convey to the client the idea that he is an important person.

The use of long and involved sentences should be avoided. Many schizophrenic persons are easily confused and have a limited attention span. Short phrases are more effective, and specific words more helpful than generalizations. For instances, *ice cream* is more meaningful than *dessert,* and *ham* is more specific than *meat*.

The nurse may be tempted to exploit the negativism displayed by some clients. She may request the client to walk backward when she assumes that he will do the exact opposite, which is the reaction actually desired. Use of negativism, however, in such activities as feeding the client and in giving medication may serve to increase his confusion and encourage complete withdrawal.

Similarly, making use of delusions and hallucinations to direct the client's behavior should be avoided. If, for instance, he hallucinates and believes that he hears the voice of his mother, the nurse may be tempted to say that his mother just told him to eat his lunch. If the client believes himself to be John the Baptist, it might seem at first that on that delusional assumption he can be persuaded to be more careful of his personal hygiene. The client will cease to trust the nurse when such symptoms are used to accomplish the nurse's purpose.

It is not helpful to try to explain away the individual's false ideas or argue with him about them. Such an approach will cause the individual to become increasingly hostile and suspicious. If one recognizes the significance of the delusion to the person and the fact that life is intolerable to him without this ego-saving device, the futility of trying to change the individual's ideas will become obvious. It is a wise plan to listen respectfully to the client without commenting on the content of his conversation.

If a client asks for a confirmaton of his hallucinations, it is better to answer truthfully, "No, Mr. Jones, I do not see the face of Christ on the wall" or "No, Mr. Smith, your face is not that of a dog." It is wise to give honest replies that focus on reality.

Meticulous honesty and fairness on the part of the nurse are of primary importance. Should the client make a request with which it is impossible to comply, a suitable answer is, "I am sorry that I am not allowed to carry out such a procedure." Once a promise is made, the nurse is obligated to carry it out. If possible, all requests and questions should be answered. If no answer is possible, the client should be informed that his request will be referred to an appropriate person who can give an answer or that the answer is truly not known.

When behaviors resulting from feelings of suspiciousness are prominent, it is important to remember that the person is essentially shy, sensitive, and unable to relate positively to others. Because he has never learned to trust, he resorts to the mental mechanisms of projection to cope with his environment and therefore places the blame for his inadequacies on people and objects about him. Hostility is frequently a dominant attitude. Insight is poor, and usually the client is convinced that he is being treated illegally or without just cause. Consequently, he may engage in threatening behavior, which can become dangerous to others if his anxiety becomes unmanageable.

Such a person rarely desires to enter group activity. As a defense, suspicious persons are usually aloof, sarcastic, and generally hostile toward everyone about them. This behavior is actually based on intrapersonal fear and anxiety, and the nurse who truly appreciates this fact will not feel personally threatened, and therefore will remain with the individual and try to allay his fear and anxiety.

Such fearful, hostile people must be approached with utmost tact and understanding. Solitary activities are more successful for them initially than are group activities.

Arguments with such individuals should be avoided, since any controversy is at once integrated into the individual's delusional system. To obtain the confidence of a paranoid person requires the patient and persistent application of tact, tolerance of his hostile attitude, and a quiet consistency in establishing a relationship with him.

Because of the schizophrenic person's extreme sensitivity and fear of being unacceptable to others, the nurse should take the initiative in stimulating his interest in social activity and recreation. It is important that the nurse know something of the client's background, and with this knowledge she can initiate conversations in which he can participate. When the client develops a feeling of trust in the nurse, participation in some recreational activity can then be encouraged. This may be accomplished by extending an invitation such as, "I need a partner for a game of table tennis; come and play with me." It may be best for the nurse alone to play a game with the client to help him feel secure. The nurse should provide opportunities for him to have some successful experiences. Gradually other participants can be added as he develops more confidence. These participants should be other clients and staff members who relate well with him and will promote his sense of being accepted. Staff members should be a stable group, and the same individuals, including the nurse, should continue this program of socialization for several weeks or even months.

One aspect of the nurse's responsibility lies in the supervision of personal hygiene and in encouraging the schizophrenic person to bathe. Suspicious persons usually take at least adequate care of their own personal hygiene. However, they may make demands such as complete bathroom privacy. It is important for the nurse to help the client take responsibility for his own personal hygiene and grooming. Clients should be encouraged and helped to look as attractive as possible, since a pleasing appearance is likely to elicit the sorely needed positive reflected appraisals of others. Nurses can initiate a positive relationship by planning to help clients with all aspects of good grooming. The services of a beautician are invaluable, and it may also be of great therapeutic benefit to have female clients arrange each other's hair. Male clients should be encouraged to shave, to keep their hair well groomed, and to dress neatly.

Planning for adequate food intake for clients is a major nursing responsibility. In the case of a client who exhibits psychomotor retardation, planning and cooking a meal may be temporarily beyond his ability. It is perfectly appropriate for the nurse to initiate such plans by helping him to prepare lists or by arranging to have his food preparation and intake supervised by others. In the case of an overactive patient, foods that are high in caloric and protein value, that require little preparation, and that can be eaten easily are to be encouraged. Milk shakes are an example of a food that meets these criteria. The nurse's interest in the client's food intake often enhances their relationship because of the symbolic link between food and security.

Persons who retreat into a fantasy world often ignore physical illness and may offer no complaints even when the condition is a painful one. Acute mastoiditis, cystitis, lung abscess, and a broken bone in the hand or foot are examples of serious disorders that have been known to exist without complaint on the part of schizophrenic individuals. The psychiatric nurse should plan to be constantly alert to the physical condition of clients.

Standing and sitting in one position for hours may be observed frequently among schizophrenic persons. Edema and cyanosis of the extremities are likely to develop. To avoid this the client should be encouraged to take some exercise, even if it is only to walk up and down a hall.

Other physical problems may result from the chemotherapy the client may receive. It is imperative that the nurse know which drugs, if any, the client is taking and plan to purposefully observe for any untoward reactions. See Chapter 22 for an in-depth discussion of common chemotherapeutic agents.

CASE FORMULATION □ A WITHDRAWN INDIVIDUAL

The following case history presents the story of a young woman who resorted to catatonic withdrawal when she could no longer cope with the problems of daily living.

Frances B. was 19 years of age when she was admitted to the hospital. The only child of missionary parents, she was born in a mission station in Africa. Her father was a quiet-spoken man, definitely ascetic and consistent in his practice of religious teachings. The girl's mother was more practical and tolerant but was dominated by her husband. They were so busy with the work of the mission that they had little time to spend with their daughter.

During the first 5 years of her life, Frances's only playmates were native children. Toward them, she had always taken an attitude of superiority. On entering a boarding school in the United States at the age of 5, she had difficulty with her classmates. She was inclined to be too critical with them and insisted on dictating to them about personal matters. In her twelfth year she had a long siege of pneumonia, after which she lost weight and was chronically anemic and undernourished. She spent long hours in prayer and wrote endless letters to her parents, most of them consisting of long quotations from the Bible. She insisted on wearing old, worn clothing to the schoolroom and bitterly criticized classmates for not doing likewise.

Although her parents returned on furlough every 5 years, they could spend only a few days with her because they had many church meetings to attend while in the United States.

Her social behavior changed somewhat in her high school years, but she made few friends. She had a dog to which she was greatly attached, and she spent most of her free time in his company, taking long walks. She showed a preference for mathematics and biblical history.

Frances entered the freshman year of college some 11 months before her admission to the psychiatric hospital. Although her scholastic record was good, she was known as a strange girl who avoided company, smiled a great deal to herself, and demonstrated no interest in the opposite sex. Her parents, while on furlough from Africa, visited her during the Christmas holidays, and her mother expressed fear that she was not emotionally well. She manifested little interest in their visit, in spite of the fact that she had not seen her parents for over 5 years.

During the commencement festivities she disappeared from the campus for several days; later it was learned that she had spent the time at an evangelical camp meeting. She remained on the campus during the summer months to take some advanced courses in mathematics. During this interval she roomed with two other young women in the house of one of the faculty members. The latter were in the habit of discussing their love affairs in her presence, and she suddenly manifested an unusual interest in their conversations. Among other things, she inquired about various matters of sex and how to approach members of the opposite sex. A few nights later she informed one of the girls that she saw the face of her future husband in the light fixture. She scrutinized the fixture for several hours, during which she sat in a trancelike state with a smile on her face. Early the next morning she spoke to a 13-year-old newsboy and informed him that she would marry him. When he made light of this proposal, she became upset, struck him in the face, and chased him down the street. Returning to her room, she tore out the light fixture, removed her clothing, and became unmanageable.

On being admitted to the psychiatric hospital, she refused to answer questions. She smiled to herself and identified the house physician as "Herbert." She insisted on having the window opened because "they are playing the wedding march." Her speech was incoherent; she was definitely hallucinating and stated that she was hearing voices that questioned her moral standards.

For the first few days she talked a great deal about a fantasized courtship in which she was the central character. She carried on a dialogue, at one time representing the lover, at another time the maiden. After this she entered a long period of silence, during which she was mute, resistive, and refused food. Occasionally she said, "If thy eye offend thee, cut it out." One evening she almost succeeded in enucleating her right eye with the thumb and forefinger of her right hand. She continued to talk incoherently, laughed a great deal, and made little attempt to keep her person clean. After several months she improved but remained withdrawn, manneristic, and untidy. Five months after her illness began, her parents returned from Africa to visit her, but she manifested no interest in them. In fact, she showed no indication that she recognized them when they came into the hospital.

Discussion of development of patterns of behavior

The case report is clearly the story of a young woman who failed to develop a stable, harmonious self-concept or to evolve an ego strong enough to resolve the conflicts between the id drives and the demands of the superego.

The history of her life experiences gives us little information about this client as a child. We do know that her father dominated both the home and the mother and placed the welfare of the mission above all else. It is quite possible that her care even as an infant was relegated to employed native women who may not have remained in the household consistently. In the development of a sense of personal security, the first 5 years of a child's life are crucial. The type of mothering person by whom the child is nurtured is of the greatest importance, especially in developing the ability to share and the ability to effectively cope with hostile, aggressive instinctual drives.

At the age of 5 years Frances B. was sent away to a boarding school. Although this was probably the best plan the parents could develop, it was apparently not helpful to the girl. Authorities believe that the fifth year of a child's life is of great significance in the scheme of psychosexual development. During this period the child is beginning to identify with the parent of the same sex, has discovered that the sexual organ is a source of pleasurable sensations, and has recognized the structural difference between the sex organs of boys and girls. As has been mentioned in a previous chapter, castration fears or concern about the loss of the penis are sources of anxiety for children of this age. A boy may be concerned for fear he will be deprived of the penis as a punishment, and a girl may fear that she was deprived of a penis because of some earlier punishment or accident. When a child in this age period is removed from the parents, he is apt to feel banished as a punishment for some transgression. Since sexual longings and fantasies have occupied some of the child's thoughts and since the child realizes that these are frowned on by the parents, it is natural for the child to feel that the banishment is related to "bad" thoughts.

Frances undoubtedly felt banished by being sent to boarding school. Because of her father's strict and rigid attitudes, it is quite likely that Frances was convinced that she was being punished. Even when parents are not a source of comfort and security for a child, the child mourns their loss when separated from them because they are the only significant reality known. Thus it is reasonable to believe that Frances passed through a period of loneliness and bereavement at being deprived from the only mothering person she knew.

Initially, children protest this separation by crying or by other aggressive acting-out behavior. After several days of hopelessness and withdrawal from activity, the child usually becomes detached and seems unwilling to resume a close relationship with any adult, even if the lost person returns. This detached attitude could be altered if the parent returned and remained with the child consistently. However, in the situation being discussed, the little girl undoubtedly developed a detached attitude toward other people and attempted to isolate herself personally to avoid anxiety resulting from fear of being cast aside and abandoned a second time. Her subsequent attachment to a dog suggested that she could not trust another person with her love and therefore gave it to an animal who made no demands and gave her unconditional devotion.

After Frances had a serious illness at the age of 12, she began to spend long hours in prayer, wrote letters to her parents filled with quotes from the Bible, and wore her shoddiest clothing to school. This behavior suggests that she felt guilt-ridden for having been ill and was seeking to gain the favor and forgiveness of her parents, who in her fantasies may have been God's representatives on earth. Undoubtedly she felt unworthy of anything better when she chose to wear old and shoddy clothing to school and again was seeking to atone for fantasized sin.

Her unusual interest in the sexual affairs of other girls of her age and the inappropriate proposal of marriage was a reactivation of the very early problem of failure to develop an integrated ego. This person developed a limited capacity to clearly evaluate the realities of the situation in which she found herself. In addition, the weak ego development made it difficult if not impossible to resolve the conflicts between the id drives (interest in sex and marriage) and demands of the superego (the incorporated standards of her parents). Likewise, she had never been able to effectively repress hostile aggressive drives and expressed these feelings freely by tearing out the light fixture.

When Frances saw the face of her future husband in the light fixture, she was exhibiting a severe mental symptom called visual hallucinations. Hallucinations are one example of the personality disintegration that takes place in individuals suffering from an active psychosis. Hallucinations, like all symptoms, meet a basic need. In this situation the face supplied an answer for her that was an outgrowth of her unconscious longings and her inability to find answers to her own sexual needs through coping adequately with the social situation.

Hallucinations are an example of being out of touch with reality. This means that the person is reacting to a stimulus from within the unconscious mind that is unrelated to the real situation. The behavior of such a person becomes extremely confusing when she reacts part of the time to stimuli from the real world and part of the time to stimuli from within her own unconscious mind.

Planning and implementing nursing care for Frances B.

The assessment data, including present behavior, past life experiences, and understanding of the underlying dynamics, lead to the development of a nursing diagnosis for Frances B. It should be clearly understood that there is usually more than one way to state a nursing diagnosis; the important ideas to remember are that (1) the nursing diagnosis should be based on a synthesis of the assessment data and (2) it should give clear direction for developing specific plans for intervention.

For Frances, we might state that this is a young woman who, because of lack of development of satisfactory relationships with a mothering one and significant others and feelings of being abandoned by these persons and therefore of being "bad," has learned to cope by withdrawing from interpersonal situations in which she might be hurt, by regressing, and by trying to atone for being bad. Her behavior also reflects her failure to develop an integrated ego and positive self-concept. The planning of nursing care for Frances, then, would be directed toward providing corrective experiences in (1) developing a satisfactory relationship with another person (initially one nurse), (2) learning not to fear the risk of being abandoned, and (3) reaching a higher level of self-esteem. Other aspects of her nursing care plan should include adequate nutrition, discouragement of regressive behavior, and protection from attempts at self-destruction.

Since it was not possible to deal with all aspects of the nursing diagnosis at once, the logical starting point in carrying out the plan was the establishment of a positive relationship with Frances. It was hoped that this relationship would lead to the development of some communication with her.

Because the nurse knew that schizophrenic persons are highly sensitive of their fear of rejection, the approach to Frances was unhurried, warm, friendly, and accepting. The nurse found it necessary to make repeated verbal overtures and to modify her own nonverbal messages to Frances before Frances was able to respond.

It was decided that the entire responsibility for the nursing care of Frances during the first weeks of her hospital experience would be assigned to a few carefully chosen nurses. This decision was made because the staff recognized that Frances needed to develop a feeling of security and to learn to trust other people. Security can be enhanced by limiting the number of individuals with whom such ill persons come in contact and by keeping their daily routines much the same for several months. In the beginning, few demands were made on Frances.

It is recognized that the attitude of the people with whom mentally ill persons come in contact during the early part of their illness has a significant effect on their recovery. Persons such as Frances require consistent acceptance, sincere interest, and constant encouragement from nurses and the other members of the professional staff.

Although communication with Frances was difficult because she used language in a highly personal way, it was important for the nurse to spend time sitting with her and talking to her even though she rarely responded verbally. The nurse used simple, uncomplicated, direct statements when talking to her.

These nursing interventions were related to the plan for development of a satisfactory relationship with a significant other, which would in turn decrease Frances's fears of abandonment. In addition, much of her behavior was symptomatic of an individual who felt unworthy and guilty, and it was obvious that Frances's self-esteem was badly shattered. Thus the nurse's efforts were focused on trying to assist Frances to develop a more positive attitude toward herself. This was partially achieved by the attention provided for her and the sincere, interested way in which it was given. Self-esteem was also enhanced through the mechanism of assisting her to improve her grooming.

Early in Frances's hospital experience it was necessary for a nurse to assume a good deal of responsibility for bathing and dressing her, but in time she was encouraged to assume more and more responsibility for this activity herself. The nurses gently suggested that she would enjoy visiting the beauty parlor. At first they accompanied her on these trips and remained with her while she was there. As Frances began to feel more secure in the situation, she was able to accept most of the responsibility for her own grooming.

The dietary intake for persons who refuse food is always of great concern. Because Frances was regressed when she was first admitted, the nurses tried to help her in feeding herself by making suggestions such as, "Pick up your fork" and "Put the food in your mouth." This plan was used because it was thought that she was unable to make the necessary decisions herself. However, it was eventually necessary to spoon-feed her. The nurses used an unhurried, relaxed manner and fed her from a tray in her own room.

During the spoon-feeding periods the nurses gave Frances many opportunities to take the spoon in her own hand and assume some of the responsibility for feeding herself during a part of the meal. After a few weeks she was encouraged to return to the dining room and take her meals with others.

The problem of self-destruction was especially distressing. Criticism and reprimands for this behavior were withheld because the nurses realized that it would confirm her opinion that she was indeed a bad person. The close personal attention Frances received when she was first admitted solved the problem of self-destruction during the early part of her hospitalization. However, she was helped to reestablish her own inner controls, and the nurse served as an external authority until Frances was able to accept responsibility for her own safety.

With such close association with the nurses, Frances eventually became dependent on them. They then realized that it was important to introduce a second client into the situation as soon as possible. This was accomplished by a second client visiting the beauty parlor with Frances and the nurse.

Recreational activities were introduced into Frances's daily routine after a reasonable amount of time in the hospital had elapsed. The nurse and a second client involved themselves with Frances in finger painting and clay modeling. These activities were chosen because they have a special appeal for regressed persons.

Nursing intervention for Frances included many of the nursing roles described in Chapter 3. The effectiveness of the nursing care plan for Frances might be evaluated by periodic reassessment and development of new nursing diagnoses. These new diagnoses will reflect a more functional state of mental health if the plan has been a sound one and if implementation has been characterized by warm and skillful use of self.

Outlook for Frances B.

Although Frances was able to learn to relate to other people in a more positive way and to move from the hospital to a girls' club, her future ability to achieve a productive adjustment is uncertain. As described in the case formulation, this individual suffered a lifetime of unsatisfactory adaptation and developed a defective prepsychotic personality. As early as the twelfth year, her behavior was so unusual as to suggest that she was mentally ill. Thus it is obvious that the illness from which Frances suffered developed slowly and insidiously and actually was the unfolding of a damaged personality. Her prepsychotic interests were limited and focused on a dog, which gave affection without making any demands, and on mathematics, which was totally intellectual in nature and did not require her to relate to other people.

The acute manifestations of the illness were precipitated by Frances's inability to handle her own unconscious sexual urges. The fact that she received psychiatric help late in the development of the illness does not improve the outlook for her future recovery. A person with Frances's problems would probably require a sheltered living situation for the rest of her life. She would probably always need to return to the hospital for treatment from time to time.

Although Frances has been described as being intellectually capable, it is unlikely that she would be able to use her abilities in some future work. She lacks the coping skills necessary to deal with the problems and difficulties related to performing a demanding intellectual task.

For several years, if not for the remainder of her life, Frances would need to be kept on a maintenance dose of one of the antipsychotic drugs. Unfortunately, such drugs can only improve psychotic behavior; they cannot reconstruct the personality.

CASE FORMULATION □ A SUSPICIOUS INDIVIDUAL

The following is the case history of an individual whose maladaptive thought processes resulted in abnormal suspicions.

> Allen T. was born of parents who were not of the same racial background. His father was an engineer and died as a result of an explosion when Allen was 10 years of age. He lived in a run-down part of the city with his mother. He made few friends among the other children who lived in that section of the city. Very early in his life he developed an interest in mechanics. He was a good student but rather aloof and decidedly sensitive. He spent his leisure hours studying chemistry and physics in the city library. At the age of 15 he had a fight in the school yard with a boy who called his mother a foul name. After this affair he had very little to do with other young people, except those who were interested in a religious mission he attended regularly.
>
> He was ascetic in his tastes, drank no liquor, did not smoke, and showed little interest in girls. On graduation from high school he worked for 2 years in a tile factory as a shipping clerk. At this time he was awarded a schloarship and matriculated in college. There his social condition did not improve, since the students avoided him and he displayed no interest in them. At the end of 2 years his scholarship lapsed, and having no resources of his own, he returned home and resumed his work with the same company that previously employed him.
>
> At the city mission during prayer meetings and on Sunday he gave long testimonials and believed that he was a promising preacher. During the absence of the regular minister in the summer he expected to be asked to serve as a substitute. When another man was called, Allen expressed his resentment openly at the next meeting and resigned from

the congregation. A few weeks later his mother died. He lived alone in a small upstairs apartment that he was able to maintain because his mother had left a small legacy. Here he secluded himself for many weeks and emerged only once a day to buy a few groceries and a bottle of milk. One day his landlady, who lived on the first floor, fearing that he was ill, climbed the stairs and knocked on the door. Receiving no answer, she obtained a key and on opening the door was struck with a baseball bat. She managed to call the police, who were compelled to use force to subdue the young man.

When interviewed at a mental health treatment center, he refused to give his name. He wore a pointed beard and a loose gown resembling a monk's robe. He said, "Yes I am an engineer—to be exact, I am God's engineer. Do not concern yourself over my real name, it has enough stigma attached to it now. No, I am not married, but I have been tried by all the lures that women possess. No, I don't use rotten liquor or filthy tobacco—I am made for higher things. My enemies follow me everywhere I go and make obscene comments about me on the walls of public washrooms. I am offered only menial positions so as to keep me penniless most of the time. They put their heads together and scheme their dastardly plans.

"See this sore [pointing to a varicose ulcer]? This is where they inducted me with their electrical currents. That is why I slept in a 'nonconductor' bed. I made it myself and suspended it from insulators fixed in the ceiling. The landlady came up to destroy my devices because the bishop of her church had ordered her to do so. The modern church is determined to destroy me because I preach the older creeds. [Proudly] Why should I not be hailed as the second Christ?"

Allen's attitude and unusual ideas remained unchanged for many months. He showed little interest in or concern for entering into activities with others. He refused to shave or have his hair cut, had little interest in recreational or occupational activities, and spent most of his time staring out a window.

Discussion of development of patterns of behavior

Unfortunately, too little is reported in Allen T.'s case history to tell us much about his early childhood relationship with his mother, but there are suggestions about the results of that relationship from which certain conclusions can be drawn.

It will be clear to almost anyone reading this history that Allen is gravely mentally ill and that he suffers from persistent and systematized delusions. In most instances this individual's behavior would be diagnosed as indicating schizophrenia, paranoid type. These delusions can be classified as delusions of grandeur ("I am God's own engineer") and persecutory delusions ("Electrical currents have been run into my body").

This young man has developed these ideas to defend himself against what he perceives as a hostile world. However, his view of the hostile world is actually a reflection of his own anger (evidenced by his striking the landlady over the head with a baseball bat).

As a child of racially mixed marriage, he was faced with a difficult social situation. Thus he likely felt that he was confronted with an essentially hostile world at school and became an isolate.

In this situation being an only child left him with no ally at home or at school. His father died when Allen was 10 years of age. Normally a child of 10 is beginning to emancipate himself from the family by seeking security and companionship from peer groups of the same sex. At this period in the child's psychosexual development he normally seeks a companion or chum with whom he can share some of his self-love. Part of the tragedy of this individual's life lies in the fact that he did not develop a chum relationship with another boy of his age and did not belong to a peer group as do most 10-year-old boys. This defect in his development may have been caused in part by the family problem with which he was faced. However, it may also have been caused by the emotional relationship that developed between him and his mother. Some authorities believe that paranoid reactions have their developmental origins in the conflicts the child experiences with the mother in the first and second years of life. If the mother is overly possessive of the son, the child's psychosexual development may never advance beyond the homosexual level. Since his father died when Allen was 10 years of age and the boy had no companions, one may conclude that his relationship with his mother was unusually close. At any rate, he sought refuge in the study of science and spent much time in a library, a place where everyone is usually welcome and no social demands are made.

At 15 years of age this individual fought with a boy who maligned his mother. This was a physical act of self-defense as well as defense of his mother. After this event his social activities were confined to attending a small city mission. People who attend missions are probably more accepting of individual differences than are most individuals. Undoubtedly the city mission was a haven for Allen, who felt that the world was a hostile, unfriendly place.

He began to develop ascetic tastes that may have been designed to assist him to be more acceptable to the mission group. He drank no liquor, did not smoke, and evidenced no interest in girls. These activities represent areas of personal life about which most religious groups have prohibitions. To live up to these rules was one way of achieving acceptance and approval in this group.

After high school graduation this intellectually capable young man, who once had an interest in the sciences, went to work in a tile factory for 2 years. This move was undoubtedly made because of an economic need, but it must have been a dull, monotonous job and a great disappointment to one with academic aspirations.

After 2 years at the tile factory he obtained a scholarship and attended college. Here again he made no friends. When the scholarship ended, he returned to the tile factory, but soon the people at the city mission noticed that he was acting in an unusual way and thought himself ready to serve as the minister at the mission. When another man was chosen, he expressed hostility and resentment and resigned from the congregation. His mother's death was added to the disappointment of having to leave college, having to return to the tile factory, and not having been recognized by the city mission as the minister that he believed himself to be.

For this lonely, rejected young man the loss of his mother represented the loss of the only close human companionship he had ever known.

He attempted to carry on and to live without working at the tile factory because his mother had left him a little money. Thus he secluded himself. This action eventually led to the incident of striking the landlady and being admitted to a mental health treatment center.

When he entered the center, he was dressed as a monk and refused to give his name. Since the world was so hostile and painful for him, he had assumed the role of a man of God and had withdrawn from it altogether. This individual, like all people, had a reason for his behavior. He struck the landlady on the head to protect himself because he believed that she had come on the order of the bishop of her church to destroy his protective devices (a nonconductor bed to avoid the electrical currents people were sending through his body). In addition, he believed that churches were persecuting him because his own mission had refused to accept him as a minister. The delusion of being God's engineer had a protective meaning for him. It provided an outlet for his mechanical interests, and since he was chosen by God to be an engineer, it was obvious that he must be excellent.

Thus, through his delusions, this individual had achieved those things he could not achieve in real life. He was unconsciously using projection (blaming others for his own shortcomings and deficiencies) to defend his ego and to establish his superiority.

In this individual we have an example of a person who was ambitious but whose strivings were continuously frustrated. His continued failure to achieve highly valued goals and the need to enhance his own self-esteem caused him to resort to very unusual and paranoid defenses. With an already faulty personality development he was unable to cope with the many anxiety-producing factors in a life filled with problems over which he had little control.

Planning and implementing nursing care for Allen T.

When Allen T. entered the treatment center, he contined to wear the loose-fitting gown in which he arrived until he voluntarily exchanged it for a business suit. His unusual garb was not discouraged because the workers realized that suspicious individuals respond negatively to an authoritarian approach and that flexibility should be maintained whenever possible.

The person who admitted Allen avoided touching him because she realized that suspicious individuals frequently misinterpret such actions and believe them to be sexual overtures. She went about the admission procedure in a calm, self-assured way in the hope that by her approach she could help him to begin to develop a trusting relationship with the staff members. She was careful to speak to him clearly and to enunciate precisely to minimize opportunities for misinterpreting her comments.

During Allen's stay in the center, the professional staff tried to be consistent in their approach to him and to be meticulously honest in answering his questions. They made a special effort to treat him with respect, since they realized that suspicious persons are easily offended. The staff avoided arguing with him about his delusions and made no comment when he stated that he was the lamb of God. They accepted the fact that he would not answer to his legal name and refrained from calling him by name. The staff at the center meticulously labeled Allen's personal belongings and were careful to see that they were never confused with those of others.

He was invited to participate in group activities but his decision was accepted without discussion when he declined. They kept a supply of recreational materials on hand, which could be used by him in his room without involving other individuals.

When Allen became hostile and falsely accused the staff of misdeeds, they accepted his sarcasm without becoming angry and avoided adopting a punitive attitude toward him. They sought to help him feel accepted and important.

Large doses of an antipsychotic medication were ordered for Allen. Interestingly, he took this medication without protest, and his delusional state began to abate within 2 weeks. The nurse assigned to give him care began a nurse-client relationship with the goal of helping him to establish a trusting relationship with another human being. The long-term goal of this relationship was to help Allen learn to test reality in a more effective manner. He was discharged from the inpatient treatment setting within a month of his admission, but continued seeing the nurse for psychotherapy and supervision of medications.

Outlook for Allen T.

Allen T. was able to achieve a modicum of social recovery from his psychosis. With the understanding support and guidance of his nurse therapist and the continuation of a maintenance dose of an antipsychotic medication, he was able to obtain a job and maintain himself in his own apartment. His social relationships remained problematic, and he had few constructive leisure time activities.

CONCLUDING STATEMENTS

1. When an individual is functioning on the basis of a grossly distorted perception of reality, he is said to be psychotic.
2. When an individual's distorted perceptions of reality result from and contribute to maladaptive thought processes, that individual may be suffering from schizophrenia.
3. Schizophrenia is one of the most serious mental illnesses with which any individual can be afflicted, and it is the most prevalent of the functional mental illnesses.
4. To be diagnosed as schizophrenic, the individual must exhibit characteristic delusions, characteristic hallucinations, or other characteristic symptoms of thought impairment accompanied by either blunted, flat, or inappropriate affect.
5. Schizophrenia is classified into five major types, depending on the predominant behavioral patterns the individual uses in his attempt to achieve security.
6. There is no conclusive scientific proof of the cause of schizophrenia, but the theory that seems to have the most relevance for nursing practice is the one that postulates that faulty interpersonal relationships in the early family relationship are a major contributory factor to the ultimate development of the illness.
7. It is believed that the development of schizophrenia is a longstanding process, although the acute symptoms may appear abruptly, usually during adolescence or early adulthood.
8. Schizophrenic persons are insecure in their relations with others, are highly sensitive, lack a sense of personal value, and have a poor self-image.
9. Schizophrenic persons direct their libidinal energies toward themselves and are thus said to be narcissistic and introverted.
10. Individuals suffering from schizophrenia seem to have lost the ability to respond normally to joy, sorrow, and fear.

11. The outlook for a person suffering from a schizophrenic reaction depends on the effectiveness of his prepsychotic personality, the nature of the onset of the illness, and the timing and nature of the treatment he receives.
12. An individualized nursing care plan, based on a nursing diagnosis that reflects an understanding of the assessment data, enables the nurse to select appropriate interventions that act as corrective experiences for these individuals and, hopefully, enable them to change their behavior. The nurse learns to assume a variety of roles in carrying out these interventions.

Suggested sources of additional information

CLASSICAL

Andrews, Dixie: Process recording on a schizophrenic hebephrenic patient, Perspect. Psychiatr. Care **1**:11-39, Nov., 1963.

Bateson, Gregory, et al.: Toward a theory of schizophrenia. In Howells, J.G., editor: Theory and practice of family psychiatry, New York, 1971, Brunner Mazel, Inc.

Bellak, Leopold, and Loeb, Laurence, editors: The schizophrenic syndrome, New York, 1969, Gune & Stratton, Inc.

Carl, Mary Kathryn: Establishing a relationship with a schizophrenic patient, Perspect. Psychiatr. Care **1**:20-22, March-April, 1963.

Chrzanowski, Gerard: Cultural and pathological manifestations of paranoia, Perspect, Psychiatr. Care **1**:34-42, Sept.-Oct., 1963.

Cook, J.C.: Interpreting and decoding autistic communication, Perspect. Psychiatr. Care **9**:24-28, Jan.-Feb., 1971.

Dunham, H.W.: Sociocultural studies of schizophrenia, Arch. Gen. Psychiatry **21**:206-214, 1971.

Field, William E., and Ruelke, Wylma: Hallucinations and how to deal with them, Am. J. Nurs. **73**:638-640, 1973.

Goodman, Lillian R., and LaBelle, Mary J.: The schizophrenic's mother, Nurs. Outlook **11**:753-754, 1963.

Gregory, D.: Rusell and I (an experience with autism), Perspect. Psychiatr. Care **9**:29, Jan.-Feb., 1971.

Kaplan, Bert: The inner world of mental illness: a series of first person accounts of what it was like, New York, 1964, Harper & Row, Publishers.

Kline, Nathan S.: Synopsis of Eugen Blueler's dementia praecox, New York, 1966, International Universities Press.

Lidz, Theodore, Fleck, Stephen, and Cornelison, Alice R.: Schizophrenia and the family, New York, 1967, International Universities Press.

Lipkin, Gladys B., and Cohen, Roberta G.: Effective approaches to patients' behavior, New York, 1980, Springer Publishing Co., Inc.

Peplau, Hildegard E.: Loneliness, Am. J. Nurs. **55**:1476-1481, 1955.

Robinson, Alice M.: Communicating with schizophrenic patients, Am. J. Nurs **60**:1120-1123, 1960.

Schwartz, Charlotte Green, Schwartz, Morris S., and Stanton, Alfred H.: A study of need-fulfillment on a mental hospital ward, Psychiatry **14:**223-242, 1951.

Schwartz, Morris S., and Shockley, Emmy L.: The nurse and the mental patient, New York, 1956, John Wiley & Sons, Inc.

Schwartz, Morris S., and Will, Gwen Tudor: Low morale and mutual withdrawal on a mental hospital ward, Psychiatry **16:**337-353, 1953.

Searles, Harold: The nonhuman environment in normal development and in schizophrenia, New York, 1960, International Universities Press.

Sechehaye, Marguerite: Autobiography of a schizophrenic girl, New York, 1970, W.W. Norton Co. & Inc.

Stankiewicz, Barbara: Guides to nursing intervention in the projective patterns of suspicious patients, Perspect. Psychiatr. Care **2**(1):39-45, 1964.

Sullivan, Harry Stack: Conceptions of modern psychiatry, Washington, D.C., 1953, W.W. Norton & Co., Inc.

Tudor, Gwen: A sociopsychiatric nursing approach to intervention in a problem of mutual withdrawal on a mental hospital ward, Perspect. Psychiatr. Care **8:**11-35, Jan.-Feb., 1970.

Ujhely, Gertrud B.: Nursing intervention with the acutely ill psychiatric patient, Nurs. Forum **8:**311-325, 1969.

Van Huben, Betty J.: Discussion of a process recording on a schizophrenic, hebephrenic patient, Perspect. Psychiatr. Care **1:**40-44, Nov., 1963.

CONTEMPORARY

Aaronson, Lauren S.: Paranoia as a behavior of alienation, Perspect. Psychiatr. Care **15**(1):27-31, 1977.

Aloi, Janice P.: Birth fantasy as a reaction to separation from the therapist, Perspect. Psychiatr. Care **15**(2):82-84, 1977.

Anders, Robert L.: When a patient becomes violent, Am. J. Nurs. **77:**1144-1148, July, 1977.

Anderson, Nancy P.: Suicide in schizophrenia, Perspect. Psychiatr. Care **11**(2):106-112, 1973.

Arieti, Silvano: Schizophrenia: the psychodynamic mechanisms and the psychostructural forms. In Arieti, Solvano, and Brody, Eugene B., editors: American handbook of psychiatry, ed. 2, vol. 3, New York, 1974, Basic Books, Inc., Publishers, pp. 551-587.

Arieti, Silvano: Understanding and helping the schizophrenic, New York, 1980, Basic Books, Inc., Publishers.

Bemporad, Jules R., and Pinsker, Henry: Schizophrenia: the manifest symptomatology. In Arieti, Silvano, and Brody, Eugene B., editors: American handbook of psychiatry, ed. 2, vol. 3, New York, 1974, Basic Books, Inc., Publishers, pp. 524-550.

Cameron, Norman: Paranoid conditions and paranoia. In Arieti, Silvano, and Brody, Eugene, B., editors: American handbook of psychiatry, ed. 2, vol. 3, New York, 1974, Basic Books, Inc., Publishers pp. 676-693.

Donner, Gail: Treatment of a delusional patient, Am. J. Nurs. **69:**2642-2644, 1969.

Fochtman, Grace A.: Disturbances in object relations in a chronic schizophrenic patient, Perspect. Psychiatr. Care **13:**1, 13-16, Jan.-March, 1975.

Geach, Barbara, and White, James C.: Empathetic resonance: a counter-transference phenomenon, Am. J. Nurs. **74:**1282-1285, 1974.

Grosicki, J., and Harmonson, M.: Nursing action guide: hallucinations, J. Psychiatr. Nurs. **7:**134, May, 1979.

Jones, Susan L.: The double-bind as a "tested" theoretical formulation—five research studies are reviewed here, Perspect. Psychiatr. Care, **15**(4):162-169, 1977.

Kent, Elizabeth: A token economy program for schizophrenic patients, Perspect. Psychiatr. Care **8:**174-185, July-Aug., 1970.

Kerr, Norine: Anxiety: theoretical considerations, Perspect. Psychiatr. Care **16**(1):36-40, Jan.-Feb., 1978.

Kerr, Norine: The destruction of "goodness" in the borderline character pathology, Perspect. Psychiatr. Care **17**(1):40-47, Jan.-Feb., 1979.

Kolb, Lawrence C.: Modern clinical psychiatry, ed. 8, Philadelphia, 1977, W.B. Saunders Co.

Lynch, Vincent J., and Lynch, Mary Theresa: Borderline personality, Perspect. Psychiatr. Care **15**(2):72-75, 1977.

Lyon, Glee G., and Hitchins, Emily A.: Ways of intervening with the psychotic individual in the community, Am. J. Nurs. **79:**490-493, March, 1979.

McArdle, Karen: Dialogue in thought, Am. J. Nurs. **74:**1075-1077, 1974.

McCown, Pauline P., and Wurm, Elizabeth: Orienting the disoriented, Am. J. Nurs. **65:**118-119, April, 1965.

Masterson, James, editor, et al.: New perspectives on psychotherapy of the borderline adult, New York, 1979, Brunner/Mazel, Inc.

Maurine, Judith T.: Regressed patients in group therapy, Perspect. Psychiatr. Care **8:**131-135, May-June, 1970.

Moser, Dorthy Hale: Communicating with a schizophrenic patient, Perspect. Psychiatr. Care **8:**36-41, 45, Jan.-Feb., 1970.

Ostendorf, Mary: Dan is schizophrenic—possible causes, probable courses, Am. J. Nurs. **76:**944-947, 1976.

Reid, Linda: Approaches to the aftermath of schizophrenia, Perspect. Psychiatr. Care **17**(6):257-259, Nov.-Dec., 1979.

Rosenbaum, C. Peter, and Beebe, John E., III: Psychiatric treatment; crisis, clinic, consultation, New York, 1975, McGraw-Hill Book Co., pp. 88-89.

Sarbin, Theodore R., and Mancuso, James C.: Schizophrenia, medical diagnosis or moral verdict? New York, 1980, Pergamon Press, Inc.

Schroder, Patricia J.: Nursing intervention with patients with thought disorders, Perspect. Psychiatr. Care **17**(1):32-39, Jan.-Feb., 1979.

Spire, Richard H.: Photographic self-image confrontation, Am. J. Nurs. **73:**1207-1210, 1973.

Steiger, Thelma B.: Shadow child, Am. J. Nurs. **73:**2080-2086, 1973.

Stewart, Barbara M.: Biochemical aspects of schizophrenia, Am. J. Nurs. **75:**2176-2179, 1975.

Thomas, M.: Trust in the nurse-patient relationship. In Carlson, C., editor: Behavioral concepts and nursing intervention, Philadelphia, 1970, J.B. Lippincott Co.

Wilson, Janet S.: Deciphering psychotic communication, Perspect. Psychiatr. Care **17**(6):254-256, Nov.-Dec., 1979.

OF PARTICULAR INTEREST

Bateson, G., et al.: Toward a theory of schizophrenia. In Howells, J.G., editor: Theory and practice of family psychiatry, New York, 1971, Brunner/Mazel, Inc.

This classic paper presents the double-bind theory of communication patterns in families of schizophrenic clients.

Ruesch, J.: Disturbed communication, New York, 1972, W.W. Norton & Co., Inc.

Communication patterns associated with various psychiatric disorders are described and analyzed according to the author's framework of communication patterns and designing appropriate interventions.

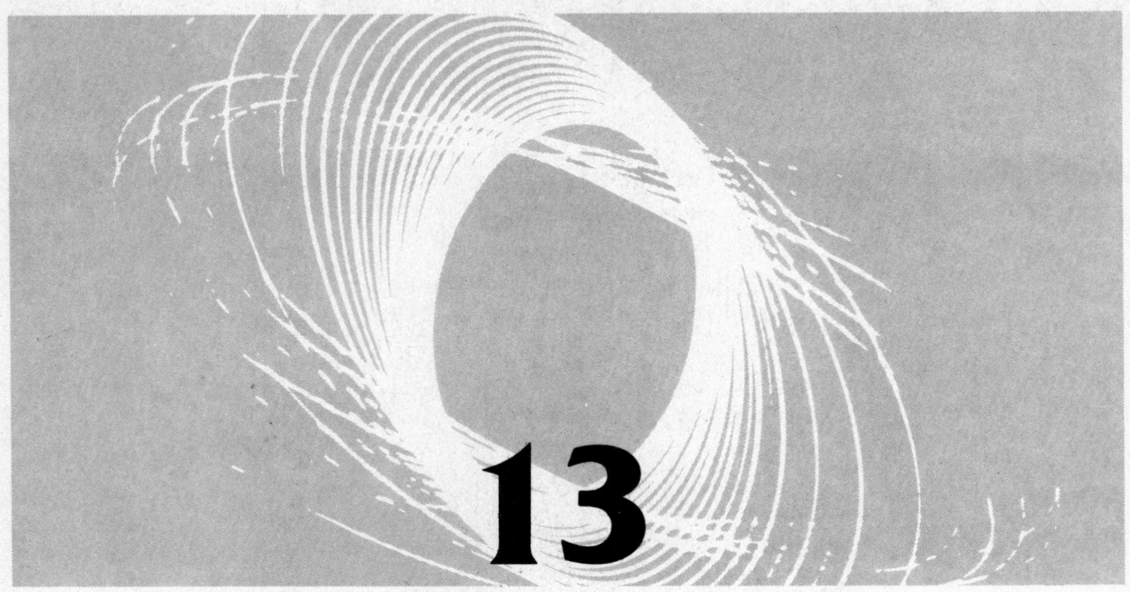

13

Behavioral patterns that reflect maladaptive mood states

- Differentiation between schizophrenic and affective disorders
- Differentiation between grief and depression
- Causative factors of affective disorders
- Nursing care of the depressed individual
- Nursing care of the elated, overactive individual
- Outlook for overactive and depressed individuals

Some individuals defend against extreme feelings of anxiety, loneliness, inadequacy, and failure by means of overactivity, elated mood, and excessive talkativeness. The elated mood may be so pronounced and sustained that the individual expresses the belief that every good thing is possible or will soon be consummated and every wish will be fulfilled. Ideas emerge in an easy, fluidlike manner; thinking seems to be effortless; memory is quickened; and the individual shows a quick but superficial wit. There is an apparent sense of self-security, and fears are pushed to the background. The individual may be aggressive, cocksure in his opinions, and ready to talk with conviction on anything and everything. The ego seems to be unrestrained, and ideas pour out so rapidly and with such ease that the tongue cannot give them full expression. Hence the individual may utter only segments of ideas and may jump from one to another in a rapid barrage. He has a quick recognition of persons and objects and a tendency to argue. The person is apt to be domineering and becomes irritable, denunciatory, and hypercritical of everything that interferes with his desire for free action. He is likely to become overactive and may extend this excessive motor excitement in every direction. When limits must be set for his behavior, he sometimes becomes noisy, belligerent, and violent. His insight is always poor. This person's interest is in the outside world rather than in himself. His ideation is concerned with his environment. In fact, the individual can almost be said to be at the mercy of his environment.

Surprising as it may seem, at another time such an aggressive, overactive individual may use quite different behavior to defend against the same bad feelings. Within a few months he may be sad, may have difficulty in thinking and expressing thoughts, and may be very slow in his physical responses, or he may exhibit agitation.

Such a person may have difficulty in formulating answers, may lose his ability to concentrate, and may be unable to choose a direct line of action. The individual may be tormented by a sense of insecurity or by ideas of remorse and self-abasement or may be overcome by a sense of guilt. He may complain of a total lack of affection and of a loss of interest in the things for which he formerly had much concern. He may feel that he is lost or being punished. Such a person may have an overpowering sense of futility, a "feeling of emptiness," and a desire to retreat from everything, to seek oblivion, and to end his life. Danger of suicide is the outstanding feature of this condition, and this alone justifies the greatest caution and consideration from the standpoint of care and treatment.

Such behavior as overactivity and elation or depression places the individual in the diagnostic category of *bipolar affective disorder*. In 1896 Emil Kraepelin identified this condition and called it manic-depressive psychosis. It the person maintains behavior marked by elation and overactivity, he is said to be in the manic phase of this illness. If the behavior is predominantly characteristic of depression, the individual is said to be in the depressed phase of this illness. When the individual's behavior moves from depression to elation or from elation to depression he is said to have a mixed bipolar affective disorder.

Although bipolar affective disorder is a common type of maladaptive mood state, many individuals suffer from an affective psychosis that expresses itself in either mania or depression. The principles stated in the following discussion are applicable to these maladaptive mood states regardless of medical diagnosis.

DIFFERENTIATION BETWEEN SCHIZOPHRENIC AND AFFECTIVE DISORDERS

It is sometimes difficult for students of nursing to differentiate between the overactivity demonstrated by some schizophrenic individuals and the overactivity that the manic individual exhibits. Both of these individuals may be physically overactive, and at times both may talk excessively. The schizophrenic individual who exhibits catatonic behavior may fluctuate from being almost stuporous to exhibiting explosive overactivity. In such a situation the individual is probably responding to inner thoughts and feelings that are not related to reality but that are threatening, upsetting, and disturbing. This type of overactivity is especially difficult to understand because there is often disharmony between the mood and the ideas expressed. The person may smile inappropriately or laugh while speaking of the disturbing thoughts that are uppermost in his mind. He may express terrifying visual or auditory hallucinations.

In contrast, the overactivity of an individual who is said to be displaying manic behavior is characterized by glib argumentative speech that may be humorous but may change quickly to sarcasm and verbal abuse. Such a person may appear to have boundless energy. He is usually irrepressible, demanding, and irritable. He frequently expresses ideas of grandeur and delusions of having great power and wealth. There is a dominant tone of euphoria even though the person may demonstrate an underlying mood of sorrow. Authorities believe that the overactivity of the manic individual is actually a defense against depression. The professional person usually finds that manic overactivity is understandable because the client maintains some contact with reality except in the most extreme examples of this illness.

Withdrawal and depression may be difficult for the beginning student of nursing to differentiate because individuals suffering from these states are usually physically inactive. However, the schizophrenic individual who is withdrawn demonstrates a disharmony of thought, feeling, and behavior. Although there may be a persistent mood, it has little apparent relationship to the situation in which the person finds himself or to his past experiences. In contrast, everything about the depressed individual conveys a depressed feeling to the observer. The way the person sits, the facial expression, the voice quality, and the ideas expressed all suggest hopelessness and a sense of impending doom. Depressed individuals remain well aware of reality, and their feelings seem understandable to individuals working with them.

Some authorities believe that the attempt to differentiate these behavioral reactions is actually an artificial and unwarranted exercise. These authorities suggest that they may be aspects of one broad disease entity.

DIFFERENTIATION BETWEEN GRIEF AND DEPRESSION

Grief is a human condition characterized by a disturbance in mood. It is a reaction that the nurse will observe frequently throughout her professional career. Grief is a normal, common, necessary reaction to the loss of a beloved individual or object to which a person is emotionally attached. The nurse may help the grieving person to cope with his sense of loss and guilt by encouraging him to talk about his feelings. The goal is to assist the individual to integrate this emotional reaction with similar experiences in his past and to learn from it.

Depression is a profound disturbance in mood that shares some characteristics with grief; however, it differs in many ways. Depression is not as common an experience as grief, but it occurs frequently. Certainly all nurses should be able to recognize the normal malfunctioning of the mechanism of adaptation to an object loss and should be able to differentiate between the normal reaction called grieving and the pathological elaboration of grief, which is called depression. The nurse needs to recognize that normal grieving should be encouraged and that it usually terminates within a few months or a year without professional help. In contrast, depression is not self-limiting, usually does not improve without professional help, and is dangerous for the individual because of the problem of suicide.

The following listing contrasts grief and depression in terms of cause, symptoms, and outcome.

Grief (bereavement)

1. Grief is a disturbance in mood that is normal, universal, and necessary in the life experience of individuals.
2. Grief is a reaction to the *real* loss of a highly valued object that may be tangible or intangible.
3. Grief is a developmentally evolved adaptive process and is closely related to the ability to develop meaningful object relationships.
4. Grief is self-limiting and gradually diminishes over a period of about a year.
5. Except in the very early, acute stage, grief is not incapacitating.
6. The three phases of normal grieving are
   a. Shock and disbelief.

Depression

1. Depression is a disturbance in mood that is a reaction to the actual, threatened, or imagined loss of a valued object, tangible or intangible. The loss, basically rooted in the individual's fantasy life, has great symbolic value. It is an overwhelming response to what the individual considers a catastrophic loss.
2. Depression is a pathological elaboration of grief. It is related to grief but is not the same.
3. The reaction of loss in depression goes beyond grief in duration and intensity. Depression is prolonged, severe, and increasingly incapacitating in all areas of the individual's life.

Grief (bereavement)	Depression
b. Developing awareness of the pain of the loss, which eventually results in crying. c. Restitution, which involves the mourning experience and eventual elevation of the memory of the lost object to a degree of perfection. (This is usually completed within a year, and new objects replace the lost ones.)	4. Depression does not enter the phase of restitution within a few weeks or months and is not self-limiting. Professional help is often required. 5. Depression represents a malfunction in the normal mechanism of adaptation to the loss of a valued object.

CAUSATIVE FACTORS OF AFFECTIVE DISORDERS

Mood deviations that are extreme enough to be categorized as either manic or depressive episodes have no specific causative factors that can be identified with scientific certainty. Many scientists believe that there is a hereditary factor operating, since 60% or 80% of these individuals come from families in which this illness has occurred.

The psychiatrists who accept the theoretical explanations of behavior that have been developed by the psychoanalytic school believe that extreme mood deviations involving elation and depression are closely related to the early feeding experiences of the infant. During this period the mother who provides food and attention is both an object of love and a source of frustration for the infant. Ambivalent feelings of both love and hate for the mothering person may be initiated in this early period and may be carried out throughout life. In adult life ambivalent feelings are directed toward the environment and the significant persons in the environment. Individuals who develop extreme mood deviations such as elation and depression are thought to be reacting to the unconscious loss of a real or fantasied love object that was incorporated at an early phase of personality development. The individual first responds as if mourning for the lost love object and eventually begins to express hostility because he feels abandoned. The aggressive, overactivity of mania is thought to be a defense against the real problem of depression.

In depression the individual is thought to turn his hostility toward himself. He feels that he is at fault, that he is responsible for the loss of the love object, and that he is unworthy; thus he hates himself. He is said to be at the mercy of a punishing, sadistic superego. Such an individual has many narcissistic love needs. His adult relationships are likely to be immature and dependent. The lifelong problems with which these individuals struggle are hostility and the feelings of guilt that the hostility precipitates when their security is threatened.

NURSING CARE OF THE DEPRESSED INDIVIDUAL

The depressed individual expresses despair, gloom, a sense of foreboding, feelings of guilt, ideas of self-depreciation, and self-accusatory delusions. The need that many inexperienced nurses feel to "cheer him up" is not helpful and often actually causes him to feel more guilty and unworthy than ever. When working with a depressed individual, such statements as, "Buck up," "Let's see you smile," or "There is a silver lining in every cloud" are not helpful. Gaiety and laughter have a tendency to make such a person feel more guilty and thus more morose. The nurse can be most helpful by being friendly in a kind, understanding, businesslike way. Attempts at changing his mood through logical suggestions are fruitless and should be avoided. Sometimes just sitting beside the person without trying to carry on a conversation is helpful. At other times it is effective to talk to him even though he may not answer. He will appreciate the personal interest being shown. Patience is the keynote in working with depressed individuals who are so greatly retarded in the spheres of thinking, feeling, and acting that every movement or word requires great effort and much time. The same question often needs to be asked more than once, and the nurse must wait patiently for the answer. A large part of the therapeutic value of the hospital situation lies in the fact that decisions can be made for the individual. Thus the nurse should avoid asking such questions as, "Do you want to take your bath now?" A more positive approach would be, "Your bath is ready now. I will help you with it."

Physical care

Since depressed individuals are retarded in thinking and action, most activity will need to be initiated for them. They are likely to develop certain distressing physical conditions because of inactivity. Some of the most common of these complications are fecal impactions, edema of the extremities, and pneumonia. Infections are frequent, and since such people tend to ignore the physical condition of their bodies, it is necessary for the nurse to be particularly alert for symptoms of physical illness.

Perhaps the most effective way of caring for a depressed person is to establish a simple daily schedule for him. Much encouragement and reassurance throughout each day will be required to help him follow the schedule.

These individuals often need to be supplied with extra clothing. They exercise very little and frequently become chilled without appearing to realize it. Vigilance in supplying sweaters, warm underwear, and warm stockings is important.

Encouraging depressed individuals to take pride in their personal appearance is part of their care. This is difficult because it is in opposition to their tendency toward self-depreciation. Careful supervision of personal hygiene with attention to supplying clean clothing and helping them dress neatly is important in developing pride in personal appearance. Women need to be encouraged to accept appointments at the beauty parlor, and men to go to the barbershop regularly. If a depressed individual is hospitalized because he is actively suicidal, it may be safer to ask the barber or beauty operator to come to the unit where the person is hospitalized, rather than to send him to the operator.

Many depressed individuals present a difficult feeding problem. It is helpful if the nurse can discover why the food is being refused. It is not uncommon for these individuals to refuse to eat because they believe they are unworthy of receiving food. Some may say that they do not deserve food because they have not paid for it. Still others seek to destroy themselves through starvation. Many of these individuals have simply lost a desire for food, along with all the other interests they formerly had in life. Inactivity also contributes to a lack of interest in food.

Finding a way to combat the depressed individual's failure to eat is dependent on the reason for which the food is being refused. If failure to eat is caused by a feeling of unworthiness or the thought that the food has not been paid for, the person may be reassured by being told that the food is prepared for the group and all are expected to eat regardless of whether they pay or not. It might be helpful to provide an opportunity for such an individual to wash dishes or to do some other simple tasks to give him a feeling of "paying" for the food.

Because such individuals are susceptible to infection, it is important that their food and fluid intake be maintained. Every method of encouraging food intake should be employed. Some suggestions include providing physical exercise, serving small, attractively prepared meals, serving foods that the individual formerly enjoyed, allowing the family to bring in food, and spoonfeeding if this seems to encourage eating. Although appetizers such as medicinal tonics, whiskey before meals, and small doses of regular insulin before meals probably should be tried, they usually have not been helpful in combating loss of appetite resulting from emotional causes.

Depressed individuals may be unable to sleep at night. Some become agitated during the night hours, and because their fears, feelings of despair, and gloom are increased, they may feel a need to pace the floor. The usual aids—warm sedative tub baths, warm milk, and some hypnotic drugs—may be of benefit to some individuals. However, some do not seem to profit a great deal from the use of these aids. Treatment with the antidepressant drugs is usually helpful.

The self-destructive suicidal individual

An individual's need to injure or destroy himself is one of the most serious problems with which the psychiatric nurse must cope. The most effective methods for dealing with this problem vary, depending on the situation and the individual. However, there are some basic principles concerning care of the self-destructive individual with which every nurse should be fully acquainted.

Self-destructive tendencies are probably coped with most effectively by developing an environment to help the individual bear the emotional pain he is suffering. Instead of removing all the potentially dangerous weapons from the environment, an attempt can be made to meet his emotional needs. This may be done by assigning a staff member, preferably a skillful psychiatric nurse, to remain constantly with the individual. The nurse helps him participate in occupational, social, and recreational activites. Subtly and appropriately ways are identified to reassure the individual that he is a worthwhile, useful human being. The acutely depressed individual should be constantly supervised, but the focus of the supervision should be to help him deal with his feelings (Fig. 13-1). The emphasis should be on supplying safe opportunities for participation in the daily routine.

It is essential that the nurse be thoroughly familiar with the self-destructive individual and constantly aware of his every activity. In fact, nurses who work with emotionally distressed individuals need to cultivate the ability to be constantly alert to

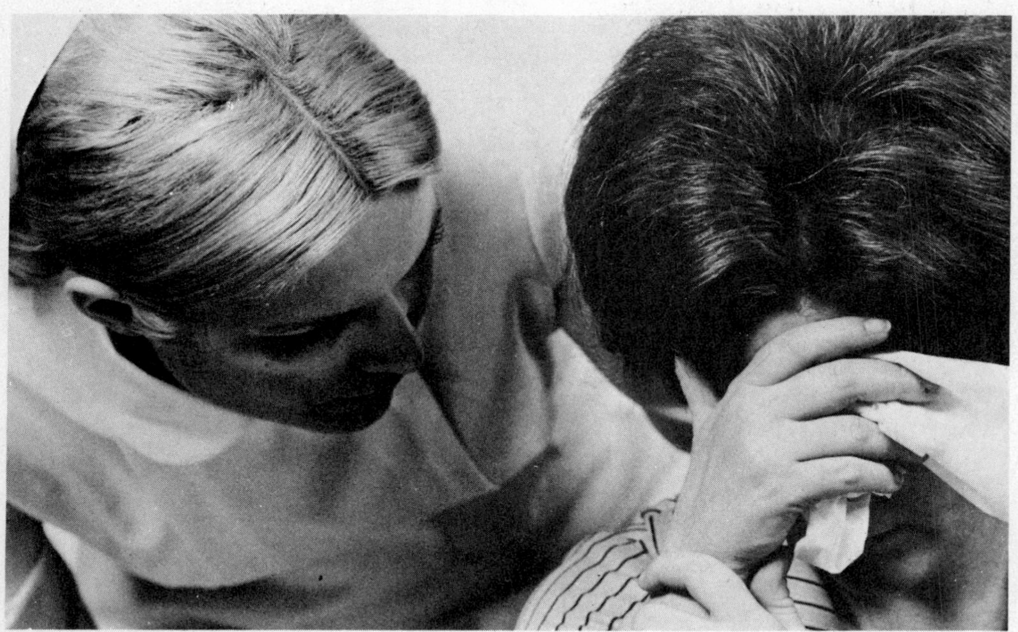

Fig. 13-1 *The focus of the nurse's work with the depressed individual is to help in dealing with feelings.*

the moods, needs, and minute-by-minute activities of these people.

"A person who talks about suicide never does it" is a common belief that every nurse should recognize as a serious fallacy. People usually talk about the thoughts that are uppermost in their minds. An individual alludes to suicide because he is thinking about it and immediately should be provided with special attention and help. Everyone involved should be made aware of individuals who are thought to have self-destructive tendencies. Special attention should be given to any individuals who look or act depressed, who make statements about life not being worth living, who suggest that they may not be around much longer, or who have actually injured themselves during a previous illness. Some authorities believe that all depressed individuals give warnings of impending suicide. Nurses need to be so well acquainted with the individuals with whom they work that they will be able to interpret the cues that are given.

It is important to understand what is being communicated through suicidal behavior. The individual may be saying that he is worthless and does not deserve to live or that life is meaningless and he does not want to live. He may be saying that he feels angry and resentful toward other poeple or toward himself, or he may be communicating that he feels so all alone that he cannot tolerate the situation any longer. In any case, his behavior is a cry for help.

A person who is depressed is at the greatest risk of suicide after his depression has begun to lift. Many nurses who show concerned care to deeply depressed individuals relax their vigilance as the person's mood begins to lift, usually as the result of the effective use of antidepressant medications. Suicide attempts at this time are common, since the individual has sufficient mental and physical energy to plan and implement a self-destructive act while still being sufficiently depressed to desire death. If individuals are able to feel that people are truly interested in them, if their needs for recognition and emotional support are being met, and if they are accompanied by workers who help them talk out the concerns, the incidence of attempts at self-destruction will be greatly lessened.

Providing activity to relieve anger and guilt feelings

Many authorities believe that depression is a problem involving hostility and anger that the individual has turned against himself. Thus it is thought that the depressed person has feelings of guilt and unworthiness that give rise to suicidal tendencies, refusal of food, inability to sleep, and loss of interest in personal appearance.

One of the methods by which a nurse may contribute to the care of some depressed individual is to provide them with tasks that will help relieve feelings of guilt. Depressed individuals have been known to ask for such menial tasks as scrubbing the floor, scouring the toilets, washing dirty socks, washing windows, or scrubbing the walls. Such tasks may provide a release for the guilt of the depressed individual and a means of atonement for real or imaginary sins. Although providing such experiences is contrary to the usual recommended treatment plan, it has proved to be of great value to selected individuals. Such work assignments for depressed persons should not be carried out without having been approved by the treatment team.

CASE FORMULATION □ A DEPRESSED INDIVIDUAL

Following is a fairly typical example of an individual who has become seriously depressed.

Carol B., 29 years of age, had been married 3 years and had one child 14 months of age. Family history revealed nothing significant, except that her father was stolid and slow-going. He had a reputation for being a pessimist but was otherwise a stable, sober individual.

Five years before marriage Carol had had a period of nervousness and depression, which lasted about 3 months. This was precipitated by an unfortunate love affair. At that time she was attending summer school at a local university where she met a young man. He had encouraged her to believe he was greatly interested in her, but at the school outing that terminated the summer session, he ignored her and danced with another girl. Carol came home, said little or nothing to her parents, and the following morning was found in bed in a stupor. She had taken 12 1-grain phenobarbital tablets. She was rushed to a hospital, given emergency treatment, and then transferred to a mental health treatment center where she remained 2 weeks.

The present attack began about 6 weeks before her second suicidal attempt. Again the onset was rather abrupt. Her husband returned home from work one evening and found her sobbing. After much urging on his part, she confessed that she was crying because she was a bad mother and a poor housekeeper. The husband naturally assured her that she was quite the contrary, but this only brought more sobbing and self-depreciation. She worried excessively about a small scar on her baby's temple that was caused by chicken pox. She accused herself of "marking" the child. The family suspected that she was merely tired from her spring housecleaning and hired a helper to come in and care for the baby. Her sister-in-law was called in to act as a companion. For 3 weeks she remained at home. She complained of inability to concentrate and prayed a great deal of the time. The well-meaning sister-in-law encouraged her by suggesting that she "snap out of it," and this merely served to agitate her. She was finally taken to her parents' home in the country. On two occasions she was found walking along the country road, and when questioned as to her destination, she merely stated that she wanted to "run away from everything." Her husband came to visit her one Sunday afternoon and took her for a car ride back into the city. She requested him to stop at their home, since she wanted some extra clothes for the baby. She went to the kitchen and, before the husband could realize what she was about to do, cut both her wrists with a carving knife. She was admitted to a short-term treatment unit in a community mental health center after receiving emergency treatment for her wounds.

On the day of admission she was able to give a clear account of her actions but responded in a dull manner. She frequently interjected the remark that she should be dead but that she was too big a coward to take her own life. She accused herself of being a rank failure and asserted that she should never have been born. She cried but did not shed many tears. She complained of a "numb" feeling in her head, of inability to sleep, and of loss of appetite. The physical examination was entirely negative.

For several days she remained indifferent and sad. She ate only when coaxed. She frequently announced that there was no sense in bothering about her, since she would die on the morrow. She never inquired about the welfare of her child and was indifferent toward her husband during visiting hours. Although she was not particularly untidy, she was rather slipshod in appearance and made no attempt to comb her hair or keep herself presentable. She took little or no interest in unit activities or in the other clients.

With her admission, chemotherapy with an antidepressant was begun. In the second week of her hospital stay, she began to show improvement. After being in the hospital for 1 month she began clamoring for discharge, insisting that she must go home to take care of her family.

She was cheerful and industrious, and in occupational therapy she was particularly adept in teaching English to a small group of foreign women.

Discussion of development of patterns of behavior

The situation in the case report presents a young woman who is demonstrating a good deal of hostility, which she has directed toward herself. Thus it must be concluded that she has introjected a harsh, punitive superego. There appears to be a conflict between the instinctual impulses of the id and the rigid controls of the superego.

The history provides little information about the present attack of depression. However, it does provide information about the first attack, which came as a result of the failure of an interpersonal relationship of great importance to her and the loss of a beloved object—a cherished lover. At that time she attempted suicide by taking an overdose of sleeping pills. This may have been an unconscious attempt to kill the introjected lover.

Authorities tell use that individuals who resort to self-destruction are frequently fixated at the oral-sadistic level of psychosexual development. During the late oral period of the child's development, the loved object (the mother or the mother's breast) is unconsciously introjected.

Later in life a loved object may unconsciously represent the original object that was introjected. When an individual attempts suicide he may be seeking relief from suffering or punishment for himself, or he may be attempting to kill the introjected person.

This young woman's child was in the toilet-training period. It is at this period in the child's development that he becomes more self-assertive and begins to defy the mother. It may be that this mother viewed as a loss the change in her child from a dependent, passive organism requiring constant tender guidance to a self-assertive individual. In a sense, she has lost a dependent organism and gained a demanding child. She may be overwhelmed with the new responsibilities brought about by the child's development. Thus she may blame herself for being a bad mother and a poor housekeeper and having caused a small scar on the baby's temple.

Her physical symptoms were those commonly found among depressed individuals: inability to sleep, loss of appetite, physical inactivity (as evidenced by sitting in a dark corner with head bowed), complaints of a numb feeling in the head, and crying without tears. Her emotional responses were also those frequently found among depressed individuals: inability to concentrate, self-accusatory ideas, suicidal ideas, feelings of unworthiness, and loss of interest in child and husband. Characteristically, she was able to give a clear account of all the experiences relating to her illness.

Planning and implementing nursing care for Carol B.

When Carol B. was admitted to the treatment center, the nursing staff believed that an accurate nursing diagnosis for the direction of care could be stated simply as "a young wife and mother who is depressed and suicidal." Her bandaged wrists and sad facial expression exemplified this acute state of feeling. Such persons require special physical arrangements and security precautions. In view of this, individual nursing care was provided for her. Nurses or other staff members with proved ability to work successfully with depressed individuals were chosen to be with her at all times until she recovered from the acute phases of the depression. They recognized the importance of showing Carol that they cared and set about to achieve this. Their goals for her care were to protect her from her self-destructive tendencies and to encourage her to discuss her feelings about the problems that concerned her.

These staff members adopted a kind, courteous, firm, hopeful attitude toward Carol. In this way they tried to convey the impression that she was not a hopeless case as she insisted. They listened carefully to everything that she said and answered her questions carefully without disputing or agreeing with her expressions of worthlessness. They accepted her silences when she did not wish to talk. They avoided using meaningless statements such as, "Cheer up" or "You know your family loves you!"

The staff members who worked closely with Carol were aware of her physical needs for food, fluid intake, and rest. They found that she ate better if served food on a tray in her room rather than going to the dining room with the other clients. If at night she wanted to sit up and talk or walk up and down the corridors, the staff member who was assigned to stay with her accompanied her in these activities.

When Carol accused herself of being a rank failure, the worker tried to help her recognize that she was improving and had demonstrated abilities and skills since coming to the treatment center. This was an attempt to improve her own self-esteem.

The staff workers made decisions for Carol until she was able to make them for herself. They tried to develop a congenital, pleasant living atmosphere for her. They encouraged her to become interested in some of the activities available in the occupational therapy department and accompanied her there whenever she felt well enough to go.

NURSING CARE OF THE ELATED, OVERACTIVE INDIVIDUAL

Individuals who are suffering from elation and overactivity require skillful and tactful nursing care. Most of these individuals are acutely aware of reality and react strongly to environmental stimuli. Because they misidentify individuals with whom they come in contact, they may express positive or negative attitudes toward a person because they are reminded of someone they once knew. Such individuals are often bitingly sarcastic and pointedly profane and vulgar. Frequently they discover a physical or personality defect about which this person, who may well be the nurse, is sensitive and delight in repeatedly calling attention to this defect. The elated mood is accompanied by extreme overactivity in both the mental and physical spheres. Such individuals are easily irritated and angered.

Whether the nurse can help elated, overactive individuals depends to a large extent on the attitude with which they are approached. The tone of voice employed by the nurse is of primary importance. A firm, kind, low-pitched voice that carries a coaxing quality probably is most effective. The nurse who uses a loud demanding tone is quickly defeated because this type of approach may provoke hostile and aggressive behavior.

It is useless to attempt to hurry the elated individual because such an approach will result in anger and hostility. Thus the attitude of having all the time in the world to accomplish a procedure will be much more effective. Quiet persuasion is one of the chief aids in getting the elated individual to cooperate.

Consistent fairness and honesty in dealing with such individuals are essential if one is to maintain rapport with them throughout a period of time. Although they deserve and must have simple, honest explanations, long discussions and explanations should be avoided, since such activities provoke irritability.

Because the elated, overactive individual's thoughts rapidly fly from one thing to another, he is described as being distractible. The skillful nurse makes use of the individual's inability to maintain sustained attention by directing his thoughts away from factors in the environment that encourage his destructive tendencies, provoke his irritability, or increase his excitement.

In dealing with overactive, elated individuals the nurse must recognize that the behavior is a result of an illness and will be replaced by socially acceptable behavior when the person is well again. The inexperienced nurse may be embarrassed by the loud talking, the vulgarity and profanity, the destructive activity, and the overt sexual behavior that is apparent. However, part of the skillful care of such a person includes understanding why he needs to behave in such a way. With understanding will come acceptance of behavior.

The psychiatric nurse who is accepting of the behavior of the elated individual will not scold or shame him for his uninhibited actions or become angered by the pointed, biting remarks because it will be understood that they are a part of his illness.

Simplifying the environment

Since all elated, overactive individuals are stimulated by environmental factors, one of the first responsibilities of the nurse is to simplify their surroundings and, insofar as possible, to provide a sedative environment for them. Because other people irritate the elated individual and provoke him to engage in an excessive amount of talking, it is wise to provide him with a single room.

The room should be as far away from other daily activities as possible and yet should be easily accessible to the nurse who needs to be constantly aware of the individual and his behavior. Pictures and colorful drapes probably should be eliminated, since they may be too stimulating and certainly may be destroyed in a burst of excitement. Unnecessary furniture such as a small table or a light chair may be used as a weapon if the individual becomes extremely irritated. Care must be individualized, depending on the degree of the individual's elation and the amount of his excessive energy. It is usually wise to limit the number of persons who come in contact with him. Only a few persons, chosen because of their patience and understanding approach, should be assigned to his care.

Controlling excessive energy

The overactive individual may react with a tremendous burst of energy for which he must find some outlet. Usually such an individual is admitted to a hospital because the outlets that he has chosen for his energy have been dangerous to him or to his family. The nurse is confronted with the task of controlling or redirecting this excessive energy into more acceptable channels.

An excellent outlet for the excessive energy of individuals who are only mildly elated is writing. Most of these people are eager to write their life stories or to disclose the deficiencies of the political system to the world and thus will readily put paper and pencil to use. Many mildly elated individuals will be content to spend hours over their manuscripts.

The physical activities provided for these individuals should require large sweeping movements, since they will become annoyed and lose interest in anything requiring fine, discriminative skills. Games such as table tennis, croquet, badminton, and medicine ball are often helpful as outlets for energy, provided there is no element of competition present. In competitive games the elated patient becomes overly stimulated and excited.

Overactive behavior is successfully controlled by chlorpromazine or one of the other phenothiazine derivatives. Recently, chronic and recurrent episodes of manic behavior in individuals with bipolar affective disorders have been controlled by oral administration of lithium carbonate.

It is unwise from a therapeutic point of view to threaten an excited individual or to suggest that he will be punished because of his nonconforming behavior. Such a maneuver usually results in increased hostility. If the individual is directed in an understanding and sympathetic way and his behavior is accepted as part of his illness, it is usually possible to redirect his energy without resorting to the use of restraints. With the advent of the psychotropic drugs, mechanical restraint of overactive persons has been practically eliminated.

The individual whose overactivity makes him dangerous

Occasionally, hospitalization is required for an individual because he is dangerous to himself or others. Intense feelings of fear, anger, hostility, or suspicion may cause individuals to strike out against other people or the environment in general. Striking out against others is dangerous. Therefore it is essential to prevent this type of behavior, if possible, and to check it if it is precipitated.

Usually an individual who strikes out against his environment does so because he is terrified. He may be afraid of what he believes others will do to him, or he may be undergoing terrifying hallucinatory experiences. If the latter is happening, the voices may be describing what physical and mental tortures are awaiting him. It is obvious that a terrified individual can be helped only by those who are in control of their own feelings and can approach him calmly. Uncontrolled fear on the part of others is extremely upsetting to emotionally ill people.

When an individual becomes terrified, a calm, quiet staff member should assist the upset individual to enter a room that is away from the center of activity. The individual should remain in the quiet room until his intense feelings of fear or anger have subsided. Someone who can be helpful and can comfort the fearful individual should remain with him until he is ready to rejoin the group.

More important than managing destructive, threatening behavior is learning to avoid it. The first step in learning to avoid problem behavior is to discover the situations that are upsetting to such individuals and to discover how to keep these from occurring. The nurse needs to learn to recognize the signs of an approaching emotional outburst and to employ measures that will help individuals to handle negative feelings without acting out against the environment. Destructive behavior on the part of terrified, angry individuals is rare in situations where an attempt is made to recognize and meet emotional needs and where the personnel recognize the importance of developing positive interpersonal relationships with mentally ill persons.

Physical care

An overactive individual often loses a great deal of weight and may become severely dehydrated. This problem is exaggerated by the fact that he frequently does not take time to eat or drink and may sleep very little. He is often oblivious to physical injury or pain. Consequently the nurse needs to be vigilantly aware of such a person's physical needs as well as his emotional ones.

Prevention of injury is one of the responsibilities of the nurse. Overactive individuals may injure themselves in a burst of elation and excitement and may disregard even such a serious trauma as a broken bone.

Keeping overactive persons warmly dressed during cold weather is sometimes difficult, since clothing may be an irritating factor. Because clothing may impede the movement of arms and legs, excited individuals may tear it off. They often appear totally unaware of body temperature and must be safeguarded against becoming chilled.

Since constipation, fecal impaction, bladder distention, or other difficulties may be present but ignored, the nurse should observe these individuals carefully.

Ensuring sufficient sleep for excited individuals is another challenge. This is important, since exhaustion and even death have been known to result from long-continued failure to sleep. Many of these individuals are so alert to all environmental stimuli that they sleep only 1 to 2 hours out of every 24. Some hypnotic drugs are helpful, but occasionally they may increase the individual's excitement. The problem of wakefulness has practically disappeared with the introduction of the phenothiazine drugs.

Excited and elated individuals may not take time to sit down to eat. In such an instance it is wise to serve food that can be carried about in the hands. Sandwiches, fruit, and cupcakes are dietary items that may be "eaten on the run." Elated, overactive individuals require a high caloric intake and should have between-meal nourishment. Nurses should not disregard the need for fluids even though water fountains are usually available; the excited individual often does not take time to drink and should have water offered to him each hour.

If the individual is served food on a tray and will take time to feed himself, the equipment on the tray should be simple and unbreakable. As in every other aspect of the care of these overactive, elated persons, the nursing procedures must be individualized to meet specific needs. In some instances the elated individual may get along well in the dining room setting. However, in most instances the elated individual is so stimulated by the dining room situation that it is more helpful if he is served on a tray in his room.

Although the individual should be encouraged to carry out his own personal hygiene, he needs to be supervised closely. Some overactive, elated individuals are too ill to assume any responsibility for their physical care and may need to have much of it done by the nurse. Other less excited individuals can take a good deal of responsibility for their own cleanliness and grooming if someone skillfully directs their activities. Such individuals may become playful and mischievous in the bathroom. Because of poor judgment these individuals have been found washing their hair in the toilet bowl, throwing water about with gay abandon, or in various other ways reducing the bathroom to a shambles. It is for this reason that such individuals should not be left alone in the bathroom.

The mouth of the overactive individual requires special attention, and lubrication should be applied to the lips regularly.

Many overactive individuals require hospitalization, at least for a short time. They are likely to swing from elation into depression and must be guarded vigilantly against the possibility of suicide as the elation subsides.

CASE FORMULATION □ AN OVERACTIVE INDIVIDUAL

Following is a fairly typical case history of an individual who was hospitalized because of overactive, elated behavior.

> Maurice H., 48 years of age, was an unmarried real estate salesman who was an only child. His mother had a mental illness at 46 years of age, which was probably depression of midlife. He had been educated in private schools and earned a college degree in business administration. During his junior year in college he failed to win a scholarship and became morose, sleepless, and nervous for a period of 2 months. A few years after finishing college he entered an auto sales contest and won first prize, a trip to Hawaii. While on this trip he became overactive and insisted on eating every meal at the captain's table, where he told obscene stories and embarrassed the women passengers. He participated in frequent brawls with the stewards and complained to the purser on the slightest provocation. On disembarking, he refused to return to his home city. He demanded the most pretentious accommodations at the hotel, and when these were unavailable, he entered into a noisy altercation with the manager that resulted in his being hospitalized because of his behavior. He remained there for 3 months and then returned to his parents' home.
>
> The present attack began about 6 weeks before he sought help. At that time he was engaged in selling real estate in a new subdivision. He became extremely active, arose early, and approached prospective clients at bus terminals, waiting rooms, and hotel corridors. He talked in such a convincing manner that he made a good sales record in the first week. He continued to send in many deposits, bragged about his sales ability, argued noisily with his fellow salesmen, and finally was arrested because he failed to pay his fare on a city bus. He then entered a damage suit against the company for $100,000. The attorney who was approached realized the absurdities of his claims and convinced him to seek help.
>
> Immediately after going to the mental health center, he demanded to see the head physician and requested permission to use the telephone. He was fairly coherent but was circumstantial in his conversation. When asked a simple question his reply was a long, rambling, and digressive account. After being continually reminded to answer the

question, he did so, only to return to another long digression. He made unreasonable demands of the personnel at the clinic and, if refused, became abusive, sarcastic, and irritable. At this time it was discovered that when a client had refused to make a down payment on a lot, he had drawn the sum out of his own bank account and had forged a signature on the sales contract. This explained his amazing sales success.

He spent much of his time while in the short-term treatment unit of the mental health clinic writing letters to the mayor, various attorneys, and influential citizens. He wrote on odd pieces of paper with pencil and in a broad, sweeping hand, underlining almost every other word and capitalizing others. Every day he met the physicians at the door of the unit and began to revile them. He particularly enjoyed arguing with the physicians, demanding evidence to prove that he was insane and consistently denying all charges of misbehavior. In a loud voice he promised to have the director of the center removed and the physicians exposed as quacks. He was suggestively lewd in his conversation with all women workers except one young woman to whom he proposed marriage.

Throughout the 4 weeks he spent in the short-term treatment unit, he was the constant focus of commotion, a chronic critic of everything and everybody about him, collecting and hoarding papers, combs, magazines, and all sorts of trash, and getting into quarrels with others. Occasionally he was very agreeable and jolly, particularly if he was allowed to do all the talking. On these occasions he was fond of reciting parodies of famous poems in a quick, witty fashion. Some of these he had not quoted since his high school days.

Although he believed that he was being abused, he harbored no other delusional ideas and at no time was he confused or hallucinatory. His intellect was keen and his memory, particularly for trivial things, remarkable, but he had no insight into his abnormal exaltation and irritability, and his judgment was poor.

Discussion of development of patterns of behavior

Elated, overactive behavior is thought by some to be an unconscious defense against depression in individuals fixated at the oral-sadistic level of psychosexual development. In very early life such individuals are thought to have sought acceptance from parents by becoming compliant, obedient, and hardworking.

Maurice H. first experienced a depression at about the age of 21 when he failed to win a scholarship in college. To him this failure to achieve a prized goal represented a failure in life, and he became depressed in an unconscious effort to punish himself as his parents might have done when he failed to fulfill some expectation of theirs. For 2 months he had typical symptoms of a mild depression. He was morose, sleepless, and nervous.

A few years later Maurice won a coveted prize in an auto sales contest. This award was a trip to Hawaii that eventually resulted in Maurice's hospitalization for 3 months because of his overactivity. In this instance the individual probably developed anxiety over the high expectations of his company. He may have reasoned that they would undoubtedly expect more and bigger sales records from him now that he had been able to achieve the award of a trip. The anxiety about being able to fulfill the future expectations of his company changed into guilt feelings that in turn caused him to feel that somehow he should be punished. To guard against the depressed feelings that arose from a sense of failure and a need to be punished, he developed overactivity and elation—the defense against depression.

Several years later he became involved again in a competitive selling activity. His unconscious need to succeed to fulfill introjected parental expectations started the chain reaction again. Thus anxiety about succeeding caused him to be concerned about the possibility of failing, and this in turn led to the depressed feelings that accompany a loss. The loss was the anticipated failure in selling, which in his own mind had already occurred. Thus the unconscious defense against depressed feelings was again used. He became expansive, overactive, argumentative, sarcastic, irritable, made unreasonable demands, and became a constant center of commotion. In a sense, he did not give himself time to become depressed because he was too busy striking out against his environment in an orally sadistic way.

Typically he was not delusional, and he did not experience hallucinations. Thus he was constantly in touch with reality. His intellect was as keen as ever, and his memory was intact.

Some inexperienced people might conclude that this man was not mentally ill. However, he was unreasonable and sometimes abusive when he did not get his own way. He also wrote letters to outside authorities because he believed he should not be undergoing treatment, and he constantly sought to expose the clinic personnel for their inefficient handling of the situation. He had no insight into his condition, and his judgment was impaired.

This mild attack of overactivity lasted for 4 weeks. At the end of this time he was able to return to his home.

This individual's mother suffered from a midlife depression. Too little is known about this situation to do more than suggest that the mother was herself fixated at the oral-sadistic level of psychosexual development, since she apparently directed hostility toward herself. This type of personality structure undoubtedly made it difficult for her to give her son the sense of security he required as an infant to develop into a well-adjusted adult. The mother's depression also raises the possibility of this individual having an inherited predisposition to an affective disorder.

Planning and implementing nursing care for Maurice H.

The nursing care plan for Maurice H. was derived from the assessment data from which a nursing diagnosis was synthesized. This was stated as "elated, overactive behavior leading to the inability to carry out activities of daily living (regarding, for example, job and nutritional status) and characterized by exaggerated responses to stimuli, verbal abuse, and extreme irritability, verging on loss of control."

The members of the staff assigned to care for Maurice were chosen carefully because his verbally hostile and physically aggressive behavior was difficult to accept. Not all staff members were able to control their feelings about his vulgar comments and understand objectively why it was impossible for him to control his behavior. In addition, he related more positively to some individuals than to others. Finally, some staff members enjoyed working with him and others did not. All these factors were considered in the choice of individuals to work with him.

The staff decided that it would be best for him to be cared for in a unit of the treatment center where a single room was available. In such a room it was possible to eliminate all but the essential furnishings. The single room was helpful in avoiding the overstimulation that might have resulted from his being assigned to sleeping accommodations where he would have been involved with other clients.

His recreational activities needed to be controlled because it was obvious that he became loud and disruptive when involved in competitive games. He became angry when he scored lower than other players in a game and accused them of cheating. These accusations usually brought on loud arguments and sometimes fights.

When it was necessary for the staff to intervene in such an altercation, they took advantage of his distractibility and subtly redirected his attention away from the argument to an activity that could be carried on in his room with only one other person, one who was able to tolerate his rapid conversation and accept his pointed criticism.

The members of the staff were careful to avoid scolding or threatening Maurice when he initiated fights with other individuals. They avoided comparing his behavior with that of other better controlled individuals or even with his own behavior on a day when he was less noisy. The staff realized that his problem behavior was part of his illness.

Maurice responded negatively to any member of the staff who attempted to speak to him somewhat sharply or who commanded him to do anything. They learned that he could not be hurried and that their approach was much more effective if they were quiet, friendly, patient, and courteous to him and used a pleasant, businesslike tone of voice. On one occasion when a staff member did order him to comply with a hospital rule, he refused and did not let the individual forget the incident.

The staff discovered that it was unwise to encourage Maurice when he was reciting or singing parodies or telling jokes. When some staff members did laugh at his jokes, he became much louder and more ribald. It was necessary for them to intervene by accompanying him to his room before he became so excited that he lost control.

In talking to this man the staff avoided getting into long, complicated discussions or giving elaborate explanations. Instead, short sentences with specific, straightforward responses to his questions seemed to satisfy him and avoided arguments.

The staff members were careful when giving him praise. They found that he sometimes turned the words of praise around and used them in a different context to refute a point they had been trying to make with him sometime previously.

They were aware of his physical needs and realized that he frequently did not eat enough. This problem arose because his attention was distracted from the food or he left the dining room early before finishing the meal. Likewise, he sometimes had dry, cracked lips because he failed to maintain his fluid intake. Maurice was weighed every week, and when his weight had dropped below a desirable point for 2 consecutive weeks, his food was served in his room on a tray. A staff member remained with him during the meal and encouraged him to eat. Removing him from the dining room served to eliminate the many distracting features present in a group. At the same time he was placed on a schedule so that fluids were offered to him every hour.

Crayons, paper, and pencils were made available to him in his room, and he was encouraged to write and sketch there in the hope that these more sedentary activities would lessen his hyperactivity. The staff members were careful to explain to him in an honest, straightforward manner why he was not encouraged to join the rest of the clients in the dining room. In like manner all other restrictions on his behavior were explained so that he could understand the reason for them and realize that he was not being rejected as a person.

After receiving appropriate amounts of the drug lithium carbonate for 2 weeks, he gained some control of his behavior and became quieter and more amenable to suggestion. The professional staff did not believe that he was well enough to leave the hospital permanently. However, at the request of his mother, he was allowed to go home at the end of 4 weeks with the understanding that he would continue taking lithium carbonate for 1 year and have the blood levels of this drug checked weekly by a physician.

Persons with episodes of overactive behavior react favorably to treatment, but recurrences are to be expected.

OUTLOOK FOR OVERACTIVE AND DEPRESSED INDIVIDUALS

For a single episode of overactivity or depression the outlook is usually good, but recurrences are to be expected. However, second and third attacks need not necessarily occur in every case. An attack of overactivity in early adult life generally means more attacks later. Depressions are more likely to occur in the later years of life.

It is never safe to predict the probable duration of any given attack, since there are great variations, and even the same individual may have both short and long periods of elation and depression. The average length for all untreated attacks of elation is about 6 months; for untreated depressive episodes it is generally longer. When depressive periods show a strong element of fear, anxiety, and hypochondriasis, the condition may endure for many years. Likewise, elation may become chronic, particularly in older individuals, if it is associated with organic changes in the brain such as arteriosclerosis. Current treatments, including maintenance levels of lithium carbonate as a preventive measure, have shortened the length of attacks in both elation and depression.

An outstanding feature of affective disorders is the fact that even after repeated attacks the intellectual capacities are rarely impaired. In the free intervals the individual is usually able to carry on his regular occupation and live an entirely normal life.

CONCLUDING STATEMENTS

1. The affective disorders are thought to have their origins in the frustrations that occur in the late oral phase of personality development.
2. Individuals who are prone to the development of affective disorders have prepsychotic personalities characterized by ambivalent, dependent, and narcissistic tendencies and have difficulty in establishing mature patterns of adult interpersonal relationships.
3. Essentially, elated, overactive individuals are venting their hostility on their environment, whereas depressed individuals have turned their hostility on themselves.
4. Depressed individuals suffer from a punishing superego.

5. Although grief and depression are both characterized by a disturbance in mood, they differ in many ways.
6. Grief is a normal, universal, necessary part of life experience that is a reaction to the real loss of a highly valued object and is self-limiting.
7. The three phases of normal grieving include shock and disbelief; developing awareness of the pain of the loss, which leads to crying; and restitution, which involves mourning.
8. Depression is a pathological elaboration of grief that goes beyond grief in duration and intensity and causes the individual to be increasingly incapacitated.
9. Depression is not self-limiting and often requires professional help.
10. Elated, overactive individuals are acutely aware of reality and react strongly to environmental stimuli.
11. Simplification of the environment is a basic principle in the care of elated, overactive individuals.
12. The task of recognizing the potentially suicidal individual and safeguarding against the possibility of injury is one of the most important responsibilities of the psychiatric nurse.
13. The depressed individual suffers from overwhelming feelings of guilt, ideas of self-depreciation, and self-accusatory delusions.
14. The prognosis for single episodes of elation or depression is good, but recurrences are to be expected.

Suggested sources of additional information

CLASSICAL

Beers, Clifford: A mind that found itself, New York, 1948, Doubleday & Co., Inc.

Bodie, Marilyn K.: When a patient threatens suicide, Perspect. Psychiatr. Care **6:**76-79, March-April, 1968.

Burgess, Ann, and Lazare, Aaron: Dual therapy by nurse and psychiatrist, Am. J. Nurs. **70:**1292-1298, 1970.

Crary, William G., and Crary, Gerald C.: Depression, Am. J. Nurs. **73:**472-475, 1973.

Engel, George L.: Grief and grieving, Am. J. Nurs. **64:**93-98, Sept., 1964.

Fallon, Barbara: "And certain thoughts go through my head. . . ," Am. J. Nurs. **72:**1257-1259, 1972.

Farberow, Norman L.: Suicide prevention: a view from the bridge, Community Ment. Health J. **6:**469-474, 1968.

Jourard, Sidney M.: Suicide—an invitation to die, Am. J. Nurs. **72:**269, 273-275, 1970.

McLean, Leonora J.: Action and reaction in suicidal crisis, Nurs. Forum **8**(1):29-41, 1969.

Parkes, Colin Murray: Bereavement; studies of grief in adult life, New York, 1973, International Universities Press.

Peplau, Hildegard: Themes in nursing situations, Am. J. Nurs. **53:**1221-1223, 1953.

Peplau, Hildegard: Mid-life crises, Am. J. Nurs. **75:**1761-1765, 1975.

Riley, Joan: Nursing intervention in depression, Perspect. Psychiatr. Care **5:**65-76, March-April, 1967.

Ruesch, Jurgen: Disturbed communication, New York, 1972, W.W. Norton & Co., Inc.

Rykken, Marjorie B.: The nurse's role in preventing suicide, Nurs. Outlook **6:**377-378, 1958.

Schagenhauf, G., Turpin, J., and White, R.B.: The use of lithium carbonate in the treatment of manic psychoses, Am. J. Psychiatry **123:**201-206, 1966.

Schneidman, Edwin S., Farberow, N.L., and Litman, R.L.: The psychology of suicide, Boston, 1970, Little, Brown and Co.

Ujhely, Gertrud B.: Grief and depression: implications for preventive and therapeutic nursing care, Nurs. Forum **5:**23-35, 1966.

Umscheid, Sister Theophane: With suicidal patients: caring for or caring about, Am. J. Nurs. **67:**1230-1232, 1967.

CONTEMPORARY

Anthony, James E., and Benedek, Therese, editors: Depression and human existence, Boston, 1975, Little, Brown and Co.

Arieti, Silvano, and Bemporad, Jules: Severe and mild depression: the psychotherapeutic approach, New York, 1978, Basic Books, Inc., Publishers.

Bahra, Robert J.: The potential for suicide, Am. J. Nurs. **75:**1781-1788, 1975.

Bigelow, Newton: The involutional psychoses. In Arieti, Silvano, editor: American handbook of psychiatry, vol. 1, New York, 1959, Basic Books, Inc., Publishers, pp. 540-545.

Boyajean, Anne: Fighting despair, Am. J. Nurs. **76:**77, Jan., 1978.

Brown, Bertram S.: What you should know about depression, Ment. Hyg. **75:**4-7, Summer, 1975.

Diller, Julie: The psychological autopsy in equivocal deaths, Perspect. Psychiatr. Care **17:**156-161, July-Aug., 1979.

Drake, Ronald E., and Price, Joseph L.: Depression: adaptation to disruption and loss, Perspect. Psychiatr. Care **13:**163-169, Oct.-Dec., 1975.

Fitzgerald, Roy G., and Long, Imelda: Seclusion in the treatment and management of severely disturbed manic and depressed patients, Perspect. Psychiatr. Care **11:**59-64, April-June, 1973.

Herman, Sonya J.: Divorce: a grief process, Perspect. Psychiatr. Care **12:**108-112, July-Sept., 1974.

Hersh, Stephen: Suicide, Ment. Hyg. **75:**24-25, Summer, 1975.

Kiev, Ari: The courage to live, New York, 1980, Lippincott & Crowell.

Knauth, Percy: A season in hell, New York, 1975, Harper & Row, Publishers.

Rosenthal, Saul H.: Involutional depression. In Arieti, Silvano, and Brody, Eugene

B., editors: American handbook of psychiatry, vol. 3, New York, 1974, Basic Books, Inc., Publishers, pp. 694-709.

Schwartz, D.A., Flinn, D.E., and Slamson, P.F.: Suicide in the psychiatric hospital, Am. J. Psychiatry **132:**150-153, 1975.

Shmagin, Barbara G., and Pearlmutter, Deanna R.: The pursuit of unhappiness—the secondary gains of depression, Am. J. Nurs. **15**(2):63-65, 1977.

Sumner, Frances C., and Gwozdz, Theresa A.: A nurse for suicidal patients, Am. J. Nurs. **76:**1792-1793, 1976.

Swanson, Ardis R.: Communicating with depressed persons, Perspect. Psychiatr. Care **13:**63-67, April-June, 1975.

Thaler, Otto F.: Grief and depression: implications for preventive and therapeutic nursing care, Nurs. Forum **5**(2):8-22, 1966.

Vollen, Karen Helon, and Watson, Charles G.: Suicide in relation to time of day and day of week, Am. J. Nurs. **75:**263, 1975.

Weiss, James M.A.: Suicide. In Arieti, Silvano, and Brody, Eugene B., editors: American handbook of psychiatry, ed. 2, vol. 3, New York, 1974, Basic Books, Inc., Publishers, pp. 743-765.

Westercamp, Twila M.: Suicide, Am. J. Nurs. **75:**260-262, 1975.

OF PARTICULAR INTEREST

Anthony, James E., and Benedek, Therese, editors: Depression and human existence, Boston, 1975, Little, Brown and Co.

This is a handy text for the student seeking to understand the origins and classifications of depressive disorders.

Kiev, A.: Somatic manifestations of depressive disorders, Princeton, N.J., 1974, Excerpta Medica Foundation.

This review of physical behaviors associated with depression is especially useful for the nurse in identifying symptoms that are related to depressive illness.

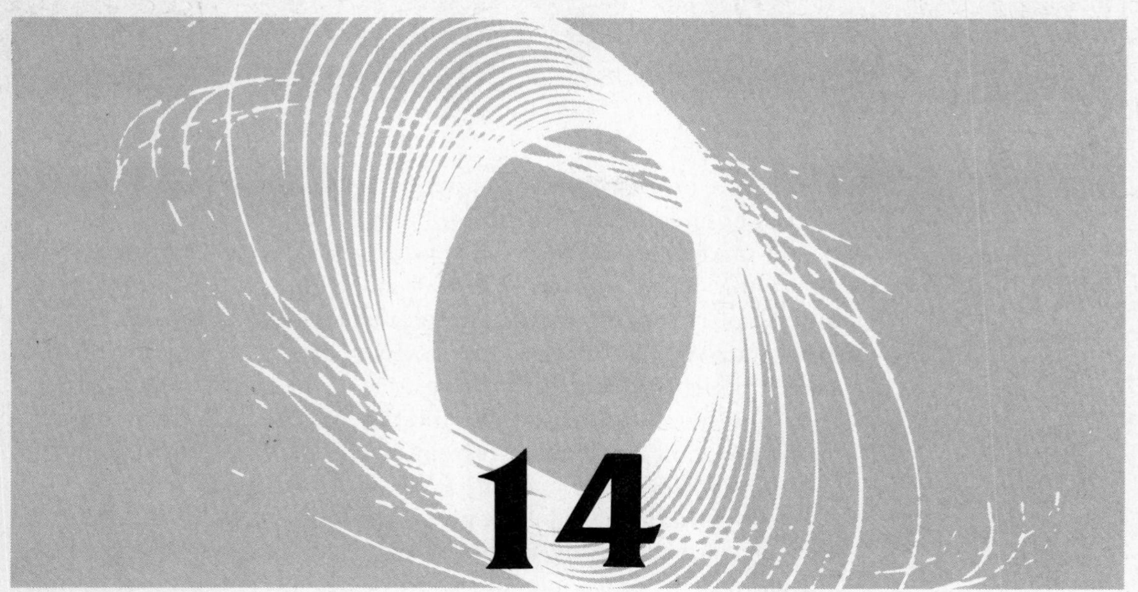

14

Behavioral patterns that reflect maladaptive efforts to control anxiety

- Anxiety disorders
- Assessment of the needs of anxious individuals
- Nursing care of anxious individuals

There is a large group of individuals whose behavior is characterized by a constant effort to gain security and to control intolerable anxiety through the use of physical symptoms that have no organic basis. Another group of individuals control anxiety by the use of repetitive, ritualistic maneuvers. All these individuals seek security by reverting to a previous level of personality development during which they were able to be comfortably dependent on others. In contrast, the individual who suffers from a psychotic reaction resorts to a retreat or flight from reality or, in the case of the overactive patient, a flight into reality.

The origin of these personality problems probably lies in conflicts developed during the early childhood experiences of these individuals. In adult life the conflict has been repressed in the unconscious mind. The repressed conflict is between two or more divergent drives or desires. The symptoms of anxiety appear because of the inability of the ego to effect a compromise between these clashing desires. The result of these unresolved conflicts may be a flight into a state of physical illness that is functional and not organic. Ritualistic behavior may have a similar origin. Each inner drive or innate trend is represented by a group of ideas, which are held together by a strong emotional bond or common feeling and are known as a *complex*. Each complex demands expression in conscious activity, and in attempting such expression it may be working at cross purposes with another equally demanding complex. Thus one often senses in the individual a struggle between the desire to express basic instinctual drives on one hand and to retain social and conventional approval on the other. In other words, a war exists in the emotional life of some individuals between the id drives and the superego restraints.

The majority of people are able to live relatively normal, anxiety-free lives through the use of various unconscious strategies or compromises. It is here that many of the mechanisms of defense discussed in an earlier chapter come into play. As has been said, if the ego is unable to achieve a compromise between the id and the superego, the tension is relieved by some individuals by converting the emotional conflict into physical illness or ritualistic behavior.

ANXIETY DISORDERS

Anxiety disorders are probably the most frequently observed manifestations of the individual's inability to deal with emotional conflicts. The threat to the conscious level of personality arises from the energy of repressed emotions such as deep-seated hostilities and resentments. Immediate external situations such as loss of social prestige or love or a threat to personal and financial security are regarded as important causative factors. Anxiety may be focused on various visceral functions, frequently to the point that one fears imminent death or physical disaster, indicating that conscious control of primary or conscious anxiety is poor, diffuse, or incomplete. The physical symptoms expressed by individuals who are exhibiting anxiety disorders may be numerous but generally center about the vital organs of the body. Tightness of the stomach, fast-beating heart, a feeling that the heart may suddenly stop, no appetite, loose bowels, and a heavy feeling in the abdomen are frequent complaints offered by the individual seeking assistance. Palpitation, a feeling of shortness of breath, compression sensations in the head, tight sensations in the throat, numbness in the extremities, and a constant feeling of exhaustion are other typical experiences reported by individuals suffering from anxiety disorders. These symptoms usually frighten the person; he cannot concentrate on his work, feels depressed, and harbors fears of sudden death or insanity. Frequently many of these symptoms appear at one time and cause the individual to respond with a panic reaction or acute fear.

Phobic disorders are characterized by specific unrealistic and inappropriate fears that are symbolic of some anxiety-laden situation in the life of the individual. In obsessive-compulsive disorders the defense against open anxiety is a preoccupation with a compelling ritual. In both these disorders the mechanisms of displacement and symbolism are the major elements and hence are being considered as essentially one entity.

A *phobia* is a specific pathological fear reaction out of proportion to the stimulus. The painful feeling has been automatically and unconsciously displaced from its original internal source and has become attached to a specific external object or situation. The phobia is an obsessively persistent form of fear that is unrealistic and inappropriate.

An increasingly common phobia is *agoraphobia,* which technically is a fear of open spaces. This fear is most often manifested by the individual expressing dread at being left alone or going out of his home. He avoids crowds and public places because he anticipates some dreadful form of collapse. Agoraphobia is particularly incapacitating because it markedly interferes with the individual's ability to live a normal life.

An *obsession* is an undesirable but persistent thought or idea that is forced into conscious awareness. The thought is charged with great but unconscious emotional significance. Such a thought may include repetitive doubts, wishes, fears, impulses, admonitions, and commands.

A *compulsion* is an unwanted urge to perform an act or a ritual that is contrary to the individual's ordinary conscious wishes or standards.

It will be noted that all these intrusive ideas and compelling urges and fears appear in consciousness as though independently self-created.

The individual who suffers from an *obsessive-compulsive disorder* is driven to think about or to do something that he recognizes as being inappropriate or foolish. There is an excessive preoccupation with a single idea or a compulsion to carry out and to repeat over and over again certain acts against his better judgment. Underlying these compulsive or obsessive states is a personality that is usually conscience-driven, sensitive, shy, meticulous, and precise about bodily functions, dress, religious duty, and daily routine.

Obsessive-compulsive disorder is a serious emotional illness because the imperative ideas so control the individual that he becomes a slave to his morbid preoccupation and can scarcely carry on his normal work and social activity. Dominating fears or phobias are the most outstanding features of this illness. The sufferer may fear dirt, bacteria, cancer, or insanity. There may be an abnormal fear of open places, narrow corridors, small rooms, running water, staircases, high places, or various animals. In fact, the phobia may be focused on anything that in some manner suggests death, disease, or disaster.

These irrational fears probably developed out of disagreeable and socially unacceptable ideas. Instead of an open anxiety or frank expression of id drives, the ideas and intense emotions attached to them are forced out of consciousness. Such repressed emotional energy attaches itself to an entirely different idea or activity and forces itself into consciousness as a tension that has little or no relationship to the original idea. The individual experiences a sense of relief after performing the compulsive act, since the symptom was developed for the purpose of relieving tension. The disorder, therefore, uses displacement and symbolization. The original conflict involving unacceptable desires is replaced by tension about something that is more socially acceptable but that functions as a symbol.

Compulsive behavior and obsessive fears are substitution devices that relieve tension arising out of a sense of guilt or a feeling of personal insecurity. Unfortunately, the relief offered by the act is only temporary, and the ritual must be repeated at frequent intervals. Relatives lose patience and attempt to "break the person of his habit." This only causes the victim to become restless, uncomfortable, and agitated because the act has become a fixed channel for the discharge of all tension arising out of his unconscious conflict.

Another type of behavior that represents maladaptive efforts to control anxiety is represented by *conversion disorder*. This disorder is a purposeful, although unconscious, psychological mode of reaction by which the individual uses a physical symptom as a disguise in an attempt to solve some acute problem or fulfill some desire, the open or conscious gratification of which is unacceptable to the individual. Conversion represents a primitive, instinctual mechanism to which a person resorts when he is incapable of adjusting through the usual methods of rational volitional activity.

The person who uses a conversion disorder unconsciously selects a set of symptoms, which are dictated by suggestion or by some previous acquaintance with persons who had the actual problem. Hence paralysis, blindness, and epilepsy are afflictions commonly presented by the person using conversion. The symptoms are physical, but no physical pathological condition can be demonstrated.

No matter what form the symptoms take, a characteristic feature of conversion is the individual's attitude of indifference toward his handicaps. There seems to be an air of contentment about the individual with conversion disorder. He seems to be more relieved than distressed, an attitude that at once suggests that he is more comfortable with the physical problem than with the mental torment.

ASSESSMENT OF THE NEEDS OF ANXIOUS INDIVIDUALS

Many health professionals who work skillfully and empathically with psychotic individuals find that they are not nearly so effective when giving care to those who express anxiety through physical symptoms or ritualistic behavior. A large part of the difficulty in dealing with anxious persons originates in an unconscious attitude toward persons suffering from these problems and in a failure to understand the true nature of the illness. Because such an individual is aware of his surroundings, is not carrying on a conversation with unseen people, and complains of physical symptoms that have no organic basis, some workers may feel unsympathetic toward him and may believe that he is "an attention getter" and that he could "snap out of it" if he really tried.

Such an attitude comes from a lack of knowledge and can destroy any possibility of the worker's being of therapeutic assistance. To achieve a more understanding attitude toward these individuals, it is important to develop some knowledge about the emotional conflicts with which the individual is struggling and the ways in which he uses the symptoms to cope with his problems.

It is important to realize that all symptoms stemming from anxiety or conversion disorders develop because of an overwhelming *unconscious* conflict and that the symptoms have great unconscious significance. The word unconscious has been stressed, since it is necessary to realize that the individual does not clearly understand why the symptom has developed nor what he is gaining by using the symptom repeatedly. He does realize that the symptom helps relieve unbearable anxiety and tension.

It is also important to realize that the discomfort and pain of which the individual complains is actually present even though there is no organic basis that can explain the existence of the symptoms. Experts are beginning to recognize that fear plays a significant role in causing pain. Since fear is prominent in the symptomatology of many anxiety-ridden people, it is not difficult to realize that they actually feel the pain of which they complain. It is important to understand that emotionally conditioned pain is as distressing to bear as is pain that results from true physical disease.

NURSING CARE OF ANXIOUS INDIVIDUALS

To make an intelligent and therapeutic plan of care, the health worker needs to understand the nature of the person's conflict and the meaning of his symptoms. Understanding the individual's needs can be achieved only through the use of the social and psychological information that is available. The plan for care and treatment should be developed collaboratively by the workers who will be involved with the individual. The type of treatment required and the goals to be established should be developed in conjunction with the individual himself. Whatever the treatment goals may be, the individual requires a consistent approach from all workers with whom he will be involved.

Although many of the specific aspects of care for these individuals will need to be planned collaboratively, there are some general suggestions that apply to the nursing care of all persons suffering from anxiety or conversion disorders.

Such individuals need a warm, friendly, empathic nurse who accepts them as people in need of help and who helps them feel that they are worthwhile human beings. Scolding or sarcastic remarks will serve only to reinforce their need to protect themselves by the use of their symptoms.

It is usually wise to listen completely and with an accepting attitude when the anxious person describes his physical symptoms. Comments should be directed toward eliciting more information about the complaints. It is important to remember that these individuals can and do become physically ill and deserve medical attention if there is any reasonable doubt about the cause of the complaint.

Some workers ignore symptoms that stem from anxiety, and in many instances this becomes synonymous with ignoring the individual himself. Since the anxious person is using symptoms to make a bid for help or love, ignoring him increases his need to use the symptoms more frequently.

Avoid asking, "How are you today?" For anxious persons this question is often an invitation for another outpouring of physical complaints. A much more helpful way to begin a conversation might be to comment on some neutral topic that is of mutual interest to both the individual and the worker.

In suggesting that an anxious person participate in some social activity, it is unwise to ask, "Would you like to go swimming with the group?" Such a question will often bring the flat answer no or a long recital about why the individual cannot possibly go. A more effective approach would be, "The group is going swimming. I hope that you will go with us." If the object is to get the individual to participate in a game of table tennis, more positive results will be obtained if the tennis paddle is placed in the client's hand by the worker, who might say, "We need one more person to play this game. Come and play." This approach is more apt to elicit participation than asking if he wishes to play.

It is helpful if the anxious individual is provided with an opportunity to succeed in the activities in which he participates. This is important because these individuals need help in building self-esteem and self-confidence. Giving deserved praise and recognition for activities performed well is one way of reassuring and encouraging them.

One of the most helpful approaches to the care of anxious clients is to assist them to develop interests outside themselves. Thus recreational and occupational therapy are significant in their treatment. Many anxiety-ridden individuals have never been able to enter into games or group activities. It is important to help them learn to play games and to participate in group activities. This provides opportunities to release tensions as well as to develop new interests. Recreational and occupational activities are usually more successful if they are focused on interests that the individual has had in the past.

The ability to encourage the anxious individual to talk about his concerns and feelings is an important aspect of his care.

The individual who is suffering from morbid fears and compulsions usually presents a challenging nursing problem. Some nurses who have no understanding of the forces that play a part in developing such symptoms may assume the attitude that the many maneuvers of the individual are ridiculous. Nurses have been known to force a phobic person to touch a doorknob even though it was well known that he was morbidly afraid of the dirt and germs he believed he would contact by touching the object. Other nurses have made it impossible for a client to get into the bathroom to carry out the handwashing rituals that were so important to him in releasing tensions and fears.

When phobic and compulsive individuals are not allowed to carry out the procedures they feel are necessary, they have no way of releasing tension. A high level of unreleased tension may culminate in a panic state. Workers should make it possible for the individual to carry out the anxiety-releasing rituals he has developed. The rituals carried on by these individuals are essential for them if they are to develop a feeling of security in the situation. Because such rituals are time consuming, time must be allowed for the individual to perform his ritualistic maneuvers.

Many workers, as well as the individual's relatives and friends, attempt to discuss the rituals reasonably in the hope of altering the behavior. This kind of pressure does nothing to help the individual and may actually cause him to feel more anxious and may increase his feeling of guilt.

Hospitalization is usually helpful for persons who exhibit severe maladaptive behavior because the environment is neutral, they are removed from the significant members of the family who may be the source of much emotional tension, and they are able to feel more secure where the routine is simple, makes few demands, and can be fairly accurately anticipated. Hospitalization on a medical unit may be unfortunate for some persons who have already focused most of their attention on physical symptoms that have no organic basis. Such individuals may become more tense, anxious, and fearful in a setting where the emphasis is placed on physical problems.

Some of the psychopharmacological agents have been helpful in reducing tension and providing the client with a degree of emotional comfort. However, the only permanent relief for persons suffering from intolerable anxiety and fear lies in discovering the basic cause of the problem and helping the individual understand the actual source of his symptoms.

There are several methods of helping individuals achieve insight and self-understanding. Most of these methods require knowledge and skill such as the psychiatrist possesses. However, well-prepared nurses are beginning to work in this area and have been successful in helping individuals through a one-to-one relationship or as discussion leaders with groups of clients. Chapters 9, 10, and 23 of this text discuss interpersonally based treatment modalities, many of which are employed in the treatment of anxious individuals.

CASE FORMULATION □ A RITUALISTIC INDIVIDUAL

The following situation is an example of how one individual began to use ritualistic behavior to defend himself against intolerable anxiety.

> Herbert B., 47 years of age, came to the community mental health center to ask for help with his problem.
>
> During his college days he had become emotionally upset and had worried excessively. His pastor was consulted, and after several conferences he was able to resume his schoolwork and graduated at the age of 21 as an accountant. He stated that he had always been very conscientious, worried a great deal about body cleanliness, and was known for his concern about keeping his room and clothing in perfect order. He was always prompt in appearing at his office and never left his desk before 5 PM. His fellow workers regarded him as very fussy, and his employer always remarked about the neatness of his desk and files—a comment that greatly pleased him. At home any irregularity in household routine upset him. His wife was fully aware of his rigid regard for rules and of his scrupulousness.
>
> Four months before he came to the center, he had been assigned the responsibility of making out the income tax report for his firm, which

dealt in stocks and bonds. This assignment was made on March 1, and he realized that he had but 6 weeks before the returns were to be filed. He worked under great pressure, and almost every day he remained in the office until late at night. With a day to spare, he entered the final figures on a roll of paper from an adding machine. Badly in need of sleep and rest, he seized this roll, thrust it into his overcoat pocket, and dashed for the midnight bus. He intended to show the slip of paper to his wife as evidence that his job was completed. On reaching his home he could not find the roll. In a frenzy he searched his clothing and ran out on the street searching the sidewalk, but failed to find it. He was put to bed in an anxious, fearful state and remained under a physician's care for several weeks.

On returning to work he found that he had developed an overwhelming compulsion. He could no longer pass a piece of crumpled paper on the floor or sidewalk without picking it up and inspecting it. During rush hour he was greatly humiliated and embarrassed by the necessity of bending over and picking up odd bits of paper. On several occasions while carrying out this compulsion he was knocked down by a hurrying passerby. A wastebasket full of discarded paper literally threw him into a panic. His only relief was obtained by waiting until after office hours when he could go over each item piece by piece. His physician recommended treatment in the community mental health center. Although he improved, the obsessive idea remained. He was well oriented, intelligent, had good insight, and otherwise appeared to be mentally normal.

Underlying this obsessive compulsive state was obviously a sensitive, overconscientious, fearful personality. The basic problem focused, in part at least, on his unresolved conflict about his role as a marital partner. This conflict was relieved to some extent by his fastidious attitude toward his body. Such problems probably originated in the attitudes that were taught during the habit-training period. The individual's wife spoke freely about the fact that their marital relations were unsatisfactory and disturbing. She had given up any hope of improving the situation by discussing it with him, since he became extremely anxious when she introduced the topic.

Herbert B.'s mother was a meticulous housekeeper who was known in her community as a fanatic about maintaining correct standards of behavior and observing religious customs.

Discussion of development of patterns of behavior and outlook

It is significant that Herbert B.'s mother was a fastidious housekeeper and a fanatic about observing religious customs and maintaining correct standards of behavior. Undoubtedly, such a mother would insist that a child achieve perfection in toilet training at a very early age. In addition, she would rear him to behave in a rigidly correct manner and would covertly encourage him to repress instinctual thoughts and desires.

A young man who at the age of 21 is known to be overly concerned about orderliness, is overly conscientious, and is worried about bodily cleanliness is already well on the road to developing compulsive symptoms to control unconscious anxiety by employing persistently repetitive acts. This behavior, like all human behavior, has purpose and meaning for the individual who employs it even though the forces producing it are unconscious. The anxiety arising from a feeling of guilt is displaced by engaging in ritualistic behavior.

In spite of Herbert's early tendencies to be upset by household irregularities, he married. He and his wife managed to work out a relationship that could be tolerated. However, according to his wife, the sexual relationship was unsatisfactory and such an upsetting topic to her husband that she avoided discussing it.

It was not until he was 47 that Herbert's symptoms became so severe that he required treatment. This was precipitated by the loss of a scrap of paper on which was recorded a final total of a complicated accounting problem he had been assigned to complete. It is interesting that he was attempting to elicit his wife's approval for a successful task accomplished. Since he did not have her approval as a sexual partner, her approval about some other aspect of life was very necessary. The loss of the paper probably represented much more than simply the loss of a list of figures. Symbolically it must have represented the loss of love and approval. This would account for his extreme fear and anxiety. The tax report had been completed before he left the office. Thus there is little doubt that a duplicate of the figures could have been found. The loss must have been symbolic of the loss of something more important and irreplaceable.

In compulsive individuals the repetitive act has a symbolic significance reminiscent of a magic ritual that is designed to eradicate the possible effect of unacceptable instinctual impulses. It also represents a type of self-punishment, since compulsive acts are recognized by the individual as being unreasonable and ridiculous. In spite of the individual's partial insight, the tension and anxiety mount until the urge to repeat the act to control the tension becomes irresistible.

Like most severely anxious individuals, Herbert was well oriented, intelligent, and intellectually normal except for his compulsive behavior. This is an example of an individual whose personality is intact except in the one area that is involved with the compulsive behavior. However, in spite of the normal aspects of his personality, he was almost totally incapacitated by the need to examine every scrap of paper.

Essentially Herbert had a lifelong history of maladaptive behavior. It became unmanageable at the age of 47. Such a severe, long-standing emotional problem requires intensive treatment. The outcome is uncertain.

CONCLUDING STATEMENTS

1. Repetitive, ritualistic behavior and physical symptoms with no organic basis are unconscious maneuvers used by the individual to gain security and to control intolerable anxiety.
2. The symptoms of anxiety rise to conscious awareness because of an inability of the ego to effect a compromise between two clashing drives.
3. Anxiety disorders are probably the most frequently observed manifestations of the individual's inability to deal with emotional conflicts.
4. Phobic disorders are characterized by specific unrealistic and inappropriate fears that are symbolic of some anxiety-laden situation in the life of the individual.
5. In the obsessive-compulsive disorder the preoccupation with a compelling ritual is the individual's way of defending himself against anxiety. The performance of the ritual provides a release of tension.
6. Conversion is a purposeful, unconscious reaction through which an individual uses a physical symptom as a disguise to solve some acute problem or fulfill some unacceptable desire.
7. All symptoms stemming from anxiety or conversion disorders develop because of an unconscious conflict and have great significance for the individual.

8. Because fear plays a significant role in pain, physical discomfort and pain may actually be present even though there is no demonstrable basis to explain the existence of the complaints.
9. Individuals who use maladaptive efforts to control anxiety behavioral patterns need a warm, friendly, empathic nurse who accepts them as worthwhile human beings who are ill and who are in need of help.
10. One of the most important aspects of the care of all anxious persons is to help them verbalize their concerns.
11. The ritualistic person should be allowed to carry out the anxiety-releasing maneuvers that are so essential to his security.

Suggested sources of additional information

CLASSICAL

Schwartz, Morris, and Shockley, Emmy Lanning: The nurse and the mental patient, New York, 1956, John Wiley & Sons, Inc.

Sullivan, Harry Stack: Conceptions of modern psychiatry, Washington, D.C., 1953, W.W. Norton & Co., Inc.

CONTEMPORARY

Abse, D. Wilfred: Hysterical conversion and dissociative syndromes and the hysterical character. In Arieti, Silvano, editor: American handbook of psychiatry, ed. 2, vol. 3, New York, 1974, Basic Books, Inc., Publishers, pp. 155-194.

Chrzanowski, Gerard: Neurasthenia and hypochondriasis. In Arieti, Silvano, editor: American handbook of psychiatry, ed. 2, vol. 3, New York, 1974, Basic Books, Inc., Publishers, pp. 141-154.

Engel, George L.: Grief and grieving, Am. J. Nurs. **64:**93-98, Sept., 1964.

English, O.S., and Pearson, G.H.J.: Emotional problems of living, ed. 3, Philadelphia, 1976, W.W. Norton & Co., Inc.

Friedman, Paul, and Goldstein, Jacob: Phobic reactions. In Arieti, Silvano, editor: American handbook of psychiatry, ed. 2, vol. 3, New York, 1974, Basic Books, Inc., Publishers, pp. 110-140.

Hadley, Alice A.H.: What is an obsessive-compulsive neurosis? In Burd, Shirley F., and Marshall, Margaret A., editors: Some clinical approaches to psychiatric nursing, New York, 1963, Macmillan Publishing Co., Inc., pp. 81-86.

Karshmer, Judith F.: The application of social learning theory to aggression, Perspect. Psychiatr. Care **16**(5-6):223-237, Sept.-Dec., 1978.

Kent, Fraser: Coping with phobias, New York, 1980, Harper & Row, Publishers.

Kerr, Norine: Anxiety: theoretical considerations, Perspect. Psychiatr. Care **16:**36-40, Jan.-Feb., 1978.

Lenefsky, Barbara, et al.: Management of violent behaviors, Perspect. Psychiatr. Care **16**(5-6):212-217, Sept.-Dec., 1978.

Mastrovito, Rene C.: Psychogenic pain, Am. J. Nurs. **74:**514-519, 1974.

May, Rollo: The meaning of anxiety, New York, 1977, W.W. Norton & Co., Inc.

OF PARTICULAR INTEREST

Kerr, Norine: Anxiety: theoretical considerations, Perspect. Psychiatr. Care **16:**36-40, Jan.-Feb., 1978.

This is a concise, relevant article discussing various theorists' conceptions of anxiety.

Roncoli, M.: Bantering: a therapeutic strategy with obsessional patients, Perspect. Psychiatr. Care **12:**171-175, Oct.-Dec., 1974.

This article is useful in discussing an approach to one particularly challenging nursing care problem.

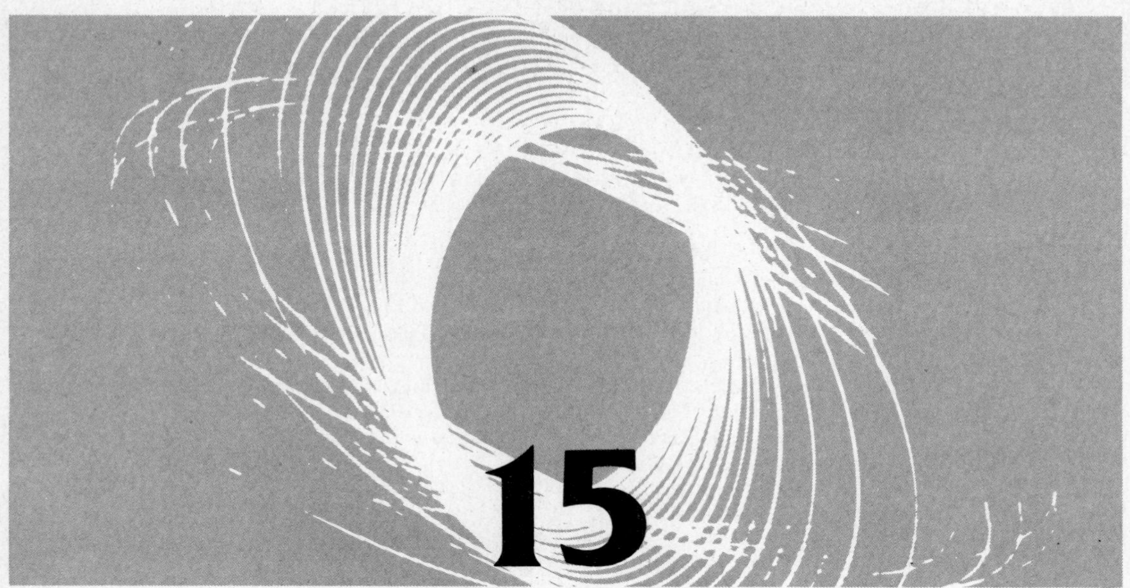

Behavioral patterns that reflect social maladaptation

- Individuals who engage in antisocial behavior
- Sexual deviation
- Individuals whose behavior is related to alcohol and drug abuse

Certain individuals engage in behaviors whose causes are even less clearly understood than behaviors that reflect maladaptive thought processes, maladaptive mood states, or maladaptive efforts to control anxiety. These behaviors are somewhat unique in that their very existence is seen as an assault on the fundamental values of society. This is not to say that the individual, his family, and his immediate associates may not suffer as a result of his behaviors; rather, the nature of the individual's behavior is such that it threatens the community at large, even though few people may have been directly involved. Behaviors that are societally offensive include antisocial acts, sexual deviances, and substance abuse.

INDIVIDUALS WHO ENGAGE IN ANTISOCIAL BEHAVIOR

Individuals who engage in antisocial acts seem incapable of conforming to social or legal standards. Many of them constitute a threat to society because of their ruthless attitude toward others and their lack of a sense of responsibility. They usually test within the normal range on an intelligence test, and some are intellectually superior. In spite of this ability, they seem incapable of making a satisfactory social adjustment. These people are usually self-centered and selfish; they lack the ability to develop lasting and meaningful relationships with other people; they possess poor judgment and insight; they do not profit by experience or punishment; and they are unreliable and lack a sense of responsibility.

Development of behavioral patterns

The reason for the inability of individuals with antisocial behavior to develop satisfactory social relationships is unknown. The defect seems to lie in the emotional and volitional aspects of the personality rather than in the intellectual areas.

In studying the longitudinal histories of many of these individuals it is apparent that they were emotionally impulsive and maladjusted children. They have apparently failed to develop a socialized superego. The personality appears to be dominated by the primitive demands of the id. The ego has failed to establish a constructive identity or to evolve socially useful adaptations and controls. In some way these individuals have failed to make a positive identification with parents or parental substitutes who could have provided the love, security, recognition, and respect that a child requires if he is to develop into an emotionally healthy individual. Failure to make a positive identification and to accept socially useful controls may have been the result of a faulty parent-child relationship. At any rate, the psychopathological forces that were initiated in the individual's early life experiences continued throughout adulthood. Thus most of these individuals seem to possess an inherent ego defect that causes them to basically distrust others and to respond to primitive id impulses regardless of society's disapproval.

Providing professional treatment

Although the current trend is to keep as many individuals as possible out of institutions, many authorities still believe that if persons with antisocial behaviors are to be treated with any hope of success, they will require institutionalization. Because their early childhood relationships with parental figures have not resulted in the development of essential ego controls or a socialized superego, an opportunity to correct this defective development must be provided. The institution should provide a friendly, accepting, humane environment, where there are firm, reasonable, consistent limits and controls placed on behavior. A permissive atmosphere is usually not helpful for these individuals. They need to be helped to develop a socialized superego, and such growth may be fostered by an organized, structured, controlled environment.

The treatment goals should include helping them to accept and use more socially approved attitudes and standards in their relationships with other people. To achieve this they must be helped to trust other people. It is hoped that this can be achieved through the development of a therapeutic relationship with one of the members of the professional treatment team. Since the psychiatrist is usually the ultimate authority in the treatment team, it would probably be helpful if the therapeutic relationship could be developed with a psychiatrist who could provide the necessary discipline.

The treatment goals can be promoted through a system of rewards and prohibitions, with socially acceptable behavior being rewarded with privileges and less acceptable behavior being responded to by the withholding of privileges.

If the antisocial behavior has developed out of negative social and cultural influences, the individual should be helped to seek a more acceptable social situation. Certainly he should be encouraged not to return to the same environment.

Nursing care plan

Sometimes the nurse feels that an individual who behaves in an antisocial way is a criminal and should be excluded from all treatment center actitivies or that he does not require hospitalization, therefore disregarding the need to establish firm, consistent limits. Either of these extremes in attitude will prove to be unsound.

Since the individual with antisocial attitudes is often attractive, above average in intelligence, and an interesting conversationalist, the nurse should avoid allowing him to gain control of the situation. It is helpful to remember that these individuals are usually clever and frequently use extremely poor judgment. They are likely to be troublemakers among other clients and have been known to organize psychotic individuals for the purpose of accomplishing their antisocial plans.

Although the nurse can be most effective if a helpful, friendly approach is used in dealing with the individual with antisocial attitudes, the nurse needs to be constantly alert to the possibility of his attempting to gain control of the situation. The clinical team should identify attitudes they believe will be most effective in dealing with this individual and should list the responsibilities that he will be expected to fulfill. When these decisions have been made, it is of primary importance for all hospital personnel to be consistent in carrying them out and in holding the individual to fulfilling his obligations.

These individuals do not profit by being scolded or lectured. Such an approach is never helpful and will serve only to arouse angry feelings. Since it is thought that these individuals learn little from experience, punishing them accomplishes nothing. Limits must be set on their behavior, since they frequently indulge in temper tantrums or destructive activities to achieve their objectives.

When the individual is demonstrating antisocial behavior, it is important to treat him in such a manner that he will know that the workers want to help him even though he cannot be allowed to continue the behavior he is exhibiting.

Individuals with antisocial attitudes need a variety of challenging activities throughout the day. They are likely to plead for special privileges, but workers should be cautious about granting such requests. Like all other individuals they should be rewarded for acceptable behavior. If possible, these individuals should be placed in situations in which they can obtain socially acceptable satisfactions. Thus success in some type of industrial therapy is ideal. It is essential to hold these individuals to fulfilling the responsibilities expected of them, since they are likely to cooperate only at their own convenience.

Because many of these individuals lack a well-developed social conscience, they usually function poorly in group activities. However, insofar as possible, it is suggested that they be helped to accept a role in some of the available group functions.

Individuals with antisocial attitudes vary greatly in emotional needs and personality limitations. Their care in the treatment center should be designed to help them with their individual problems and to make it possible for them to cultivate a more socially acceptable approach to living.

Due to the personality characteristics of the antisocial individual that result in behavior that is superficially pleasing, workers misjudge this group of persons more often than any other with whom they come in contact. Inexperienced workers are likely to feel that a perfectly normal person is being detained for treatment without justification; if a worker experiences this feeling, it would be wise to consult with a more experienced health professional for clarification.

CASE FORMULATION □ AN INDIVIDUAL WITH ANTISOCIAL BEHAVIOR

The following story was adapted from a newspaper account of the antisocial behavior of a young adolescent.

A 15-year-old youth was arrested for breaking into and robbing 18 Catholic churches. In addition to these robberies he admitted burglarizing several homes in the area of the city in which he lived.

This boy had been abandoned on the steps of a large hospital when he was an infant. He was found by a kindly woman who took him to her home and cared for him. She was a member of a Catholic church and chose to name the boy after the priest of the church she attended. After 10 years the foster mother reported that "he went bad" and was sent to a Youth Study Center where psychiatric help and rehabilitation were attempted. The child never returned to live with his foster mother. Instead, he lived with anyone who would offer him bed and board for a few days. He was arrested at the office of a community organization, which he said was his home. At that time he had several 1000 dollars in a paper bag hidden among his possessions.

Discussion of development of patterns of behavior

Although no other information was available, this story demonstrates rather clearly many of the characteristics of an individual who because of his behavior is said to possess antisocial behaviors. Although we know nothing about his foster mother or the relationship that she established with him, we can be sure that until he was 10 years old he was taken to church regularly and taught the basic beliefs of the church. It is interesting to speculate about why he turned against the church with which he was affiliated. It is possible that the church symbolized his foster mother and her teachings, which he rejected. It is safe to suggest that in some way he was unconsciously striking out against his foster mother when he attacked the church that she respected and loved.

Certainly this boy failed to develop a socialized superego. Thus his behavior was dominated by instinctual demands that included the amassing of money, which symbolizes power. Money also made it possible for him to indulge many of his fantasies. It is not possible to know what ego identity this adolescent had developed, but we do know that he failed to develop a constructive identity and had not incorporated socially useful controls. Like other individuals who are said to possess antisocial behaviors, he seemed incapable of conforming to social or legal standards. Even though he was treated at the Youth Study Center, he did not profit by this experience and thus it can be said that in this situation he was not able to profit by experience. He appeared to lack a sense of responsibility.

The situation demonstrates the reason why for many years such behavior was thought to result from a constitutional defect within the makeup of the individual. Antisocial behavior is usually exhibited early in life. It is difficult to identify a reasonable explanation for its occurrence.

This boy was abandoned by his own parents. To some this may suggest that they too were lacking in the ability to accept responsibility and to conform to social or legal standards. Some people might conclude that this young man inherited a defective personality. However, current theories of personality development would not support this belief. Instead, the search for the basic problem would focus on the relationship that existed in the family situation where this young man lived during his first 10 years.

Planning and implementing nursing care

It can readily be seen that treatment of this boy was challenging, since his conflict obviously lay in the emotional and volitional areas of life. His antisocial personality developed very early and progressed rapidly.

A friendly, accepting, humane environment is the only type of situation in which personality defects can be corrected. However, at the same time, such an individual requires firm, consistent, reasonable controls. The treatment goals would include helping this young man to accept and use more socially approved behavior in relation to other people and society's institutions. Success in achieving these goals is problematic at best and depends on the ability of the treatment team to identify and work with the healthy aspects of the individual's personality.

SEXUAL DEVIATION

According to the psychoanalytical explanation, sexual deviations are the result of failure to outgrow some infantile or preadolescent manner of obtaining sexual pleasure. The sexually deviant individual is one who continues to get sexual satisfaction by immature methods throughout adult life.

The normal sexual development in the human being is a slow and complex psychobiological process. As Freud has postulated, the sexual instinct passes through several stages of growth, and an arrest or fixation at immature levels may cause serious distortions of the total personality.

The various sexual deviations are, therefore, malconditionings or incomplete expressions of the psychological accompaniments of sexual activity. Apart from the explanations offered by the psychoanalysts, little is known about the cause of most deviations in sexual behavior. In general, society looks with antipathy and disfavor on individuals who practice sexual deviations, and in some instances expresses violent resentment. Although the legal attitudes toward sexual deviation are becoming more rational, there are laws on the statute books of some states to punish sex offenders, even when their sexual acts are carried on with consenting adults. Many of these individuals are unfortunate victims of a distorted psychosexual development. These legal implications are probably based on mid-Victorian attitudes and a failure to understand the origin of sexual deviations. They may also be related to society's concerns about a threat to normal propagation and successful survival of the race. Sex variants tend to repeat their particular deviation even after experiencing cruel, inhuman punishment and suffering.

Development of sexually deviant patterns of behavior

As more psychological understanding of the personalities of individuals who have failed to achieve a mature psychosexual development is achieved, there is a growing belief on the part of specialists that the psychopathology underlying their problems is basically related to otherwise uncontrollable anxiety. Usually sexual deviation is only one manifestation of a deep-seated emotional maladaptation of long duration. All individuals who use a deviant outlet to achieve sexual satisfaction exhibit a pattern of behavior that is repeated compulsively without reason or logic. It is not a substitute for normal heterosexual relations but is carried on to meet a specific unconscious need, which the individual himself does not understand.

The following is an example of such behavior. A respected

middle-aged married citizen of a small midwestern town was arrested for *voyeurism* (for being a Peeping Tom). He admitted that for most of his life he had been peeping at night into the bedroom windows of his neighbors. Unfortunately he was not apprehended for many years, and when he was finally caught, the anger of the townspeople was so great that he and his family were forced to leave the community.

In addition to voyeurism, some of the other sexual perversions include pedophilia, fetishism, transvestism, and exhibitionism. A brief explanation of each follows.

Pedophilia is the technical word used to describe adult males who demonstrate a pathological sexual interest in children. This situation usually occurs when the adult male feels inadequate sexually and is afraid to approach an adult female for fear of being rejected or of being sexually inadequate. Thus the individual approaches a child sexually in the unconscious hope that he will be accepted by a less discriminating person. His behavior is apt to frighten the child, who usually cries out for help. The cry frightens the offender, who may flee. Unfortunately, some offenders have injured or killed the child to keep from being apprehended.

Fetishism occurs in men who may unconsciously fear genital heterosexual contact due to castration fears that developed early in life. For these men sexual feeling is attached to some inanimate object that may have belonged to a woman for whom the individual once developed admiration, or the object may simply have a female association. The fetish may be a glove, a shoe, a girdle, or some other very personal feminine object. Since contact with the object usually leads to orgasm, the use of the fetish is a substitute for genital heterosexuality.

Transvestism occurs when an individual has a deep-seated urge to dress in the clothing of the opposite sex. In some persons this urge may be one of several manifestations of a profound personality disturbance involving homosexuality with a paranoid ideation.

Exhibitionism occurs when the individual has an uncontrollable urge to exhibit the genitalia to others, usually members of the opposite sex. This symptom is thought to occur in persons who are defending themselves against guilt and fear of punishment arising out of unconscious incestuous wishes. For example, the male exhibits the penis to reassure himself that it is still intact and that he has not been punished for his incestuous desires. Exhibition of the genitals may also serve to demonstrate sexually aggressive feelings.

Homosexuality

Although there are a variety of sexual deviations, the one that receives the most attention in our modern culture is homosexuality. It involves sexual attachment and love for a person of the same sex. There is a wide range of homosexual behavior in both men and women. According to the statistics revealed by the armed services and draft and induction boards, it occurs frequently.

Today most psychiatrists accept the theory that the basic cause of this emotional problem lies in the early childhood experiences of the individual. It is essentially an arrest in the individual's psychosexual development. Homosexuality is often attributed to excessive domination by the parent of the opposite sex or by fixation on siblings of the same sex. In extreme forms, the evidence of homosexuality is clearly shown in the tendency to take on the manners, dress, and vocational interests that normally belong to individuals of the opposite sex. This is, however, not a universal rule, the milder degrees of homosexuality are intermixed with manifestations of natural heterosexuality. In the homosexual male, for example, an effeminate body may or may not be present, and frequently the physique may be definitely athletic and suggestive of masculinity.

Many individuals with a homosexual orientation carry on well-adjusted, productive lives. They bitterly resent the theory that homosexuality develops out of negative early childhood experiences. Recent studies of a large group of homosexuals have shown that many are capable of carrying on effectively in the business and professional world without being handicapped by disrupting symptoms. Earlier studies focused attention on poorly adjusted homosexuals who had sought psychiatric help.

When confronted by a situation in which denied homosexual

longings can no longer be repressed or when threatened by open exposure of their psychosexual orientation, persons whose homosexual desires are latent may react violently with behavior described as *homosexual panic.* This reaction may take on the proportions of a true psychosis. However, it is usually of short duration unless it appears as a prelude to schizophrenia. Homosexual panic occurs in the individual whose homosexual desires are latent. It often occurs when the individual is compelled to live in intimate contact with a group of individuals of the same sex.

Latent, unconscious homosexual impulses that are unacceptable to the superego may become the basis for paranoid ideas through the process of reaction formation.

Changing attitudes toward sexually deviant behavior

In the past the individual who failed to reach psychosexual maturity and who satisfied his sexual drive by using one of the sexual deviations was referred to as a sexual psychopath or sexual deviate. Historically, some nations have looked on sexual deviation entirely as a moral and legal problem. Partially because of their heritage of the English moral code, Canada and the United States adopted this attitude. Now there is reason to believe that a beginning understanding of the psychological causes of sexually deviant behavior is developing. Some positive changes in attitude can be observed in the treatment of these individuals by the courts, professional people, and law enforcement officers. Today there seems to be a beginning recognition of the fact that individuals who display sexually deviant behavior may suffer from a personality defect caused by an arrest in psychosexual development. This deviation probably came about through no fault of theirs but rather because of faulty parent-child relationships. For example, sons may unconsciously identify with the female role when brought up by overprotective mothers or in homes where there is no father or in situations in which the father is an awesome, threatening figure. Thus these boys may grow up rejecting the male role and emotionally embracing the less threatening role of the woman.

Although there are many homosexual women in the United States, their sexual choice has never caused the negative reaction that the sexual choice of men has elicited. The development of homosexuality in women is also thought to develop out of the family situation.

At least one nation, Great Britain, has adopted laws that permit homosexual activity between consenting adults. Many experts believe that adult homosexuals should not be hounded by the police and punished by jail sentences, as some states in the United States have permitted in the past.

Everyone agrees that children and adolescents should be safeguarded against seduction by a sexual deviate. Many of the laws relating to homosexuality were originally enacted as a safeguard. The entire legal question about sexual deviation is currently being reviewed in many nations. Certainly this is a difficult question that needs rethinking in the United States.

Recently, homosexuals or "gay people" in the United States have joined forces to improve their legal status. Their struggle has been assisted by the civil rights movement. They are slowly achieving equal rights in the areas of housing and jobs. They have been successful in persuading the American Psychiatric Association to eliminate homosexuality as a diagnostic category.

Prevention and treatment

Sexually deviant behavior is difficult to treat successfully because the problem arises out of the individual's personality structure. By the time an individual comes to the attention of professional workers who can provide treatment, the personality structure has developed. The individual seeks sexual satisfaction in a deviant way because his psychosexual development has been arrested or has regressed to an immature and less threatening level. Thus sexually deviant behavior is a deeply ingrained part of the individual's personality. In addition, he has little understanding of it, and since it temporarily satisfies his sexual needs, he is loathe or unable to substitute more mature behavior.

One treatment method now available that may be able to assist the individual to make a profound alteration in his personality adaptation is psychoanalysis. This treatment is expensive, involves a great deal of time and personal commitment on the part of both the individual and the analyst, and consequently is available only to a limited number of people. Success is entirely dependent on the sincere interest of the individual in changing his sexual orientation. Although individuals who practice sexually deviant behavior are interested in avoiding involvement with the legal authorities, they are not always interested in profoundly altering their sexual orientation.

If competent psychiatric treatment is available, if the individual is highly motivated to change his lifelong pattern of adaptation, and if he is prepared to continue therapy for a prolonged period of time, some positive changes in sexual orientation may be achieved.

Some individuals who practice sexually deviant behavior are sentenced to prison terms because some aspect of their behavior is considered damaging to the morals of others. Prison environments have a negative influence on these individuals. In spite of this, it is sometimes necessary to confine some of them in corrective institutions if they have committed serious social offenses.

When an individual who exhibits sexually deviant behavior requests psychiatric help and willingly accepts treatment, some authorities believe that it is therapeutically valuable to admit him to a psychiatric treatment situation. In this way the individual's therapist can supervise his environment. Another advantage of hospitalization is that it removes the individual from the environment in which sexually deviant behavior was his mode of expression. In time, with competent psychiatric help, the individual may be able to redirect his sexual and aggressive drives so that his personal and social functioning may be improved.

Currently, "gay" individuals are encouraging the attitude of recognizing and publicly admitting that their choice for a sexual relationship is someone of the same sex. This is referred to as "coming out of the closet" and is undoubtedly a move toward more positive mental health for these people. For those who do recognize and accept their sexual choice, treatment is not indicated.

Sexually deviant behavior, like all human problems with a psychological origin, should be prevented so that treatment will be unnecessary. An important step in prevention is effective sexual education for all children. Currently, much discussion is being carried on throughout the United States concerning sex education. The arguments focus on who should provide it and where it should be given. Some lay people are attacking the efforts that have been made in some schools to provide adequate sex education. The schools introduced this instruction because there was evidence that sex education was not being adequately provided elsewhere. Certainly children require accurate and complete sexual information if they are to develop wholesome, mature attitudes. Most authorities agree that such information can be taught most effectively in schools by individuals who are educationally prepared to provide such information. Most people also agree that this teaching should be reinforced and elaborated by the parents in the home.

Not only is adequate sex education essential, it is also necessary to provide positive parent-child relationships and a healthy family environment in the early formative years for children to achieve mature psychosexual development. Because children identify sexual roles at an early age, they need the presence of both parents in the home to establish an identification with the parent of the same sex. Thus the family pattern established in homes is crucial to the healthy emotional development of children. During their formative years they need guidance from wise parents in redirecting aggressive impulses into constructive and socially acceptable channels.

It would be helpful if early corrective experiences could be provided for children who seem to be developing social reactions that vary greatly from those expected from others of their peer group.

Meeting the needs of individuals with sexually deviant behavior

When an individual suffers from arrested psychosexual development, his total personality is affected. Thus immature behavior in many aspects of living can be expected from an individual who uses an immature way of expressing sexual needs. He may sulk, demand special attention, display many dependent needs, use provocative behavior, blame others for his situation, or become sarcastic and hostile toward the staff.

The clinical workers should collaborate in identifying the

most appropriate ways to deal with the behavior such an individual presents. Certainly the workers should avoid identifying with the client or reinforcing his negative behavior by giving nonverbal approval to it.

Sometimes workers behave as if the individual who has a history of sexual deviation is a social outcast. When they harbor such feelings, they inevitably treat the person in a cold, unfriendly manner. Such feelings on the part of a member of the professional treatment team tend to destroy much of the therapeutic effect the group is attempting to achieve. Such attitudes suggest that the individual holding them fails to realize that the sexually deviant person is not entirely responsible for his problem.

Sexually deviant individuals deserve a friendly, accepting climate in which they are treated with respect and consideration. In addition, they require the establishment of firm limits that are fairly and consistently enforced. Since the nurse has a good deal of responsibility for developing the climate in the treatment situation, her understanding of the client's problem and her attitude toward him are of major importance. He needs to have a well-planned schedule of daily activities available so that he can avoid lethargy and boredom. He needs help in becoming an active participant in some aspects of the planned schedule of activities.

CASE FORMULATION □ AN INDIVIDUAL WITH ARRESTED PSYCHOSEXUAL DEVELOPMENT

A young man, 20 years of age, was admitted to a mental health treatment center because of a handwashing compulsion, feelings of unreality, and because he feared that he would kill his mother.

He was an unplanned baby, born after his parents had been married for 12 years. His father frankly stated that he wanted a girl and paid no attention to the child until he was old enough to walk. The child never seemed content in his mother's arms and pushed her breast away from the first time it was offered to him. As he grew older, he bit and scratched her.

When the individual was 5 years old, his father died. He became overly attached to his mother and shared her bed until he was 11 years old. During these years he would scream for his mother if she were out of sight. He frequently called out to her, "Mama, are you all right?"

His mother began drinking heavily after the father's death and often relegated his care to a neighbor woman. At age 11 responsibility for his care became more than the mother could manage, and she sent him to live at a boys' boarding school. This decision made him desperately unhappy, and he pled with her not to send him away. During these years he was sent to a boys' camp during the summer months. This was seen by him as banishment. He especially disliked the camp because he did poorly in all sports. About the time he was in the eighth grade, his mother became interested in remarrying. He told her that he would kill himself if she did.

As he grew older, his relationship with his mother became progressively more strained. When he was 16, in the hope of improving the situation, his mother allowed him to remain at home and attend high school. Instead of responding to this decision with pleasure, his anger toward his mother increased, and he began calling her a liar and other derogatory names.

During his sixteenth year he had his first homosexual experience, during which he participated in anal intercourse as the passive partner. After this first experience he participated frequently in homosexual relations. Although he enjoyed the physical pleasure derived from this activity, it also caused him to feel ashamed, guilty, and angry. The handwashing compulsion as a ritualistic protection against his bad thoughts and deeds developed soon after he began engaging in mutual masturbation and anal intercourse. It relieved his anxiety and guilt feelings.

Discussion of development of patterns of behavior

In studying this young man's life history it seems clear that he spent his years at home seeking approval from his mother. After his father's death, he became very good and docile in the hope of winning his mother's acceptance and love. Until puberty this boy dedicated himself to being his mother's "good little girl." At puberty his behavior changed because he was in great conflict. His conflict appeared to be based on his fear of behaving like a man sexually and being punished for being sexually dangerous to women (especially his mother) or renouncing his masculinity and being humiliated by being treated like a woman (when accepting the role of passive partner during anal intercourse with a man). His conflict between his fear of injuring someone if he behaved like a man and of acting like a woman and being humiliated resulted in an inability to make decisions or to function effectively. The handwashing ritual, like all symptoms, fulfilled an important purpose in his life. In addition to relieving tension, it kept his hands from harming others.

This young man was rejected by both his father and mother. He lost his father at the age of 5 years, which is a crucial time in a child's life. It is not unusual for children of that age to fantasize that they were responsible for the loss of the absent parent. During his formative years he slept with his mother. Undoubtedly, his close contact with his mother aroused sexual feelings and gave rise to sexual fantasies. When he was banished at 11 years of age to the boarding school, he may have felt that it was a punishment because of his "bad" (sexual) thoughts. He had no male parent with whom to identify and after whom to pattern his behavior. An attempt to adapt by accepting the feminine role resulted in guilt and frustration.

Planning and implementing nursing care

Admission to a short-term treatment center where the environment is quiet and calm probably would be the best immediate plan for this individual. The neutral environment would be helpful in lowering his anxiety level. However, the plan would not include keeping him in the center for more than a few weeks, since responsibility for his actions must eventually be accepted by him and not by an institution. During the time that he is in the treatment center, the workers should give him plenty of time to carry out the handwashing rituals without disapproving of them verbally or by attitude. At the same time, he should be encouraged to direct his energies into satisfying occupational activities and group recreation.

Only workers who are sincerely interested in this individual should attempt to work closely with him. When workers are genuinely interested, they will be able to be patient and understanding, to reassure him, and to help him to express his feelings. In this way he may begin to understand his own behavior and identify the source of his conflicts.

Since he did not experience a positive mature relationship

with either his father or mother, corrective experiences may be provided in therapy sessions in which both men and women therapists are involved. These sessions should be continued as frequently as needed when the individual establishes a living situation outside the treatment center and away from his mother.

Workers should avoid discussing his handwashing compulsions or trying through logical reasoning to encourage him to give them up. They were developed as a defense against intolerable anxiety and guilt and will be relinquished only when they no longer serve the original purpose.

Outlook for this client

This individual will be able to find sexual satisfaction with a woman if, through therapy, he is able to resolve his conflicts and fears about the sexual roles of men and women.

Obviously this person's early personality development was defective, and homosexuality was only one of several pathological symptoms that he developed. In evaluating his future, it is unrealistic to expect psychiatric help to provide him with a well-integrated personality. Psychotherapy can give him some relief from his most painful symptoms and help him cope more effectively with his emotional problems.

INDIVIDUALS WHOSE BEHAVIOR IS RELATED TO ALCOHOL AND DRUG ABUSE

There are many chemical substances that, when taken internally, cause unusual mental reactions. Not all of them are taken intentionally. Some are given as medication to which there is an individual sensitivity, and still others may be absorbed slowly without the knowledge of the individual. Examples of the latter form of poisoning are lead and manganese encountered in industry and the inhalation of exhaust fumes from automobiles. When excessive amounts of many drugs are absorbed or allowed to accumulate slowly in the blood, delirium, loss of memory, and stupor may result.

Far more common are the mental reactions caused by the intentional and habitual use of drugs such as alcohol, barbiturates, bromides, and morphine, which deaden the senses and provide a temporary escape from anxiety. Unfortunately, individuals who abuse alcohol and drugs are often rejected by society, and many nursing personnel carry this cultural attitude with them as they perform their professional activities. Individuals who rely on the emotional support of external factors such as alcohol and drugs are unquestionably emotionally inadequate, fearful, lonely people who are in desperate need of help. The subtle rejection conveyed to the individual when the worker actually believes that he is unworthy simply reinforces his low self-image. Thus it would be better for the worker to be reassigned to a different kind of responsibility if a wholehearted acceptance of the alcoholic or addicted individual and the provision of a positive attitude of understanding and genuine interest are not possible.

Alcohol dependence

People are said to be alcoholics when their intake of alcoholic beverages is so great that it interferes markedly with their work performance and their functioning as responsible citizens.

Alcohol dependence may take many forms and has many causes. One individual may be a chronic alcoholic, which means that he drinks excessively and is incapacitated most of the time. Another person may be referred to as a periodic or cyclic alcoholic, which means that he drinks excessively during certain periods of his life but during other periods may not drink at all. A third type of alcoholism is exhibited by an individual who drinks large quantities of alcohol daily over a period of years. At first he may not seem to be seriously affected by this overindulgence. Slowly and insidiously, physical, mental, and emotional deterioration occurs. Eventually this person may be described as suffering from alcoholic deterioration. No matter what type of alcoholism is being considered, the problem is thought to have its basis in some emotional conflict, frustration, or feeling of inadequacy. Alcohol makes it possible for the individual to escape temporarily from overwhelming emotional or social problems.

In general, those individuals who take alcohol to excess do so because they are unhappy, distraught, and maladjusted and because alcohol furnishes them a temporary release from the stresses of living. Most alcoholics are fundamentally unstable, sensitive, self-indulgent people, and many of them are suffering from a poorly developed sexual identity. Alcohol not only offers a surcease from feelings of inferiority but also provides an occasion for conviviality and sympathy and provides a temporary and false sense of ease and security. Inhibitions are weakened, and repressed desires may be freely expressed. Excessive alcoholic intake sometimes precipitates a psychotic reaction. Its effects are not uniform and may bring to the surface many different reactions, some of these apparently determined by racial, social, and temperamental factors that vary with each individual.

Understanding the alcohol-dependent individual. Each alcoholic is a unique individual with problems that are characteristically his own. Consequently, the treatment and care of the alcoholic individual begins with the understanding of his personality and the problems from which he has a need to escape. Many alcohol-dependent individuals use alcohol in somewhat the same way that psychotic individuals use psychotic symptoms. That is, alcoholics escape from reality through alcohol, whereas some psychotic individuals escape from reality through the use of their symptoms. When some alcoholics are deprived of alcohol, they may substitute psychotic symptoms such as withdrawal from reality, depression, or a paranoid reaction.

Sometimes alcohol is used to cover symptoms of mental illness. Thus some people who are labeled as alcoholics are actually suffering from a depression or anxiety state. Such persons are clearly in need of the care and treatment usually provided in a mental health treatment center.

Many alcoholics are described as having oral personalities. This suggests that they are fixated at an early stage of emotional development. This early stage of emotional development is called the oral-dependent period and is characterized by infantile emotional reactions. Such individuals receive many of their emotional satisfactions from the intake of food and fluids by mouth. They find it difficult to function as independent adults and unconsciously want to be dependent on a strong person, much as they once were on a mother figure. Such adults are difficult to help because they may have faulty personality structures and a limited amount of ego strength. For this reason some therapists are reluctant to accept alcoholics for treatment. Some mental health treatment centers have adopted a policy of refusing admission to alcoholics because experience has shown that many of them respond poorly to treatment. On the other hand, some centers have concentrated on the treatment of the alcohol-dependent individual. Alcoholism is such a serious social and health problem that the United States Public Health Service is encouraging the establishment of centers to develop more effective methods of treating this condition.

Treatment. Several treatments have been developed in an attempt to help alcoholics function without alcohol. One of these is called the *aversion treatment*. This treatment, which is rarely used today, consists of allowing the individual to drink a good deal of his favorite alcoholic beverage, after which an emetic drug is administered. In a few minutes the person becomes acutely nauseated and spends approximately an hour vomiting and retching. The treatment is administered two or three times a week until the individual develops such an aversion to alcohol that he begins to gag at the sight of the alcoholic beverage toward which the aversion has been developed. This treatment does not help the individual solve any of his basic emotional problems, although some therapists have combined the treatment with psychotherapy. The aversion treatment does keep some individuals away from alcohol for several months, and some are able to give it up permanently. Many individuals substitute some other form of emotional support for alcohol and may begin the use of drugs, particularly the barbiturates, after giving up the use of alcohol.

The drug disulfiram (Antabuse) has been used successfully to treat some alcohol-dependent individuals. It functions something like the aversion treatment in that the individual who takes a specific amount of disulfiram daily will become nauseated when he takes even a small amount of alcohol. This drug is helpful as long as the individual is under close supervision and takes the drug regularly. Away from supervision some individuals stop taking the drug. The drug is considered to be dangerous in some instances, and a few individuals have suffered untoward reactions from it.

Although alcoholism is one of the major mental health problems in the United States today, few specific ways of helping alcohol-dependent persons have been identified.

Every alcoholic drinks for a reason. That reason is fundamentally an inability to adjust to certain demands of adult living or an attempt to cope with the anxiety resulting from a basic defect in personality development.

The primary treatment for the alcoholic is to aid him in coping with life's responsibilities without having to resort to the use of alcohol. This generally means a long period of helping the individual to identify the source of his conflicts and reeducation in how to cope with them more effectively. The success of this reeducation depends to a large extent on the individual's personal motivation.

Rehabilitation. The magnitude of the problem of alcoholism in the United States is demonstrated by the fact that it has now become the fourth largest health problem. Today it follows cardiovascular disease, cancer, and mental illness in the ranking of health problems set forth by the United States Public Health Service. Rehabilitation of individuals who suffer from this condition is difficult and often inadequate. This situation exists primarily because too few communities have recognized and accepted full responsibility for offering aid to individuals with this problem.

As a result of shortsightedness on the part of many communities, there were until recently a limited number of facilities for treating alcohol-dependent persons. This is remarkable in view of the magnitude of the problem, which affects almost all age groups. The incidence of alcoholism in children, adolescents, and women has dramatically increased. The stereotype of the alcoholic being the male laborer (or executive) is no longer accurate.

The stigma attached to alcoholism has been one of the chief causes for the attitude of disinterest toward the problem. Until recently this disinterest has blocked the way toward a more adequate approach to the treatment and rehabilitation of individuals suffering from alcoholism. For generations both professional and lay people have dismissed the alcoholic as a person for whom little could be done. They believe that he was socially and morally incapable of giving up the habit and assuming a more responsible way of life. Alcoholism, like mental illness, has been one of the human problems to which many taboos have been attached. Thus both of these tragic social and health problems failed to receive serious scientific attention until recently. Today there is more professional help available for persons who are mentally ill than for those who suffer from alcoholism.

Actually, the problems of mental illness and alcoholism are not so unrelated as they appear to be at first glance. Recently much has been written and said about alcoholism being a disease. This designation is probably not entirely accurate. Some authorities believe that the purpose of promoting the idea that alcoholism is a disease is to remove it from the category of punishable crimes and to place it in the health field, where it can be treated by medical measures. Alcoholism is more accurately thought of as a behavioral syndrome in which the drinking is symptomatic of physiological, psychological, social, and economic stresses on the individual.

The first step in rehabilitating the alcoholic is to discover the reasons that underlie his personal problem. Hand in hand with this task is that of encouraging the individual to accept the fact that he is an alcoholic, that he is unable to control his life without the help alcohol provides, and that he needs assistance to cope with this problem. Discovering the reasons that underlie the need for alcohol frequently requires the combined work of a team of professional workers, including the social worker, the psychologist, the psychiatrist, and the nurse. Each alcoholic is an individual with a severe personality maladaptation caused by problems that are uniquely his own. Thus it becomes necessary to know a great deal about the individual's family relationships, his psychological makeup, and his emotional health before a decision can be made concerning the treatment and rehabilitation methods appropriate for him.

Significant help for the alcoholic requires some outside intervention to enable him to establish an emotional reorientation to the world. He must be helped to shift his emotional tensions and pressures in such a way as to achieve satisfactions from life without having to seek release of tensions from alcohol.

This formula for helping the alcoholic is deceptively simple. In reality it is extremely difficult to assist an individual to establish an emotional reorientation to the world. To date, few therapists or rehabilitative institutions have been successful in helping alcoholics achieve these goals. Part of the reason for the difficulties that have been experienced has to do with the fact that many alcoholics have strong unconscious dependency needs. The need to depend on a strong person, as they once did on a mother figure, may be met by some of the situations that are precipitated by alcoholism.

A perceptible change in the attitude of both lay and professional people toward the problem of alcoholism has been noticeable during the last few decades. There has been an increase in clinics in this country that have as their major purpose the treating of alcoholics. More hospitals of a general nature have designated beds for use by patients who are suffering from alcoholism. Within the last few years there have been many statewide conferences focusing on the problems of prevention and treatment of alcoholism. These conferences were organized in the hope that the public health agencies might take the lead in solving this national problem.

Industrial management and alcoholics themselves have created two strong national forces that have provided much of the impetus for this change in attitude. Industry has come to recognize alcoholism as one of the primary reasons for the loss of manhours on the production line. This loss of the worker's time and efficiency has become such a significant factor in the economic health of the nation that the leaders in industry have begun to seek answers to the problem through the medical services that industry normally provides. Thus industrial physicians and nurses have been alerted to their role in the prevention and treatment of alcoholism. Clinics have been developed to cope with the problems of these individuals. Some industries have added therapists to their medical staffs. Help has been sought from members of Alcoholics Anonymous. This organization has provided a great impetus in this country to better understanding, treatment, and rehabilitation for alcoholics.

Alcoholics Anonymous was founded in 1935 by two alcoholics and usually admits to membership only individuals who are themselves alcoholics. It has had a dramatic development and today numbers more than 160,000 members throughout the world. Alcoholics Anonymous offers the alcoholic answers to his emotional needs because it uses the psychological principles that have been recognized as being effective in helping troubled people. Alcoholics Anonymous also has two affiliated groups. One is for the teenaged children of alcoholics and the other is for their spouses.

Because membership is limited to individuals who themselves have been unable to control the problem of alcohol, members have a good deal of sympathy, patience, and understanding for each other. They work in teams of two or three and call on known alcoholics who are in need of help. Through the program of the organization they are able to meet the alcoholic's dependency needs by seeking him out, encouraging him, helping him find a job, accompanying him to meetings of the organization, and giving him a sense of personal value and worth. Membership requires that each individual admit that he is powerless over alcohol and is in need of help from a power greater than himself. He searches out his own past errors and, having admitted them to another human being, undertakes to make amends for them. He strives to follow a simple code of living that eventually becomes a philosphy of life. The organizational meetings include testimonials by the members concerning their struggles with alcohol and their eventual triumph.

Alcoholics Anonymous offers an experience in group participation and the use of group support. This organization is able to assist its members to develop a new emotional orientation toward life and to begin to meet the problems of life without the aid of alcohol. Many physicians refer alcoholic patients to this organization for help. Most social agencies work closely with Alcoholics Anonymous, and it is generally accepted as the most helpful approach to the problem of alcoholism available at this time. The following life story of one member will serve to point up the effectiveness of the work of this group.

CASE FORMULATION □ AN ALCOHOL-DEPENDENT INDIVIDUAL

Mr. White, a successful 34-year-old shoe salesman, was the father of four children ranging in age from 2 to 10 years when his wife was killed in an automobile accident. When this tragedy struck the White family, they were living in a modest home they had started to purchase. Mrs. White's parents lived in the same neighborhood and were able to help Mr. White with the care of the children. However, he was responsible for their total care after he came home from work each evening and all day on Saturday and Sunday. In addition, he found that he had to plan meals, direct the housekeeper who came in for a few hours each day, and make many decisions that were entirely new to him about the care of the home and the children. Mr. White missed the golf games he had formerly enjoyed on Sunday afternoons. In many ways he felt overwhelmed by the responsibility of being both mother and father to four children. He felt lost without the advice and counsel he had grown to seek and expect from his wife.

In spite of his apprehension, he planned ways to make it possible for him to carry this added responsibility. At first, neighbors and fellow workers were concerned and asked often about how things were going. Occasionally someone invited the family out for a meal so that once in a while he was relieved of having to prepare the evening meal. However, in a few months people began to take his tragic plight for granted and no longer seemed concerned about him or his family.

It was about 6 months after the death of Mrs. White that he began stopping at a bar for a drink after work. Soon he found that the companionship in the bar was so pleasant that he lingered longer than he should and drank more than he had intended. Frequently the children were crying when he arrived home because they were hungry and there was no one at home to prepare the evening meal. The 10-year-old daughter did all she could and eventually began assuming the responsibility for cooking supper. This made it possible for Mr. White to spend many more evenings away from home and frequently to return inebriated. Soon his paycheck began to dwindle. He no longer worked efficiently, and his commissions decreased. Eventually he was fired from his job. Things grew progressively worse for the White family. After Mr. White lost his job, the unpaid grocery bills began to accumulate. The housekeeper stopped coming. Mr. White drank more and more to ease his anxiety, loneliness, and feelings of guilt.

Two members of Alcoholics Anonymous knocked on the front door one evening when Mr. White was lying on the couch sleeping off the latest bottle of whiskey and the children were finishing a meager supper of cereal and milk. When the knock came, the 10-year-old daughter opened the door somewhat fearfully. She answered the questions about the grocery bills and her father's job. The visitors explained that they planned to find a home for the children until Mr. White was well enough to care for them. They told her that they were planning to place her father in a hospital for a few days until he felt like working. These plans were carried out. The children were placed in a foster home, and Mr. White was admitted to a general hospital in which Alcoholics Anonymous maintained a unit for the use of their members who were in need of physical care. He remained in the hospital for 2 weeks. During this time he received vitamin therapy and a normal diet. Members of Alcoholics Anonymous visited him regularly and discussed his problems. They talked about the ways in which the organization could help him. When he was ready to leave the hospital, friends from Alcoholics Anonymous helped him find a job, and for a few days they accompanied him to and from work. They also began taking him to the organizational meetings where he became interested in other men who needed help with problems much like his own. As time went on, Mr. White was able to reestablish his home and to resume the care of his children. Eventually he remarried and was able to establish a home from which he received the emotional satisfactions that he needed. Thus he was helped to give up alcohol permanently.

Discussion of the case formulation

The story of Mr. White is an example of how a social force (Alcoholics Anonymous) entered the life of an individual in trouble and, by using the efforts of its members, effected a shift in the emotional tensions and pressures in his life. This shift resulted in the eventual reestablishment of Mr. White's emotional equilibrium and his complete rehabilitation.

Drug dependence

According to John E. Ingersoll, former director of the U.S. Bureau of Narcotics and Dangerous Drugs, the "abuse and misuse of narcotics and dangerous drugs has reached epidemic proportions in this country. A significant segment of the American community is involved in at least the occasional use of drugs. This constitutes a serious threat to our national health." The use of drugs, especially by adolescents, has become so prevalent and of such concern to the nation that articles are featured on the subject in almost every newspaper and magazine.

Many authorities believe that the legal approach to the drug problem in the United States should be revised. Unfortunately, there seems to have been little carry-over learning from the experience the nation had with the Volstead Act in the early 1920s when an attempt was made to outlaw alcoholic beverages. It seems clear that a repeat of that period of disregard for the law is being experienced now that an attempt is being made to stop the flow of marijuana into the United States through the enactment of laws. More recently, some states have lessened the punishment for possessing or using small amounts of marijuana.

Dr. Stanley Yolles, former director of the National Institute of Mental Health, estimated that between 12 and 20 million people in the United States have used marijuana at least once and that 50% of the students on college campuses located on the east and west coasts have tried marijuana at least once. These comments testify to the widespread concern currently being expressed in the communication media throughout the nation concerning the use of drugs in the United States.

In 1969 Professor Hardin Jones of the Donner Laboratory at the University of California in Berkeley estimated that the consumption of drugs was rising in the United States at the rate of 7% a month. By 1973 the drug problem had begun to level off. Unfortunately, many young people began to substitute alcohol for the drug of their choice when it became difficult to obtain.

Most of the users of drugs do not come to the attention of physicians or nurses. Those who require treatment are usually individuals who have taken drugs because of unresolved conflicts, depressed feelings, seriously disturbed basic personalities, or other unresolved psychological disorders. Effective treatment is focused not only on helping them cope with the drug problem but also on resolving their basic personality disturbance.

Effects of morphine or morphine derivatives. The habitual use of morphine or one of the morphine derivatives or pharmacological substitutes (heroin, codeine, dihydromorphinone [Dilaudid], metopon, meperidine [Demerol]) is generally found in individuals who are unstable, emotionally immature, and lacking in the capacity to face reality. Very few of them have actually acquired the habit from thoughtless overmedication by a physician, although many addicts claim this to be the cause of their problem.

These drug-dependent individuals usually resort to skillful lying and other clever forms of deceit to conceal the habit from others and to obtain the drug through illegal channels. Heroin is the addict's drug of choice in the United States, probably because in this country it is more easily obtained than morphine and is more potent than other narcotics.

The victim of opiate or heroin addiction must live close to his source of supply, which means that he is compelled to associate with the people who smuggle it into the country and who sell the drug.

The drug produces a temporary state of well-being; troubles appear to be trifling and remote; and there is a comfortable sense of complete relaxation. The addict feels "normal," which means that he feels as if his basic needs have been met. He feels sexually satisfied, full of food, free from anxiety and pain, and is not concerned with a feeling that he should fulfill aggressive strivings. Ever-increasing amounts are necessary to produce this exhilaration, so that the chronic morphine or heroin user may require as much as 15 to 20 grains daily. Unfortunately, when the effects wear off and sufficient amounts are not immediately available, certain *withdrawal symptoms* promptly appear. Tears, sneezing, coryza, yawning, great irritability, and restlessness become quickly evident. Within 24 hours this is followed by abdominal cramps, vomiting, and diarrhea. To these distressing symptoms are added headache, sweating, and pains in the muscles and joints of the lower extremities. Finally, on the third day of abstinence the nervous irritability is so pronounced that the individual becomes hysterical, noisy, and threatening; he frequently throws and destroys objects within his reach. Within a week, however, all these painful withdrawal reactions disappear.

Most chronic users of morphine or heroin are undernourished, either because they have anorexia or because they have insufficient funds to purchase enough food. Opiate or heroin addiction does not cause mental deterioration, but the treatment that addicts receive from society causes them to deteriorate socially. Contrary to general opinion, the addict is not a fiend or a criminal. He is in fact an inadequate, immature individual who shrinks from authority and commits crimes only to obtain money to buy the drug. Whenever a drug-dependent individual obtains an adequate dose, he may expose his addiction with an abnormal euphoria and contentment or even a sleepy languor. The pupils may show a telltale "pinpoint" constriction, and in most instances the arms and thighs are scarred or pigmented by the hypodermic needle.

Effects of withdrawal of morphine, its derivatives, or synthetic substitutes. Until recently it was thought to be absolutely necessary to treat the addict in a closed institution to prevent the concealed continuance of the habit. Currently, dozens of treatment centers treat drug-dependent individuals, especially heroin addicts, on an outpatient basis. These centers usually provide the drug methadone as a replacement for heroin.

Withdrawal of morphine or its derivatives has been made more humane through the use of methadone, which is a substitute for the opiate on which the individual is dependent. The use of methadone has been a somewhat controversial method of treating drug addiction. This is partially because of the fact that methadone has been declared to be a narcotic by the Federal Bureau of Narcotics. However, some authorities believe that the use of methadone with former heroin addicts holds the best hope for halting their criminal activities and for making them self-supporting citizens. It has been used more or less successfully with large groups of heroin addicts in several large cities.

In the use of methadone the individual loses his dependency on morphine or one of its derivatives by becoming addicted to the "substitute," methadone. The user then requires regular doses of methadone daily.

This treatment has at least two advantages: (1) it is relatively inexpensive—an individual can be maintained on methadone for a few cents a day and (2) an individual who is on methadone does not lose his ability to function normally—he can usually hold a job and function as a responsible citizen. Today most large cities have methadone clinics where several hundred individuals go to receive the daily dose of methadone. Most clinics require proof that the individual is not continuing to use heroin by producing a urine specimen free of the drug. Methadone as a treatment for heroin addiction continues to be controversial, but because of its advantages it is used widely.

Chlorpromazine has been helpful in relieving tension states that occur when narcotics are being withdrawn. Severe withdrawal symptoms can be avoided with proper medical management. Unless the individual who is dependent on morphine or one of its derivatives is highly motivated to give up the habit, he is likely to return to it after treatment. Sooner or later most of these individuals gravitate into the habit of seeking their former associations, visiting old haunts, and finding life more tolerable by resuming the drug and the artificial sense of security it affords.

Effects of barbituric acid dependence. There are many preparations of barbituric acid, of which barbital (Veronal) is the most frequently employed. Most of the barbiturates tend to accumulate slowly in the tissues, particularly when taken for the relief of emotional tension or insomnia or when administered to control a noisy, psychotic patient. These drugs are frequently taken in enormous single doses by unstable people with the intent of committing suicide.

Early stages of intoxication are initiated by muscular incoordination with ataxia, dizziness, nystagmus, slurred speech, and sluggish mentality. The person acquires many bruises by falling or stumbling against walls and furniture. In more profound barbituric acid intoxication, there are varying degrees of stupor, speech is incoherent, memory is defective, and hallucinations may appear. When aroused, the person is usually very irritable and resistive. He presents the symptoms of a person suffering from delirium. Recovery may be slow and may leave in its wake a mild degree of permanent brain damage.

Treatment consists of withdrawal of the drug. Prolonged bed rest, saline cathartics, and a high-calorie diet are the best restorative measures. In cases of deep coma, hypotension, shallow breathing, and subnormal temperature, more drastic measures must be taken. Artificial respiration and hemodialysis by the artificial kidney are effective means of clearing barbiturates from the blood.

Effects of amphetamine dependence. Amphetamines are called *speed* in the language of the modern drug users and are the most widely used of the really dangerous drugs. They are drugs that have been legitimately used in small doses under medical supervision to treat depression and curb appetite. They are known medically as Benzedrine, Desoxyephedrine, and Desoxyn. Individuals who take these drugs solely to become "high" take from 6 to 200 times the daily dose usually prescribed by a physician. The effect of such large doses is to elevate the blood pressure, sometimes to dangerous levels. Such large doses have been known to cause immediate death. This fact accounts for the current saying among drug users that "speed kills."

Individuals who use the amphetamines feel that these drugs sharpen their physical and sexual reactions and increase their confidence. Thus a period of frantic activity results from the ingestion of large amounts of amphetamine. This is followed by a great letdown in which the fatigue and depression are so tremendous that the addict is apt to seek release by taking the drug again. Chronic use can lead to a schizophrenic-like psychosis or massive, irreparable brain damage that may result in death.

Effects of LSD (lysergic acid diethylamide) dependence. LSD is a drug that was originally used for research into the causes of schizophrenia. Ingestion of reasonably small doses of LSD produces temporary hallucinations and other schizophrenic-like symptoms. Mescaline and psilocybin are related substances found in nature. Mescaline is an alkaloid derived from a plant that grows wild in the southwestern part of the United States and in Mexico.

LSD is referred to as *acid* by members of the subculture of drug addicts. It is 4000 times as strong by weight as mescaline. The user experiences waves of color, and vibrations seem to pass through the head. Reality gives way to intense hallucinations. Individuals have been injured because LSD causes them to imagine that they can fly or engage in other miraculous stunts. Users take massive doses that sometimes bring to the surface long-repressed mental conflicts and psychotic reactions, which may continue even when the drug wears off.

Marijuana intoxication. Until recently, marijuana was an easily obtained and relatively inexpensive drug. It is a crude preparation from the whole *Cannabis sativa* plant, which grows wild in Mexico and is easily cultivated in the United States. It is usually absorbed into the body through the smoking of cigarettes called *reefers.* Hashish is prepared by scraping resin from the tops of the hemp plant. The active ingredient in both marijuana and hashish is tetrahydrocannabinol, with hashish being much more potent.

Inhalation of marijuana causes a state of exhilaration or euphoria. Under its influence the user feels light in body, as if he were floating through space, and the general behavior is not unlike a mild mania. Marijuana is not an aphrodisiac, but it can lower inhibitions and intensify sexual pleasure. It seems to make many users temporarily passive, in contrast to alcohol, which frequently releases aggression. Marijuana affects the individual's sense of time but not his motor and perceptual skills. Users become psychologically dependent on it but may not become physically addicted as with morphine.

Currently a great deal of attention is being given to marijuana by the government because its use has risen dramatically. Official arguments have been carried on in the press concerning the relative dangers of marijuana and the appropriate penalties that should be or should not be levied against people who use it. Unfortunately, there is a limited amount of research on which to base a scientific, unbiased judgment concerning the immediate dangers of smoking marijuana or the eventual outcome of long-term use of this drug. Many of the research findings have been contradictory. Certainly the present laws controlling its use are inequitable, as well as widely unenforceable.

Self-help for drug-dependent individuals. Some drug-dependent individuals who have been able to give up the habit, like cured alcoholics, have developed a method for helping others suffering from drug dependence. In many large cities there are institutions that are much like halfway houses. They are usually under the direction of a trained professional worker, who may have one or two other professionally trained people to assist him. Most of the therapy as well as the other work required to keep the place functioning is done by the drug-dependent individuals who are there to be helped or by those who have been helped and who stay on to make a contribution to the work.

In these situations, drug-dependent individuals who sincerely want to stop the drug habit live with other people struggling with similar problems. The house is usually organized along the lines of communal living, with each person accepting a share of the work necessary to keep the house liveable and to prepare the meals. Several group sessions are carried on each week, during which members of the group are supportive to each other but are very straightforward in demanding that the group members face their rationalizations, evasions, personal problems, and social deceptions. If a member returns to drugs, he is expected to leave the group. This realistic but supportive approach has apparently helped many drug-dependent individuals to give up drugs and return to school or to a job.

Rehabilitation. Until a few years ago the U.S. government maintained one treatment center at Lexington, Kentucky. It was called the National Institute of Mental Health Clinical Research Center. In such a specialized hospital, everything possible was done to help drug-dependent individuals break their habit and become useful, productive citizens. Many individuals were treated at Lexington several times. Unfortunately, the personality of some drug addicts is so faulty that they are not able to function without the emotional support the drug provides.

Many communities have organized facilities for treating individuals who suffer from this problem. As in all situations that involve the emotional life, it is necessary to discover why this kind of unusual emotional support is needed and then attempt to supply the support in more positive ways while at the same time helping the individual to give up the drug.

Some authorities believe that a more realistic approach to the problem of drug addiction would be to supply each drug-dependent individual with a minimum weekly supply of the drug to which he is addicted. This practice, it is argued, would make the illegal traffic in drugs unprofitable. It is thought that this practice of supplying a small amount of the drug to the addict each week would aid in cutting down the crimes that addicts now commit to obtain drugs. It would make it possible for the addict to purchase adequate food and maintain his physical health at an optimum level instead of denying himself food to purchase the drug, as he frequently has done in the past. The major thrust toward rehabilitation of the heroin addict in today's society is the methadone treatment discussed earlier.

Much more study and research must be done on drug addiction before a more effective approach to treatment and rehabilitation can be made.

CASE FORMULATION □ A HEROIN-DEPENDENT INDIVIDUAL

This 24-year-old individual began using marijuana and then heroin when he was a junior in high school. This occurred when his 14-year-old girl friend refused to date him any longer. About the same time, he was sent by his mother, who lived in New York City, to attend high school in a distant southern city because his parents were getting a divorce.

According to the individual, marijuana made him feel excited, stimulated, and happy. Everything seemed more pleasant, and he enjoyed his daydreams. He was also sexually stimulated by the drug. About the same time, he tried taking barbiturates, which made him sleepy. Because he did not enjoy their effect, he did not continue them. He got drunk a few times, but alcohol failed to produce the calmness and contentment he was seeking. Since marijuana did not completely fill the bill either, he was convinced that his willpower would be great enough to keep him away from the drug when he wanted to be free of it.

He first took heroin in the vein. Among drug-dependent individuals this method is referred to as the *main line* method. He described feeling a "flash," which was accompanied by a flush of blood from the abdomen to the head and a feeling of "happiness." Although the "flash" passed away, a constant feeling of euphoria remained. For the first time in his life he experienced a feeling of deep contentment. He said, "It didn't affect my intellect, only my emotions. I was happy and content." From that time on he took heroin to assist him in facing any situation that caused him to be tense or anxious. Heroin helped him feel independent of his mother and reduced his nervousness when he was out with a girl. Although heroin gave him a feeling of contentment, it lessened his sexual desire and made it impossible for him to reach a sexual climax.

After the individual discovered the contentment heroin could achieve for him, he became involved in crimes to support his drug habit. As his need for larger and larger quantities of heroin grew and his habit became more costly, his crimes became more frequent and more serious. His mother repeatedly intervened to keep him out of jail by paying his fines. He entered several colleges but because of his drug habit was never able to stay in any of them for more than a semester.

Finally the individual tried to withdraw himself from heroin. He thought he could achieve this alone, since he had been withdrawn twice before in treatment centers. He was not able to accomplish his goal, and finally at 24 years of age signed himself into a treatment center in the hope of stopping the drug habit so that he could return to college. He had set for himself the goal of becoming an engineer.

The individual was extremely hostile toward his mother and referred to her as a physical woman but not a mother. The reasons for his hostility seemed obvious when reviewing the family history. His parents were married when the mother was 16 years old. He was their first child, and his mother reminded him frequently that his birth had been traumatic for her. During his formative years his father suffered from tuberculosis and spent many months in a tuberculosis sanitarium. When the individual was 3 years of age, his mother focused much attention during his bath on his genital hygiene. As he grew older, she allowed him to observe her dressing and bathing but scolded him if he evidenced interest in her body. He began heterosexual experiences at the age of 16 years and homosexual activity at age 18.

Discussion of the case formulation

This young man was highly intelligent and tested in the superior range on an intelligence test. When he became motivated to give up drugs, his only hope for achieving a more socially productive adaptation lay in his acceptance of and cooperation with a treatment center for drug-dependent individuals. It was obvious that his psychosexual development had been defective because of his rejecting, seductive mother and the frequent absence of a father figure from the home. His original experimentation with drugs and alcohol and sex may have been an expression of rebellion against an ambivalent mother who banished him in high school but who continuously intervened on his behalf with the police.

CONCLUDING STATEMENTS

1. Behaviors that are societally offensive include antisocial acts, sexual deviances, and substance abuse.
2. Individuals exhibiting antisocial behavior seem incapable of conforming to social or legal standards of living and lack a sense of responsibility.

3. The defect from which individuals with antisocial behaviors suffer lies in the emotional and volitional aspects of their personalities.
4. Individuals with antisocial behaviors are thought to have failed to develop constructive identities or socially useful adaptations and controls and are dominated by the primitive demands of the id.
5. Individuals with antisocial behaviors are treated most successfully in a situation that provides an organized, structured, controlled environment.
6. Treatment goals for individuals with antisocial behaviors include helping them to accept more socially approved attitudes and standards in their relationships with other people.
7. Individuals with antisocial behaviors need to be rewarded with praise and recognition for acceptable behavior.
8. Sexually deviant behavior develops as a result of a failure to substitute mature sexual behavior for infantile or preadolescent ways of obtaining sexual pleasure.
9. Usually, sexually deviant behavior is only one manifestation of an emotional problem of long duration.
10. Sexually deviant behavior is difficult to treat successfully because the problem arises out of faulty interpersonal experiences early in life.
11. Successful treatment for the sexually deviant individual requires a competent therapist, a highly motivated client, and a long period of time for treatment.
12. No matter what type of alcoholic dependence is being considered, the problem is thought to have its basis in some emotional conflict, frustration, or overwhelming feeling of inadequacy.
13. The treatment and care of the alcohol-dependent individual begins with understanding his personality and the problems from which he has a need to obtain relief.
14. The primary treatment of the alcohol-dependent individual is to aid him in meeting life's responsibilities without using alcohol as an escape. This generally means a long period of reeducation.

15. Morphine or heroin dependence does not cause mental deterioration as does addiction to alcohol, but the treatment that addicts receive from society causes them to deteriorate socially.
16. Unfortunately, many nurses and other workers approach the treatment of the alcoholic and addicted individual with the same rejection that is meted out to such individuals by society in general.
17. Alcohol-dependent individuals are almost universally in need of physical rehabilitation and a nutritional regimen designed to restore their physical stamina.
18. The permanent rehabilitation of alcohol- and drug-dependent individuals is greatly influenced by their personal motivation to be free of their dependence.
19. Methadone maintenance clinics are one of the major approaches being made today in the rehabilitation of the individual addicted to heroin.

Suggested sources of additional information

CLASSICAL

Barbee, Evelyn L.: Marijuana a social problem, Perspect. Psychiatr. Care **9:**195-199, Sept.-Oct., 1971.

Caskey, Kathryn K., Blaylock, Enid V., and Wauson, Beryl M.: The school nurse and drug abusers, Nurs. Outlook **18:**27-30, Dec., 1970.

Condon, Alice, and Roland, Arelene: Drug abuse jargon, Am. J. Nurs. **71:**1738-1739, 1971.

Dannels, Joann C.: Homosexual panic, Perspect. Psychiatr. Care **10:**106-111, July-Sept., 1972.

Fort, Joel: Comparison chart of major substances used for mind alteration, Am. J. Nurs. **71:**1740-1741, 1971.

Kimmel, Mary E.: Antabuse in a clinic program, Am. J. Nurs. **71:**1173-1175, 1971.

Kromberg, Carol J., and Proctor, Judith Betz: Evaluation of a day program, Am. J. Nurs. **70:**2575-2577, 1970.

Lion, John R., editor: Personality disorder: diagnosis and management, Baltimore, 1974, The Williams & Wilkins Co.

Lipkin, Gladys B., and Cohen, Roberta G.: The addicted patient. In Effective approaches to patients' behavior, New York, 1980, Springer Publishing Co., Inc. pp. 124-127.

Morgan, Arthur James, and Moreno, Judith Wilson: Attitudes toward addiction, Am. J. Nurs. **73:**497-501, 1973.

Pearson, Barbara A.: Methadone maintenance in heroin addiction, Am. J. Nurs. **70:**2571-2574, 1970.

Randell, Brooke Patterson: Short-term group therapy with the adolescent drug offender, Perspect. Psychiatr. Care **9:**123-128, May-June, 1971.

Underwood, Patricia R., and Davis, Anne J.: Clutter, crowding, chaos—and therapy in a young drug unit, Perspect. Psychiatr. Care **9:**211-216, Sept.-Oct., 1971.

Yolles, Stanley F.: The drug scene, Nurs. Outlook **18:**24-26, July, 1970.

CONTEMPORARY

Burkhalter, Pamela K.: Nursing care of the alcoholic and drug abuser, New York, 1975, McGraw-Hill Book Co.

Butz, R.H.: Intoxication and withdrawal. In Estes, N.J., and Heinemann, M.E., editors: Alcoholism: development, consequences, and interventions, St. Louis, 1981, The C.V. Mosby Co.

Carruth, Beatrice F.: Modifying behavior through social learning, Am. J. Nurs. **76:**1804-1806, Nov., 1976.

Chafetz, Morris E., Hertzman, Marc, and Berenson, David: Alcoholism: a positive view. In Arieti, Silvano, and Brody, Eugene B., editors: American handbook of psychiatry, ed. 2, vol. 3, New York, 1974, Basic Books, Inc., Publishers, pp. 367-392.

Chavigny, Katherine: Self-esteem for the alcoholic: an epidemiologic approach, Nurs. Outlook **24:**636-639, 1976.

Dambacher, Betty, and Hellwig, Karen: Nursing strategies for young drug users, Perspect. Psychiatr. Care **9:**201-205, Sept.-Oct., 1971.

Detzer, Eric, Carlin, Albert S., and Muller, Bart: Detoxifying barbiturate addicts: hints for psychiatric staff, Am. J. Nurs. **76:**1306-1307, 1976.

Dickinson, Sister Corita: The alcoholic an unperson? Nurs. Forum **14:**194-203, 1975.

Ditzler, Joyce: Rehabilitation for alcoholics, Am. J. Nurs. **76:**1172-1175, 1976.

Estes, Nada J.: Counseling the wife of an alcoholic spouse, Am. J. Nurs. **74:**1251-1255, 1974.

Foreman, Nancy Jo, and Zerwekh, Joyce V.: Drug crisis intervention, Am. J. Nurs. **71:**1736-1739, 1974.

Fortin, Mary L.: A community nursing experience in alcoholism, Am. J. Nurs. **80:**113-114, Jan., 1980.

Fultz, John M., et al.: When a narcotic addict is hospitalized, Am. J. Nurs. **80:**478-482, March, 1980.

Gross, Mary Jane: Changing attitudes toward homosexuality, Perspect. Psychiatr. Care **16:**70-75, March-April, 1978.

Haglund, R.M.J., and Schuckit, M.A.: The epidemiology of alcoholism. In Estes, N.J., and Heinemann, M.E., editors: Alcoholism: development, consequences, and interventions, St. Louis, 1981, The C.V. Mosby Co.

Horowitz, June A.: Sexual difficulties as indicators of broader interpersonal problems (as reflected in psychotherapy groups), Perspect. Psychiatr. Care **16**(2):66-69, March-April, 1978.

Huberty, David J., and Malmquist, Jeffrey D.: Adolescent chemical dependency, Perspect. Psychiatr. Care **16:**21-27, Jan.-Feb., 1978.

Johnson, Vernon E.: I'll quit tomorrow, San Francisco, 1980, Harper & Row, Publishers.

Lawrence, John C.: Homosexuals, hospitalization, and the nurse, Nurs. Forum **14**:305-317, 1975.

Levine, Martin P., editor: The sociology of male homosexuality, New York, 1980, Harper & Row, Publishers.

McDermott, Sister Raphael: Maintaining the methadone patient, Nurs. Outlook **18**:22-26, Dec., 1970.

McNiff, Martha A.: Nursing in a psychiatric prison service, Am. J. Nurs. **73**:1586-1587, 1973.

Mann, George: Recovery of reality: overcoming chemical dependency, San Francisco, 1980, Harper & Row, Publishers.

Marmor, Judd, editor: Homosexual behavior: a modern reappraisal, New York, 1980, Basic Books, Inc., Publishers.

Mitchell, Carol Edgerton: Assessment of alcohol abuse, Nurs. Outlook **24**:511-515, 1976.

Mueller, John F.: Treatment for the alcoholic: cursing or nursing? Am. J. Nurs. **74**:245-247, 1974.

Nelson, Karin: The nurse in a methadone maintenance program, Am. J. Nurs. **73**:870-874, 1973.

Nyswander, Marie: Drug addiction. In Arieti, Silvano, and Brody, Eugene B., editors: American handbook of psychiatry, ed. 2, vol. 3, New York, 1974, Basic Books, Inc., Publishers, pp. 393-403.

Pillari, George, and Narus, June: Physical effects of heroin addiction, Am. J. Nurs. **73**:2105-2108, 1973.

Raymond, Janice G.: The transsexual empire, Boston, 1980, Beacon Press.

Roache, Margaret Olson: Humanistic learning, Am. J. Nurs. **74**:1453-1456, 1974.

Rouslin, Sheila: A psychoanalytic view of homosexuality: an interview with Joseph Geller, M.D., Perspect. Psychiatr. Care **16**:76-80, March-April, 1978.

Seixas, F.A.: The course of alcoholism. In Estes, N.J., and Heinemann, M.E., editors: Alcoholism: development, consequences, and interventions, St. Louis, 1981, The C.V. Mosby Co.

Smith, Thomas M.: The dynamics in time-limited therapy with methadone-maintained patients, New York City V.A., Perspect. Psychiatr. Care **16**(1):28-33, Jan.-Feb., 1978.

Socarides, Charles W.: Homosexuality. In Arieti, Silvano, and Brody, Eugene B., editors: American handbook of psychiatry, ed. 2, vol. 3, New York, 1974, Basic Books Inc., Publishers, pp. 291-315.

Tripp, C.A.: The homosexual matrix, New York, 1976, W.W. Norton & Co., Inc.

Yearwood, Alma C., and Hess, Susanne K.: How can an alcoholic change in 28 days? Am. J. Nurs. **79**:1436-1438, Aug., 1979.

OF PARTICULAR INTEREST

Estes, N.J., and Heinemann, M.E., editors: Alcoholism: development, consequences, and interventions, St. Louis, 1977, The C.V. Mosby Co.

The authors provide a comprehensive literature review on the problem of alcoholism. It is an excellent resource regarding various aspects of the problem.

Mann, George: Recovery of reality: overcoming chemical dependency, San Francisco, 1980, Harper & Row, Publishers.

This is a complete report on the nature, effects, treatment, and prevention of chemical dependency. It includes personal histories and the latest information on diagnostic and treatment methods for alcoholism and other dependencies.

Symposium on alcohol and drug abuse, Nurs. Clin. North Am., Sept., 1976.

Chemical dependency is the focus of several articles in this collection. It is useful in providing the reader with several relevant perspectives on the problem.

SECTION FIVE

Therapeutic interventions for individuals whose maladaptive behavioral patterns are age associated

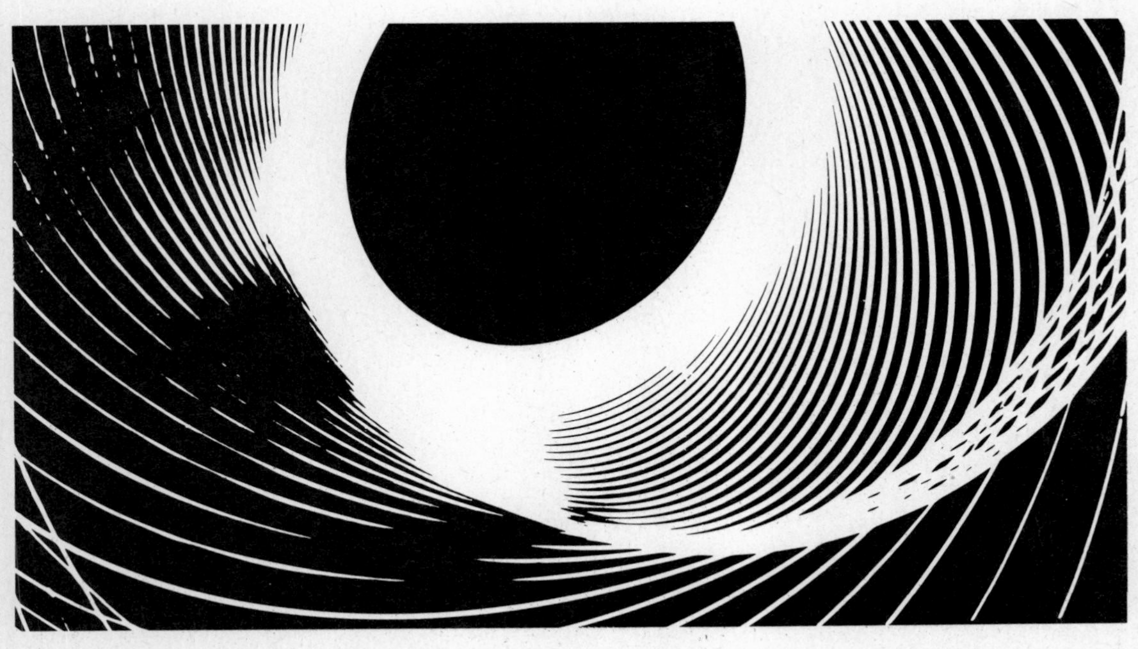

Section Five focuses on the nursing care of emotionally disturbed children and adolescents, individuals who have faulty intellectual development, and the elderly. As population groups, these persons have unique identifiable needs that are closely related to their developmental stages. Hence the reader is well advised to review Chapter 4, Personality: Its Structure and Development, prior to studying this section.

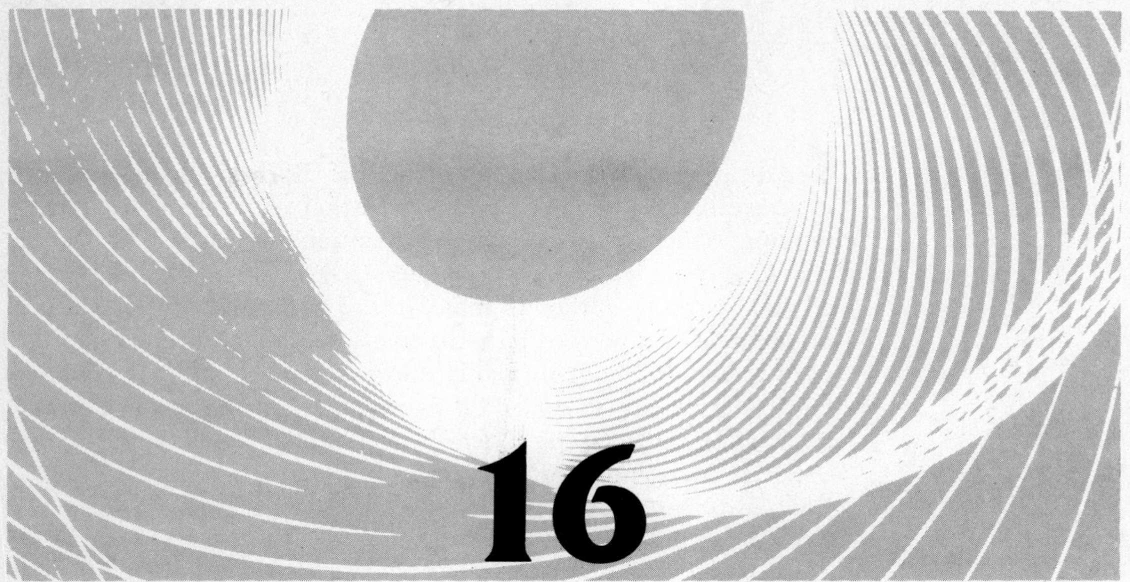

16

Maladaptive behavioral patterns associated with childhood and adolescence

- Historical background of the study of emotional disturbances in children
- Causes of emotional disturbance among children and adolescents
- Understanding parents of emotionally disturbed children
- Emotionally disturbed children
- Behaviorally disturbed children
- Behaviorally disturbed adolescents

The treatment of emotional disorders of children and adolescents is recognized as an area of specialization in both medicine and nursing. Thus it deserves more attention than can possibly be provided in a textbook devoted primarily to the field of adult psychiatric nursing. Although many of the basic principles useful in understanding and dealing with emotionally disturbed adults apply to emotionally disturbed children, there are special problems and concerns in this aspect of psychiatry that require additional knowledge and training. There is even less agreement among authorities concerning the cause, prevention, and treatment of emotional problems in children than there is concerning similar problems involving adults.

Although behavioral disturbances in children such as thumb sucking, enuresis, and temper tantrums indicate the presence of emotional problems, these symptoms do not necessarily connote the severity of fundamental personality limitations usually associated with the term *mental illness*. Mentally ill children, such as autistic children, suffer from severe fundamental personality defects, whereas those having behavioral disturbances are more likely to exhibit symptomatology reflective of an inability to cope with a current stressful situation. Therefore children exhibiting less severe emotional problems will hereafter be referred to as *behaviorally disturbed*, and children suffering from the more severe fundamental personality problems will be referred to as *emotionally disturbed*.

Certainly an understanding of normal personality growth and development is essential before beginning a study of emotional problems in children. Thus it is suggested that before reading any further the student review Chapter 4, which deals with personality development.

HISTORICAL BACKGROUND OF THE STUDY OF EMOTIONAL DISTURBANCES IN CHILDREN

Interest in child psychiatry has developed rapidly in the last half century. Before 1920 many authorities believed that mental illness was limited to adults. The occasional emotionally disturbed child who came to the attention of physicians was thought to be a clinical curiosity. There is no mention of children in the classic treatise on psychiatry by Emil Kraepelin, a famous German psychiatrist. This book was published in Leipzig in 1904 and is studied even today. In 1912 Boston Psychopathic Hospital, now Massachusetts Mental Health Center, became the first psychiatric hospital in the United States to accept children in an outpatient clinic. The first written report concerning the existence of childhood schizophrenia was published by H.W. Potter in the *American Journal of Psychiatry* in 1933. Although this article precipitated much controversy among psychiatrists at the time, the existence of a schizophrenic-like psychosis in children is almost universally accepted today.

CAUSES OF EMOTIONAL DISTURBANCE AMONG CHILDREN AND ADOLESCENTS

Some authorities believe that the rapid rise of emotional problems among children and adolescents in today's society is related in some way to the fundamental problems and insecurities that have developed in many American homes in the twentieth century. Others go so far as to suggest that the phenomenal rise in emotional problems among children may indicate that there is a breakdown in the structure of the American family, the basic institution in this culture. Certainly the current high divorce rate, with the resultant loss of one parent or the sharing by the children of the homes of two parents; the rise of the practice of babysitting, in which children are frequently cared for by a variety of individuals, many of whom are minimally competent to deal with children; the increasingly technological nature of our culture; and the relative relaxation of moral and religious standards are all factors that may provide many children with home lives that seem unsafe and insecure to them.

Other possible factors cannot be ignored in considering the increase of emotional problems among children and adolescents. One of these may be the greater demands put on children and adolescents by members of a sophisticated and technologically oriented society.

Genetic and physiological factors that may contribute to the development of emotional problems of children and adolescents are the subject of much current research. As is the case with emotionally ill adults, the incidence of mental illness in children is greater in families that have a history of mental illness. Furthermore, it is not unusual for a mentally ill child to have siblings whose emotional development is quite normal. Both these phenomena can be plausibly explained by interpersonal and environmental factors, but physiological and genetic influences cannot be ignored.

Emotional problems of childhood and adolescence are not distinct and well-defined clinical entities. While there is no universal agreement as to their cause, studies suggest that an emotionally healthy climate within the family is essential if children are to develop into mentally healthy adults. Thus it seems reasonable to look to the early parent-child relationships, especially the quality of the mothering that the child receives, for insight as to why children do or do not achieve the psychosocial maturational levels exhibited by emotionally well children.

Among the most important attitudes children learn as a result of their earliest experiences with a mothering person is to trust others and the environment. This ability to trust is a basic ingredient in the development of a well-integrated personality. It develops as a result of the way in which the mothering person responds to the infant's very earliest need for food, comfort, cuddling, and attention. The responses experienced by the infant to these needs establish the basis for the mother-child relationship, which is profoundly influential in the child's total personality development. If the ability to trust does not develop, it is reasonable to conclude that all was not well in the very earliest experiences with which the child was involved. Unless the child is handled with patience and love, the habit-training period is another time in the growth of the child that is fraught with potential emotional problems. At this time the child learns that refusing to cooperate in the toilet-training efforts of his parents provides him with a powerful method for controlling the situation. If the parents respond with rigid and harsh treatment to the child's first experiment in exerting his own will, a situation involving conflict is apt to arise.

Likewise, as the child develops physically, emotionally, and intellectually, he advances from one phase of development to another. More is expected of him in each phase. Each phase presents the child with potential emotional conflicts somewhat unique to the phase through which he is passing. The key to the situation and to successful personality development is found in the relationships the child and the parents are able to develop and maintain and the effectiveness with which the child is guided through each of the several phases of development.

UNDERSTANDING PARENTS OF EMOTIONALLY DISTURBED CHILDREN

Because parents have been intimately involved in the personality development of the child, nurses and physicians sometimes behave as if the parents are to blame for the child's emotional problems. This blaming attitude is expressed by many professional workers more often than they realize. Parents usually feel guilty and apologetic in the face of the many searching questions that are asked when they seek professional assistance for their child. These feelings on the part of parents are understandable. However, professional workers could be much more helpful if they approached the parents with the understanding that within their limitations most parents do the best they can in meeting the responsibilities of childrearing. Parents usually strive to be successful in rearing healthy children even though their personality structures and emotional conflicts may not always promote success. In addition, it is well known that parents respond differently to individual children; one child may thrive in a home under one type of parental care and another child may not be able to tolerate the same situation. An individual child may not be constitutionally able to develop a normal, healthy personality in a given situation with parents possessed of dispositions contrary to the temperament of the child.

By the time parents have sought professional help for an emotionally disturbed child, the interpersonal interactions between the parents and child probably have been unsatisfactory for some time. Thus the parents are understandably distressed by the situation and require the same support and understanding that is provided for individuals undergoing excessive stress in any situation.

Because the child's future is to a considerable extent determined by the emotional health of the parents and by the complex forces interacting within the family group, the parents are usually involved in the total treatment program for the child. Most authorities agree that this approach is required if effective help is to be provided. Improvement in the child's behavior may depend on alterations in the parents' attitudes and approaches. Thus parents are usually included in the treatment plan as much as the child and may be seen by the same therapist or by a second therapist. Whatever decisions are made about the final treatment plans, the parents are usually as much recipients of psychotherapeutic care as the child himself.

EMOTIONALLY DISTURBED CHILDREN

Children who suffer from severe fundamental personality limitations are usually referred to as being mentally ill. In most instances their behavior is so obviously atypical that parents and professionals alike agree that a problem exists; however, the determination of a specific diagnosis may be difficult. For example, it is well known that some children who were originally diagnosed as being mentally retarded were actually mentally ill.

Psychoses of childhood

Childhood psychoses are thought to develop in children who have not yet reached puberty as a result of the interaction between a constitutionally susceptible child and an environmental situation psychologically incompatible with the needs of the child. Children who have experienced some organic brain damage or sensory deprivation are thought to develop a psychosis more readily than children without one of these physical problems. However, this illness frequently occurs in children who apparently have not been subjected to any damaging physical insults.

Although psychotic children display a broad spectrum of behavioral patterns, most of them have some or all of the following behaviors: autistic withdrawal, failure to develop language or to use communicative speech, failure to develop according to the normally expected developmental pattern, use of repetitive mannerisms, impairment of ego functioning, failure to develop a clearly defined body image, lack of sexual identity, and inability to perceive time and space accurately. The older the child is when he develops the psychosis, the more nearly the symptoms approximate those found among adult schizophrenic individuals.

Under the broad category of childhood psychosis there are two rather clearly identified patterns of behavior that carry the descriptive names *early infantile autism* and *symbiotic infantile psychotic syndrome.* Early infantile autism was first described in 1943 by Dr. Leo Kanner, a psychiatrist at Johns Hopkins University. The symbiotic infantile psychotic syndrome was first described by Dr. Margaret S. Mahler in 1956. Although both these clinical entities were controversial when introduced, they are fairly widely accepted today. Children suffering from either of these are withdrawn from reality and have a severe disturbance in the area of self-identity.

These two syndromes are widely believed to be clearly related to the early mothering experiences the child has received. *Infantile autism* is usually recognized by the end of the first year of age and not later than the second year. It occurs more frequently in boys than in girls. The child is thought to be fixated at, or regressed to, the earliest developmental period of his life when he has not yet differentiated himself from the mother's body, the breast or bottle, and the blanket and other inanimate objects in his immediate world. Thus the mother is not a representative of the outside world to the child and apparently has not been perceived as a separate entity. Since the child has not been able to use the mother in relating to the world, he is incapable of forming a relationship with any person and thus is emotionally unresponsive to human contact. Bruno Bettelheim, a famous child psychoanalyst, accepts the theory that the basic cause of the autistic child's problem is parental rejection. It should be noted, however, that some theorists, notably Dr. Lauretta Bender, believe that the causative factors in the development of early infantile autism are primarily physiological in nature, although the resultant behavior is psychologically reinforced by the mothering person.

Many autistic children come from homes in which the parents are highly intelligent and economically and professionally successful. The parents are often focused on achieving recognition in the areas of their scientific and academic interests. The family life is such that little genuine mothering is provided for the child. In reporting the child's problems the parents usually comment that he does not talk and is obsessively attached to some inanimate object such as a doll or teddy bear. He usually plays alone with this inanimate object for hours. He may display temper tantrums if his environment is altered in the slightest way. Thus the child creates a small world restricted to himself. Although his parents sometimes seek professional help because they believe he is mentally retarded, the autistic child frequently displays flashes of intelligence. He seems devoid of emotional ties and appears to have chosen to use autism as a defense against the outside environment, which demands an emotional response he is incapable of making.

In some children's units in large institutions it is not unusual to observe 20 to 40 autistic children, all under the age of 10 years. Most of them are nonverbal or communicate through the use of a functional sign language. They appear to live in an emotional vacuum. Many of these children resort to aggressive hurting acts directed toward themselves. These acts may include head banging, hand biting, or other behavior that is self-mutilating. Some of these children appear to be acutely unhappy and cry pitifully. Many of them exhibit temper outbursts or other frantic behavior. This behavior, which is almost incomprehensible to adults, appears to help the child gain some concept of his body and its boundaries and thus achieve some sense of identity. Heroic steps are sometimes necessary to safeguard these children against their own self-destructive behavior. These steps may include the use of protective clothing such as football helmets.

The child who displays behavior classified as the *symbiotic infantile psychotic syndrome* apparently has been able to progress somewhat further toward achieving normal personality development than has the autistic child. He is thought to have progressed to the maturational level at which he was able to recognize his mothering one as a separate individual differentiated from himself. At this point he was able to make use of his mother to satisfy his needs. Unfortunately, for reasons not clearly understood, the symbiotic child was unable to continue the process of separation from the mother when he reached the age at which the development of some autonomous functions were expected. As he developed physically, his emotional ability to differentiate himself from his mother became less and less effective until he was confronted with a situation that demanded a level of adjustment greater than he was able to achieve.

Such a situation is thought to have been the precipitating factor in the child's psychotic break but was not the cause. Separation of the child from the mother may occur, for example, when she must be hospitalized, when he must be enrolled in a nursery school, when he is hospitalized, or when a sibling is introduced into the family. Any of these real-life events may cause the child to panic and break with reality because of the threatened loss of the oneness with the mother, which the child has not been able to abandon.

The symptoms of the symbiotic infantile psychotic syndrome are usually recognized by the parents between the second and the fifth year. The child often appears agitated, has temper tantrums, seems to be panic-striken, hallucinates, and distorts reality in a bizarre way. For these children, reality is unbearable, and thus autistic withdrawal becomes a defensive maneuver.

Providing corrective experiences for emotionally disturbed children

General goals of treatment for all emotionally disturbed children include providing opportunities to develop a concept of self, to develop more appropriate object relationships, and to experience and work through or to relive those phases of personality development that were missing, distorted, negatively experienced, or hurriedly passed through.

The symbiotic psychotic child may profit by the special therapeutic environment provided by treatment centers geared to the child's special needs. For example, substitutes for the unhealthy symbiotic relationship with the mothering one are provided for the child.

Although the autistic child rejects contacts with others, it is thought that he may profit from individual therapy because his greatest task is to learn to relate to others. Since he avoids bodily contact, cuddling or holding such a child is not helpful and may actually repel him. His attention and interest must be obtained through the use of other methods that will be pleasantly stimulating. One such method that has experientially been found to be helpful is the use of music.

The problems of the autistic child have been brought to the attention of the general public through numerous television programs and magazine articles. This media coverage often has been initiated by the National Society for Autistic Children, which was founded in 1965 by parents of autistic children. The media reports tend to describe the successful use of the principles of reinforcement therapy (operant conditioning) in altering the behavior of the autistic child. The therapist rewards the child with praise and candy when a specific aspect of his behavior is considered normal for his age. After many weeks or months of repeating the reward-praise reinforcement of normal behavior, the child's autistic behavior may be replaced by the more normal behavior that has been reinforced. A part of reinforcement therapy may include negative reinforcement if the child reverts to autistic behavior. The therapist may reproach the child with a forceful "No!" or even punish him to discourage autistic behavior.

Special emphasis should be placed on communicating verbally and nonverbally with the autistic child even though his response may be unintelligible. Most mothers talk to their very young children even though the children cannot respond because they have not yet achieved the use of verbal language. Likewise, talking to the autistic child about the environment and the happenings of the day may be helpful even though he does not appear to respond. A soft, warm voice, a friendly facial expression, and other nonverbal ways of responding positively to the autistic child may be effective in communicating genuine concern and interest to him. It has been suggested that the child's attention should be "engaged by consciously echoing and imitating his vocal and motor behavior. Eventually, through imitation and identification the child is led to more advanced communication and relatedness."*

The symbiotic child needs help in gradually developing independence. Opportunities should be provided through which the

---

*From Spurgeon, Ruth: Nursing the autistic child, Am. J. Nurs. **67:**1418, 1967.

child can learn to recognize himself as an independent person apart from his mother. He needs to be encouraged and supported whenever he attempts to perform any aspect of his own daily physical care such as dressing or feeding himself.

Instead of placing the autistic child in an institution for treatment, it is becoming increasingly common for him to be treated while remaining in the home. This plan may be less disturbing to both the parents and the child. If this is to be the treatment plan, it is absolutely essential that the therapist develop a close working relationship with the parents, especially the mother. The therapist will require some feedback about the child's behavior at home. In addition, when the therapist is helping the child to relive some phases of development, his behavior may regress. He may revert to taking milk from a bottle or to soiling himself. Thus the mother must understand the treatment approach and why regressed behavior may occur. Equally important are the changes that need to be made in the attitude of the mother toward the child, which may be achieved if she works with the therapist in attempting to alter her child's behavior.

In view of the increasing number of disturbed children being treated in the home, a significant role for the public health nurse is emerging, especially in regard to working to support and reassure other family members.

Play therapy is almost universally employed in the treatment of children with emotional problems. Its use is based on the knowledge that play is the medium through which children normally express themselves. Therapists use the child's play as a means of gaining insight into his unconscious feelings and attitudes about life as he is experiencing it. Play therapy has the additional function of enabling some children to work through some of the problems they are experiencing. The therapy room is furnished with a variety of toys and other equipment the child may choose to play with. The therapist remains in the playroom with the child and spends time in getting acquainted with the child and in developing a relationship of trust. The therapist observes the child carefully and listens attentively to his comments. If the therapist and the child have developed a relationship of trust, the therapist may ask the child to tell something about the meaning of the play in which he is engaging. Usually a complete dollhouse and a family of dolls are part of the equipment in a play therapy room. This equipment is purposefully included because the way the child plays with the family of dolls provides insights into the relationships the child is experiencing with the members of his own family. Since the child's emotional life revolves around the members of his family, these insights are significant.

When children are questioned about spanking or punishing one of the child dolls excessively, one learns much about the punishment the child has experienced or fantasizes that he should have experienced. Children sometimes try to destroy an offending child doll or one of the adult members of the doll family. When asked to talk about these occurrences, the child may explain some of his unconscious fears or his feelings toward a sibling or a parent. Thus play therapy helps the therapist and the child to communicate with one another. Even when the child is essentially nonverbal, much can be learned from observing the child at play.

It is important that the form of play therapy chosen be appropriate to the developmental level at which the child is functioning. For example, finger painting and other forms of artwork may be used in therapy. This type of activity may appeal more to some children than does playing with toys. This is especially true in the case of an older child. Much can be learned from the child's choice of color, the choice of topic to be featured in the artwork, and the story the child may tell about the painting when it has been completed. Finger painting is one of the substitute activities that may be provided for children who have not successfully passed through the habit-training aspect of personality development.

BEHAVIORALLY DISTURBED CHILDREN

Identifying behaviorally disturbed children

It is sometimes more difficult to identify behavioral disturbances among children than among adults because children are actively involved in a dynamic growth process that produces constantly changing behavior. Although children with behavioral disturbances may not be able to complete each developmental task successfully, their behavior, like that of normal children, shows rapid modifications.

When children are slow to walk or talk or to develop any of the other physical, intellectual, or social achievements on which the judgment of normal development is based, the advice of a pediatrician should be sought. If the child's development continues to lag, professional help should be requested from a child psychiatrist. Evaluation of developmental progress should be based on a thorough study of the child and his family. A developmental history is required, as well as a complete physical and psychological examination. An understanding of the parents' attitude toward their life together and toward their child should be acquired through an in-depth study of the family. Some evaluation of the response of the child to his parents is important. The information required to understand the essential difficulties involved in the development of the child's behavioral disturbance may include the shared knowledge of the parents, other key relatives, neighbors, teachers, the family physician, and others.

Behavioral disturbances of childhood

As has been stated earlier, there is little agreement among child psychiatrists concerning the nomenclature appropriate for identifying the types of disturbances from which children suffer. Because even the normal child is easily influenced by all types of environmental changes and has a poor tolerance for variations in his emotional climate, some of the behavioral disturbances of childhood have been classified under the title of anxiety disorders.

Anxiety disorders include such behavior as nail biting, thumb sucking, enuresis, soiling, masturbation, and tantrums. They are behaviors usually used by a child to express unmet needs or unconscious unmet strivings. Thus some of these habits are developed by the child in an attempt to comfort or reassure himself in tense, lonely, or frightening situations. Others are used to express rebellion or anger at parental figures as they handle the situation perceived as stressful by the child. Children are rarely admitted for institutional care because of one of these behaviors and can usually be treated while remaining in their homes.

A second group of behaviors called *conduct disorders* includes truancy, stealing, destructiveness, cruelty, sexual offenses, and the use of alcohol. Although these behaviors usually appear in older children, they are also expressions of unmet needs, of anxiety and tension, or of anger and rebellion. Children who use one or more of these behaviors usually have a distorted perception of the world and have experienced unsatisfactory family relationships throughout their total personality development. As in other childhood disturbances, a complete understanding of the child and his family is required before treatment is attempted. These behavioral disturbances may be expressions of a severely disturbed child and may require long-term treatment.

Other behaviors indicative of problems in the emotional life of children include tics, habit spasms, somnambulism, stammering, overactivity, and phobias. Like the others that have been discussed, they are defenses against anxiety. Some of them, especially tics and stuttering, may be examples of conversion.

Older children might first exhibit emotional problems in behavioral patterns that interfere with school or social adjustment. Examples include the overconforming child who is not able to relate on a child's level to other children, the child with an emotional problem manifested by a reading disability, and the bright child who because of a need to use patterns of withdrawal gives the appearance of having limited intelligence.

Psychophysiological disorders include feeding difficulties (chronic anorexia, food faddism, recurrent vomiting, obesity), difficulties of coordination (writing dysfunctions), respiratory dysfunctions (asthma, rhinitis), lower bowel dysfunctions (colitis, constipation), and others. Each of these psychophysiological disorders presents a complex of symptoms that originally were used by the child to defend against unbearable tension resulting from some interpersonal conflict usually existing within the family. If the situation has continued over a long period of time, as so often happens in asthma, colitis, or anorexia, the behavior becomes progressively more complex, and the relationship to the original conflict becomes somewhat obscure. All these conditions are difficult to treat and require close collaboration among appropriate professional workers who deal with the family situation. The emotional conflict underlying any one of these disorders is usually long standing and is deeply significant to the child.

Providing corrective experiences for behaviorally disturbed children

Providing therapeutic care for disturbed children is one of the most challenging tasks a nurse or a child care worker can undertake. Yet it is one that these workers must meet, since it is they who are most likely to have both initial and sustained contact with these children, particularly as they function in guidance centers and community mental health treatment centers. The behavior of children with emotional problems is frequently more baffling and more difficult to understand than the behavior of emotionally ill adults. If the care provided for disturbed children is to be therapeutic, it must be based on the individual needs of the child. The nurse, like all other individuals working with disturbed children, will find it necessary to study the child and the symptoms he displays to identify his immediate needs and to respond to them in a realistic and helpful way. In so doing, an attempt is made to offer the child experiences that can correct, in some measure, the negative experiences that have been a part of his life.

As the nurse and the child care worker understand that the behaviors the child exhibits are symptoms of more basic problems, they will learn to be sensitive in the manner in which they respond to the disturbed behavior. There is no question that the disturbed behavior requires a response; however, if this becomes the primary focus of intervention, one runs the risk of reinforcing the behavior with the result that it may not only continue but actually worsen. Rather, the goal should be an attempt to discover the nature of the underlying problem, and the intervention should be directed toward its resolution, not merely toward the obliteration of the symptom. For example, it is commonly known that attempts to stop a child from nail biting are generally unsuccessful when this behavior is the sole focus of concern. To intervene on a level more basic than the presenting symptom, the nurse and the child care worker need to work collaboratively with the therapist, the pediatrician, and the social worker.

Since many of these children are highly sensitive to their environment and the people who are a part of it, nurses and child care workers need to examine their feelings, attitudes, and behaviors in an attempt to understand their own reactions to the child.

In this way they can modify their behavior for the benefit of the child. A good rule to follow in dealing with the behavior of disturbed children is to look for cues the child is expressing through his behavior and to respond naturally and appropriately.

Disturbed children require attention and guidance in the same areas of personal care that mothers usually provide. Thus the adult working with disturbed children will need to be involved actively in the child's bathing, toileting, feeding, dressing, and play activities. In addition, these children require organization and supervision in a variety of play activities, protection from potentially dangerous situations, and, at times, appropriate limit setting. Like normal children, each disturbed child is unique and occasionally needs special understanding and attention. It is a demanding task to respond as a wise adult to all the situations that may arise from the activities of daily living. The cooperation of all the nurses and other child care workers involved in the situation is required to assist each child to express his needs and find satisfying ways of meeting them.

Sometimes disturbed children, like all children, need to be held, cuddled, rocked, or comforted. Such an activity is clearly a part of the role of the nurse and necessitates a good deal of knowledge, sensitivity, and mature judgment to realize when and how much of such gratification is therapeutic for each child.

When admission to a treatment center is recommended for disturbed children, it is done in the hope that the climate of the center will provide greater opportunities for ego development than can be provided elsewhere. Thus the goal for the treatment of every child is the development of a climate that will encourage the adaptive aspects of the child's ego so that he will experiment with methods for coping with the environment and for developing more effective ways of dealing with people.

Disturbed children are frequently unclear about simple aspects of reality and need to have repeated clarification about these confusions. Thus the nurse-child interactions should logically focus on the reality of the situation, with emphasis being placed on verbal communication about reality matters.

Inappropriate response to environmental stimuli is a frequent problem for the disturbed child. The nurse needs to help the child recognize more appropriate responses to stimuli. Opportunities should be provided for him to test and use these new responses.

Consistency in dealing with any child is of major importance and is especially necessary in providing care for disturbed children. When several people are involved in providing care for children, consistency is difficult to achieve but is nonetheless important. Assuring a consistent approach depends on adequate communication among all people involved. Thus frequent staff meetings involving all the adults who come in contact with the child are essential. Every adult involved must understand what approach is being made to each child, why it has been adopted, and what it is expected to achieve. Repeated clarification of the treatment goals for each child is essential. Each worker must have frequent opportunities to share with the group personal experiences in caring for the child. Thus all workers will be equally aware of the child's progress, and inconsistencies in the treatment approach can be eliminated.

Disturbed children sometimes become hyperactive and exhibit destructive behavior. Establishing and enforcing reasonable limits for children is an important responsibility for all child care workers. It may be necessary to restrain these children to avoid injury to themselves or to others. Restraint can best be accomplished by holding the child firmly until the outburst has subsided. Assuring the child that the staff is not frightened by his behavior may be reassuring to him because the child may fear his own angry feelings. It may also be reassuring to the child to tell him that he will not be allowed to hurt himself or other people.

The nurse or the child care worker frequently has an opportunity to talk with the parents of disturbed children. Most parents of disturbed children are themselves working with a therapist and thus have opportunities to discuss their concerns and anxieties. However, the nurse is frequently the most available professional person to whom they can turn to share the concerns that may have arisen or to ask advice about some aspect of behavior the child has developed. The nurse's interest in their child and willingness to listen to their fears and doubts are therapeutic for the parents.

In addition, many workers have had the experience of finding that when they focus on the family in assisting them to explore and resolve familial conflicts, the child's disturbed behavior improves. The theoretical basis for this phenomenon is that the family is a system and that the disturbed behavior used by the child is seen as a symptom reflecting dysfunction within the family unit. As the family unit becomes more functional, the child is likely to have more of his needs met and to feel more secure and therefore has less need to use disturbed behavior. I had the experience of working therapeutically with the mother of an asthmatic child and after a series of visits with the mother learned that the child's asthmatic attacks decreased in frequency and severity without my ever having met the child. One of the possible explanations of this occurrence, simplistic as it may be, is that as the mother's needs were more fully met, she was able to be more supportive to the child.

Another important function of the nurse that cannot be overemphasized is her role in providing anticipatory guidance to families to prepare them for the behaviors that can be expected of the child as he progresses through each developmental stage. Many parents, particularly mothers, feel most comfortable in sharing their concerns with a nurse. Appropriate reassurances and instruction can be of inestimable value in helping parents to provide acceptance and guidance for an emotionally disturbed child. In addition, appropriate anticipatory guidance of parents may play an important role in the prevention of behavioral disturbances in children who are basically healthy.

BEHAVIORALLY DISTURBED ADOLESCENTS

Identifying behaviorally disturbed adolescents

Adolescence is the term applied to the period of life roughly between the ages of 12 and 21, when many emotional and personal crises occur. During this period the individual exerts a great deal of effort to control impulses and desires that come about as a result of biological maturation. In addition, the adolescent strives to become independent and to be emancipated from parents. Thus the adolescent is torn between devotion to family members and the need to depend on them and the conscious and unconscious need to reject them as a means of establishing independence.

The adolescent is constantly engaged in an intrapsychic struggle in an attempt to develop a new psychological equilibrium. The outcome of this struggle depends to a large extent on successful achievement of the developmental tasks that must be accomplished during the earlier years of life. The strength of the individual's early ego development is tested during the adolescent years. The number and severity of emotional problems of adolescents continue to increase. This is especially true in relation to suicide and mental illness.

Adolescence is a period when individuals normally experience fluctuations in behavior, instability of emotional equilibrium, and rapid changes in mood. A few adolescents actually become emotionally disturbed and develop the characteristic symptomatic behavior of schizophrenia, including bizarre ideation, hallucinations, withdrawal, ideas of reference, and feelings of unreality.

Adolescents may also develop depression or any one of the other behavioral maladaptations that have been described elsewhere in this text. Treatment of major emotional problems among adolescents requires the use of the same psychiatric skills as those used for adults who suffer from these illnesses.

Some young people may be admitted to a mental health treatment center in an emotionally disturbed state indistinguishable from a true psychotic episode. The adolescent may hallucinate or be highly suspicious. However, the symptoms prove to be temporary, and the situation clears after a few weeks of treatment. In this instance it is likely that the adolescent has reacted to a particularly stressful situation. The neutral environment of a treatment center diminishes the emotional stress that is upsetting the individual and helps in gaining control and in reconstituting the personality. Such a situation is thought to have been caused by the inability of the individual's ego to cope with the conflicting social and personal pressures that are present in the lives of all adolescents.

Treatment of adolescents requires collaboration among the therapist, the child care workers, the school, the nurse, the family, and the social worker in identifying the individual's problem and in helping him to cope with it.

Providing corrective experiences for behaviorally disturbed adolescents

Even healthy adolescents experience fluctuations in behavior, instability of emotional equilibrium, and rapid changes in mood. Nurses who attempt to work with emotionally disturbed adolescents need an in-depth understanding of the normal behavior of persons in this stage of development to be able to differentiate between normal and abnormal responses.

Since adolescence is a period of transition from childhood to adulthood without clearly demarcated parameters along the way, the first step in planning care is to assess the developmental level of the individual and avoid making assumptions based solely on chronological age.

A major developmental task for the adolescent is the establishment of an identity that is separate from that of his family. The normal adolescent conflict between independence and dependence is greatly heightened in emotionally disturbed adolescents, resulting in even greater emotional lability. There are a number of ways in which the individual attempts to resolve this conflict, many of which are acted on simultaneously.

One common mode of adjustment, also evident in normal adolescents, is the development of a fierce group cohesiveness and loyalty; the group's norms are substantively different from the perceived norms of authority figures and parents. This strong attachment to a peer group substitutes for the security previously experienced in the family setting, thereby enabling the adolescent to move away from the family with some degree of safety.

Group activity among adolescents is normally accompanied by a great deal of physical roughhousing. The nurse needs to be aware that the emotionally disturbed adolescent has decreased impulse control and that the roughhousing, which began as horseplay, can easily become a traumatic acting-out experience for all concerned. The sensitive and experienced nurse will intervene by setting limits before it reaches this point. While a feeling of loss of control produces anxiety for persons in any stage of development, loss of control is extremely frightening for the disturbed adolescent whose grasp on reality is relatively tenuous. Because a feeling of loss of control for these persons may result in even greater personality disintegration, it should be avoided at all costs. In a sense, the nurse acts as an alter ego for the individual or group when she sets limits, even though in doing so she may be perceived as an interfering and punitive authority figure.

Group activity among adolescents should be encouraged because it serves a number of very important functions for the adolescent, such as facilitating emancipation from parents, establishing identity, and developing social skills. The nurse must be knowledgeable and skillful in dealing with both structured and unstructured groups. The nurse who is experienced in working with adolescents will find that pressure from the peer group is the most effective means of facilitating behavioral changes in members of the group. Therefore it is wise to learn to work with and through the group to accomplish therapeutic goals for individual adolescents.

Adolescents use testing behavior in an attempt to establish an equilibrium between dependency and independency. This testing behavior takes place in both one-to-one interactions and in group situations and is directed at the situation as well as at other people. Therefore the environment should be consistent, secure, and supportive, in the sense that all rules should be made explicit from the beginning, should be fair and reasonable, and should be consistently enforced. Although the adolescent will inevitably rebel against any restrictions, a lack of them will greatly contribute to his sense of insecurity. The importance of limit setting that is clear and consistent but nonpunitive cannot be overemphasized.

Another task of adolescent development is the establishment of a satisfactory heterosexual relationship. Disturbed adolescents seem to have particular difficulty with this task, probably because of unsatisfactory resolution of earlier developmental tasks. Therefore it is quite common for the disturbed male adolescent to act in an inappropriate, provocative manner in approaching the young female nurse and for the female adolescent patient to engage in similarly inappropriate behavior when approaching young male attendants, nurses, and interns. These behaviors, on the one hand, provide the staff with a valuable opportunity to help the individual develop more socially acceptable skills in relating to peers of the opposite sex. On the other hand, behavior that is sexually provocative often elicits in young staff members feelings related to some of their own unresolved problems. Some staff members even act sexually provocative with adolescent clients, although on an unconscious level. Therefore self-awareness is critically important if the nurse is to be successful in assisting the disturbed adolescent to make the treatment setting a learning experience that will be of value in the future. Because behavioral patterns are not permanent at the time of adolescence, the treatment setting provides an opportunity to test a variety of patterns of behavior as the adolescent learns to become an adult.

Older staff members may be viewed as parental authority figures and can expect to be the recipients of hostility from disturbed adolescents. As long as the staff members can remain objective and avoid personalizing verbal assaults, this experience can be a meaningful one for the individual as he learns that anger and disagreements do not inevitably destroy relationships or people and that people who have different beliefs and frames of reference can genuinely care about each other. It should be remembered that, for the disturbed adolescent, rebelling against staff members is immeasurably safer than rebelling against or disagreeing with parents. It is hoped that, as the adolescent gains more ego strength, he will be able to confront his parents in a constructive and mature way, using the practice he has experienced with staff members.

Physiologically, adolescents are experiencing a major growth spurt that has a number of physical and psychological implications. Their nutritional needs are great, partly because of a dramatic increase in motor activity. All adolescents, especially those experiencing emotional disturbances, require a great deal of physical space in which to discharge energy. The workers should provide for this need within the limitations of the physical environment. One concrete suggestion is to keep the chairs in the group therapy session further apart than would be necessary when conducting group therapy with adults. It is also possible that the adolescent's need for space is symbolic of his intermittent need to create emotional distance so as to establish his independence. At the same time, the adolescent needs to feel assured that he is not being abandoned or being forced into young adulthood until he is able to deal with the crucial decisions required by that stage.

Because the challenges of dealing with disturbed adolescents seem to be unique and to change from day to day, there is much controversy among authorities as to whether special treatment settings should be operated solely for adolescents or whether adolescents should be part of the regular treatment setting for emotionally disturbed adults. There are convincing arguments for both positions, the former allowing for a more consistent, homogeneous treatment approach, whereas the latter is believed by its proponents to more closely approximate the world of reality in which the adolescent must learn to function.

Treatment of adolescents whose initial symptom is the use of hard drugs is even more poorly understood than the more general emotional problems of this age group, and it is very common for treatment centers to have special units solely for these individuals. Because this has become a highly specialized area of study, it is suggested that students refer to current journal articles on the subject. It is interesting to note, however, that current statistics show that in young people there is an increasing return to the use of alcohol, as opposed to other drugs, to cope with anxiety. The significance of this apparent trend is yet to be understood.

CASE FORMULATION □ A BEHAVIORALLY DISTURBED ADOLESCENT

Jennie, a 15-year-old girl, was referred to the community mental health center by her school counselor with the approval of her mother. She came to the center willingly and described herself as being unhappy, upset, and without friends. The school counselor was concerned about Jennie, who had entered the school as a new student only a few months earlier. Her concern focused on the following problems: Jennie had made no friends, was receiving failing grades, was absent from school about half the time, and was involved in almost no school clubs or extracurricular activities.

Jennie talked freely to the nurse at the mental health center and stated that she could not study because she did not sleep well at night. She described some of the nightmares that frightened her and kept her awake. Their content often featured an older man who molested her sexually.

In discussing her family she spoke of the frequent fights between herself and her mother over her mother's drinking and her mother's boyfriend. About a year ago Jennie's mother and father separated, and they were in the process of getting a divorce when she came to the clinic. After her parents separated, her father moved to another city and rarely found time to come back to visit with his three children, of whom Jennie was the oldest. She blamed her mother for the separation and the move from their old neighborhood and the school she had attended all her life.

Jennie's two brothers had become her responsibility since her mother's interest in her boyfriend had increased. Thus Jennie was expected to supervise her younger brothers, get their meals, and do the laundry. With this amount of work expected of her, Jennie stated that she was too tired to attend school more than half the time. Jennie's brothers did not follow her directions and resented her attempt to supervise them. Thus there was conflict between the children in this family with no adult to act as a buffer between them.

There was a family dog, which actually belonged to Jennie's brother. However, Jennie fed him and gave him more attention than did either of her brothers. Jennie stated that the dog loved her more than he did anyone else in the family and was the only member of the family who cared about her.

Her mother's boyfriend was a large, middle-aged taxi driver who teased Jennie a good deal. She told the nurse that she disliked him intensely and said that she was afraid of him. In addition, she did not want anyone taking her father's place in the home, since she loved her father very much.

Jennie was somewhat smaller in stature than most girls of her age. Her breasts had not yet begun to develop, and she was extremely sensitive about this fact. She viewed her flat-chested appearance as a serious defect that made her different from other girls. Likewise, she had not yet begun to menstruate, which increased her belief that she was different and lacking in feminine appeal. Unfortunately, Jennie was not physically attractive because her hair was dull and unkempt and her complexion sallow. She had never had a date with a boy, and she felt rejected by both boys and girls in her class.

Jennie's mother was invited to come to the clinic to discuss the treatment plans for her daughter. She found it difficult to arrange a convenient time, since she held a part-time job. However, she finally kept the appointment and gave much the same information about the family situation as did Jennie. However, the mother stated that the conflict between the children was due to Jennie's attempt to boss her brothers. She felt that Jennie's resentment of her boyfriend was the cause of many of their disagreements and declared that her dates were none of her daughter's business. According to her mother, Jennie was her father's favorite child, but he did not deserve her devotion.

Jennie's developmental history, according to her mother, was uneventful except that she had been enuretic until the age of 9. This problem reappeared after the separation of the parents and was present even now. Her mother also reported that Jennie had responded to discipline by having temper tantrums. This began when she was being toilet trained and continued until she was 9. Although she no longer has what could be described as temper tantrums, she does fly into rages. These rages seem to be related to the mother's boyfriend and the approaching divorce. The mother stated that, because of her job and home responsibilities, she had not been able to work with the school counselor.

Discussion of development of patterns of behavior

Jennie is having difficulty adjusting to the present factors impinging on her life. Her mother, who may be an immature woman, has not provided Jennie with the love and support she required to develop the ego strengths and defense system necessary for her to cope with the challenges confronting an adolescent. Jennie and her mother have been in serious conflict since her infancy; the temper tantrums and enuresis appear to have been an expression of anger and frustration directed toward the mother and an attempt to control the situation and achieve some autonomy. Her father, who did provide her with love, was separated from the family, and the reappearance of the enuresis when he left home suggests a revival of the childhood feelings toward her mother, since Jennie blames her mother for this loss. The most recent deprivation occurred when the family moved to a new neighborhood, which made it necessary for her to enter a strange school and develop new relationships—something she had always found difficult. To add to all these problems, Jennie's mother began dating and drinking with a man who was frightening to Jennie and who threatened to take her father's place. Jennie felt overwhelmed by the responsibilities of the housework and the care of her younger brothers. Many adolescents develop self-esteem because they perform well at school, are socially successful with peers, and have many outlets for excess energy through extracurricular activities. Since Jennie was not successful in any of these areas and had not even developed the physical characteristics of a woman, she felt different, unloved, and close to emotional collapse.

Jennie's nightmares have undoubtedly increased by the introduction into the family of her mother's boyfriend, who is frightening to her. However, her dreams of being molested sexually may suggest that she is unconsciously in rivalry with her mother for the taxi driver's sexual attention. Her rages are an attempt to cope with her feelings of rejection and are directed at her mother for saddling her with too much responsibility, for banishing her father, for withholding love, for failing to give her approval, and for introducing a new, unwanted man into the family.

To some extent Jennie's problems at school are a reflection of the turmoil at home. However, her inability to make friends is a long-standing problem that has existed since childhood. Jennie's failure to involve herself in the activities of her peer group developed as a result of her fear of competition and her lack of self-confidence. Her slow sexual development has reinforced her concern about being different and inadequate.

Nursing care plan

1. After a physical examination to determine Jennie's status in relation to her retarded sexual development, institute treatment, if indicated, as well as a program of sexual education. In this way Jennie can be helped to understand her body and anticipate eventual normal menses and breast development.
2. Encourage good grooming to improve her attractiveness and thus her self-esteem.
3. Encourage involvement in group therapy sessions with other adolescents in which age-related concerns are discussed frankly.
4. Work toward helping Jennie establish a trusting relationship by treating her with dignity and respect and by listening carefully to whatever she has to say. Accept her opinions without moralizing.
5. Assist Jennie to direct anger and hostility into more socially acceptable activities.
6. Encourage participation in appropriate age-related occupational and recreational activities.
7. Encourage independent functioning by establishing fair and

reasonable limits and by consistently enforcing them. Praise her when she functions independently and wisely.

8. Include Jennie in decisions about her care and treatment, and keep her informed in relation to her progress.
9. Help her to discuss her feelings and concerns and assess them realistically.

Outlook for Jennie

Jennie has many emotional needs that are not being met at home. In view of her mother's attitudes toward her daughter, the best approach to helping her to cope with the many problems in her life would be admission to a residential treatment center where a consistent, supportive relationship with caring adults would be available, appropriate group activities with other adolescents could be developed, more effective external controls could be learned, and self-esteem could be improved. If such a treatment situation were available and if significant individuals in her life were involved in the treatment plan, she could be helped to complete the unfinished developmental tasks of earlier stages of growth. Her response to these therapeutic efforts would be more success in school and with her peers. Unless her mother could be helped to alter her attitude in a positive way, Jennie would probably continue to maintain a basically hostile attitude toward her.

CONCLUDING STATEMENTS

1. The treatment of emotional disorders of children and adolescents is recognized as an area of specialization in both medicine and nursing.
2. There is even less agreement among authorities concerning the cause, prevention, and treatment of emotional problems of children than there is concerning similar problems among adults.
3. Understanding normal personality growth and development is essential before one can understand emotionally disturbed children.
4. Causes of the increase in the numbers of children with emo-

tional problems are obscure but are probably related to some of the basic problems in our culture.

5. Childhood emotional disturbances are not distinct and well-defined clinical entities, and there is no universal agreement as to their cause.
6. An emotionally healthy climate within the family is essential if children are to develop into mentally healthy individuals.
7. The ability to trust is a basic ingredient in the development of a well-integrated personality and is learned by infants during their earliest mothering experiences.
8. Each phase in personality development presents the child with more pressure to conform and thus more opportunity to develop emotional conflicts.
9. Parents respond differently to individual children; one child may thrive in a home where a second child may be unable to tolerate the situation.
10. Improvement in the child's behavior may depend on alterations in the parents' attitudes and approaches. Thus parents usually work with a therapist at the same time that the child is being treated.
11. Childhood psychoses are thought to develop as a result of the interaction between a constitutionally susceptible child and an environmental situation psychologically incompatible for the child.
12. Most children afflicted with a childhood psychosis have one or all of the following symptoms: autistic withdrawal, failure to develop language or to use communicative speech, failure to develop according to the normally expected developmental pattern, use of repetitive mannerisms, impairment of ego functioning, failure to develop a clearly defined body image, lack of sexual identity, and inability to perceive time and space accurately.
13. Early infantile autism and symbiotic infantile psychotic syndrome are two fairly clearly identified childhood psychoses and are believed to be clearly related to the failures during the early mothering experiences received by the child.
14. General goals of treatment for all emotionally disturbed chil-

dren include providing opportunities to develop a realistic concept of self, to develop more appropriate object relationships, and to work through or relive phases of personality development that were imperfectly experienced.

15. Because learning to relate to others is the greatest task of the autistic child, he is thought to be able to profit from individual therapy.
16. The symbiotic infantile psychotic child may profit from the special therapeutic environment provided by treatment centers for children in which substitutes for the unhealthy symbiotic relationship with the mother are made available to the child.
17. The symbiotic infantile psychotic child needs help in gradually developing independence.
18. Play therapy is used as a means of gaining insight into the child's unconscious feelings and attitudes, as a means of communicating with the child, and as a means for working through the child's problems.
19. Many behavioral disturbances adopted by children are attempts by the children to comfort or reassure themselves in tense, lonely, or frightening situations and to defend against anxiety.
20. If the care and treatment provided for disturbed children is to be therapeutic, it must be based on the individual needs of the child.
21. The child with a behavioral disturbance will benefit more from the nurse's efforts to discover the nature of the underlying problem and to assist in its resolution than if the focus is on the specific symptoms exhibited by the child.
22. Nurses and child care workers need to examine their feelings, attitudes, and behavior in an attempt to understand and modify their behavior for the benefit of the child.
23. Disturbed children require attention and guidance in the same areas of personal care as mothers usually provide for children.
24. Sometimes disturbed children, like all children, need to be held, cuddled, rocked, or comforted.

25. Nurse-child interactions should focus on the reality of the situation, with emphasis on communication about reality matters.
26. Consistency and the establishment and enforcement of fair and reasonable limits in dealing with all children are of major importance and are critical in dealing with disturbed children.
27. If the family of a disturbed child is assisted in developing a more emotionally healthy climate, the child will have more of his needs met and feel more secure, thereby having less need to resort to abnormal defenses.
28. Because of the labile, rapidly changing nature of normal adolescents, the nurse needs an in-depth understanding of the normal behavior of persons in this stage of development to be able to differentiate between normal and abnormal responses.
29. A major developmental task for the adolescent is to establish an identity separate from that of his family.
30. Peer group cohesiveness and loyalty are normal for all adolescents and have therapeutic potential for disturbed adolescents.
31. A therapeutic environment for the disturbed adolescent should be consistent, secure, and supportive in the sense that any rules should be fair, reasonable, explicit, and consistently enforced.
32. Disturbed adolescents have poor impulse control, which requires consistency in limit setting.
33. The nurse needs much self-understanding to deal therapeutically with behavior that is hostile and provocative.

Suggested sources of additional information

CLASSICAL

Ackerman, Nathan W.: Child and family psychiatry today: a new look at some old problems, Ment. Hyg. **47**:540-545, 1963.

Axline, Virginia M.: Dibs—in search of self, New York, 1976, Ballantine Books, Inc.

Bowlby, John: Separation anxiety; a critical review of the literature, J. Child Psychol. Psychiatry **1**:251-269, 1961.

Bowlby, John: Maternal care and mental health, ed. 2, World Health Organization Monograph Series No. 2, Geneva, 1965, World Health Organization.

Caplan, Gerald: Prevention of mental disorders in children: initial explorations, New York, 1961, Basic Books, Inc., Publishers.

Fagin, Claire M., editor: Readings in child and adolescent psychiatric nursing, St. Louis, 1974, The C.V. Mosby Co.

Freud, Anna: The psychoanalytic treatment of children, ed. 4, New York, 1971, Shocken Books.

Gregory, Diane R.: Russel and I; an experience with autism, Perspect. Psychiatr. Care **9:**29-31, Jan.-Feb., 1971.

Kanner, Leo. Child psychiatry, ed. 4, Springfield, Ill., 1979, Charles C Thomas, Publisher.

Middleton, Agnes B., and Pothier, Patricia C.: The nurse in child psychiatry—an overview, Nurs. Outlook **18:**52-56, May, 1970.

Pothier, Patricia C.: Individual therapy with a mute autistic child, Perspect. Psychiatr. Care **5:**124, 134, May-June, 1967.

Redl, Fritz: Controls from within, New York, 1965, The Free Press.

Redl, Fritz, and Wineman, D.: Children who hate, New York, 1965, The Free Press.

Spitz, René A.: Hospitalism. An inquiry into the genesis of psychiatric conditions in early childhood in psychoanalytic study of the child, vol. 1, New York, 1945, International Universities Press, p. 53.

Spurgeon, Ruth: Nursing the autistic child, Am. J. Nurs. **67:**1418, 1967.

Turner, Ruby: A method of working with disturbed children, Am. J. Nurs. **70:**2146-2151, 1970.

CONTEMPORARY

Bentz, Willard K., and Davis, Ann: Perceptions of emotional disorders among children as viewed by leaders, teachers, and the general public, Am. J. Public Health **65:**129-132, Feb., 1975.

Blackwood, R.O.: Operant control of behavior, Akron, Ohio, 1972, Exordium Press.

Brown, Daniel G.: Behavior modification with children, Ment. Hyg. **56:**22-30, Winter, 1972.

Caplan, Gerald: Child and adolescent psychiatry. In Arieti, Silvano, editor: American Handbook of psychiatry, ed. 2, vol. 2, New York, 1974, Basic Books, Inc., Publishers, pp. 3-397.

Casoly, Rose Marie: Affective development in a psychotic boy, Perspect. Psychiatr. Care **9:**34-37, Jan.-Feb., 1971.

Clark, Carolyn C.: Psychotherapy with the resistant child, Perspect. Psychiatr. Care **15**(3):122-125, 1977.

Clark, Deborah, and Long, Kathleen A.: Nurses as health educators with emotionally disturbed children. Perspect. Psychiatr. Care **17:**167-175, July-Aug., 1979.

Closurdo, Janette S.: Behavior modification and the nursing process, Perspect. Psychiatr. Care **13:**25-36, Jan.-March, 1975.

Cook, Judith C.: Interpreting and decoding autistic communication, Perspect. Psychiatr. Care **9:**24-28, Jan.-Feb., 1971.

Crowdes, Nancy E.: Group therapy for preadolescent boys, Am. J. Nurs. **75:**92-95, 1975.

Feingold, Ben F.: Hyperkinesis and learning disabilities linked to artificial food flavors and colors, Am. J. Nurs. **75:**797-803, 1975.

Freeman, Thomas: Childhood psychopathology and adult psychoses, New York, 1976, International Universities Press, Inc.

Fremont, Theodore S., and Seifert, David: What you should know about hyperactivity, Ment. Hyg. **60:**11-13, Summer, 1976.

Friedman, Allison L., Juntti, M. Jeanette, and Scoblic, Mary A.: Nursing responsibility in child abuse, Nursing Forum **15**(1):95-112, 1976.

Hart, Nancy A., and Keidel, Gladys C.: The suicidal adolescent, Am. J. Nurs. **79:**80-84, Jan., 1979.

Hecht, Murray: Children of alcoholics are children at risk, Am. J. Nurs. **73:**1764-1767, 1973.

Hyde, Naida D.: Play therapy: the troubled child's self encounter, Am. J. Nurs. **71:**1366-1370, 1971.

Joint Commission on Mental Health of Children: Crisis in child mental health: challenge for the 1970's, New York, 1970, Harper & Row, Publishers.

Kalisch, Beatrice J.: Nursing actions in behalf of the battered child, Nurs. Forum **12**(4):365-377, 1973.

Kessler, Jane W.: Psychopathology of childhood, Englewood Cliffs, N.J., 1966, Prentice-Hall, Inc.

King, Dorothy A.: Anorexic behavior: a nursing problem, J. Psychiatr. Nurs. **71:**11-17, May-June, 1971.

Light, Nada: Differentiation in a pre-adolescent, pre-psychotic child, Perspect. Psychiatr. Care **15**(2):78-81, 1977.

Liu, Aimee: Solitaire, Philadelphia, 1980, J.P. Lippincott Co.

Lore, Ann: Adolescents: people, not problems, Am. J. Nurs. **73:**1232, 1234, 1973.

McDonagh, Mary Jo: Operant conditioning effective in reducing enuresis and encopresis in children, Perspect. Psychiatr. Care **9:**17-23, Jan.-Feb., 1971.

Melton, Janet Howell: A boy with anorexia nervosa, Am. J. Nurs. **74:**1649-1651, 1974.

Mindek, Laurie: Sex education on a psychiatric unit, Am. J. Nurs. **74:**1865-1868, 1974.

Novack, Alvin H., Bromet, Evelyn, Neill, T. Kerby, Abramovitz, Robert H., and Storch, Susan: Children's mental health services in an inner city neighborhood, Am. J. Public Health **65:**133-138, Feb., 1975.

Olson, Robert J.: Index of suspicion: screening for child abusers, Am. J. Nurs. **76:**108-110, 1976.

Piche, Judith C.: Tell me a story, Am. J. Nurs. **78:**1188-1193, July, 1978.

Pratt, Sandra J., and Fischer, Joel: Behavior modification: changing hyperactive behavior in a children's group, Perspect. Psychiatr. Care **13:**37-42, Jan.-March, 1975.

Savino, Anne B., and Sanders, R. Wyman: Working with abusive parents; group therapy and home visits, Am. J. Nurs. **73:**482-485, 1973.

Schmidt, Mary P. H., and Duncan, Beverly A. B.: Modifying eating behavior in anorexia nervosa, Am. J. Nurs. **74:**1646-1648, 1974.

Smith, Linda F.: Communicating with young children: an experiment with play therapy, Am. J. Nurs. **77:**1963-1965, Dec., 1977.

Steiger, Thelma B.: Shadow child, Am. J. Nurs. **73:**2080-2086, 1973.

Taylor, John: The hyperactive child and the family: the complete what-to-do handbook, New York, 1980, Everest House.

Tiedt, Eileen: The adolescent in the hospital: an identity-resolution approach, Nurs. Forum **11:**(2):120-140, 1972.

Volmut, Joyce A.: Fantasy in the nursing of children, Perspect. Psychiatr. Care **17**(5):211-217, Sept.-Oct., 1979.

Wilbur, Cornelia, and Aug, Robert: Sex education, Am. J. Nurs. **73:**88-91, 1973.

OF PARTICULAR INTEREST

Fagin, Claire M., editor: Readings in child and adolescent psychiatric nursing, St. Louis, 1974, The C.V. Mosby Co.

This excellent book outlines the role of the nurse in relating therapeutically with adolescent clients and makes use of clinical examples to assist the reader in application.

Kessler, Jane W.: Psychopathology of childhood, Englewood Cliffs, N.J., 1966, Prentice-Hall, Inc.

This book discusses the various emotional illnesses related to childhood and outlines recommendations for therapeutic intervention.

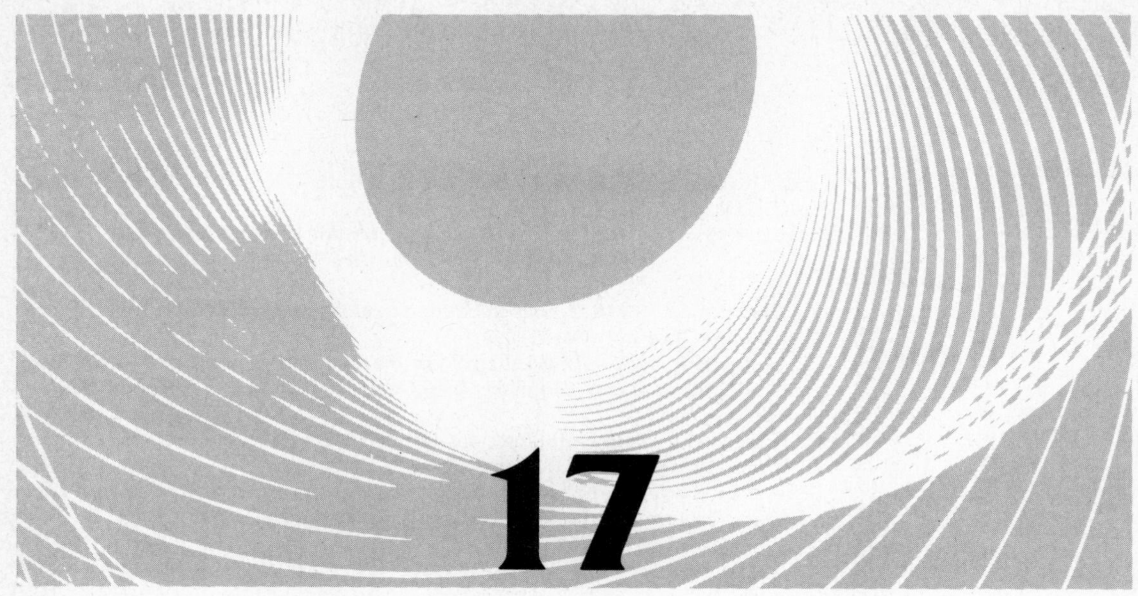

17

Maladaptive behavioral patterns associated with faulty intellectual development

---

- Mental retardation leading to faulty intellectual development
- Identifying the needs of individuals with faulty intellectual development
- Improving the emotional climate for individuals with faulty intellectual development

MENTAL RETARDATION LEADING TO FAULTY INTELLECTUAL DEVELOPMENT

A grasp of several areas of scientific knowledge is required to develop an adequate understanding of the cause and prevention of mental retardation and the treatment of individuals who are mentally retarded. Understanding the broad scope of this problem may encompass aspects of one or more of the following areas of learning: medicine, sociology, psychometric testing, genetics, nutrition, psychiatry, neurophysiology, education, and community planning. Effective prevention and treatment of mental retardation require a multifaceted approach directed toward correcting many inequities in the living situation of several million citizens. Thus adequate discussion of mental retardation requires more attention than is possible in one chapter of this text.

Some experts suggest that such a large and important social problem should not be introduced if adequate attention cannot be provided for it. Others point out that mentally retarded individuals frequently require psychiatric help and are sometimes housed in institutions that have been organized for the care and treatment of the mentally ill. These facts suggest that a textbook of psychiatric nursing should include some of the essential information about the cause, prevention, and treatment of mental retardation. It also seems clear that information about faulty intellectual development should be included in the pediatric nursing course, since problems related to it are usually identified during the individual's early childhood.

Definition

The term *mental retardation* is used to describe a condition in which the individual's intellectual and social development have been partially or completely arrested in the early years of life. If the intellectual development is relatively normal before adolescence and stops sometime after its onset, mental retardation is not an appropriate designation.

There is little agreement about the appropriate terminology by which to designate individuals whose mental and social development has been incomplete. The American Psychiatric Association and the American Association on Mental Retardation both prefer mental retardation. The older terms *idiot, imbecile,* and *moron* are used infrequently today.

Causes

Although the cause of mental retardation is unknown in approximately 75% of the individuals so diagnosed, some specific conditions are known to be accompanied by or result in mental retardation.

There are some known inherited abnormalities of brain development resulting from specific metabolic defects that result in mental retardation. Some of these diagnostic entities fall under the heading of *lipoidoses* and include the following:

1. Amaurotic familial idiocy or Tay-Sachs disease, which results from the accumulation of ganglioside in the central nervous system. The disease is transmitted by a single recessive gene and is frequently found in families of Ashkenazim Jews who emigrated from Northern Europe. The child becomes progressively more apathetic and develops muscular weakness. Death usually occurs before the age of 3 years.Through genetic counseling this disease can be eliminated.
2. Niemann-Pick disease, which results from deposits of sphingomyelin in the nervous system as well as in the reticuloendothelial system. This condition is transmitted as a recessive gene and manifests itself symptomatically by the time the child is 6 months old. This condition is accompanied by spasticity, abnormal movements, tremor, and convulsions. The child becomes progressively more disabled, with an intellectual retrogression. Death usually occurs by the third year.
3. Gaucher's disease, which has a clinical picture much like that of Niemann-Pick disease, with the child suffering a rapid downhill course.
4. Metachromatic leukodystrophy, which results in a progressive impairment of the brain function and death by the age of 6 years.

Another inherited abnormality that results in defective brain development results from specific metabolic defects in relation to the use of amino acids. This condition is called *phenylketonuria* and is caused by a disturbance in protein metabolism. It is inherited from parents carrying a recessive gene. Unless it is treated very early in the child's life, severe mental retardation occurs, with tremors, cortical atrophy of the frontal lobe, dwarfism, and failure to develop speech. The treatment is to restrict phenylalanine in the diet, which requires a special formula for the infant.

Galactosemia is an abnormality in carbohydrate metabolism inherited as a recessive trait. It produces a profound disturbance in growth and development and leads to mental retardation unless recognized and treated early. The treatment is to eliminate milk and to provide soybean or casein hydrolysate substitutes.

Gargoylism or *Hurler's disease* is probably caused by a generalized enzymopathy resulting from the deposit of a mucopolysaccharide in almost all organs and connective tissue of the body. The child develops a stunted body, a protruding forehead, a saddle nose, coarse features, and other grotesque bone changes as well as mental retardation. Death usually occurs before the age of 16 years.

Mongolism or *Down's disease* is a condition transmitted by a recessive gene. The child's somatic cells have 47 chromosomes instead of the normal 46. The abnormality is found within the twenty-first chromosome. It is estimated that from 3 to 4 infants out of each 1000 are born with mongoloid features. About 5% to 10% of these children actually suffer with the severe symptoms of Down's syndrome. These children develop an intellectual capacity that rarely exceeds 50 and often is as low as 15 or 20. There is no specific treatment for this condition.

A few children exhibit mental retardation because of an unfavorable condition that existed during fetal life. Some of the conditions that may result in mental retardation include (1) eclampsia, (2) Rh blood incompatibility, (3) toxic drugs in the mother's blood, (4) rubella infection early in the life of the fetus, and (5) syphilis infection.

Environmental or traumatic factors during or after birth may result in the development of a mentally retarded infant. The situations that may result in a retarded child include (1) difficult labor resulting in cerebral trauma, (2) brain damage at birth caused by hemorrhage into the brain tissue or anoxemia of the brain, (3) encephalitis caused by a virus from one of the early childhood diseases such as measles, scarlet fever, or chickenpox, and (4) prematurity, which increases the infant's vulnerability to all stressors.

A particularly tragic cause of mental retardation in survivors is Reye's syndrome. This syndrome is a severe viral illness that produces liver dysfunction and subsequent cerebral edema. It occurs as a sequela to what usually is a mild upper respiratory infection in a previously normal child. The child's "cold" seems to run a normal course, but a few days after his apparent recovery he becomes acutely ill, rapidly going into a coma. Many of these children die, but those who survive are often moderately to mildly retarded due to the brain damage incurred.

At least two endocrine disorders result in mental retardation unless replacement therapy is introduced very early in the child's first year. These conditions are *cretinism,* which is caused by hypothyroidism, and *Fröhlich's syndrome,* which is a result of a pituitary gland dysfunction.

Only about 25% of all the mental retardation in this country has been caused by the several possible factors just discussed.

A few children appear to be mentally retarded but are able to achieve at a normal level on intelligence tests. Such a situation in which the child has an apparent inability to cope with learning situations, lacks interest in his environment, and fails to respond appropriately in social situations is thought to result from a long-standing emotional deprivation. It may be that the child has been so emotionally and culturally deprived within the family and school that to a large extent he has ceased to involve himself intellectually or socially with his environment.

The cause of mental retardation in the majority of the individuals who are diagnosed as being retarded is obscure. It occurs much more often among children born into families who are described as living in poverty than among families who have an adequate financial income. In such families, because of financial limitations, prenatal care is frequently poor or entirely absent, inadequate nutrition is often the rule, and infants are likely to receive a limited amount of handling, cuddling, and intellectual stimulation from overworked mothers who have too many children and too many responsibilities. Thus authorities believe that the prevention of mental retardation among children of socially and financially deprived families requires a total effort from government and social agencies to provide the conditions necessary for the normal growth and development of children. This means that mothers must have adequate prenatal and obstetrical care. Adequate care during this period is the first step in preventing abnormal fetal development and prematurity, which frequently result in faulty intellectual development.

Better housing is essential. More opportunities must be provided for children to engage in intellectually stimulating play activities. Adequate diets for these families are necessary to ensure the physical health of children and make it possible for them to participate in family and community activities. Parents need to be helped to understand the psychological and social requirements of their children and how these essential aspects of normal development can be supplied. More adequate educational programs are necessary and must be available for children at an earlier age if those who are potentially capable at birth of developing into intellectually and socially effective individuals are to achieve at their highest possible level.

Identification

The diagnosis of mental retardation should be made only after a multifaceted assessment of the individual has been carried out. This should include a study of his physical, social, cultural, educational, vocational, and emotional capacity. However, the determination of mental retardation leans heavily on the results of a battery of psychometric tests from which a definitive score is derived. Although authorities continue to call attention to the limitations and weaknesses of the several psychological tests currently in vogue, intelligence testing continues to be one of the major tools in categorizing individuals in relation to intellectual functioning. Such categorization is useful for many practical reasons, especially in planning educational and training programs.

A score called the intelligence quotient (IQ) is calculated by use of a formula in which the mental age (MA) is divided by the chronological age (CA) and multiplied by 100. The mental age is determined by calculating the results of answers to questions on one of several psychometric tests. Therefore the formula is

$$IQ = \frac{MA}{CA} \times 100$$

Several IQ classifications have been suggested that may be helpful in providing guidance for the establishment of educational programs.

Level of retardation	IQ
Committee on Mental Retardation, U.S. Department of Health and Human Services	
Profound	Below 20
Severe	20-35
Moderate	36-52
Mild	53-68
World Health Organization	
Severe subnormality	0-19
Moderate subnormality	20-49
Mild subnormality	50-69
American Psychiatric Association	
Severe—requires complete protective care	Below 50
Moderate—requires special training and guidance	50-70
Mild—borderline; may be trained to be economically productive in limited situations	70-85

Scope of the problem

It is estimated that there are 200,000 individuals who require institutional care in the United States because of mental retardation. It is also estimated that 225,000 retarded children are enrolled in the special classes now being offered by the public schools in this country. Some authorities estimate that about 3% of the children born each year in the United States will not achieve the intellectual development of a 12-year-old.

Most of the individuals who are mentally retarded are physically indistinguishable from the rest of the population, but they are severely limited in their ability to cope economically and socially in this highly complex society. Because of their handicaps they are mentally and emotionally vulnerable to many environmental events and constitute a high-risk group.

In February 1963 President John F. Kennedy delivered a message to the Congress of the United States calling attention to the fact that mental retardation is a major national problem. As a result, more attention was focused on this problem by the government, and financial aid to the states to improve programs for the mentally retarded was made available.

IDENTIFYING THE NEEDS OF INDIVIDUALS WITH FAULTY INTELLECTUAL DEVELOPMENT

Mentally retarded children are first of all children, with essentially the same needs as other children. The difference lies in the rate at which mentally retarded children are able to achieve the levels of maturational development, their ability to grasp new ideas, their ability to handle frustration, their ability to deal with other people socially, and their educational attainment.

Likewise, mentally retarded adults have the same basic needs as other adults. The ways in which these needs can be fulfilled are altered by the degree of the mental retardation with which the individual must cope. Mental retardation drastically affects the individual's ability to deal effectively with others in a social situation.

Most individuals with IQ ratings of less than 25 are too retarded to benefit from educational programs on even the simplest level. These individuals require personal care not unlike that provided for infants. They also need to be safeguarded against ordinary physical danger.

Those with IQ ratings of 25 to 50 are usually able to benefit from habit training, and given repetition and patience can be taught to master simple motor skills. Thus individuals in this group can be expected to learn to toilet themselves, keep themselves clean, and feed themselves.

The group whose IQ ratings range from 50 to 70 are classified as educable and, in addition to having those abilities expected of the previous group, can profit from a simple educational program. Some of these individuals can be taught to perform uncomplicated tasks through which they may become economically useful. A general guiding principle in dealing with all mentally retarded individuals is to encourage the use of their intellectual abilities at the highest possible level but at the same time to avoid pressuring them to achieve at a level that is clearly beyond their capacities.

The individual's level of mental retardation dictates to a large extent where he can be cared for most effectively and the program from which he can receive the greatest benefit. All programs of care should be highly individualized. The goal of treatment for each mentally retarded individual should be to assist him to achieve at the highest level of intellectual and social functioning possible for him.

Importance of the parent-child relationship

Because mentally retarded children have essentially the same emotional needs as other children, they too need the experience of a warm parent-child relationship. Retarded children have a greater chance of developing their intellectual and social potential if they are nurtured within a family, at least during the preschool years. No longer is institutional placement considered the only solution for a family when a child has been diagnosed as being mentally retarded.

When the child reaches school age, it may become apparent that the best possible plan for him is to live at an institution among other children with whom he can compete successfully. Even if the child spends most of the week at a special school, it is important for him to return to his family for weekend visits and on holidays. This is the ideal solution if the family is warm, accepting, and loving toward the child.

Parents need help in accepting a mentally retarded child and in providing the affection, security, and approval all children require if they are to develop a stable personality. Unfortunately, parents may feel ashamed of a retarded child and develop a sense of failure in relation to him. The child may be rejected, emotionally deprived, and coerced to achieve beyond his abilities.

Parents need support and guidance if a retarded child is to be successfully reared at home. They need encouragement in allowing the child to develop at his own rate without being overly protected, rejected, or forced to achieve beyond his potential. One significant way in which the nurse can make a contribution to improving the care of mentally retarded children is to help parents cope with their feelings and work toward meeting the needs of their children.

In spite of all efforts, there are families who cannot accept a mentally retarded child as part of the group. In such a situation a foster home placement is probably the most appropriate solution. If this solution is not possible, institutionalization in a hospital or school designed to care for mentally retarded individuals would be the logical answer.

No matter where the child lives, he needs to be cared for by warm, friendly people who understand his handicap and who will work with him intelligently and helpfully. Mentally retarded children, like all other children, need love, respect, patience, and clearly established and sensibly enforced limits on behavior. If it is decided that the child will profit most by living in an institution, the establishment must provide a substitute for the home and family of which he may be deprived.

Educational and training programs are essential parts of the daily regimen of all mentally retarded individuals who can benefit from them. Some of the more successful agencies operate much like private day or boarding schools, with the curriculum including personal habit training, instruction in personal grooming and social skills, lessons in activities designed to fill leisure time hours, and help in improving interpersonal relations. In addition, those children who can profit by more formal education attend classes organized for various age and maturational levels. Educators, with special preparation in teaching the mentally retarded, guide the children in developing simple reading skills, the ability to make change, do simple sums, budget small amounts of money, and the other educational knowledge essential for independent living. Manual skills are also taught to individuals who are capable of performing them. These educational tasks must be geared to the aptitudes of the individuals involved in the program. The aim of such a program is to equip the individual with the knowledge, vocational skill, and social effectiveness required to live as independently as possible.

Some mentally retarded children who suffer from severe physical defects as well as mental deficiency may require throughout their lives the personal care usually provided for a very young child. On the other hand, some individuals who are less handicapped may become self-supporting in the community. It has been estimated that approximately one half of the mentally retarded individuals who are admitted to an institution for care and training are eventually able to live in the community.

Institutional facilities

Many of the essential elements of an effective institution have already been mentioned. These include (1) employees who are warm, friendly, and knowledgeable about the needs of the handicapped individuals with whom they work, (2) an educational program that aims to help each individual achieve his highest intellectual and social potential, and (3) the provision of a homelike atmosphere for the individual who is deprived of home and family by being institutionalized.

Thus friendly, homelike living quarters, dining rooms, and sleeping dormitories should be available. A well-developed recreational program with a variety of activities designed to appeal to many different interests, ages, and maturational levels is important. Opportunities for participation in a variety of group experiences, including musical activities, dances, sports, movies, and television viewing, should be a part of the activities program. A library should be provided with colorful reading material chosen to appeal to the levels of the intellectual abilities of the individuals living at the institution.

Although many mentally retarded individuals are admitted as children, their problems frequently require long-term institutional care. Because of this, individuals may remain in the same institution for years. Thus access to a barber shop and a beauty parlor is a necessary part of the institutional offerings. Mentally retarded individuals need to be assisted to look as well groomed and attractive as possible.

Opportunities for individuals who can profit by work assignments should be available. Through appropriately assigned work, mentally retarded individuals can gain a sense of usefulness by performing meaningful tasks that make a significant contribution to the total work of the institution. Such work assignments should be rewarded appropriately with a cash payment. This does more than almost any other form of recognition to help the individual develop a sense of being useful.

Treatment procedures to meet physical and emotional needs

Care and treatment for the mentally retarded person should be based on an accurate evaluation of the individual's assets and capacities and the concomitant physical, emotional, and psychological problems present. Thus specific medical conditions must be treated with the appropriate therapeutic agents. Nutritional and metabolic conditions must be corrected by providing the required diet and the therapeutic measures necessary to eliminate the metabolic disequilibrium. Surgical procedures should be performed when they are indicated, especially in the case of the orthopedic deformities frequently seen in individuals who have been confined to a bed or wheelchair. Replacement therapy in such conditions as cretinism should be undertaken. All these procedures require an institutional staff of professional individuals who are capable of providing the necessary therapeutic measures. These procedures are designed to assist mentally retarded individuals to achieve the highest possible level of intellectual, physical, and social functioning.

Unfortunately, for many severely mentally retarded individuals, the ability to cope with the environment or to achieve at a higher level is not greatly improved by specific treatments. Instead, these individuals require the kind of environment that provides for their special physical and emotional needs.

Some mentally retarded individuals are aware of their limited abilities and are troubled by their inadequate coping patterns. They may believe that they are a great disappointment to their families and become guilt ridden and depressed. Many of them suffer from the same anxieties, frustrations, and psychotic symptoms found among individuals in other situations. Such emotional problems appear frequently among mentally retarded individuals and require the same kind of professional help that would be provided in other settings.

The psychotropic drugs may be useful in helping mentally retarded individuals control behavior that is disturbing to others. The phenothiazine derivatives are the drugs frequently chosen for this purpose and have proved to be helpful in quieting overactive, boisterous, excited mentally retarded individuals.

Because the occurrence of mental illness is high among mentally retarded individuals the institution must provide some professional workers who are prepared to deal therapeutically with disturbed people. Unfortunately, many psychiatrists question the value of providing psychotherapy for such handicapped individuals. This is because they are sometimes thought to have difficulty relating to others and are limited in their ability to learn from experience. However, it has been demonstrated that selected individuals from the mentally retarded population can profit from having a therapeutic relationship with a helping person. This person may be a psychiatrist, a clinical psychologist, a psychiatric nurse, or a social worker. It is important that the therapeutic sessions be held regularly, that they focus on reality-oriented material, that the length of the session be timed to coincide with the limited attention span of the individual, and that the helping person respect and like the retarded individual. In addition, unless the helping person is highly skilled, supervision should be sought from an experienced psychotherapist.

Group therapy is another way of providing emotional help for mentally retarded individuals. This approach has many of the same advantages for them as for individuals in any group therapy experience. In addition, it provides a peer group with whom the individual can relate and by whom he can feel accepted. Group therapy for the mentally retarded must be more structured than the technique usually employed, more specific limits need to be established, and the focus needs to be placed more on action than on ideas. A nurse with some knowledge of and experience with group therapy can make an important contribution in the field of mental retardation by providing leadership for group therapy sessions for these handicapped individuals.

One successful technique in the treatment of the mentally retarded is called *operant conditioning*. This is a method of motivating the mentally retarded to modify their behavioral patterns in the direction of that which is considered socially desirable.

This technique is based on B.F. Skinner's theories, and it focuses on changing or modifying the individual's response to the environment by reinforcing certain desirable patterns of behavior or eliminating undesirable patterns. This is done by rewarding the individual for demonstrating specific behavioral patterns considered desirable.

In the language of the technique, behavioral patterns may be modified by operant conditioning or by operant extinction. A positive reinforcer is used to reward desirable behavior. Thus something that the retarded individual enjoys or that is meaningful to him is forthcoming when the approved behavior emerges. This reward can be praise, approval, food, or social privileges. Frequently candy has been used successfully as the reinforcer. It is also possible to use what is referred to as a negative reinforcer. A negative reinforcer might be the rewarding of desirable behavior by the removal from the environment of something the individual dislikes. Thus such actions as the extinguishing of a bright light or of a loud, unpleasant noise or the removal of the individual from a very cold or very hot room might be classified as negative reinforcers. The third way of reinforcing desirable behavior according to the operant conditioning technique is by the use of an adverse response to the behavior. Thus the individual would receive disapproval or punishment for the use of behavioral patterns that are not considered to be acceptable or desirable. In most situations punishment as a negative reinforcer has not been successful.

To use the operant conditioning technique successfully, the members of the institutional staff working with the individual whose behavioral patterns are to be the focus of attention must agree on the desirable behavioral pattern they wish to reinforce, the reinforcer to be used, and the way in which it is to be applied. Consistency in the approach is important.

Operant conditioning was chosen as the method of approach to a retarded, adolescent girl who soiled her bedding each night, failed to attend to her personal hygiene and grooming, and offended others because of a body odor. The hospital staff decided to encourage maintaining a dry bed, combing the hair, and bathing. Initially they focused on keeping the bed dry. Thus the girl was rewarded with candy and with praise each morning when she was found to have a dry bed. If it was wet, no comment was made and no candy was provided. At first the bed was dry only occasionally, but after several weeks of rewarding her on the dry days, the bed remained dry most of the time. In like manner, personal grooming and bathing were encouraged and rewarded with praise and candies. After months of consistent work, this young girl was dry every night, was appropriately groomed, and no longer had an offensive odor.

As this example demonstrates, operant conditioning technique can be useful in eliminating undesirable behavior as well as motivating socially acceptable behavior. The use of this technique may provide the answer to the ever-present problem of setting limits for the behavior of the mentally retarded and for helping them to achieve behavior that conforms to socially acceptable standards.

IMPROVING THE EMOTIONAL CLIMATE FOR INDIVIDUALS WITH FAULTY INTELLECTUAL DEVELOPMENT

Mentally retarded individuals as a group are at the mercy of the people who organize and staff the institutions where they spend many years. Many nonprofessional workers are employed to provide the large amount of individualized personal care and supervision required by retarded individuals in every aspect of the activities of daily living. This fact presents the nurse with the opportunity to accept a major role in improving the care of the mentally retarded by teaching and directing the care given by the nonprofessional workers. Through teaching by example, as well as in more formal situations, the nurse can instill positive attitudes among the workers toward their handicapped charges. They can be helped to understand the basic needs of handicapped individuals and develop ways of meeting those needs. The nurse can demonstrate the importance of respecting the mentally retarded and giving them praise and encouragement. To a large extent the nurse is responsible for the emotional climate of the institution.

The nurse's role with mentally retarded individuals also includes giving expert nursing care to those who present challenging nursing care problems and demonstrating nursing care to less skillful workers. In addition, the nurse may develop innovative ways of coping with some of the unique physical and emotional needs of these individuals.

The nurse works closely with the clinical psychologist in developing and carrying out decisions about the use of the techniques involved with operant conditioning. The nurse should accept responsibility for providing counseling sessions for selected individuals. However, because there are so many areas in which the nurse's expert knowledge and guidance are crucial in improving the care of the mentally retarded, it is necessary for her to establish priorities in determining areas in which her services can provide the greatest therapeutic impact on the total situation.

Probably the most significant role the nurse accepts in the care of mentally retarded individuals is that of the mothering person. In this role the nurse becomes the significant helping person in the lives of both the young children and the individuals who have been institutionalized for a longer period of time. Through her consistent presence in the situation and her conviction that mentally retarded individuals are worthwhile human beings, the nurse provides emotional support and security for these deprived individuals. There is probably no situation in which the nurse can play a more significant role in altering the situation positively than in an institution where mentally retarded individuals are cared for.

CONCLUDING STATEMENTS

1. Effective prevention of mental retardation and early treatment of individuals with faulty intellectual development require a multifaceted approach directed toward correcting many inequities in the lives of several million citizens.
2. Mental retardation is a condition in which the individual's intellectual and social development have been partially or completely arrested in the early years of life.
3. The specific cause of mental retardation is unknown in 75% of the individuals who are diagnosed as being handicapped in this way.
4. The known causes of mental retardation include genetically inherited conditions, unfavorable conditions during fetal life,

endocrine disorders, specific metabolic defects, and traumatic factors that may occur after birth.

5. The prevention of mental retardation among children of socially and financially deprived families probably requires an all-out effort by government and social agencies to provide the many conditions necessary for the normal growth and development of children.
6. The diagnosis of mental retardation should be made only after a multifaceted assessment of the individual has been made.
7. Most individuals who are mentally retarded are physically indistinguishable from the rest of the population, but they are severely limited in their ability to cope in a highly complex society.
8. Mentally retarded children are first of all children, with essentially the same needs as other children.
9. Individuals with an IQ rating of less than 25 require complete protective care and usually do not profit by even the most simple educational program.
10. Individuals with IQ ratings of from 25 to 50 are usually able to benefit from habit training and can master simple motor skills.
11. Individuals with IQ ratings of from 50 to 70 are classified as educable and can be taught to perform simple, uncomplicated tasks.
12. A guiding principle in dealing with mentally retarded individuals is to encourage the use of their intellectual abilities at the highest possible level but to avoid pressuring them to achieve at a level that is clearly beyond their capacities.
13. Retarded children have a greater chance of developing their intellectual and social potential if they are nurtured within a family.
14. Parents need support and guidance if a mentally retarded child is to be successfully cared for at home.
15. No matter where the retarded child lives, he needs to be cared for by warm, friendly people who understand his handicap and who will work with him intelligently and helpfully.
16. The aim of the educational programs provided for mentally

retarded children is to equip them to live as independently as possible.

17. Care and treatment for the mentally retarded individual should be based on an evaluation of his assets and capacities and concomitant physical, emotional, and psychological problems.
18. Emotional problems appear frequently among mentally retarded individuals and require psychiatric help.
19. Some of the psychotropic drugs are useful in helping mentally retarded individuals control behavior that may be disturbing to others.
20. Selected mentally retarded individuals can profit from a therapeutic relationship with a helping person.
21. The technique called operant conditioning has greatly improved the treatment of the mentally retarded by reinforcing desirable patterns of behavior or eliminating undesirable patterns.
22. To a large extent the nurse is responsible for the emotional climate of the setting in which she is employed.
23. Probably the most significant role the nurse accepts in caring for mentally retarded individuals is that of the mothering person.

Suggested sources of additional information

CLASSICAL

Barnard, Kathryn: Teaching the retarded child is a family affair, Am. J. Nurs. **68:**305-311, 1968.

Bourgeois, Theodora L.: Reinforcement theory in teaching the mentally retarded: a token economy program, Perspect. Psychiatr. Care **6:**116-126, 136, May-June, 1968.

Buck, Pearl: The child who never grew, New York, 1950, The John Day Co., Inc.

Fackler, Eleanor: The crisis of institutionalizing a retarded child, Am. J. Nurs. **68:**1508-1512, 1968.

Patterson, E. Gene, and Rowland, G. Thomas: Toward a theory of mental retardation nursing—an educational model, Am. J. Nurs. **70:**531-535, 1970.

Skinner, B.F.: Science and behavior, New York, 1965, The Free Press.

Wright, Margaret M.: Care for the mentally retarded; scope of the problem, Am. J. Nurs. **63:**70-74, Sept., 1963.

CONTEMPORARY

Anderson, Camilla M.: Minimal brain damage, Ment. Hyg. **56:**62-66, Spring, 1972.

Barnard, Kathryn E., and Erickson, Marcene L.: Teaching children with developmental problems: a family care approach, ed. 2, St. Louis, 1976, The C.V. Mosby Co.

Bellam, Gwendoline: The nursing challenge of the child with neurological problems, Nurs. Forum **11**:396-418, 1972.

Berni, Rosemarian, and Fordyce, Wilbert: Behavior modification and the nursing process, ed. 2, St. Louis, 1977, The C.V. Mosby Co.

Blackwood, R.O.: Operant control of behavior, Akron, Ohio, 1972, Exordium Press.

Brown, Daniel G.: Behavior modification with children, Ment. Hyg. **56**:22-30, Winter, 1972.

Clayton, Bonnie C., and Vaughn-Cole, Beth: The light switch as a developmental tool, Perspect. Psychiatr. Care **15**:76-77, 1977.

Closurdo, Janette S.: Behavior modification and the nursing process, Perspect. Psychiatr. Care **13**:25-36, Jan.-March, 1975.

Etters, Lloyd E.: Adolescent retardates in a therapy group, Am. J. Nurs. **75**:1174-1175, 1975.

Geiger, Jane, Sindberg, Ronald M., and Barnes, Charles M.: Head hitting in severely retarded children, Am. J. Nurs. **74**:1822-1825, 1974.

Hyde, Naida: Behavior theory and therapy in mental retardation, Am. J. Nurs. **74**:883-886, 1974.

McDonagh, Mary Jo: Is operant conditioning effective in reducing enuresis and encopresis in children? Perspect. Psychiatr. Care **9**:17-23, Jan.-Feb., 1971.

Maxwell, Jane E.: Home care for the retarded child, Nurs. Outlook **19**:112-114, 1971.

Mori, Waltraut: My child has Down's disease, Am. J. Nurs. **73**:1386-1387, 1973.

Pratt, Sandra J., and Fischer, Joel: Behavior modification: changing hyperactive behavior in a children's group, Perspect. Psychiatr. Care **13**:37-42, Jan.-March, 1975.

Roberts, Mary Jo, and Canfield, Marcia: Behavior modification with a mentally retarded child, Am. J. Nurs. **80**:679-680, April, 1980.

OF PARTICULAR INTEREST

Hagarty, J.R.: Psychological assessment of the mentally handicapped, Nurs. Mirror **143**:59, 1977.

The special merits of this article are in the area of assessing strengths and weaknesses of the mentally handicapped individual. The emphasis is on nursing assessment in conjunction with psychological assessment.

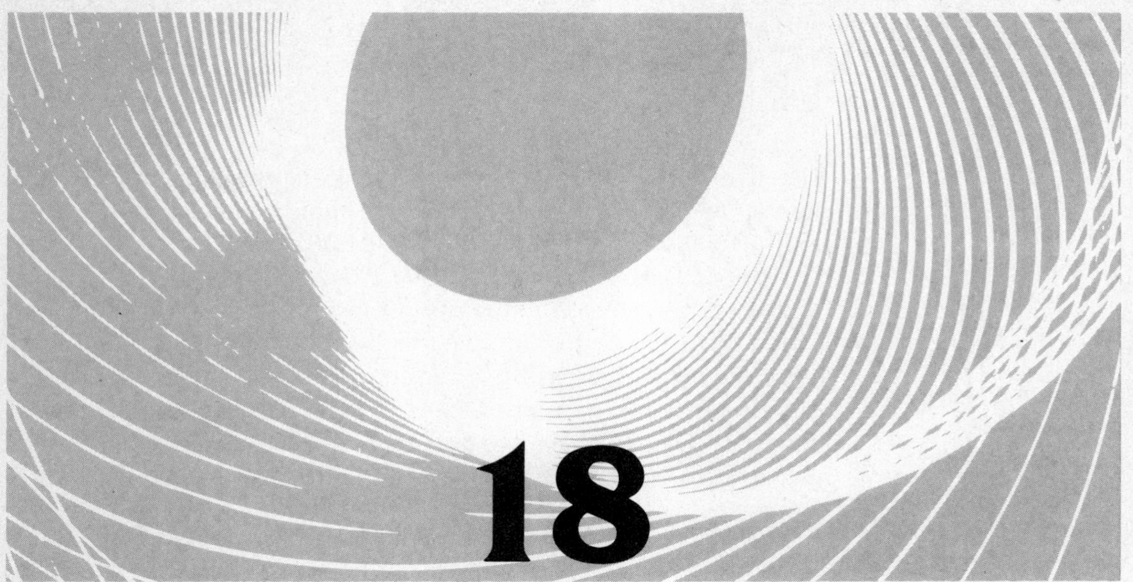

18

Maladaptive behavioral patterns associated with aging

- Life review
- Loneliness
- Loss and grief
- Suspiciousness
- Depression
- Confusion

The size of the U.S. population over 65 is growing rapidly. The number of persons aged 65 years and older increased from 3 million in 1900 to 22 million in 1979. Currently 1 in 7 persons is over 65 years of age, and soon it will be 1 in 5 persons.

Old age is part of the life cycle continuum, not one stage separated from the rest of life. People become more like themselves as they age. In other words, they continue the adaptive responses that they have integrated into their personality in earlier years. However, they still have the potential to learn and grow. Survival with esteem—not mere physical survival—is the goal of the aged person.

The most common type of maladaptive behavioral pattern associated with aging is technically called *senile dementia.* The simple form of this illness is said to result in a gradual and orderly development of the following symptoms:

1. Loss of memory for recent events—the happenings of today are hazy, whereas minute details of events of early life are readily recalled.
2. Increased difficulty in comprehension—important events are no longer significant if they do not touch directly on the life of the individual.
3. Tendency to reminisce—dwelling on the life and achievements of early years occurs, with a desire to recount them frequently.
4. Intolerance of change—an alteration in routine is likely to precipitate tension and irritability.
5. Disorientation—the year is frequently forgotten and then the day of the month, but the day of the week, which more directly dictates the routine of the individual's life, is generally retained.
6. Restlessness—there is a desire to be up and about, to travel from relative to relative, sometimes resulting in the individual's getting lost.
7. Insomnia—there is a tendency to get up in the late hours of the night or early morning and to wander aimlessly about the house.
8. Failure of judgment—an aversion to taking on new respon-

sibilities and a tendency to withdraw into apathy and indifference occur.

To view these symptoms in isolation from the cultural context in which they occur is to artificially separate emotional problems from the stressors that are likely to cause their development. To separate emotional problems from social problems is a mistake with any age group, but to do so with the aged is to completely misunderstand the process of aging in our society.

The aged are beset by the same social problems as the young, but their options for dealing with such problems are more limited. An example is economic inflation where the value of savings and pensions is eroded and where there are very few opportunities for employment even if an older person were physically able to hold a job. In our society the elderly as a group are poor. Certain groups—the American Indian and blacks—have over 75% of their elderly below the poverty level. Poverty not only deprives persons of an opportunity to have their basic needs met, but it also deprives individuals of a powerful social tool in that it takes money to look one's best and to attend many social functions.

Another example of a social phenomenon that has an impact on the elderly is the change from stable, small communities to mobile, large urban centers. This change affects people of all ages and often results in a feeling of powerlessness. Older persons in particular are left without family to help mediate the bureaucracies necessary to survival in an industrialized society. The result often is a sense of alienation and worthlessness.

The accelerating rates of social change, as well as technological change, have subjected human beings to an unprecedented need to make adaptations. The ability of the elderly to make these adaptations is dramatically impeded by a society that puts no value on age. Simple cultures value older persons because it is this group that passes on the legends of the culture. In contrast, in an industrialized society mythology that remains important is written down, printed, and sold. Therefore, in an industrialized society characterized by the nuclear family and printed and electronic communication media, there is no role for the elderly. In a society such as this it is obvious that the achievement of Erikson's psychosocial task of aging—the achievement of ego integrity versus despair and disgust—might be difficult to achieve, especially since the negative views of society toward aging have often been internalized by the elderly themselves.

It is important for all concerned citizens to confront and challenge the events in the culture that support devaluation of the aged. If health care personnel, particularly nurses, are to promote the mental health of the elderly, it becomes imperative for them to understand the interplay between the inevitable characteristics of the aging process and the characteristics of the culture, the combination of which may very well result in the symptomatology associated with senile dementia.

LIFE REVIEW

Life review is the process of thinking about the meaning of one's life. Most authorities believe that life review is a near universal occurrence as older persons face the prospect of impending death. On the one hand, life review facilitates achieving closure to one's life. On the other hand, it leads to personal growth by bringing unresolved crises to consciousness, allowing them to be talked about at length in such a way as to lead to their resolution.

The life review process involves almost obsessive reminiscence—remembering the significant events, people, and places in the past that helped to shape and provide meaning to the individual's life. When an individual is engaged in life review, he finds this to be an all-engrossing task. Small wonder that there is little interest in the events of the present, while the events of the past are recalled and recounted in minute detail.

Since it is likely that all elderly people reminisce whether alone or with another human being, it is vital that the nurse facilitate this process as a means of providing interpersonal feedback. Furthermore, planning for nursing intervention will become more individualized to the needs of the client if the life review process is used both as an aspect of assessment and as a means for intervention. For example, at the very least, the nurse giving care to an elderly person must allow time to actively listen to his reminiscences and provide appropriate feedback.

LONELINESS

More than any other group, aged persons often experience loneliness. Moustakos states the following:

> Elderly citizens in our society are particularly affected by the social and cultural changes and by the separation, urbanization, alienation, and automation in modern living. There is no longer a place for old age, no feeling of organic belonging, no reverence or respect or regard for the wisdom and talent of the ancient. Our elderly citizens so often have feelings of uselessness, so often experience life as utterly futile. Old age is fertile soil for loneliness and the fear of a lonely old age far outweighs the fear of death in the thinking of many people. Loss of friends and death of contemporaries are realities. The mourning and deep sense of loss are inevitable, but the resounding and lasting depression which results and the emptiness and hopelessness are all a measure of the basic loneliness and anxiety of our time.*

To combat the loneliness of the elderly, nurses need to reach out consistently to the older person. Five minutes daily for 5 days is a louder message of concern and caring than is 20 to 30 minutes once in a while. Attempts to involve the older person in a relationship must be persistent. Nurses need to be aware of their own feelings of loneliness that may be triggered by the loneliness they sense in the older person. Younger nurses in late adolescence often experience profound loneliness as they seek their own identity and thus often want to move away from others who are experiencing loneliness. Therefore the withdrawal of the older person may evoke a mutual feeling of withdrawal in the nurse. The nurse must be conscious of her own feelings and aware of her needs when she is tempted to withdraw from the older person.

LOSS AND GRIEF

When a major interpersonal loss occurs, physical changes that the individual had not been previously aware of are often brought to awareness and perceived as losses. This phenomenon, in turn, intensifies the significance of the interpersonal loss. For example, it is not unusual to hear an elderly woman remark, "If my husband had died 10 years ago, I could have managed this house by myself, but now I'm not physically able to keep the place up."

---

*Moustakos, Clark: Loneliness, Englewood Cliffs, N.J., 1961, Prentice-Hall, Inc., p. 26.

The need to grieve for losses may not be seen as necessary by the older person, and grieving may be avoided because of the pain associated with this process. Many aged persons develop physical problems rather than grieving, thereby directing their attention and the attention of others away from the loss and its attendant emotions to the somatic concerns. Consequently, the crisis of the loss is not resolved.

The older person's limited energy level and hesitance to get in touch with pain and resentment allow him to deal with these feelings only in small, manageable doses. The nurse must observe for signs that the older person has had enough for now. The willingness to return again and again to the painful area both by the nurse and by the older person provides for the resolution of the crisis. One 89-year-old man who had experienced a major illness was talking about the loss of his mother when he was 7 years old. He paused and said, "There are losses that everyone expects as they go through life and those you get through. However, there are losses that you feel that, in some way, you caused or that it was your fault, and those are much harder to bear. And the worst losses are those that refresh old wounds—they bring the pain of other losses to the surface. These are very hard losses to bear."

The nurse can be most effective in helping the elderly person resolve his grief about a major interpersonal loss by

1. Assisting the person to accept the pain of the loss by validating that it is appropriate to feel pain with losses.
2. Encouraging the expression of sorrow and sense of loss by commenting on nonverbal communication, such as a shaky voice or teary eyes.
3. Facilitating the expression of hostility by viewing it as a sign of the older person's feeling of vulnerability.
4. Facilitating the expression of guilt. When the person says, "If only I had done . . . ." it is helpful if the nurse restates this comment by saying, "I sense you blame yourself for. . . ." Only if the person is able to acknowledge that he feels guilty can the reality of the situation be explored.
5. Assisting the older person to talk about the person who has died. Asking questions about how they met and the experi-

ences they shared is most facilitative of helping the bereaved person to relive meaningful experiences.

The process of grieving over a major interpersonal loss may take as long as 2 years in the elderly. Signs that the individual is beginning to resolve his grief in a healthy way include indications that he is beginning to see himself as separate from the deceased person. The most common indicator of this differentiation is a movement away from talking about "we" to referring to "I." In addition, the healthy resolution of grief is indicated by behaviors indicating adaptations to an environment that acknowledges the absence of the deceased person. For example, the widow who disposes of her husband's clothing in order to use his closet for storing her sewing materials has made a constructive environmental adaptation that acknowledges the death of her husband. Finally, the person who is successfully resolving his grief over a major loss is able to form new relationships that are mutually satisfying and rewarding.

SUSPICIOUSNESS

Extreme suspiciousness or outright paranoia is frequently encountered in older persons, particularly in those individuals who were not trusting in their earlier years. When this personality structure is compounded by the hearing and sight losses that accompany aging, the person is likely to misinterpret others and his environment and conclude that the world and the people in it are hostile. To be sure, all persons experience instances in which they have been the object of hostility or discrimination, but the suspicious elderly person overgeneralizes these isolated events so that his view of the environment becomes consistent with his preconceived ideas of persecution.

The necessity for change that accompanies relocation sets a fertile stage for the onset of a paranoid reaction in the elderly. The following case illustrates such a situation.

> Mrs. Daniels is a 75-year-old widow who has lived by herself in the inner city apartment she shared with her husband until his death 5 years ago. Mrs. Daniels's daughters who live in the suburbs became increasingly concerned about their mother's safety in the inner city. They prevailed on her to move and finally, after 6 months, were able to convince

her that she would be better off living in a newly constructed apartment complex for senior citizens that was in a better section of the city. Shortly after she moved, Mrs. Daniels began to suspect that people were stealing her belongings. She also began hearing voices that told her they were going to "get her" in retaliation for the way she had behaved when she was a child. Mrs. Daniels told her daughters about these experiences. The community mental health nurse was called in to assess the situation.

Since Mrs. Daniels had no history of unwarranted suspiciousness, the nurse correctly assessed that her paranoia was precipitated by the move. She explained to Mrs. Daniels that she was now living in a new area of the same city, that her apartment was different, the neighborhood was different, and the people were different from those she was used to. The nurse then helped Mrs. Daniels set up her new apartment as nearly like the old one as possible. She put up pictures so that Mrs. Daniels could see them from her chair as she used to. The nurse instructed Mrs. Daniels in how to routinize all her daily activities; for example, she should rise and go to bed at the same times every day and go to the same checkout clerk at the same supermarket at the same time every day. This seemingly rigid routine was established as a quick and efficient means of simultaneously providing structure and helping Mrs. Daniels familiarize herself with her new surroundings. Both structure and familiarity increase an individual's feeling of control, and subsequently feelings of disorientation and suspiciousness are often diminished.

Mrs. Daniels was instructed by the nurse not to tell her daughters or her new friends anything about her fears or her experiences of people stealing from her or talking about her. If she was asked about her problems, she was instructed only to say that she was fearful because of the new place. This intervention was designed to prevent other people from personifying Mrs. Daniels as "crazy" and thereby reinforcing her paranoid behavior by having that expectation of her.

The nurse continued to visit Mrs. Daniels daily for periods that ranged from 15 minutes to 1 hour. By the end of 2 weeks, Mrs. Daniels was no longer overtly suspicious, she did not hear any voices, and she expressed increased pleasure in her new home.

In summary, appropriate nursing intervention goals when working with older persons who are exhibiting unwarranted suspiciousness include reducing the individual's anxiety level by establishing a relationship with him, helping him to restructure his environment to maximize his sense of control, and minimizing his sight and hearing deficit by the use of prosthetic devices or by adapting the environment to better accommodate the sensory loss. Throughout all of these interventions, the consistent presence and availability of the nurse is of inestimable value in helping the aged person give up his feelings of suspiciousness.

DEPRESSION

On the whole, depression goes unrecognized in the older person both by the person and by the health care workers. The physiological symptoms of depression—constipation, slow movements, and insomnia—are usually expected signs of age, so they tend to be ignored. Apathy and lack of interest in the environment are characteristics of depression in the aged but are stereotypically viewed by most persons as characteristic of the aging process itself.

There is a decided increase in the severity and the number of depressions in the aged and a close relationship between physical illness and depression. The aged seem better able to tolerate the loss of a loved one or their prestige rather than their loss of physical health. The nurse who helps older persons maintain and sustain an interest in controlling those factors that keep them healthy, such as diet, helps to prevent depression.

Suicide prevention is an important aspect of nursing care when working with the depressed elderly (see Chapters 13 and 26). The creation of a significant relationship with the aged person is still the greatest deterrent to suicide. Nurses must also be aware that some elderly, physically ill persons are unwilling to see any alternative except death. The fear of the process of dying, experiencing unremitting pain, being alone, and not being in control of their lives are frequently cited factors in the choice of suicide as an alternative. Several life-threatening methods used by older people are refusal of medication, failure to follow prescribed medical regimes, and refusal to eat or drink.

In addition to intervening therapeutically on an individual basis with the elderly depressed person, group activities are often very useful in helping to alleviate depression. While traditional group psychotherapy is rarely appropriate, remotivation groups and other quasi-social, task- oriented groups have been successfully used by nursing personnel in helping the depressed older person.

CONFUSION

Dealing creatively with aged persons who are confused is a challenge for nurses. When confusion is sudden and acute, the assessment process includes determining the cause of the confusion. However, confused persons are in obvious need, and often the nurse must take some action before a thorough assessment is able to be made. In this case, the nurse makes an attempt to orient the confused person by introducing herself and proceeding in the least threatening manner to elicit only the information needed to help with the immediate problem. For instance, the nurse might say, "My name is Miss Jones. You seem afraid of something on the wall, Mrs. Smith. Would you tell me what is frightening you?" During the ongoing assessment process it is important to note when the individual is more confused. Some persons have long periods when they are mentally clear. Oncoming darkness or being alone for long periods may precipitate or intensify confusion in an aged person.

An index of risk for precipitating confusion in elderly persons is the amount and rate of change they have experienced. Living alone after having had a partner for most of a lifetime is a time of high risk for confusion. Sleeplessness, restlessness and agitation, and changes in medications associated with any of these behaviors may precipitate a confused state.

Hospitalization for any reason is also a time of high risk for confusion and therefore an appropriate time for the nurse to begin preventative intervention. While all persons have a need to know what is going to happen to them when they are hospitalized, when aged persons are hospitalized, knowledge and support are critical to the prevention of confusion and to keeping the elderly person accessible to intervention when confusion does occur. Demands placed on elderly persons who are hospitalized should be kept to a minimum. Young technicians need to learn that x-ray films, blood tests, and other tests cannot be hurried because this sets up a situation where the older client feels highly anxious, incompetent, and out of control.

As the older person loses the ability to hear all tones accurately and communication becomes a problem, there is a greater risk of his not perceiving the reality of a given situation. Neurological status should be thoroughly assessed in acute confusion and periodically assessed in chronic confusional states. Of course vital signs, electrolyte balance, and blood urea nitrogen level are baseline assessments for any person who has a sudden onset of confusion. Prevention of confusion and early intervention with individuals who are confused are cardinal principles to follow with elderly persons. Remembering that the elderly person has adaptive responses to shut others out, one should make persistent efforts to maintain contact. If possible, a calm, consistent, persistence over a period of time is the best therapy, although this is not always possible. All staff members should be aware of basic strategies of care. For example, the elderly individual should be approached slowly to avoid startling him. He should be called by name at all times, and the nurse should use her name often. Elderly persons who close their eyes often are not asleep. The nurse needs to get as near as possible to keep good eye contact at the person's level. Touch contact should be initiated carefully and gently, perhaps by taking the individual's hand at first. If he pulls away, attempts to establish touch contact should be made later.

Lighting should be strong without glare, and natural light is preferable to artificial light. Elderly persons should have eyeglasses, hearing aids, and any other needed support appliances readily available. All unnecessary stimuli should be closed out when the nurse is trying to engage the confused elderly person in a conversation. If the person is frightened, someone should stay with him. This is where a member of the family could be very helpful if this person understands what is expected and receives some positive reinforcement.

Basic reality orientation is very helpful and should be part of the therapeutic relationship from the beginning. For instance, the nurse might say, "You are in the hospital for your broken hip, and in a few minutes we're going to help you sit in a chair where you can watch the Mike Douglas Show." It is important to keep the routine in the hospital as near to the home life-style, if this is possible. The more the life-style is changed, the greater the risk of confusion. Medications, especially those for control and sedation, should be used with caution, and systematic monitoring for response to treatment should be frequent.

Whatever the elderly person is able to do alone should be encouraged and help given only to ensure success with the task. Food should be set up so that the older person can see it and smell it. The confused elderly person often needs to be told what the food is. If he is not eating well, high caloric drinks offered frequently help to maintain nutrition. The nurse should encourage the family to help with nutritional problems, since they may know and be able to supply some favorite foods.

Family members may be very helpful if they are taught how to deal with the individual who is confused. The family should be made aware that it is not helpful to withhold information from the aged, confused person. Sometimes family members and staff members think they are sparing the older person's feelings; however, in reality, the person most often knows that something is amiss but does not know how to deal with the mixed communication and becomes *more* confused, often acting bewildered. During acute confusional states, individuals need to know what day it is, where and when the meals are served, where the bathroom is, and what time of day it is—morning, afternoon, or evening.

It is truly a fine thing to see a nurse model creative care of a confused elderly person. Often she must use her whole being to explore the meaning of the behavior of a confused individual and to respond in a way that is helpful and dignified to him. Modeling excellence in terms of caring for aged, confused persons is the best way to teach staff and families.

CONCLUDING STATEMENTS

1. The most common type of maladaptive behavioral pattern associated with aging is technically called senile dementia. However, if health care personnel are to promote the mental health of the elderly, they must understand the interplay between the inevitable characteristics of the aging process and the characteristics of the culture, the combination of which may very well result in the symptomatology associated with senile dementia.
2. Life review is a nearly universal occurrence in older persons as they face the prospect of impending death. Nurses need to facilitate this process as a means of providing interpersonal feedback.
3. More than any other group, aged persons often experience loneliness. Nurses need to be aware of their own feelings of loneliness that may be triggered by the loneliness they sense in the older person.
4. The elderly are subject to an inordinate number of losses to which they adapt in varied ways.
5. The need to grieve for losses may not be seen as necessary by the older person and may be avoided because of the pain associated with this process.
6. The nurse can be most effective in helping the elderly person resolve his grief about a major interpersonal loss by
   a. Assisting the person to accept the pain of the loss by validating that it is appropriate to feel pain with losses.
   b. Encouraging the expression of sorrow and sense of loss by commenting on nonverbal communication, such as a shaky voice or teary eyes.
   c. Facilitating the expression of hostility by viewing it as a sign of the older person's feeling of vulnerability.
   d. Facilitating the expression of guilt.
   e. Assisting the older person to talk about the person who had died.
7. Suspiciousness or outright paranoia is frequently encountered in older persons, particularly in those who were not trusting in their earlier years.

8. Appropriate nursing intervention goals when working with older persons who are exhibiting unwarranted suspiciousness include reducing the individual's level of anxiety, helping him to restructure his environment to maximize his sense of control, and using appropriate measures to minimize his sight and hearing deficits.
9. In addition to the nurse's intervening therapeutically on an individual basis with the elderly depressed person, group activities are also very useful in helping to alleviate depression.
10. An index of risk for precipitating confusion in elderly persons is the amount and rate of change they have experienced.
11. When aged persons are hospitalized, knowledge and support are critical to the prevention of confusion and to keeping the elderly person accessible to intervention when confusion does occur.

Suggested sources of additional information

CLASSICAL

Austin, Catherine L.: The basic six needs of the aging, Nurs. Outlook **7:**138-141, March, 1959.

Bancroft, Anne Vandermay: Now she's a disposition problem, Perspect. Psychiatr. Care **9:**96-102, May-June, 1971.

Browne, Louise J.: Reality therapy for the geriatric psychiatric patient, Perspect. Psychiatr. Care **10:**135-139, July-Sept., 1972.

Burnside, Irene Mortenson: Grief work in the aged patient, Nurs. Forum **8:**416-427, 1969.

Burnside, Irene Mortenson: Group work among the aged, Nurs. Outlook **17:**68-71, June, 1969.

Burnside, Irene Mortenson: Gerontion: a case study, Perspect. Psychiatr. Care **9:**103-109, May-June, 1971.

Burnside, Irene Mortenson: Loneliness in old age, Ment. Hyg. **55:**391-397, 1971.

Burnside, Irene Mortenson: Touching is talking, Am. J. Nurs. **73:**2060-2063, 1973.

Burnside, Irene Mortenson: Listen to the aged, Am. J. Nurs. **75:**1801-1803, 1975.

Goldfarb, Alvin I.: Responsibilities to our aged, Am. J. Nurs. **11:**78-82, Nov., 1964.

Hulicka, Irene M.: Fostering self-respect in aged patients, Am. J. Nurs. **3:**84-89, March, 1964.

Levine, Rhoda L.: Disengagement in the elderly—its causes and effects, Nurs. Outlook **17:**28-30, Oct., 1969.

Mead, Margaret: The right to die, Nurs. Outlook **16:**20-31, Oct., 1968.

Sink, Susan Mary: Remotivation; toward reality for the aged, Nurs. Outlook **14:**26-28, Aug., 1966.

Stone, Virginia: Give the older person time, Am. J. Nurs. **69:**2124-2127, 1969.

Yalom, Irvin D., and Terrazas, Florence: Group therapy for psychotic elderly patients, Am. J. Nurs. **68:**1690-1694, 1968.

CONTEMPORARY

Alfano, Genrose J.: There are no routine patients, Am. J. Nurs. **75:**1804-1807, 1975.

Botwinick, Jack: Aging and behavior; a comprehensive integration of research findings, New York, 1978, Springer Publishing Co., Inc.

Bowe, Frank: Rehabilitating America, New York, 1980, Harper & Row, Publishers.

Bozian, Marguerite W., and Clark, Helen M.: Counteracting sensory change in the elderly, Am. J. Nurs. **80:**473-478, March, 1980.

Brink, T.L.: Is TLC contraindicated for geriatric patients? Perspect. Psychiatr. Care **15:**129-131, 1977.

Bumagin, Victoria E., and Hirn, Kathryn F.: Aging is a family affair, New York, 1980, Lippincott and Crowell.

Burnside, Irene Mortenson: Nursing and the aged, New York, 1976; McGraw-Hill Book Co.

Burnside, Irene Mortenson: Psychosocial nursing care of the aged, ed. 2, New York, 1980, McGraw-Hill Book Co.

Busse, Ewald W., and Pfeiffer, Eris, editors: Mental illness in later life, Washington, D.C., 1973, American Psychiatric Association.

Butler, Robert N., and Lewis, Myrna I.: Aging and mental health: positive psychosocial approaches, ed. 2, St. Louis, 1977, The C.V. Mosby Co.

Callahan, Catherine L.: The 1971 White House Conference on Aging, Nurs. Outlook **20:**96-99, 1972.

Carty, Rita: Patients who cannot hear, Nurs. Forum **11**(3):290-299, 1972.

Chamberlin, Adaline B.: Providing motivation, Am. J. Nurs. **78:**80, Jan., 1978.

Cumming, Elaine, and Henry, W.E.: Growing old: the process of disengagement, New York, 1979, Basic Books, Inc., Publishers.

Diekelmann, Nancy: Emotional tasks of the middle adult, Am. J. Nurs. **75:**997-1001, 1975.

Dodson, Fitzhugh, and Reuben, Paula: How to grandparent, New York, 1980, Lippincott and Crowell.

Dresen, Sheila E.: Staying well while growing old: autonomy; a continuing developmental task, V, Am. J. Nurs. **78:**1344-1346, Aug., 1978.

Dupuis, Pamela H.: Old is beautiful, Nurs. Outlook **18:**25-27, Aug., 1970.

Frenay, Sister Agnes Clare, and Pierce, Gloria L.: The climate of care for a geriatric patient, Am. J. Nurs. **71:**1747-1750, 1971.

Gage, Frances Boland: Suicide in the aged, Am. J. Nurs. **71:**2153-2155, 1971.

Galton, Laurence: The truth about senility—and how to avoid it, New York, 1980, Lippincott and Crowell.

Gresham, Mary L.: The infantilization of the elderly: a developing concept, Nurs. Forum **15:**195-210, 1976.

Hirschfeld, Miriam: Care of the aging holocaust survivor, Am. J. Nurs. **77:**1187-1189, July, 1977.

Kalish, R.A.: Late adulthood: perspectives on human development, Monterey, Calif., 1975, Brooks-Cole Publishing Co.

Limandri, Barbara J., and Boyle, Diana W.: Instilling hope, Am. J. Nurs. **78:**78-79, Jan., 1978.

Lipkin, Gladys B., and Cohen, Roberta G.: Effective approaches to patients' behavior, New York, 1980, Springer Publishing Co., Inc.

McMordie, William R., and Blom, Sharon: Life review therapy: psychotherapy for the elderly, Perspect. Psychiatr. Care **17**:162-166, July-Aug., 1979.

Moritz, Derry A.: Understanding anger, Am. J. Nurs. **78**:81-83, Jan., 1978.

Niland, Maureen: Understanding the elderly, Nurs. Forum **9**:273-289, 1972.

Putnam, P.A.: Orienting the young to the old, Nurs. Outlook **22**:519-521, 1974.

Schwab, Sister Marilyn: Caring for the aged, Am. J. Nurs. **73**:2049-2053, 1973.

Sink, Susan Mary: Remotivation: toward reality for the aged, Nurs. Outlook **14**:26-28, Aug., 1966.

Vladeck, Bruce C.: Unloving care, New York, 1980, Basic Books, Inc., Publishers.

Whitehead, J.A.: Psychiatric disorders in old age; a handbook for the clinical team, New York, 1974, Springer Publishing Co., Inc.

Wilkiemeyer, Diana S.: Affection: key to the care for the elderly, Am. J. Nurs. **72**:2166-2168, 1972.

OF PARTICULAR INTEREST

Busse, E.W., and Pfeiffer, E.: Behavior and adaptation in late life, ed. 2, Boston, 1977, Little, Brown & Co.

Assessing mental functioning of the elderly individual is an important facet of this collection of articles on gerontology.

Butler, Robert N., and Lewis, Myrna I.: Aging and mental health: positive psychosocial approaches, ed. 2, St. Louis, 1977, The C.V. Mosby Co.

This text is an excellent resource for evaluating the biopsychosocial functioning of the elderly individual. It is especially valuable for initial assessment of the individual and for community- and institutionally-based treatment.

SECTION SIX

Therapeutic interventions with individuals whose maladaptive behavioral patterns are associated with physiological alterations

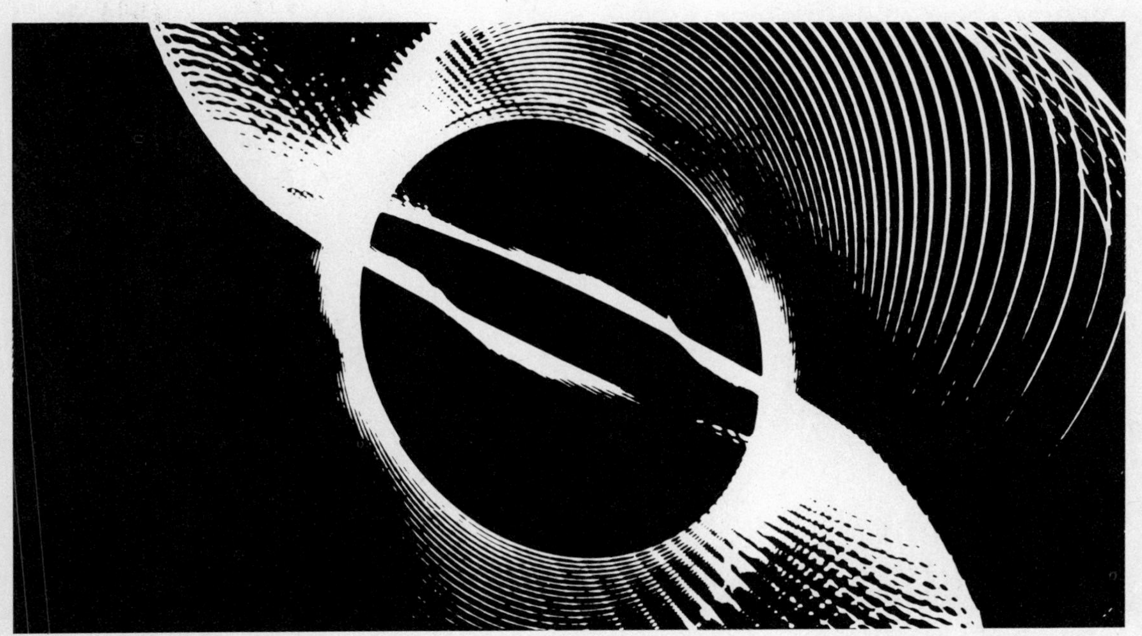

Section Six presents a discussion of those behavioral responses that are associated with physiological alterations, either as etiological agents, as concomitant factors, or as responses to emotional conflict. The inclusion of these topics reflects the belief in the holistic nature of human beings and the professional commitment of nursing to address the emotional, social, and physical needs of all persons.

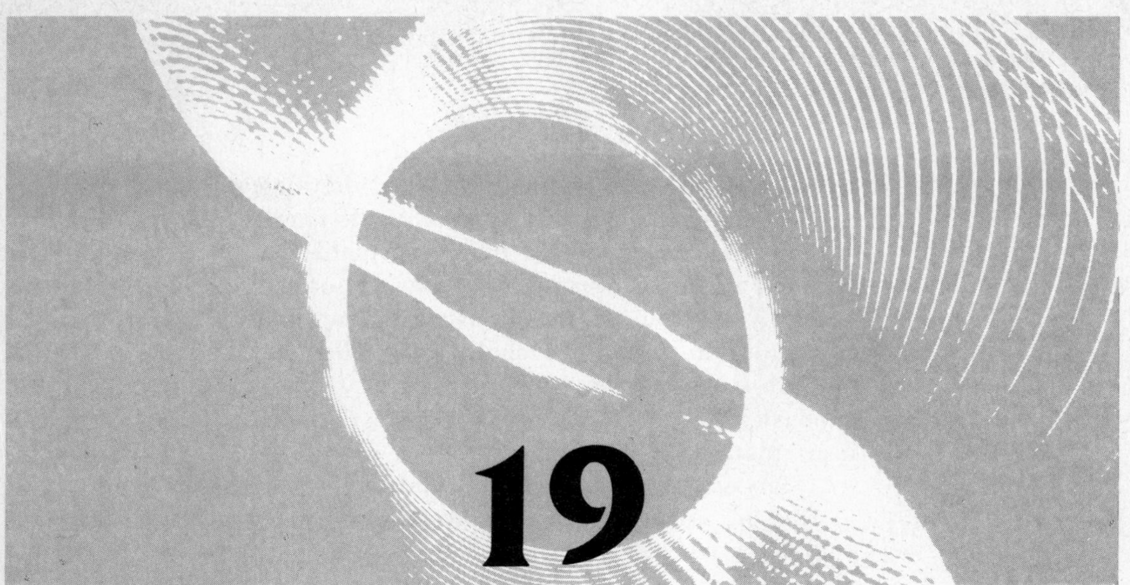

19

Behavioral patterns associated with toxic and organic mental disorders

- Delirium
- Reversible organic mental disorders
- Irreversible organic mental disorders

The human brain is sensitive to a wide range of disorders. Their effect causes the person to respond with varying degrees of behavioral disturbances. As a highly specialized organ, the brain requires an unfailing amount of oxygen and has an elaborate blood supply that cannot be seriously disturbed without creating physical, emotional, and psychological problems. Like other organs of the body, the brain suffers whenever some systemic disease or physical insult disseminates poisons, damages tissues, or impairs circulation.

Physical and behavioral syndromes that result from these stressors are known as *organic mental disorders,* a term implying that the mental alterations exhibited have a physiological cause. In addition to personality changes, organic mental disorders are reflected by alterations in the cognitive functions of perception, orientation, memory, level of consciousness, and verbal, spatial, and numerical ability. Disturbances may involve one or a combination of these functions, and the degree of impairment may vary dramatically. When impairment is in more than one function, the syndrome often appears as a dramatic, florid clinical picture.

Organic mental disorders can best be categorized according to their reversibility. The reversible or acute disorders occur as neurochemical and electrical responses to specific stressors. The symptomatology exhibited by individuals suffering from these disorders is dramatic but recedes in response to immediate treatment or removal of the stressor. Irreversible or chronic disorders result from trauma, chronic infection, or cerebrovascular disruptions that affect the cerebral cortex. The ensuing tissue damage is irreversible, but early diagnosis and treatment can arrest the progression of the disease. Irreversible organic mental disorders can occur at any age, but they are most often seen in the elderly.

Prior to a discussion of reversible and irreversible organic mental disorders, it is necessary to discuss the symptom of delirium, since it can accompany either of these disorders.

DELIRIUM

Delirium is a term that has been used for centuries to describe a wide variety of disorders affecting the functioning of the brain.

The term has now come to be accepted as descriptive of a set of symptoms and not as a separate diagnostic entity. Delirium can occur in both reversible and irreversible organic mental disorders and is characterized by dysmnesia and attention disturbances that in turn lead to disorientation and emotional disturbances. Neurological findings include headache; dysarthria; electroencephalogram (EEG) abnormalities characterized by slow waves; coarse, irregular tremors; and sudden nonrhythmic, nonpatterned, gross muscle contractions in a resting posture.

The delirium may be mild or severe. It implies some degree of clouding of consciousness. In the severe forms there are vivid visual hallucinations. The delirious individual may see terrifying images of animals, human faces, dancing objects, or merely flashes of light. There may also be illusions and hallucinations of touch, as if insects were crawling over the body and the environment. These are perceived as *real* to the individual and are therefore extremely frightening to him.

The nurse should remember that delirium may be of fleeting occurrence. It may last but a few minutes and be followed by a lucid period and frequently may be manifested by merely a frightened look or a muttering of a few unintelligible words.

The symptoms of delirium vary greatly among individuals and show marked fluctuation even within a given situation. The individual's mood may be depressed and apathetic or excited and agitated. The most characteristic affective state is that of bewilderment and fear. Thinking is greatly disorganized and disconnected. The characteristic irritability is exaggerated by darkness, which makes accommodation to reality especially difficult. Irrespective of the specific clinical picture, many delirious persons lapse into "terminal sleep" lasting from 12 to 24 hours after which their recall of the episode is foggy or entirely obliterated.

Suggestions concerning nursing care for delirious individuals

Irrespective of the cause, the delirious individual is critically ill and requires constant and understanding care. His fluid and electrolyte balance must be maintained, and his condition should be closely monitored for dehydration and fluid intoxication.

Feeding should begin with high-calorie fluids, and as rapidly as the person can tolerate them, semisolid and solid foods should be added. Water in ample quantities should be given at frequent intervals, particularly if the fever is constant and dehydration is present. A cool sponge bath in bed may induce sleep. The skin is usually dry and hot and should be closely watched for abrasions and pressure spots. Cold cream applied to the lips prevents fissuring. The mouth and tongue should be cleansed several times a day. The individual should be protected from complications such as secondary infection, cardiac dysfunction, and hyperthermia.

Attempts should be made to control the client's anxiety and agitation by structuring the environment. Reality orientation may be facilitated by use of bright night lights, calendars, and familiar objects. Excessive stimulation should be avoided. A physician may order medication to assist the client in reducing his anxiety and agitation. Phenothiazine derivatives may be useful in all delirium states except those resulting from the seizure disorders or withdrawal from central nervous system depressants. Phenothiazine derivatives are contraindicated in these instances because they lower the seizure threshold.

The delirious individual should be secluded in a quiet room, and visitors should be limited to one or two members of the family or very close friends. Restraint should be avoided. Instead, this individual should receive constant supervision to avoid injury to himself or others.

Insofar as possible, all procedures and treatment should be carried out at one time. It is important to keep in mind that the person should be subjected to a minimum amount of stimulation and that rest is a most essential part of the care of an individual who is in a toxic condition, restless, and delirious.

Various etiological factors may result in delirium. These include a febrile state, impaired capillary function, exhaustion, vitamin imbalance, toxicity, interference in the reticular-activating system, and factors related to the individual's age, overall health state, and general constitution. In any case, it is essential that the stressor be identified so that immediate specific treatment can be instituted.

Recovery from any systemic condition that causes delirium is necessarily slow. Relapses into a confusional state are not uncommon. Except for some simple forms of occupational therapy, exercise and mental concentration are contraindicated for several weeks after the acute illness.

Following is a discussion of two commonly seen causes of delirium.

Delirium associated with acute infectious diseases

Very young children, chronic alcoholics, and elderly people develop delirium very quickly if an infection is severe and the fever is very high. Delirium is more likely to occur at night. If an individual with a high fever becomes restless, tires easily, and seems to have difficulty in grasping simple statements, one should be on guard and suspect an impending delirious state. The delirious individual wanders in speech content, seems dreamy, dazed, and apprehensive, may fumble with the bedclothes, and generally looks about in a bewildered manner. He may not clearly recognize persons, or he may look at his visitors with apparently unseeing eyes. If the delirium deepens into stupor or coma, the condition is undeniably grave.

Occasionally the delirium resulting from an acute infection may include agitation and sudden irritability. The individual may even climb out of bed and walk about in a confused manner.

Treatment. It is obvious that the treatment of delirium is essentially the treatment of the etiological factor. Bed rest and seclusion from external stimulation are essential. Delirium in the presence of very high fever may be controlled by giving sodium salicylate or aspirin. This will usually bring the temperature down. Because delirium may be an expression of vitamin deficiency, the administration of 10 to 50 mg of vitamin B_1 daily may be effective in eliminating the symptoms of delirium.

Delirium tremens

Delirium tremens is an acute reaction to the withdrawal from a heavy and consistent intake of alcohol for a period of several weeks without an adequate intake of food. In an individual who has been a chronic alcoholic for several years, delirium tremens may be precipitated by a head injury or a surgical procedure without the individual's having taken alcohol at the time of its appearance. Delirium tremens consists of confusion, excitement, and delirium. It is usually of relatively short duration and does not cause a profound and permanent change in the personality.

The delirium is preceded by loss of appetite, restlessness, and insomnia. Slight noises cause the patient to jerk with fear, and moving objects lead to great excitement and agitation. Gradually, consciousness becomes clouded, friends are no longer recognized, and designs in the wallpaper appear as insects or crawling animals. The person becomes terrified. Imaginary threads are picked off the bedclothing, and nonexisting insects are felt and seen on the skin. There is a ceaseless fumbling and picking movement of the fingers and hands. The face has an anxious or terrified expression, and the eyes are bloodshot. The skin is moist with perspiration; the tongue and lips are tremorous. The pulse is rapid and weak, and there is always some elevation of temperature.

The death rate in delirium tremens is high: 10% to 15% of these persons die. Heart failure and bronchopneumonia are the most frequent causes of death. Autopsy reveals an edematous brain.

CASE FORMULATION □ AN INDIVIDUAL WITH DELIRIUM TREMENS

The following history furnishes an example of how such a problem can develop.

> Mark M., aged 29 years, was admitted to the hospital from a boardinghouse where he was found suffering from delirium tremens. He was unmarried, worked intermittently as a dock laborer, and shared his room with a fellow worker with whom he often drank at a nearby saloon. He had been drinking excessively for 3 weeks. The day before admission he was excitable and quarrelsome and accused his roommate of throwing sand down his neck. During the night he mumbled to himself, rolled about, and fell out of bed. He claimed a dozen dogs were looking in at the window. Toward morning he was stuporous, shaky, and incoherent.
>
> On admission he was put to bed. He wore a terrified expression on his face. Constant supervision was necessary. He picked incessantly at the bedclothes. He was able to mumble his name, but little more. During short lucid moments he said he had been drinking too much and asked for another "shot." He insisted that he saw leering faces on the

walls and that there was a leopard under the bed. He was dehydrated and feverish; his eyes were bloodshot; and his gaze shifted constantly from one corner of the room to another.

Twelve days after admission his sensorium cleared. He was able to give a clear account of his past but remembered nothing of the first 10 days of his hospital experience. In fact, he was greatly puzzled to find himself in a hospital bed and inquired into the identity of the institution.

REVERSIBLE ORGANIC MENTAL DISORDERS

Reversible organic mental disorders are severe illnesses. However, their effects can be reversed if prompt specific treatment is instituted. Another major factor in determining the reversibility of these disorders is the individual's general state of health. The following are common stressors leading to reversible organic mental disorders.

Transient cerebrovascular impairment is often implicated in the development of reversible mental disorders, especially in the elderly. Cerebrovascular impairment includes ischemic attacks, cerebrovascular accidents, and multiple small infarcts in the circulatory system of the brain. The latter are of a relatively mild nature with little lasting effect.

Common endocrine imbalances that may lead to reversible organic mental disorders include hypothyroidism and hyperthyroidism, hypopituitarism, adrenal disease, and hypoglycemia. These endocrine disorders are usually readily amenable to medical intervention.

Infectious processes such as epidemic encephalitis may lead to a reversible organic mental disorder, although it is not unusual for this disorder to become irreversible. Psychoses with epidemic encephalitis are probably caused by a virus infection of the brain. In the acute phase the individual is delirious and feverish and often complains of diplopia. These symptoms are usually followed by a long period of lethargy that may last for several days and in rare instances for several months. In adults the symptoms that usually become progressively more severe include gradual spasticity of the limbs, constant tremor of the hands, a masklike expression, and drooling of saliva. This condition is called *Parkin-*

son's syndrome. The mental disturbances are usually secondary to the individual's muscular rigidity and general physical helplessness. Irritability, moroseness, frequent bodily complaints, and insomnia are the most common features. True mental deterioration rarely occurs except in very advanced cases.

There are a number of medications available that help to control the symptoms of stiffness, fatigue, and drooling. Sedatives are helpful for irritability and insomnia. The nursing care of the person with the chronic form of encephalitis requires patience, understanding, and thoughtful guidance. Mild exercise should be alternated with long periods of bed rest. The individual should be encouraged to feed himself, even though the procedure requires an extra amount of time. The food should be solid, because the patient has difficulty in swallowing soups or semisoft material. Because of constant tremor, the person suffering from Parkinson's syndrome should not be hurried, and much patience is essential on the part of the nurse when she assists him. Occupational therapy is recommended when the tremor is mild and the medical treatment provides muscular relaxation.

Internal toxins, such as elevated urea nitrogen in the blood, and external toxins, such as drugs and alcohol, are often offending agents that can lead to reversible organic mental disorders.

Finally, accidental or surgical trauma of the brain and brain lesions is a common cause of organic mental disorders that may be reversible. The degree of impairment experienced by the individual with a brain tissue injury or lesion is determined by the amount of tissue damage and the location of the injury or lesion. Early diagnosis and treatment of many brain injuries and lesions can prevent lasting damage.

Individuals suffering from reversible organic mental disorders are characteristically disoriented, perhaps in all three spheres of time, place, and person. Thought disorganization leads to poor judgment and decreased decision-making ability. Misinterpretation of reality is common, since the individual commonly experiences illusions and hallucinations. These may also precipitate violent or assaultive behavior. The individual's mood state is highly labile, and his behavior may be socially inappropriate, such as playing with food, undressing, and making sexually provocative movements toward another person.

The death rate of persons suffering from reversible organic mental disorders is approximately 10%, if not treated early. Some of those who survive may develop an irreversible mental disorder.

IRREVERSIBLE ORGANIC MENTAL DISORDERS

Irreversible organic mental disorders may begin with a severe, acute illness. In other instances the onset of the impairment is insidious. In either event, the effects are irreversible, although progression can sometimes be delayed with treatment.

Physiological stressors that may lead to brain cell deterioration and thus to symptoms of irreversible organic mental disorders include toxins, such as those that result from chronic liver or kidney disease; severe and prolonged vitamin B deficiency, as characteristically seen in alcoholism; infection, as seen in syphilis; inadequate oxygenation of the brain, as seen in cerebral arteriosclerosis; and direct brain cell damage or deterioration due to trauma, hereditary factors, or idiopathic causes. Seizure disorders may also lead to an irreversible brain cell deterioration, although the mechanisms by which this occurs are not clearly understood.

The individual suffering from an irreversible organic mental disorder characteristically becomes disoriented in all three spheres in the order of time, place, and then person. The fluctuations in the individual's mental acuity often become a source of embarrassment to him during periods of mental clarity. The memory loss is especially noted regarding immediate and recent memory, while remote memory may be intact. This memory deficit results in frequent misidentification of people in the immediate environment. The memory loss also may result in confabulation, which should not be mistaken for intentional deceit. The individual's mood is labile and impulsive, resulting in socially inappropriate behavior. This may be seen as the individual's attempt to reach out for assistance and identity confirmation. Restlessness and agitation are especially severe during the evening hours, a phenomenon called "sundown syndrome." This may be a result of the decreased daylight, leading to increased disorientation and fear. The individual resists change and coercion, and therefore the establishment of a routine that is effective in accommodating the necessary activities of daily living is often helpful.

Following is a discussion of the most commonly encountered irreversible organic mental disorders.

Behavioral disorders associated with chronic alcoholism

Korsakoff's psychosis. In some respects, Korsakoff's psychosis, a form of alcoholism first described by Sergei S. Korsakoff in 1887, is an acute alcoholic reaction. It is regarded as evidence of brain damage because it results in a certain degree of personality change and blunting of intellectual capacity. In this condition the individual may appear to be delirious, but more accurately the picture is one of memory defect concealed by falsification. The person has a memory gap for recent events and fills in these gaps with confabulations. In addition, there is peripheral neuritis with tingling of the extremities, and in severe cases there may be wristdrop and footdrop.

Characteristically, there are pronounced changes in the brain cells, as well as degenerative disease of the peripheral nerves. All these disturbances result from a prolonged deficiency of vitamin B, particularly niacin. Treatment with thiamine, niacin, brewer's yeast, and a vitamin-rich diet of milk, fruit, and meat may restore the individual to nearly normal physical and mental health.

Alcoholic deterioration. Alcoholic deterioration is the end result of prolonged and excessive drinking and is essentially a chronic disorder. The onset is gradual, and a personality change, which becomes evident earlier to the family than it does to friends or co-workers, occurs slowly. The individual lacks perseverance, becomes maudlin, and is careless in regard to grooming. He will not tolerate any criticism of his drinking and becomes touchy and irritable. He uses rationalization to explain his drinking. His capacity for work suffers greatly, and he not only neglects his family but also becomes dependent on them for support. Chronic alcoholic degeneration represents one of the most common and serious social tragedies that affect family life. Its influence may extend to many innocent individuals, particularly children, on whom it may leave a deep psychological impression.

General paresis or meningoencephalitic syphilis

General paresis, or meningoencephalitis of syphilitic origin, is caused by a progressive syphilitic infiltration of the brain tissue that results in a degeneration of nerve elements and produces typical neurological and mental disturbances. Since the use of penicillin in the treatment of early syphilis, paresis has become relatively uncommon.

General paresis, or tertiary syphilis, develops within 2 to 20 years after the first stage of the syphilitic infection. It is much more frequent in men. Before adequate treatment was developed, about 10% of all admissions to mental hospitals carried the diagnosis of general paresis.

The early signs of this disease are so insidious in appearance that they may be unrecognized even by intimate friends until an acute episode of some kind occurs. This may be a seizure, or the full-blown symptoms may appear only after an injury to the head. Gradual changes in personality are the principal features of the very early phase. The individual becomes forgetful in keeping appointments, is careless of his grooming, and shows a general deterioration of his ability to perform in socially approved ways. Judgment becomes poor, and there is a tendency to evade important issues and to show a smug indifference or apathy to critical problems. General loss of mental acuity is covered by shallow rationalizations, by outbursts of irritability, and by moods of depression or elation.

In the complete mental picture of a person suffering from general paresis, a feeling of grandeur is frequently the most outstanding symptom. Delusions of wealth or power and euphoric ideas about the future may be freely expressed. The basic personality of the individual influences his reaction to meningoencephalitic syphilis, and some may be depressed rather than elated. Memory defects are prominent, and irritability is easily evoked when attempts are made to control the expansive ideas. The mood is unstable, and the person laughs and cries easily.

The physical signs are equally typical. The pupils are irregular. There is marked tremor of the lips and tongue. The speech is seriously affected—words are slurred, syllables or even words are omitted, and certain phrases are incomprehensible. Writing is likewise affected. Tendon reflexes are usually overactive. Incontinence of urine and absence of the tendon reflexes generally indicate that the syphilitic process has involved the spinal cord. This form of the disease is called *taboparesis*.

Laboratory tests are most valuable in confirming the diagnosis. Unless the person with general paresis is radically treated with large doses of penicillin, the outcome is a progressive degeneration of mind and body. Death usually occurs within 6 to 8 years after the mental symptoms appear. These individuals have little resistance to infection. Although late syphilis has almost disappeared, it is feared that it will reappear because of the significant increase in early syphilis and a recent trend not to seek treatment because it is so readily available.

Behavioral disorders associated with cerebral arteriosclerosis

Many individuals between the ages of 50 and 65 years suffer from a circulatory disturbance called arteriosclerosis, which is characterized by a narrowing or an obliteration of the lumen of the blood vessels that provide the brain with nutrition and oxygen. In like manner, the heart and kidneys may also be deprived of an adequate flow of blood. When the blood vessels are thrombosed by an accumulation of patches or plaques of fatty and calcified material, the resulting impairment of cerebral function is technically called *atherosclerosis* but is more commonly known as *arteriosclerosis*.

Although arteriosclerosis is not necessarily related to the aging process, it seems to be affected by that process. Thus there has been a tremendous increase in the numbers of individuals who have developed this condition during the last 50 years, since the life span of the general population has been increasing.

Arteriosclerosis may begin rather insidiously with fatigue, headache, dizziness, loss of the ability to concentrate, and diminution of physical and mental acuity. Sometimes the individual appears to be undergoing a personality change, and previous negative personality traits seem to become more prominent. Episodes of confusion or excitement may be an early symptom. During such episodes the individual is likely to be restless and incoherent and may be confused. Emotional outbursts of crying or laughing are common, and the individual may become irritable, quarrelsome, jealous, or suspicious. The memory is usually impaired, but this varies with individuals. At night the individual is likely to become anxious, fearful, bewildered, and sometimes difficult to control. Suppressed hostile attitudes may be released.

As time progresses, the arteriosclerotic individual begins to neglect his personal hygiene and his appearance. His judgment becomes defective. The content of his thinking is a reflection and exaggeration of his former rationalizations and personality defenses.

The person with arteriosclerotic changes is aware of the early stages of his deterioration and is distressed by the decline in his physical and mental capacity. He may become anxious, depressed, and hopeless.

The cardiac and renal complications as well as the cerebrovascular disturbances resulting from an inadequate blood supply contribute to the physical problems and the death of individuals suffering from arteriosclerosis.

Unfortunately, there is little definitive information about the cause and prevention of cerebral arteriosclerosis. The treatment involves a carefully regulated life, which includes an occupational activity that is pleasant without being too demanding, and an appropriate drug to assist in reducing restlessness, confusion, insomnia, excitement, and aggressive behavior. Some medical authorities discourage the use of the barbiturates, which tend to increase confusion. They instead recommend chlorpromazine in carefully controlled amounts.

Providing nursing care for individuals suffering from a psychosis due to cerebral arteriosclerosis. There is nothing that can be done to reverse an advanced arteriosclerotic process. However, some drugs are now available that dilate the walls of the cerebral blood vessels and may assist such individuals to think more clearly. Some physicians believe that small amounts of alcohol serve to improve the circulation, and they order it for individuals once a day. Nicotinic acid given regularly may also be of some assistance in improving cerebral functioning.

Sedative drugs should be avoided, although some of the antianxiety drugs such as diazepam may be helpful in enabling the individual to sleep through the night.

Such individuals require a quiet environment in which they can feel safe and secure. Nurses who work with such people should enjoy caring for them. Nurses need to be content to establish limited goals that include helping these individuals to be as comfortable and happy as possible. Adequate nutrition must be maintained, as well as physical cleanliness and grooming.

Some of these individuals will participate in and enjoy simple, repetitive occupational therapy activities. They may enter into recreational activities that are appropriate from the standpoint of their physical limitation.

CASE FORMULATION □ AN INDIVIDUAL WITH AN ORGANIC MENTAL DISORDER

Mrs. Steffan, a 77-year-old widow, was the mother of one middle-aged daughter, Ruth, who was a professional woman and away from home a great deal. Mrs. Steffan was attractive, petite, and socially charming. She accompanied Ruth to social affairs and smiled and laughed at the proper times, although she did not attempt to carry on a conversation with anyone. It was not until after Mrs. Steffan's devoted husband of 55 years died suddenly that Ruth realized how dependent her mother had been on him and how serious her mental problems were. It became clear that he had supervised her constantly, including standing by her side when she cooked and directing her every action. After he died, Mrs. Steffan no longer had dinner ready when Ruth returned home at night. If she attempted to prepare a meal, she failed to turn off the gas when the food was cooked, and thus the meal was ruined. She could not read a recipe, collect the necessary ingredients, or follow the directions.

Without her husband to supervise her, Mrs. Steffan often wandered out of the house and down the street. She could not find her way back to her home, and when Ruth returned from work, she had to search for her mother, sometimes for several hours. It soon became clear that Mrs. Steffan could not stay alone, so her daughter began staffing the home with friends, relatives, and employed helpers. If someone was not able to arrive at the home early in the morning to relieve her by taking over

Mrs. Steffan's supervision, Ruth could not leave and was late for work. Likewise, she had to be home by 5 PM in the evening to relieve the afternoon caretaker. This schedule jeopardized Ruth's functioning on the job and curtailed her social life drastically.

Mrs. Steffan had many irrational fears. Because of fear of fire, she insisted on unplugging every electrical appliance in the house and on placing every newspaper and magazine in the bathtub before she retired. She insisted on sleeping with Ruth because she feared that someone would enter the house at night and injure her.

Probably the most upsetting behavior was that of putting Ruth's pocketbook away in places where it could not be located for several days. On one occasion she placed it in the large freezer in the basement, which was opened infrequently. At another time she placed it in an old suitcase that had not been used for years.

Although Mrs. Steffan was noted for her pleasing personality, she began to express irritation at some of the necessary restrictions that Ruth and the several other individuals who assisted in her care had found it necessary to impose. She began to throw food onto the floor if she disliked what was served to her. She watched for chances to slip out of the house and go shopping alone, although she became lost as soon as she reached the corner of the next street. She became quite skillful at eluding the individual who was staying with her. Sometimes it was necessary to ask the police for help in locating her.

Mrs. Steffan developed a strong dislike for a neighbor who stayed with her frequently. She was sarcastic with this woman and refused to cooperate with her in any way, although she had once enjoyed staying with her. Mrs. Steffan began to ask for her daughter and refused to believe that Ruth was her daughter. She said, "My daughter is a little girl with long blonde curls and you are keeping her from me." As the months passed, Mrs. Steffan began pleading to go home, saying that the house in which she and Ruth lived was not her home, although she had occupied it since she was a bride.

Mrs. Steffan had once been meticulous about her personal cleanliness. For years she had insisted on having her hair and nails done professionally and applying makeup each day. Suddenly she began to refuse to bathe or to allow anyone to help her bathe. She no longer kept her hair combed and resisted attempts from others to arrange it. As time progressed, she became more garrulous and talked continuously, although her thoughts were bizarre and were not related to current happenings. Her irritability increased, and she often had what some people described as temper tantrums. She began getting up at night and wandering about the house. This disturbed Ruth's sleep and was dangerous because she was unsteady on her feet and often complained of dizziness. Her restlessness at night was the behavior that finally made Ruth decide that she could no longer care for her mother adequately at home.

She searched for, and finally found, an appropriate nursing home where the care was acceptable and the expense was within her means. Mrs. Steffan did not object to being taken to the nursing home and appeared to accept the workers there as well as she had those who cared for her at home.

Discussion of the case formulation

Mrs. Steffan was suffering from a psychosis due to cerebral arteriosclerosis. In her situation the blood flow to the brain was diminished due to the constriction of the lumen of the cortical vessels by fatty deposits in the vessel walls. Thus functioning capacity of the cortical cells in the brain was diminished. As the arteriosclerotic condition progressed, Mrs. Steffan's ability to function mentally became increasingly impaired. Because Mrs. Steffan was an elderly woman, her physical ability also deteriorated at the same time.

Even though a psychosis due to cerebral arteriosclerosis is essentially a physical problem, the individual's premorbid personality has a profound effect on the behavior that is exhibited. Undoubtedly, Mrs. Steffan had suffered advanced cerebral arteriosclerosis before her husband died. However, his loss was a severe emotional blow to this woman who had undoubtedly been extremely dependent on him during their lifetime together. Her irrational fears, her prolonged interest in her appearance, and her need to cling to her daughter suggest that she was always a somewhat dependent, self-centered person who had never developed the ability to cope with life independently.

Traumatic mental disorder

Traumatic mental disorder implies that the individual has received a definite brain injury, which has resulted in either brain contusion, laceration, or compression or damage to the cerebral blood vessels. The impact to the head has been sufficiently severe to produce varying degrees of surgical and traumatic shock. The brain responds to injury as does any large visceral organ such as the stomach, intestines, or liver. Hence the person is not only rendered unconscious but also becomes very pale and cyanotic and has shallow, irregular respiration and a feeble, rapid pulse. The pupils are usually widely dilated, different in size, and respond poorly to light. Vomiting of a projectile type may occur within a short time after the injury.

Bleeding from a large vessel, particularly an artery, causes a rapid rise in intracranial pressure. The spinal fluid may be grossly bloody.

Individuals with severe brain laceration or slow bleeding within the cranial cavity may often appear to be normally conscious and alert. However, this may not be a clear consciousness but a condition called *automatism*. In this state the person appears to be answering questions correctly and coherently, but on closer inquiry it will be discovered that he is not aware of having been injured, his insight is poor, and he gives a falsified or garbled account of the accident. He may also be abnormally elated or facetious. After recovery is complete, he will recall none of this immediately posttraumatic experience.

When the individual does recover from the immediate effects of the trauma, he not only fails to recall the events that followed the time of the injury but also fails to remember events and experiences that occurred several hours or days before the time of the accident. This is called *retrograde amnesia*. Some authorities regard this symptom as a better criterion of brain damage than the duration of the period of unconsciousness.

Posttraumatic deterioration or encephalopathy. Even after apparently complete recovery from severe brain injury, gradual degeneration of brain cells and overgrowth of glial tissue may develop over a period of several years, and the individual may deteriorate mentally.

Encephalographic changes that confirm the clinical signs of chronic intellectual deterioration can be detected. The brain rhythm is irregular, with slow brain wave activity.

Seizures may appear in the person with a traumatized brain as late as 5 years after the injury. Marked personality changes display themselves through a greatly altered personality, emotional instability, and outbursts of rage that are contrasted against a general mood of indifference. Memory defects can be demonstrated, as well as inability to focus attention on productive work.

In addition to seizures, the person suffering from posttraumatic brain deterioration may also be subject to recurring attacks of automatism. The individual may have "wandering states" or may have explosive outbursts of violent and homicidal behavior that are not recalled when normal conduct is resumed.

Treatment and nursing care. The treatment and nursing care of the individual with psychosis or "personality change" following severe brain damage is largely a matter of sensible, understanding management. It is better that such individuals occupy quiet quarters. Emotional demonstrations of any sort should be avoided as much as possible. Simple forms of occupation that make little demand for sustained physical or mental effort do much to keep the individual contented and free of wide mood swings.

Huntington's chorea

Huntington's chorea is a hereditary disease involving the brain. It was first described by an American physician in 1872. The symptoms usually develop in the middle years of life, with twitching of the face and purposeless movements of the trunk and limbs. In severe cases these movements become so pronounced and constant that the individual can no longer feed or dress himself. There is frequently evidence of slow intellectual deterioration and personality changes expressed by irritability and outbursts of temper. Occasionally the individual expresses ideas of reference and delusions of persecution. Attempts at suicide are common because individuals become aware of the hopelessness of their condition. There is no specific treatment for this disease.

Seizure disorders

The term *epilepsy* is to be avoided because it suggests a stigma that is unwarranted. The most common feature of all seizure disorders is a lapse of consciousness of varying duration that is accompanied by changes in motor, sensory, and visceral functions. In brief, seizures are disturbances in the electrophysiology of the brain, and the symptoms depend on which areas of the brain are producing abnormal electrical discharges. A vast amount of new knowledge has been gained through study of the brain with the EEG.

The *grand mal seizure,* perhaps the most common type, and certainly the most disturbing, is a generalized discharge from all parts of the brain that causes a sudden and complete cessation of consciousness associated with alternating extension (tonus) and flexion (clonus) of all four limbs, respiratory arrest with cyanosis, biting of the tongue, foaming at the mouth, and occasionally incontinence. After each seizure there is usually a short period of mental clouding and agitation. When such seizures appear in rapid succession, the condition is known as *status epilepticus.* In grand mal seizures the EEG tracings show diffuse, symmetrical, slow brain wave activity.

Since seizures are a symptom, the grand mal seizure may be caused by brain injury, tumors, toxins, or infections, but by far the greatest number of these generalized attacks have an unknown cause. They may first occur in early infancy but more often appear in puberty and endure throughout adult life.

The *petit mal seizure* and its variants consist of momentary lapses of consciousness marked by a staring or blank expression with some deviation of gaze in an upward direction. These spells sometimes appear in early childhood as often as 100 times a day but may be so fleeting as to escape the attention of parents and teachers for several years. They may disappear in early adult life. The EEG usually shows a striking three-per-second spike and dome configuration.

Perhaps the most interesting seizures from the psychiatric standpoint are the so-called *psychomotor attacks,* because individuals suffering from this type of disorder exhibit a wide variety of psychic phenomena. In EEG studies the abnormality is a random spike that appears to be in one or both temporal lobes. The most common lesion is a small area of degeneration believed to be caused by birth injury. The warning sign (or aura) is often a peculiar sensation ascending from the gastric area associated with an intense feeling of fear, or it may be a familiar and unpleasant odor or taste. There is rarely a complete loss of consciousness; instead the individual seems to be reacting to some situations in his past in what seems to be a bizarre manner and performs inappropriate acts such as undressing in public. These acts are known as automatisms. Occasionally during an attack the individual reacts with smacking of the lips, lip licking, chewing, gulping, and excessive salivation. The function of memory is also involved, and in one type the individual undergoes strangely familiar experiences or dream states referred to as *déjà vu*. When consciousness is restored, the individual does not recall the content of his dreams except to state that they were familiar.

Jacksonian seizures are caused by specific focal lesions in the cerebral cortex. They are partial seizures involving only one side of the body, beginning in one hand, arm, or leg.

Treatment. Treatment for seizure disorders is possible through the use of a large number of anticonvulsant drugs. However, each person responds differently, and treatment must be highly individualized. Some of the side actions of these drugs may be health hazards, such as depression of bone marrow function, ataxia, and mental stupor.

Most effective, particularly in grand mal and psychomotor attacks, are phenytoin, primidone, mephenytoin, and phenobarbital. Trimethadione or paramethadione is usually prescribed for petit mal seizures, but evidence that these drugs are highly specific is lacking.

The nurse needs to understand the emotional problems of the person who is subject to unpredictable seizures. The numerous restrictions imposed by the condition, such as being deprived of driving a car, swimming, or working with machinery, the ever-present possibility of a seizure in the schoolroom, factory, or a public place, and the onerous necessity of regular and unrelenting medications that often dull the senses, may lead to an irritable state with bouts of depression, rebellion, and hysteria that at times overshadows the disease itself.

CONCLUDING STATEMENTS

1. Like other organs of the body, the brain suffers whenever some systemic disease or physical insult disseminates poisons, damages tissues, or impairs circulation. Physical and behavioral syndromes that result from these stressors are known as or-

ganic mental disorders, a term implying that the mental alterations exhibited have a physiological cause.

2. Organic mental disorders can best be categorized according to their reversibility.
3. The symptoms stemming from reversible organic mental disorders recede in response to immediate treatment or removal of the stressor.
4. The brain tissue damage that results from irreversible organic mental disorders cannot be corrected, but early diagnosis and treatment can arrest the progression of the disease.
5. The treatment of delirium is essentially the treatment of the etiological factor. Irrespective of the cause, the delirious individual is critically ill and requires constant skilled care.
6. Transient cerebrovascular impairment, endrocrine imbalances, infectious processes, internal toxins, and brain injury and lesions are commonly implicated in the development of reversible organic mental disorders.
7. Irreversible organic mental disorder may begin with a severe, acute illness. In other instances the onset of the impairment is insidious. In either event the effects are irreversible, although progression can sometimes be delayed with treatment.

Suggested sources of additional information

CLASSICAL

Duran, Fernando A., and Errvon, Gerald D.: Perpetuation of chronicity in mental illness, Am. J. Nurs. **70:**1707-1709, 1970.

CONTEMPORARY

Bruya, Margaret A., and Bolin, Rose Homan: Epilepsy: a controllable disease. I. Classification and diagnosis of seizures, Am. J. Nurs. **76**(3):388-392, March, 1976.

Bruya, Margaret A., and Bolin, Rose Homan: Epilepsy: a controllable disease. II. Drug therapy and nursing care, Am. J. Nurs. **76**(3):393-397, March, 1976.

Burgess, Ann Wolbert, and Lazare, Aron: Psychological disturbances resulting from pharmacological, medical, surgical, and neurological conditions. In Psychiatric nursing in the hospital and community, Englewood Cliffs, N.J., 1976, Prentice-Hall, Inc., pp. 317-330.

Foreman, Nancy Jo, and Zerwekh, Joyce: Drug crisis intervention, Am. J. Nurs. **71:**1736-1739, 1971.

Fowler, Roy S., Jr., and Fordyce, Wilbert E.: Adapting care for the brain-damaged patient, Am. J. Nurs. **72:**1832-1835, Oct., 1972.

Fowler, Roy S., Jr., and Fordyce, Wilbert E.: Adapting care for the brain-damaged patient, Am. J. Nurs. **72:**2056-2059, Nov., 1972.

Hayter, Jean: Patients who have Alzheimer's disease, Am. J. Nurs. **74:**1460-1463, 1974.

Hinkhouse, Ann: Craniocerebral trauma, Am. J. Nurs **73:**1719-1722, 1973.

Hirschfeld, Miriam J.: The cognitively impaired older adult, Am. J. Nurs. **76:**1981-1984, 1976.

Morris, Magdelena, and Rhodes, Martha: Guidelines for the care of confused patients, Am. J. Nurs. **72:**1630-1633, 1972.

Preston, Tonie: When words fail, Am. J. Nurs. **73:**2064-2066, 1973.

Wells, Robin W.: Huntington's chorea: seeing beyond the disease, Am. J. Nurs. **72:**954-956, 1972.

OF PARTICULAR INTEREST

Field, W.E., and Ruelke, W.: Hallucinations and how to deal with them, Am. J. Nurs. **73:**638, 1973.

This article discusses the development of auditory hallucinations through predictable stages and suggests interventions appropriate for each.

Trockman, G.: Caring for the confused or delirious patient, Am. J. Nurs. **78:**1495, 1978.

Behaviors characteristic of the delirious patient are described in this article, and relevant nursing interventions are outlined.

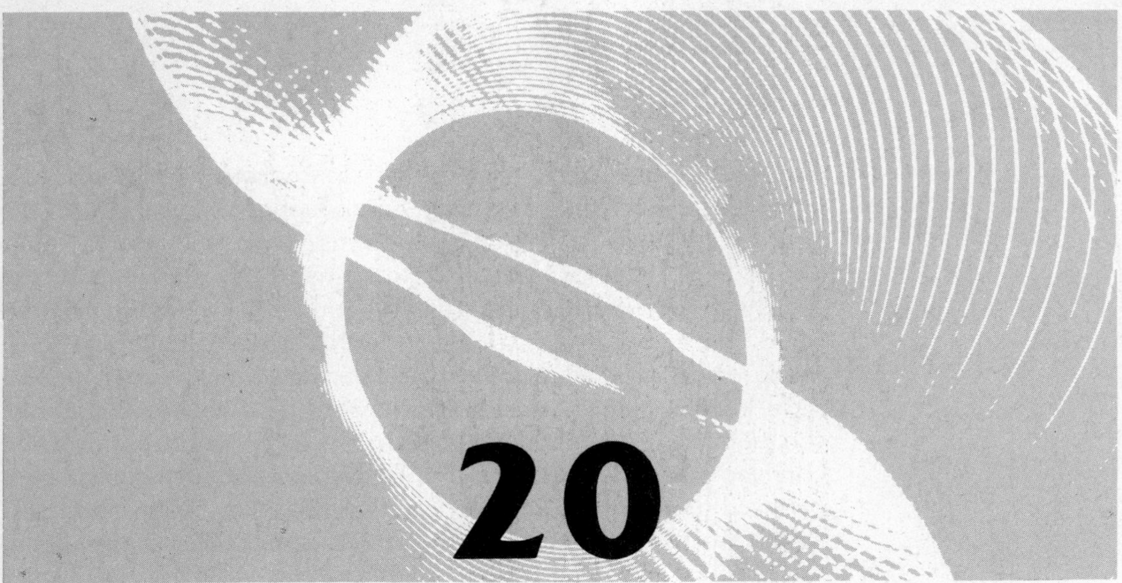

20

Physiological responses that reflect psychological maladaptation

- Theories of development
- Gastrointestinal system
- Cardiovascular system
- Respiratory system
- Integumentary system
- Musculoskeletal system
- General guidelines for nursing care of individuals with psychophysiological disorders

The phenomenon referred to as *somatization* is a process whereby an individual's feelings, emotional needs, or conflicts are manifested through physical symptoms. This process inevitably occurs when the emotional state is intense and supports the widely accepted belief that the functions and reactions of the mind and body are inextricably related. Medical historians have found evidence that even from the earliest times human beings have known that there is a relationship between the mind and the body. Beliefs about the nature of this relationship have changed over time, however. For example, some primitive people believed that deviant behavior and physical illnesses were caused by the invasion of the individual by evil spirits. This belief led to the practice of trephination, in which holes were bored into the skull of the afflicted person to facilitate departure of the evil spirit. Accompanying this surgical procedure were elaborate rituals performed by a revered member of the community known as a priest, a witch doctor, or a shaman. This procedure was sufficiently successful to justify its continued use over many centuries. Modern authorities believe that the socially sanctioned unconditional trust in the healer was the primary factor in reversing the disease process. The importance of this factor in the healing process is still seen as basic to effective intervention, whether it be physical or psychological.

Other beliefs that have supported the mind-body relationship were that deviant behavior and some forms of physical illness were caused by sinning of the individual and that a physical imbalance of body fluids or humors caused emotional problems.

Psychophysiological disorders are more complex than the previously cited examples of the mind-body relationship. These disorders are believed to have an emotional cause, to affect one body system, and to involve innervation of the autonomic nervous system. Affected individuals present a physical illness in which there is evidence of organic alteration. They are often acutely ill and in fact may have life-threatening exacerbations of the illness.

In the past this group of illnesses was referred to as psychosomatic illnesses. Unfortunately, this term has been incorrectly incorporated into the language as meaning that the physical illness is not real but rather is a product of the person's imagination designed to elicit attention and sympathy. No belief could be further from the truth, and the health care team must never assume that persons with these disorders are not really sick or are merely looking for attention through their physical symptoms.

Early beliefs about the mind-body relationship attempted to postulate a singular cause of either physical or behavioral malfunction. None of these early theories took the broad view of humans as interrelated systems in which alterations in one component inevitably result in compensatory alterations throughout the entire system. This is the view currently held by most authorities. As discussed in Chapter 21, emotional reactions to physical illness are universal and range from mild anxiety to severe emotional disturbance. The nature and degree of the individual's reaction to a physical illness are determined by the interrelationship of a number of variables, including the person's degree of mental health, the nature of his personality structure, and the nature and severity of the illness and its treatment.

Another phenomenon that illustrates the mind-body relationship is that of conversion reaction, which is briefly discussed in Chapter 14. The reader will remember that conversion reactions are manifested through physical symptoms that have no demonstrable organic basis and about which the individual is characteristically indifferent. These symptoms clearly have as their cause a severe emotional problem that needs to be alleviated before the physical symptoms will disappear.

When the somatization process is sustained and organic changes occur, the individual is said to have a psychophysiological disorder. Although it is important for the nurse to be aware of the emotional concomitants of all physical illnesses, it is imperative that she have some understanding of the etiological dynamics of those physical illnesses believed to be psychophysiological disorders. Only with this understanding will the nurse be able to provide care designed to meet the individual's needs.

THEORIES OF DEVELOPMENT

Although there seems to be consensus among authorities regarding the major role a person's emotions play in the development of certain physical illnesses, the exact nature of that role is not yet determined. One widely accepted theory postulates that repressed conflicts are stimulated by intrapsychic or interpersonal events and lead to an overall increase in the individual's level of anxiety. An automatic physical concomitant to an increase in anxiety is innervation of the autonomic nervous system. In other words, the person who is anxious becomes physically ready to engage in flight or fight. However, since the emotional conflict that serves as the basis for the anxiety and the subsequent physical response is unconscious, the individual has no outlet for the physical response, as would be possible if the conflict were conscious or if the danger were external. Consequently, the state of physical readiness for flight or fight does nothing to resolve the underlying emotional conflict. Should this phenomenon be sustained, a cyclical pattern is established. This pattern results in physiological alterations such as a peptic ulcer, which is caused by increased gastric acid secretion and gastric hypermotility as compensatory to the initial decreased gastric acid secretion and hypomotility caused by the flight-fight reaction. As the individual perceives physical discomfort, it is not unlikely that his anxiety will further increase, thereby compounding the problem. The originator of this theory is a physician named Franz Alexander, whose works on the subject remain classics in the field.

A second theory postulates that there are personality types that are particularly prone to the development of certain physical illnesses. An example of this theory is the designation of a specific personality type that is considered to place the individual in a high-risk category for myocardial infarction. These persons are seen to be highly competitive, overly ambitious, and denying of any needs for dependency. This personality syndrome is manifested by hard work, aggresive behavior, and a great deal of risk taking as a means of getting ahead. These persons frequently have many individuals dependent on them, but no one on whom they feel they can depend.

A third theory places emphasis on the symbolism of the illness. For example, a person who unconsciously feels a great deal of rage at significant others and the environment in general but for whom expression of this rage is not acceptable may develop ulcerative colitis. Since ulcerative colitis is an illness in which the person has frequent bowel movements requiring, at the very least, alterations in his and others' activities, one might say that he is symbolically defecating on those around him, a very hostile act indeed.

A fourth theory is referred to as organ weakness. This theory postulates that all humans have one body system that is relatively less healthy than are the others. If a person has underlying unconscious problems that interfere with his effective functioning but at the same time has sufficient ego strength so that a flight from reality is not necessary, this person may develop a physical illness as a means of coping with the unconscious problem, and the type of physical illness developed will be determined by the body system that is most physiologically vulnerable.

Regardless of which theory or combination of theories proves to be correct, they all have several concepts in common, the understanding of which will prove invaluable to the nurse in caring for persons with psychophysiological disorders. Following are these concepts:

1. Persons who develop psychophysiological disorders have *unconscious* emotional conflicts that increase their anxiety and interfere with their effectively meeting their needs.
2. The physical illness is a result of or an expression of this unconscious conflict and serves as a means of lowering the anxiety level.
3. The physical illness is real in that there are demonstrable organic changes that may be life threatening.

It is also generally accepted that the onset of the psychophysiological illness is associated with a real or perceived stressful life event. The physical symptoms occur as a response to this stress and mask the emotional turmoil with which the person cannot cope, thereby achieving the primary purpose of lowering anxiety. In our society, however, the individual also may experience unexpected and unintended benefits from the illness. These benefits may be such things as having one's dependency needs indirectly met, receiving attention and special consideration, or being relieved of responsibility. These benefits are *secondary gains,* which tend to unconsciously reinforce the pattern of somatization.

It is beyond the scope of this text to discuss each of the psychophysiological disorders in depth. The student should be aware that there are many excellent references available from which much may be learned about each of these disease entities. Discussion in this chapter will be limited to the ones most commonly encountered in general nursing practice and that are illustrative of different body system involvement.

GASTROINTESTINAL SYSTEM

Peptic ulcer is a syndrome that is very common in a highly industrialized society such as the United States. The diagnosis of peptic ulcer encompasses both gastric ulcers and duodenal ulcers, although there is evidence that emotional factors play a larger role in the development of duodenal ulcers, which tend to occur more in men than in women and in younger age-groups. Duodenal ulcers stem from sustained gastric hypermotility and marked increase in gastric secretions, which eventually erodes the lining of the stomach. Clinically, the individual complains of epigastric pain that occurs within 1 to 4 hours after the last meal and is relieved by eating or by taking antacids. If alterations in diet and the taking of nonprescription remedies do not help, the person is likely to seek medical help, since the pain becomes severe enough that it cannot be ignored. Hospitalization may be necessary, either to establish the diagnosis through testing or for treatment. Although medical treatment is always conservative if possible, the presence of bleeding or intractable pain may indicate the need for surgical removal of the affected part of the stomach or severance of a branch of the vagus nerve. Unfortunately, when this occurs, it is not uncommon for the individual to subsequently develop another even more severe form of psychophysiological disorder.

The personality characteristics of a person who develops a peptic ulcer are that of a person who sees himself and is seen by others as strong, independent, hard working, and unemotional. Despite their occupational successes, these persons are tormented by feelings of not having done well enough and constantly strive to achieve even higher goals. Authorities believe that underlying these behaviors are strong dependency needs that are in conflict with the individual's self-image and therefore cannot be directly expressed. If these needs are met, it is a result of fortuitous accident rather than goal-directed behavior.

The initial onset of the illness as well as subsequent exacerbations tend to be precipitated by stressful life events that bring the dependency-independency conflict closer to the surface of consciousness. One man experienced his first episode of duodenal ulcer attack at the time of his marriage when he left his parents' home to establish with his wife a home of their own. Despite the fact that he married an attractive, caring woman whom he loved very much, the very act of marriage abruptly changed his role from that of son to that of husband, or symbolically from child to adult. The first gastrointestinal episode was successfully treated through diet modification and medication, and the symptoms subsided. The second attack occurred after the birth of their first child, a son, 4 years later. Once again, it can be seen that the birth of a child, particularly a son with whose infantile dependency the father may have identified, put increased pressure on this man to act as a strong, responsible adult while simultaneously decreasing direct opportunities to have his dependency needs met. As in the previous attack, conservative medical treatment was successful in alleviating the ulcer symptoms, although they were more severe and took longer to disappear than in the initial episode. It is interesting to note that when their second child, a daughter, was born 4 years later, no exacerbation of ulcer symptoms occurred. The third and most severe episode of ulcer symptoms took place about a year after this man's father died. The father died as a result of bowel cancer, which was treated by colostomy and radiation, but which nevertheless metastasized. During the course of his illness, the father moved in with his son and daughter-in-law because of his increased need for physical care and supervision. Although the daughter-in-law provided most of the care, the son frequently willingly helped, especially with more personal tasks such as bathing. The father died in the home, and during the following year the son was deeply involved in settling his father's complex estate. It was after this task was completed that he once again experienced ulcer symptoms that were so severe that surgical removal of two thirds of his stomach was ultimately required. It can be conjectured that the death of this man's father was unconsciously seen by him as the ultimate proof of his adulthood, which he was not able to withstand because he maintained a large reservoir of unmet dependency needs, and his father's death symbolically cut off all hope of having these needs met.

Although peptic ulcer is a common form of gastrointestinal psychophysiological disorder, other illnesses such as ulcerative colitis or chronic constipation are also seen as having a strong emotional cause.

CARDIOVASCULAR SYSTEM

A health problem of increasing incidence, particularly among black Americans, is that of essential hypertension. Essential hypertension is a sustained elevation of systolic and diastolic arterial blood pressure in the absence of any of the demonstrable known causes of arterial hypertension. Although persons suffering from essential hypertension may remain asymptomatic for years, if the syndrome is sustained, organic alterations, particularly renal damage, may occur. Often the acceleration of the disease with resultant complications occurs in conjunction with life crises. It is believed that huge amounts of repressed rage that have no acceptable outlet are the emotional dynamics underlying the development of essential hypertension. The mental mechanism used by the individual is usually denial, since the person also has a need to conform with the expectations of others, especially authority figures, as a means of meeting his dependency needs. Feeling and expressing rage is therefore highly anxiety producing, and the individual often has a calm, placid exterior. The frequency of occurrence of essential hypertension in the black population has led investigators to explore genetic factors simultaneously with cultural factors as major etiological predeterminants.

RESPIRATORY SYSTEM

A major psychophysiological disorder affecting the respiratory system is bronchial asthma. Bronchial asthma is caused by bronchial obstruction that does not interfere with inspiration but causes difficulty in expiration. This results in the characteristic asthmatic wheeze that sounds so similar in all patients that it is almost diagnostic. The underlying cause of the bronchial obstruction may be an infectious process, an allergic reaction, or an idiopathic bronchospasm. When an underlying disease process such as a bacterial infection is present, other symptoms such as an elevated temperature and white blood count are also present and require treatment if the asthmatic episode is to be alleviated. There are some instances, however, when there is no demonstrable physiological cause for the asthmatic episode, and it is here that emotional factors are believed to play a major etiological role in the occurrence of the illness.

The personality characteristics of the individual who suffers from asthma seem to include strong dependency needs directed toward the mother or mother figure, with simultaneous anger toward this individual, which elicits unconscious fears of abandonment. In fact, some psychoanalytically oriented authorities claim that the characteristic asthmatic wheeze is a symbolic cry for the mother. During an acute asthmatic attack the individual is a clinging, dependent person whose behavior is justified to himself and others on the basis of the life-threatening symptoms. Therefore it is not uncommon for the dependency needs of the person to be met during the acute episode, but unfortunately these temporary episodes of need fulfillment do little to alter the underlying personality dynamics, and thus future episodes are not prevented. Continued episodes of asthma result in pulmonary changes that may not be reversible and affect the vital capacity of the person's respiratory system.

INTEGUMENTARY SYSTEM

The integumentary system serves a unique function in the ego psychology of an individual in that it is the only body system that is equally visible both to the person and to others. Because of this, the skin represents the self to others in the environment. An awareness of this fact is reflected in such sayings as, "He's too thick- [or thin-] skinned" or "You can't tell a book by its cover."

The skin is richly endowed with sense receptors for pain, pressure, and temperature sensations. As a result, many emotional states are reflected in skin changes—the blush of embarrassment and the paling that accompanies fear are examples. These common skin changes are received by others as nonverbal clues to the emotional state of the individual, frequently despite verbal reassurances to the contrary. In healthy interpersonal relationships, the skin acts as a friendly ally in communicating to others what is being felt and therefore enhances the probability of having the individual's needs met. When the skin is involved in a psychophysiological disorder, however, it becomes a means of self-disclosure representing the individual's unconscious conflict between a repressed emotion and the simultaneous need to have this emotion be known and responded to.

There are numerous dermatological conditions that can cause a person severe discomfort, either in the form of itching, pain, or disfigurement. Although in many instances their exact cause is unknown, an amazing number of these maladies respond well to the treatment of a dermatologist who may try a number of remedies before finding one that seems to help. Although not denying the positive benefits of the physical treatment received, many authorities believe that the major benefit is achieved from the sustained, concerned interest in the individual and his illness that is frequently shown by dermatologists and that indirectly helps to meet the person's immediate needs. Exacerbations of skin rashes and severe itching are closely related to occurrences of stressful life events to which these persons seem to respond without undue emotional upset but rather react by somatization on which they and others can focus their concern. Many psychiatrists believe that skin somatization is one of the most primitive ego defenses available and therefore are very cautious in pursuing aggressive physical and psychological treatment unless the individual is in great pain or unable to carry out activities of daily living. The rationale underlying this conservative approach is that if the person is enabled to give up this defense without a considerable increase in ego strength, he might be forced to resort to the more serious and incapacitating defense of mental illness.

MUSCULOSKELETAL SYSTEM

The most common and severe form of psychophysiological disorder that affects the musculoskeletal system is rheumatoid arthritis. This disease results in marked organic damage and affects not only the joints but also other tissues. Its onset may occur at any age, and it affects females more frequently than males. The personality characteristics of persons affected by this disease almost universally include masochistic, self-sacrificing behavior, which is in response to a rigid, punitive superego and a weak ego organization. Their family background frequently gives evidence of maternal deprivation, leaving them with a great many unmet dependency needs. Prior to becoming ill, these individuals indirectly express their emotional needs by being helpful and kind, willing to do almost anything for others, and thereby receiving positive feedback from their social system. Under usual circumstances, therefore, their dependency needs are minimally met through environmental and interpersonal support, allowing them to remain healthy until such time as this support is withdrawn. Many individuals report that an event such as the death of a spouse or the loss of a job immediately preceded the initial onset of the illness.

Treatment of these persons is exceedingly complex. Many of them reflect their emotional conflict by denying the severity of their illness and either refuse treatment or are unreliable in following the treatment regimen. Conversely, there are some who quickly become highly dependent on family, friends, and health care personnel despite the fact that their symptoms may be only mildly debilitating.

GENERAL GUIDELINES FOR NURSING CARE OF INDIVIDUALS WITH PSYCHOPHYSIOLOGICAL DISORDERS

The care of persons suffering from psychophysiological disorders is usually directed by a physician whose emphasis is on the reduction of physical symptoms and the prevention of further organic damage. However, because of the nature of the illness, close collaboration with a psychiatrist is often necessary. Once the acute physical symptoms have abated, the psychiatrist may continue to treat the individual on an outpatient basis in an attempt to help the person deal with underlying emotional problems. The nurse is usually involved in providing care during those times when the person is hospitalized for an exacerbation of the illness or in follow-up care in the home. During her involvement, the methods used by the nurse in carrying out physical care are often pivotal factors in enhancing or impeding the overall treatment goals. The following are some suggested guidelines that should be considered in the nursing care plan for persons with psychophysiological disorders.

The nurse must fully understand and accept the fact that these persons are physically ill and that their symptoms may reach life-threatening proportions. The nurse must not convey the attitude that she believes the individual would get better if he merely exerted more control over his emotions. During acute episodes of the illness, meeting the physical needs of the client is of primary importance, even if in so doing the nurse is supporting dysfunctional emotional adaptation. For example, a couple whose tension-laden relationship exacerbates the wife's physical symptoms should not be encouraged to discuss their relationship during the acute episode of the wife's illness.

Most physical illnesses, regardless of cause, present a potential threat to the person's perception of himself as an independent adult. In the case of persons with psychophysiological disorders, there often are underlying conflicts between dependency and independency needs, and the imposed dependence that results from the illness may stimulate a high degree of anxiety in the client. In such instances the nurse can be helpful if she meets the individual's needs for dependence in an indirect way while simultaneously acknowledging his status as a responsible adult. An example of such an intervention is the nurse who wisely addresses the client with a peptic ulcer as Mr. Smith instead of John. At the same time, Mr. Smith's dependency needs can be indirectly met by the nurse's administering the prescribed Sippy diet instead of leaving the milk or cream at the bedside or asking the client to ring his call light every half hour so that she can bring the medicine. By spontaneously making frequent contact with the client the nurse is indirectly saying that she is willing to take care of him without his having to assume the responsibility of asking for help. It should be noted that the administration of oral medication or food, especially milk, has great symbolic significance, since eating is the vehicle through which people have their dependency needs first met.

Many persons are not aware of the interpersonal resources available to them within their social system. Persons with psychophysiological disorders can often benefit from help in identifying already existent interpersonal resources and in enlarging their social network, thereby increasing the possibility of having their emotional needs met by a larger variety of people.

The nurse has many opportunities to engage in conversation with the hospitalized person. She can be of emotional assistance to him if she encourages him to talk about his feelings. It must be understood, however, that many of the client's feelings are unacceptable to him and therefore acceptance of him and his feelings by the nurse is of primary importance. As in communicating with any client, the nurse is most helpful when she is accepting and nonjudgmental. Reflecting or restating what the client has said is an appropriate communication technique to employ, since a direct interpretation may be very threatening and raise the client's anxiety level and perhaps thereby increase the severity of his physical symptoms.

As is true of any client, the person suffering from a psychophysiological disorder can be helped to feel in control of his situation by adequate explanations of what he can expect to experience during diagnostic and treatment procedures. Some clients, however, become increasingly anxious if they are given too much information, and their dependency needs are best met by trusting in the judgment of their physician and nurse. Therefore the amount and nature of information offered to the client should be primarily determined by an assessment of his anxiety level. Certainly the client's questions should be answered, but the degree of elaboration necessary should be gauged by his response to the answer rather than by the nurse's need to engage in health teaching.

The secondary gains achieved by the individual as the result of his being physically ill need to be minimized once the acute episode has passed. The nurse can be instrumental in working with him to strengthen or develop coping mechanisms that do not involve somatization.

Working with the client's family is necessary to aid them in understanding the complexity of his illness and its treatment. The effect of the family on the client and the effect the client and his illness have on the family is a process that is often explored in family therapy under the guidance of a skilled therapist.

CASE FORMULATION □ AN INDIVIDUAL WITH ASTHMA

Martha B. was a 10-year-old girl who had suffered from asthma since the age of 2. Although respiratory infections always precipitated an asthmatic attack, there were many instances of asthmatic episodes that were unaccompanied by an infectious process. Martha was the only child of an attractive 29-year-old woman who had never married and was not sure who Martha's father was.

Since the age of 16, Martha's mother had engaged in prostitution and had become pregnant several times. For reasons that were not clear, at the time she was pregnant with Martha, she decided not to have an abortion as she had done on previous occasions. After Martha was born, the mother set up housekeeping in an apartment, which she furnished with the child's needs in mind. Martha's mother was so successful in her occupation that she no longer was a streetwalker but rather made appointments with her customers by telephone and therefore had advance notice as to when she would not be home. At those times she left Martha with her grandmother, a warm, kind woman who seemed unaware of her daughter's activities. When Martha and her mother were together, they seemed to enjoy each other and have a mutually satisfying relationship. When Martha began school, it became quickly evident that she was an intelligent child who strove hard to please the teacher. Her report cards showed her to be an excellent student, which pleased both the mother and grandmother. Martha's school attendance was somewhat erratic, however, because of the increased frequency of asthmatic attacks and the necessity for the mother to leave Martha with her grandmother who lived outside the school district and had no car to take Martha to school. The event preceding Martha's latest and most severe asthmatic attack was a telephone call to Martha's mother late one evening from a prosperous businessman who requested the mother to accompany him on a business trip to another country, for which she would be paid a large sum of money. If she agreed, however, she would have to leave that very evening and would be gone for an indeterminate amount of time. Martha's mother believed that she could not refuse such a lucrative offer, and, since Martha was already asleep, she telephoned the grandmother and asked her to come to the apartment rather than waking Martha and taking her to the grandmother's house. The grandmother agreed and arrived by taxi shortly therafter, whereupon the mother left for the airport. The following morning, Martha awakened and was very surprised to find her grandmother in her mother's bed. The grandmother's explanation about where the mother was and how long she would be gone was vague, since she herself did not consciously understand the situation but was pleased at her daughter's opportunity for earning a great deal of money from which she would undoubtedly also benefit. Martha left for school but by 10 AM began to experience an asthmatic attack that was so severe that the school authorities rushed her to the emergency room of the local hospital, at which point the grandmother was notified. Martha was admitted to the pediatric unit in a highly anxious state, manifested by a great deal of crying, gasping for breath, and motor restlessness. She was placed in an oxygen tent and promptly curled up in one corner of the bed, turning her back to the nurse. The nurse attempted to administer the prescribed oral bronchodilator, which Martha refused to take, becoming increasingly agitated as the nurse increased her efforts to administer the medication. The desperate crying and flailing around in the bed obviously increased Martha's respiratory difficulties and the nurse's anxiety, so the nursing supervisor was consulted. Quickly assessing the cyclical nature of the situation and understanding the psychodynamics, the nursing supervisor sat the grandmother in the easily available rocking chair, lifted Martha out of the oxygen tent, and placed her in the grandmother's arms with instructions to her to rock Martha and speak soothingly to her. The grandmother was more than willing to comply with this request, and within less than 15 minutes Martha was sufficiently calm that it was possible for her to take her medication.

Discussion of development of patterns of behavior

Martha's family situation contained all the elements sufficient for the development of idiopathic asthma. It can be conjectured that Martha's mother was in fact a very immature person lacking in self-esteem who engaged in prostitution as one means of reinforcing her feelings of worthlessness. If this were true, it is likely that her decision not to terminate her pregnancy with Martha was an unconscious attempt to provide herself with a consistent person who would need and value her. Unfortunately, this rarely succeeds, since children require more attention and love than they can give during their formative developmental periods. Martha undoubtedly felt that her mother's frequent absences were a result of some failing on her part, while at the same time she experienced much anger at her mother for not providing her with the emotional support she needed. Ironically, the grandmother seemed able to meet some of these needs in Martha, although her relationship with her own daughter was not growth producing, as evidenced by their lack of communication. It would not be surprising if Martha were unable to benefit from the attention given her by her grandmother because she unconsciously realized that this attention was really intended for her mother and displaced onto her by the grandmother. In other words, the relationship between Martha and her grandmother might have been perceived by Martha as a means by which her mother and grandmother could work on their own relationship, and therefore the positive effects on Martha would have been attenuated. Martha made attempts to please her mother and therefore attain and retain her love, but although her mother's pleasure at Martha's performance in school was evident, her mother's living situation interfered with even this avenue of achievement.

Nursing care plan

Neither the nurse on the pediatric unit nor the nursing supervisor had much time to explore much of Martha's previous life experiences, since the great need, initially, was to relieve Martha's acute physiological symptoms by administration of medication. Both these nurses, however, knew that a child with asthma is usually part of a family system that does not meet many of his emotional needs and that creates huge dependency needs coexisting with feelings of anger toward the mothering one. Since an appropriate *initial* nursing diagnosis for Martha can be stated as "severe dyspnea, probably related to somatization of dependency needs and feelings of anger, resulting in severe anxiety and physiological disequilibrium," the nursing supervisor decided that an appropriate plan would be to decrease the anxiety, which would in turn decrease the physiological disequilibrium. Since mothering and dependency needs are related to asthma, a specific nursing intervention would be to provide physical cuddling, rocking, and comforting words. This intervention results in secondary gain, which is usually to be avoided. In this instance, however, it reduced Martha's anxiety and dyspnea so that medication could be given and so that a therapeutic relationship with the nurse could begin.

Subsequent nursing interventions for Martha would be related to conveying acceptance, gaining trust, encouraging Martha to talk about her feelings, and involving Martha, her mother, and grandmother in family therapy.

Long-term outcome criteria against which nursing care would be evaluated include a decrease in frequency and severity of Martha's asthmatic attacks and a lack of development of other psychophysiological disorders in any members of this family system.

CONCLUDING STATEMENTS

1. The phenomenon referred to as somatization is a process whereby an individual's feelings, emotional needs, or conflicts are manifested through physical symptoms.
2. Human beings have known since the earliest times that the functions of the mind and the body are inextricably related.
3. Psychophysiological disorders are physical illnesses that are believed to have an emotional cause, to affect one body system, and to involve innervation of the autonomic nervous system.
4. The person experiencing a psychophysiological disorder may be acutely ill and have life-threatening exacerbations of the illness.
5. There are a number of theories that attempt to explain the underlying dynamics of psychophysiological disorders. All these theories have the following concepts in common:
   a. Persons who develop psychophysiological disorders have unconscious emotional conflicts that increase their anxiety and interfere with their effectively meeting their needs.
   b. The physical illness is a result of or an expression of this unconscious conflict and serves as a means of lowering the anxiety level.
   c. The physical illness is real in that there are demonstrable organic changes that may be life threatening.
   d. The onset of the illness is associated with a real or perceived stressful life event.
6. Secondary gains are the unexpected and unintended benefits the person receives as a result of his illness that unconsciously reinforce the pattern of somatization.

7. Peptic ulcer, essential hypertension, bronchial asthma, many skin disorders, and rheumatoid arthritis are examples of common psychophysiological disorders.
8. The nurse can be most helpful to these persons by
   a. Skillfully meeting the person's immediate physical needs.
   b. Conveying an accepting, nonjudgmental attitude by understanding that the physical distress the individual is experiencing is not under his control.
   c. Meeting the person's dependency needs in an indirect way while simultaneously acknowledging him as a responsible adult.
   d. Helping the person to use and enlarge his interpersonal resources.
   e. Encouraging the person to talk about his feelings.
   f. Providing appropriate explanations of diagnostic and treatment procedures.
   g. Minimizing the secondary gains achieved by the individual once the acute episode of the illness has passed.
   h. Working with the person's family to aid them in understanding the complexity of his illness and its treatment.

Suggested sources of additional information

CLASSICAL

Alexander, Franz: Psychosomatic medicine, New York, 1954, W.W. Norton & Co., Inc.

Dunbar, Flanders: Emotions and bodily changes, New York, 1954, Columbia University Press.

CONTEMPORARY

Bahnson, Claus Bahne: Epistemological perspectives of physical disease from the psychodynamic point of view, Am. J. Public Health **64:**1034-1040, 1974.

Bragg, T.L.: Psychological response to myocardial infarction, Nurs. Forum **14:**383-395, 1975.

Cassell, John: An epidemiological perspective of psychosocial factors in disease etiology, Am. J. Public Health **64:**1040-1043, 1974.

Ciseaux, Annie: Anorexia nervosa: a view from the mirror, Am. J. Nurs. **80:**1468-1469, Aug., 1980.

Claggett, Marilyn S.: Anorexia nervosa: a behavioral approach, Am. J. Nurs. **80:**1471-1472, Aug., 1980.

Davis, Marcella Z.: Socioemotional component of coronary care, Am. J. Nurs. **72:**705-709, April, 1972.

Eisenman, Elaine P.: Primary care in a mental health facility, Nurs. Outlook **24**:640-645, 1976.

Fagerhaugh, Shizuko Yoshimura: Mental illness and the tuberculosis patient, Nurs. Outlook **18**:38-41, Aug., 1970.

Grossniklaus, Daurice M.: Nursing interventions in anorexia nervosa, Perspect. Psychiatr. Care **18**:11-16, Jan.-Feb., 1980.

Jackson, Bettie: Ulcerative colitis from an etiological perspective, Am. J. Nurs. **73**:258-261, 1973.

Lambert, Vickie A., and Lambert, Clinton E.: The impact of physical illness and related mental health concepts, Englewood Cliffs, N.J., 1979, Prentice-Hall, Inc.

Lego, Suzanne: The golden cage: the enigma of anorexia nervosa, Perspect. Psychiatr. Care **17**:232-237, Sept.-Oct., 1979.

Liu, Aimee: Solitaire, Philadelphia, 1980, J.B. Lippincott Co.

Richardson, Thomas F.: Anorexia nervosa: an overview, Am. J. Nurs. **80**:1469-1471, Aug., 1980.

Syme, S. Leonard: Behavioral factors associated with the etiology of physical disease: a social epidemiological approach, Am. J. Public Health **64**:1043-1045, 1974.

Wittkower, Eric D., and Warnes, Hector: Psychosomatic medicine: its clinical applications, New York, 1977, Harper & Row, Publishers.

OF PARTICULAR INTEREST

Liu, Aimee: Solitaire, Philadelphia, 1980, J.B. Lippincott Co.

This book describes a young woman's triumph over anorexia nervosa, including the developmental impact of adolescence.

Wittkower, Eric D., and Warnes, Hector: Psychosomatic medicine: its clinical applications, New York, 1977, Harper & Row, Publishers.

This useful text has an especially good series of articles on the major physiological manifestations of psychological maladaptation.

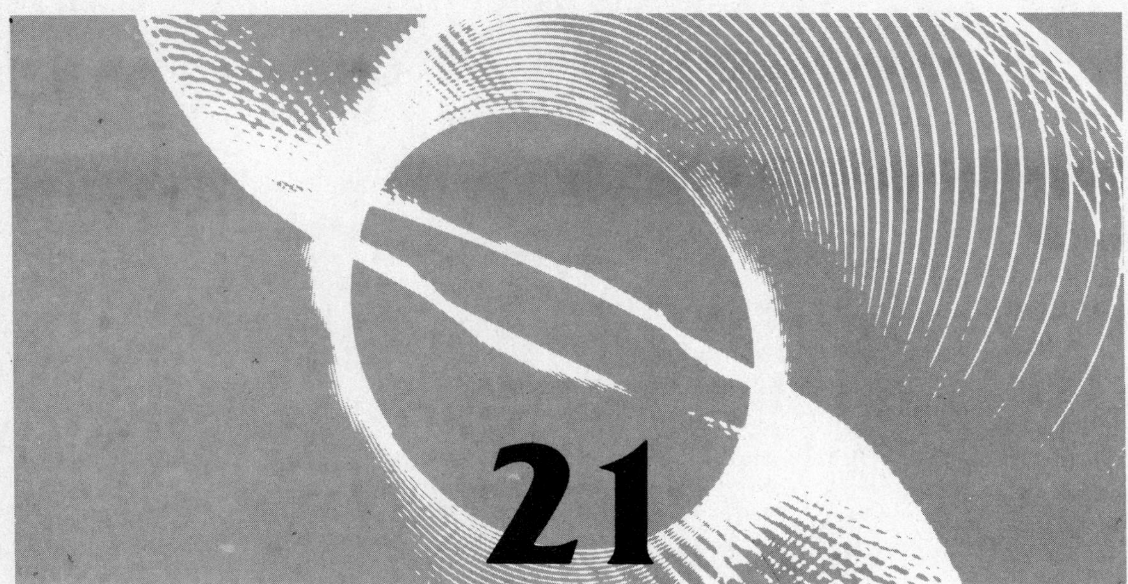

Improving nursing care for the physically ill

- Emotional reactions precipitated by the use of mechanical devices
- Emotional reactions precipitated by organ transplants
- Emotional reactions precipitated by the loss of a body part
- Emotional reactions precipitated by cardiac surgery
- Emotional reactions precipitated by an untoward obstetrical experience
- Emotional reactions precipitated by an abortion
- Emotional aspects of death and dying
- Self-help groups

The reader will recall the previously stated belief that sound interpersonal skills are foundational to all nursing practice. This belief implies that knowledges and skills regarding interpersonal relationships should be an integral part of the nurse's entire educational program. Nevertheless, it is apparent that all too often the emotional needs of the physically ill are given little attention and that student nurses frequently look to their psychiatric nursing experience to provide them with direction in giving more comprehensive care to the physically ill. Therefore this chapter is devoted to helping the nurse develop an understanding of some common emotional needs of the physically ill individual, although no situation in this chapter can be discussed in depth.

Physically ill individuals display a variety of feelings, which may include intense anxiety, hostility, depression, elation, fear, anger, and sorrow. These are the same feelings that may be expressed by the mentally ill. Perhaps one of the few differentiations that can be made between the reactions of these two groups is the presumed ability of the physically ill to maintain conscious control of behavior and to use better judgment than do individuals who are mentally ill. However, even these expected differences are not always observed.

Placing psychiatric units in general hospitals has been one attempt to eradicate the traditional artificial boundaries between the needs of individuals who are mentally ill and those who are physically ill. Increased awareness of the psychophysiological nature of many illnesses is another manifestation of the recognition by health care professionals of the interrelatedness of the mind and body.

There is growing dissatisfaction with the nursing care provided in general hospitals in the United States. Studies of these dissatisfactions point up the fact that only a few of them are related to the physical care given. The large majority of complaints have to do with failure of professional nurses to establish satisfying interpersonal relationships with individuals receiving their services. The nurse is frequently said to lack warmth, to fail to give individuals a feeling of being important human beings, to fail to listen empathically to the concerns of individuals being cared for, or to fail to ask enough questions to gather the necessary data to make wise decisions about individual needs.

Listening to individuals, helping them feel they are important, and demonstrating a caring attitude do make heavy demands on the professional nurse's already limited time. However, the understanding and emotional support that physically ill individuals deserve and are demanding is omitted more often because the nurse does not understand the character of the emotional needs of the individuals and how to provide the help they require, rather than because time is not available to give this type of care.

It is often more difficult and more challenging to recognize and cope with the emotional needs of the physically ill than it is to work effectively with the emotional needs of the mentally ill. Because part of a mentally ill individual's problem is his lack of emotional control, he sometimes expresses needs openly and directly. The emotionally ill individual's needs may be difficult to understand, but their existence is obvious. Because he is said to be mentally ill, the nurse realizes that part of the task is to help him cope with his emotional problems. In contrast, the physically ill individual usually tries to control his feelings and to solve his own problems. Nurses frequently expect this individual to cope with his own emotional problems. They sometimes fail to recognize that in addition to his need for physical care, the physically ill person needs the same acceptance, understanding, and concern as does the mentally ill person (Fig. 21-1).

The very occurrence of a physical illness that is serious enough to warrant hospitalization causes an interruption in the normal life-style of the individual and his family. As a result, some degree of stress is produced with which the individual and his family may or may not be able to cope successfully. In addition, any physical illness for which hospitalization is necessary forces the individual to assume a dependent role that may be disturbing to him. Although the society's view of masculinity and femininity is becoming less stereotyped, a dependent role is still seen as particularly problematic for men who are often expected to portray an

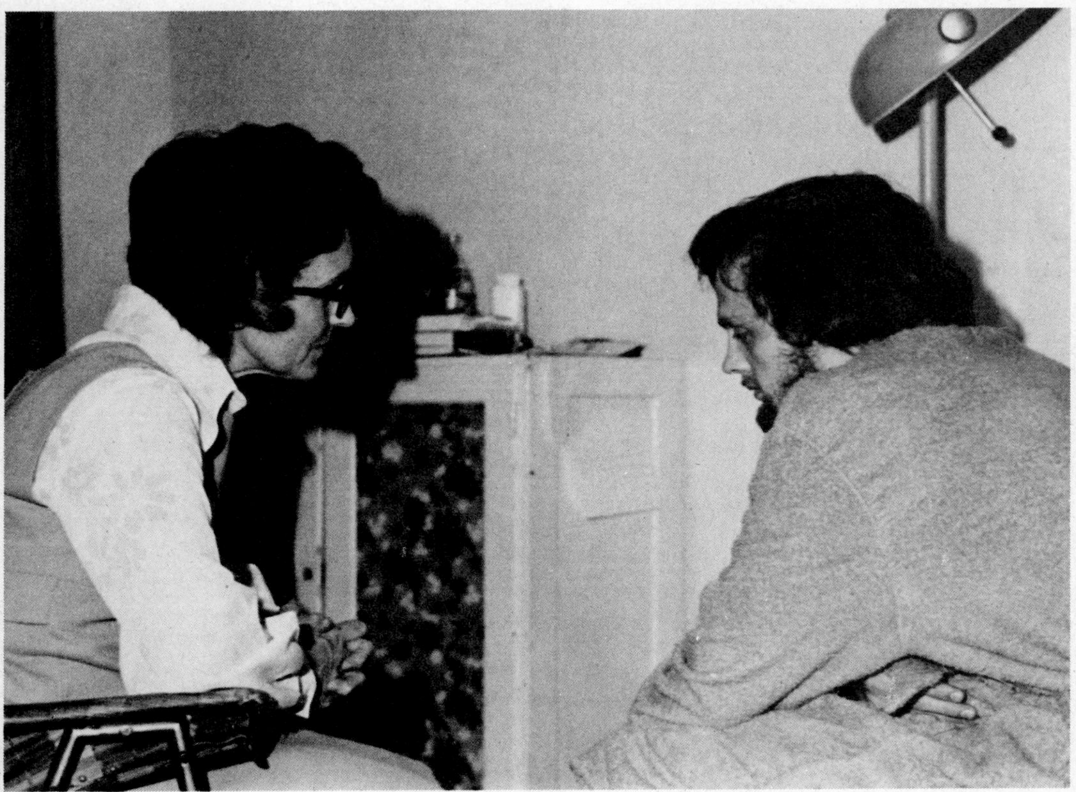

Fig. 21-1 *The physically ill person needs the same acceptance, understanding, and concern as the mentally ill person.*

image of strength and independence and who may see physical illness as an expression of weakness. Inability to accept the forced dependency required in many hospitals is one reason for the uncooperative behavior of some individuals.

The modern hospital is a highly organized creation of a mechanized world. Regardless of the nature of the illness that brings the individual to the hospital, he is expected to submit to a variety of procedures without always understanding what they are or why they are being done. He often believes they are being performed without his consent or without his having been given any explanation about them. Many procedures that seem commonplace to health professionals, such as enemas, catheterizations, and intravenous injections, may be viewed by others as intrusions into their bodies. Not only may the individual have no understanding of the reasons for the procedure, but he may also feel that he has lost control over his body. At the same time, he frequently is covertly given the message by personnel that he should be thankful to them for performing these procedures. This conflict may result in an increase in his anxiety level, which, paradoxically, decreases the effectiveness of the procedure itself. Therefore it is imperative for the individual's physical and emotional well-being that the nurse provide him with an opportunity to explore his feelings about the procedure as well as giving him an appropriate explanation of its nature.

Although the individual may have signed an operative permit, he is not likely to realize that this may cover a variety of tests and procedures before the actual operation is undertaken. The physician may have explained the preoperative tests, but the anxiety level of many individuals is so high that they are unable to comprehend what the physician is saying. Even when individuals are able to concentrate on the physician's words, they do not always understand the full meaning of them, and the preoperative procedures may still come as a shocking surprise. It is not difficult to understand that a newly admitted surgical patient may be frightened and feel that he has lost his identity. Such a situation could be eased if nurses understood the importance of giving reassurance, if they could identify the basis for the anxiety, and if they were skillful in giving emotional support. Sometimes reassurance requires only a few minutes of time spent listening, answering questions, and recognizing that the individual is a unique human being who is reaching out for understanding and help.

Sometimes the results of hospital procedures, especially surgical procedures, precipitate an emotional crisis. Such a crisis is overwhelming for a person who has already developed the feeling that he is lost, forgotten, and reduced to a childlike state of dependence in the hospital. These feelings may actually impede his recovery and may cause him to view his hospitalization as an extremely traumatizing experience.

EMOTIONAL REACTIONS PRECIPITATED BY THE USE OF MECHANICAL DEVICES

Currently the developments in biomedical science have provided several life-sustaining devices that make it possible to prolong the lives of many individuals who would be doomed to death otherwise. Among these devices are kidney dialysis machines and cardiac pacemakers.

The kidney dialysis machine is likely to produce a more profound emotional response from the individual than the pacemaker. The individual who must rely on a kidney machine recognizes how dependent he is on the device for life itself. He also becomes aware of the fact that his activities are circumscribed by his need to be attached to the machine for 8 to 10 hours, two or three times each week. This schedule interferes with his work, his ability to make a living, his social life, and his family life.

Dependency on a mechanical device to sustain life in the case of both the pacemaker and the kidney dialysis machine creates anxiety in almost all individuals who are so involved. It causes many individuals to feel dehumanized and to be concerned about the maintenance of their personal autonomy. In addition, the individual may be resentful and angry, or he may be depressed and respond by being tearful, disinterested in his surroundings, and uncommunicative. On the other hand, the individual may express his anger and frustration at the situation by speaking sharply to the nurses or to his family. He may express fear by demanding constant attention and that the nurse remain with him at all times. He may express his disturbed emotional feelings by being critical of the hospital or clinic where he must go for the dialysis. He may fear that the device will fail to function properly and thus end his life abruptly.

Pacemakers do not interfere with the individual's activities as much as do kidney dialysis machines, but they sometimes cause great anxiety and fear, since it is possible for them to cease to function properly without giving adequate warning. Individuals who must rely on either of these devices realize they will never be completely well again and must look forward to a long-term reliance on mechanical assistance.

Because the kidney dialysis machine must be attached to the individual so often, a permanent arteriovenous shunt is frequently implanted in an arm or leg to provide access to an artery or vein whenever necessary. Individuals with these shunts have been known to tear them out, causing the loss of a great deal of blood. This action is usually considered to be a suicidal gesture, since the rate of suicide is high among individuals who resent their dependence on kidney dialysis machines.

Family members have been taught to operate portable dialysis machines and thus free the individual from constantly returning to a hospital or clinic to have his blood cleansed. However, this practice makes it necessary to teach a family member to operate the machine and to require that the family member be available when the treatments are scheduled. This amount of dependence on another person is also cause for hostility and resentment among some individuals and has not provided the solution to the time-consuming kidney dialysis procedure that it was originally intended to do.

Individuals who must rely on mechanical devices often feel that they have lost control of their bodies and of their destinies. This may lead to a loss of confidence and self-esteem. Such a loss of confidence results in behavior that requires emotional support and understanding.

In summary, the life-saving biomedical devices that are currently available are capable of improving the physical health of the individual but do not always improve emotional health. Specifically, those individuals who must rely on kidney dialysis machines are chronic worriers. They worry about all the daily problems of living that confront everyone. They require nurses who are not only skilled in understanding and coping with their physical needs but who can understand that their behavior is sometimes an expression of anger, fear, and depression brought on by their resentment of being dependent for life on a mechanical device and being unable to control the situation. They require a great deal of reassurance and emotional support.

EMOTIONAL REACTIONS PRECIPITATED BY ORGAN TRANSPLANTS

Until recently, organ transplants were viewed by medical scientists as providing a viable alternative for individuals with seriously damaged organs, especially hearts and kidneys. Unfortunately, the inability to effectively control the problem of tissue rejection has resulted in some surgical centers discontinuing experimentation in cardiac transplants altogether, and in others curtailing the number of kidney transplants performed. Undoubtedly, the problem of tissue rejection will be conquered sometime in the future, but the answer is not yet available.

In addition to the problem of tissue rejection, the difficulty in identifying and obtaining an appropriate organ donor has slowed progress in the treatment of individuals awaiting such surgery.

Almost from the initiation of organ transplant surgery, it was recognized that providing an organ for an individual from the body of another could be an emotionally disturbing experience, both for the person donating the organ and the recipient. Thus psychiatric evaluation of the donor as well as the recipient was begun soon after some of the earliest kidney transplants were performed. Since there were more individuals awaiting transplant surgery than there were appropriate organs available, it was possible to choose the organ recipients carefully. Thus those who were thought to be able to accept an organ from another individual without becoming emotionally disturbed were chosen. Likewise, donors should be stable individuals before agreeing to supply an organ for another. One mother who donated a kidney to a son was heard to shout at him, "What do you expect from me? Wasn't it enough that I gave you life? Do you also demand a part of my body?"

Organ transplant procedures are long and involved surgical techniques. Individuals who are the focus of such procedures are aware of their physical condition and that they are seriously ill. They realize that without a transplant their lives would end within a short time and that the only hope for the future lies in the replacement of the damaged organ. Thus they are willing to undergo the procedure even though they recognize the seriousness of the situation and the possibility that the organ may be rejected. These individuals are understandably fearful of what the future will bring. Although many of the recipients of such surgery have been able to cope successfully with their anxieties and fears, a few have responded with full-blown psychiatric reactions. There are few situations in which an individual is placed under so much tension as when he undergoes an organ transplant. Nurses working with these individuals need to be sensitive to their emotional difficulties, to be realistically reassuring, and to provide as much emotional support as the individuals require. The individual should be encouraged to discuss his concerns and fears about death, dependency on others, and loss of self-esteem. The nurse needs to express concern for the individual and interest in his future welfare.

EMOTIONAL REACTIONS PRECIPITATED BY THE LOSS OF A BODY PART

Every person has a mental image of his own body that is called the *body image.* This body image may be realistic or it may be part of the individual's wish-fulfilling fantasy about himself. To a large extent, an individual functions within the boundaries of this unconscious image. A young man once said in a hopeless voice, "I can never marry. What woman would want a man with one short leg?" This man's body image was so misshapen and ugly that he could not accept it. Because he could not accept his own body, he was convinced that no one else could. He was especially convinced that no woman could want him as a marriage partner. Although he was reasonably attractive, his reaction to all aspects of life was in keeping with this attitude of being worthless and of having an unacceptable body.

Some people maintain an unrealistic image of themselves that was realistic at an earlier period in their lives. For example, it is not uncommon to hear a large, matronly woman ask a saleswoman for a size 12 dress. Without making a comment the understanding clerk brings out the required large size and helps the customer try on the garment.

Surgical removal of a breast or the uterus is among the most emotionally disturbing surgical procedures that women must face. It is unfortunate that many nurses have not been helped to understand the meaning these experiences have for some women and have not been assisted in helping with the feelings precipitated by such surgical procedures.

Although people respond in highly individual and unique ways to the same surgical procedures, almost all women unconsciously feel that they have been mutilated by a breast amputation or the removal of the uterus. If given an opportunity after such a surgical procedure, many women will express feelings about not being a whole woman or about being of less value to the world than they were before the operation. They may express fears about losing the acceptance of their marital partners.

Many women pass through a period of mourning for the lost part of the body. Nurses need to understand the realistic reasons that underlie the frequent tears shed by women hospitalized in a gynecological unit of the hospital and should accept this as an expression of a normal emotional response about an extremely upsetting experience. Crying is probably one of the most helpful ways of expressing grief. Unfortunately, some women cannot cry about this kind of problem. Instead, they sometimes repress their feelings of despair and sadness and respond in other ways that may be more difficult for the nurse to understand and cope with. After breast surgery one individual turned her face to the wall, refused to see any visitors, and requested that even her husband be excluded from the room.

Sadness and mourning may be expressed in a reaction that appears to an observer as an outburst of anger. The individual may respond as does a child when something of value is taken away. This response may be an expression of underlying depression, but the external reaction is one of anger at having lost something that was highly valued. Another frequent response to such a surgical loss is an unconscious feeling on the part of the woman that she is being punished for some real or fantasized transgression that may have occurred years before. This feeling may lead the woman to respond as if she were unworthy of attention from friends or relatives.

The possible reasons for the many emotional reactions to breast amputation and hysterectomy are as varied as the women who require these procedures. The important thing for the nurse to remember is that these experiences are difficult for women to accept, that individuals respond to them in highly individual ways, depending on their life situation and personality, and that the nurse needs to demonstrate an understanding and caring attitude about the woman and her feelings.

Good physical care is always the first place to start in meeting the emotional needs of physically ill persons. Ways in which the nurse can demonstrate a caring attitude about the individual include an unhurried approach, attentive, perceptive listening, and anticipation of physical needs before it is necessary for the individual to ask for care. It is also important that the nurse not respond to the client's anger with an angry response. The nurse will not be tempted to respond in an angry manner if she understands the frustration and fear that is the basis for the client's outburst. Likewise, she will not attempt to minimize the client's concerns by using hollow phrases such as, "Tomorrow will be a better day."

Women are not the only people who are unable to accept an altered body image. All individuals who submit to disfiguring surgery of any type have a variety of fears that focus on their concern about being acceptable to other people, especially to their sexual partners. Operations involving amputation of a leg or disfiguring facial surgery are especially difficult for individuals to accept. However, it has been noted that people are able to accept body mutilation more readily when the location is such that it is evident to everyone. This phenomenon may result from the fact that something that is obvious must be recognized and talked about. Some individuals refrain from mentioning a problem that is hidden under clothing. They are therefore burdened with a tremendous amount of unresolved sensitivity for years. Perhaps the much joked about American habit of discussing one's operation and exhibiting the surgical scar at social gatherings has some psychologically healing attributes. It is therapeutic to help individuals discuss the way they feel about the surgical procedure they have experienced.

Nurses should avoid censuring individuals who blame the surgeon for their disfigured bodies. It is a natural human response to relieve anxiety by blaming someone else for an unhappy situation that the individual cannot control with his usual defenses.

One example of this kind of reaction was a man who was hospitalized for plastic reconstruction of a thumb that was lost in an accident involving high-voltage electricity. After several skin grafts and months of hospitalization, the man was disturbed when he saw the reconstructed thumb. It was many times larger than a normal thumb and was covered with short hair because the skin graft had been taken from the patient's thigh. He had expected a normal-looking thumb and had looked forward to having a functioning hand as a reward for the long period of boring hospitalization. He was bitterly disappointed and disgusted at the appearance of the thumb. He remarked to the nurse, "Look at that! It's obscene. I am going to sign myself out of this hospital and have my own doctor cut this thing off." The nurse reported this reaction to the head nurse who said, "He should be ashamed of himself for criticizing his doctor, who is the best plastic surgeon in this part of the country. The doctor has worked terribly hard on that thumb."

The individual did leave the hospital against medical advice. He was angry and disappointed. If someone had explained that the surgeon planned to shape the thumb to normal proportions after the body had established effective circulation to the new tissues, he might have been helped to wait for a few more weeks for the surgeon to complete the delicate and tedious work. Unfortunately, the nurse with whom the client had developed a positive relationship did not know enough about plastic surgery to use the opportunity to be helpful at the time when he needed reassurance. This incident highlights the importance of the nurse's possessing and using scientifically correct knowledge concerning the nature of the illness and treatment.

A colostomy is another emotionally disturbing experience for individuals. In our culture the emphasis placed on cleanliness and fastidiousness in personal hygiene creates a serious conflict for those who find it medically necessary to resort to a colostomy. Cultural attitudes toward toileting, which are taught early in a child's life, sometimes cause the adult to rebel at the thought of caring for a colostomy. Probably no surgical procedure has the potential for presenting individuals with more emotional and social problems than does a colostomy. Although hundreds of individuals have been able to adjust successfully to a colostomy, the nurse should not forget that the person who is just beginning to cope with the problems presented by the loss of normal bowel function has many hurdles ahead of him. Individuals who have undergone a colostomy worry about their acceptability to their friends and their sexual partners. Persons who have received support in working through their feelings about their colostomies report that they have been able to maintain satisfying sexual relations. Unfortunately, others find that it becomes emotionally impossible for them to do so.

It is helpful if individuals with a colostomy are encouraged to express their feelings, attitudes, and questions about their condition. Individuals are not helped by nurses who insist on the light, gay approach and refuse to involve themselves in serious conversation about these problems. The person with a colostomy deserves a nurse who will give his situation thoughtful, sympathetic, realistic consideration.

Such procedures as colostomy operations are performed only when they are necessary to save the individual's life. The nurse cannot alter the problems that such an operation presents, but she can help the individual to talk about the problem, to accept the reality of the situation, and to learn all he can about his condition so that he can handle it as effectively as possible. The following clinical report illustrates the effect that a colostomy can have on some fastidious people.

> A fastidious man who understood English poorly entered the hospital with a diagnosis of far-advanced carcinoma of the rectum. He had suffered a great deal before coming to the hospital and was grateful when surgery relieved the pain. A colostomy opening was established. His physical recovery was rapid. When he was discharged, he left many gifts for the hospital staff. In every way he appeared to be happy and grateful. The surgeon had attempted to explain the seriousness of the problem to the patient before surgery. The hospital staff believed that the man understood the nature of his operation and the need for a permanent colostomy. One week after discharge he returned to the surgical clinic and requested admission to the hospital to have the colostomy

> opening closed. Again the surgeon explained the nature of the operation and the permanent character of the surgery. The individual left the clinic without appearing to be upset. The next day the newspapers carried a notice of his suicide.

The problems experienced by this individual undoubtedly grew out of his language handicap and his attitude toward the importance of physical cleanliness. Although his response to the colostomy was unusual, many individuals will admit that in the beginning of their experience with a colostomy, they occasionally wondered if life was worthwhile under such circumstances. Of particular significance in this situation was this individual's lack of expression of any negative feelings. If the health care personnel truly understood and appreciated the huge emotional significance of a colostomy, they would have viewed this man's behavior as an untoward response and could have intervened in a way that might have prevented his suicide.

Surgical operations on the male genitourinary tract sometimes cause severe emotional conflicts. Occasionally such an operation precipitates a psychotic reaction. The following clinical report presents an example of such a situation.

> A middle-aged gentleman who was a devoted church member was admitted to a surgical unit because of symptoms of prostatic hypertrophy. A successful operation was performed to relieve the distressing symptoms. Within 1 or 2 days he was complaining of the suggestive pictures on the walls of his room, which he said the hospital authorities had placed there for the purpose of tormenting him. The nurses were confused by these complaints because no pictures were hanging in his room. A psychiatrist was called to talk with the individual who told the psychiatrist that the annoying pictures were of young, nude women. The gentleman stated that a man of his principles should not be surrounded by such lewd art.

The psychiatrist concluded that the individual was not able to accept the fact that a man of his social standing would indulge in such an active fantasy life dealing with sexual material. To relieve his own anxiety about his unconscious sexual longings, which were dramatically brought to light by his complaint about the nude pictures, he unconsciously used the mechanism of projection. It was much more acceptable to him and safer from the standpoint of self-esteem to blame the hospital for hanging nude pictures around the room than to accept the explanation that the pictures represented his own fantasies.

This unusual reaction was undoubtedly precipitated by the surgical procedure, but it would not be accurate to say that the procedure caused the response. During most of this individual's life he probably had exerted a great deal of emotional energy to repress unacceptable sexual thoughts. The emotional crisis presented by the surgical experience was apparently enough to make it impossible for him to continue to keep his unacceptable thoughts repressed.

EMOTIONAL REACTIONS PRECIPITATED BY CARDIAC SURGERY

Individuals respond to life-threatening situations uniquely, depending on the coping mechanisms that have been developed and the attitude of personal security they maintain. In view of this, it is difficult, if not impossible, to predict how a specific individual will respond to any surgical procedure, especially one that is potentially as dangerous as cardiac surgery.

No matter how well the individual appears to be anticipating the procedure, the nurse must realize that cardiac surgery is a major crisis and that the person is struggling to control feelings of anxiety and fear. He cannot avoid being concerned about the possibility of death and the separation from family and friends.

Individuals who have accepted the fact that they must undergo cardiac surgery have come to this decision after months or years of cardiac symptomatology. They may have been semi-invalids because of these symptoms, or the surgery may have been planned in the hope of preventing future invalidism. Thus the individual's fear of the outcome of the procedure is coupled with his anticipation of great improvement in his health in the immediate future.

The nurse who is assigned to the individual before cardiac surgery should be prepared to anticipate any number of reactions, depending on the individual's personality. He may deny the seriousness of the situation and avoid discussing it. This attitude probably suggests that he finds it difficult to bear the burden and thus copes by avoiding the topic. A different person may discuss his fears, may become tearful, and, by identifying many personal needs, may insist that the nurse stay with him. A third individual may appear to be angry and sarcastic and may be critical of the way the nurse performs the necessary nursing procedures. Each of these individuals deserves a calm, empathic nurse who is a good listener and who understands that the emotional response the individual is exhibiting is his way of coping with a situation that presents him with a personal crisis. The nurse should encourage him to express his feelings and concerns and should respond to his questions in an honest, straightforward manner without alarming him. The individual deserves to be assured that he will be cared for by a team of physicians and nurses who are knowledgeable, skillful, and deeply interested in his welfare and comfort.

After the surgical procedure the individual will be helpless and dependent for a short time. As he becomes aware of his dependence on others and on mechanical devices, he may respond in a variety of ways. He may be depressed and hopeless or angry and sarcastic. The postsurgical response is dependent to a large extent on the coping mechanisms the individual has used in the past.

Just as in the presurgery period, these patients require a quiet, calm, reassuring nurse who listens carefully to their comments and encourages them to express their anxieties and concerns. Reassurance is essential for these individuals, as is focusing on the reality of the improvement they are making.

Only nurses who are sensitive, caring people who can gain the patients' confidence should be assigned to work with these individuals.

EMOTIONAL REACTIONS PRECIPITATED BY AN UNTOWARD OBSTETRICAL EXPERIENCE

Many nurses choose to work in obstetrics because the obstetrical unit is said to be a happy place. In talking about their work, obstetrical nurses frequently emphasize the great happiness of mothers and fathers when a new baby is born. It is true that there is much happiness among new parents, but nurses should not overlook the fact that there are a few new mothers who are emotionally distressed and in great need of understanding and reassurance because they have delivered imperfect babies or their babies have failed to survive. Young mothers who deliver imperfect babies may be as troubled as mothers whose babies are stillborn. Death is an accomplished, final fact that a mother can be helped to accept and occasionally to understand. Death of a new baby will undoubtedly precipitate sadness and grief in the mother, as well as questions about her adequacy as a woman. However, our culture has provided some ways of helping people handle these feelings. Funeral services provide culturally sanctioned opportunities for the expression of grief. Families and friends offer emotional support at such a time. Some mothers can console themselves by looking forward to a second child.

Production of perfect babies has traditionally been thought to be one of the most important tasks performed by women. When a woman fails in this effort, she sometimes wonders about her effectiveness and her intrinsic value. Therefore mothers of imperfectly formed babies or premature infants are frequently distressed by doubts concerning their own adequacy as women and by guilt about their responsibility for the existence of the problem. It may surprise some nurses to learn that almost all mothers whose babies are born prematurely or congenitally imperfect respond with questions that reflect concern about themselves. They ask questions such as, "What did I do to cause this?" or "Why has this happened to me?" Since the cause of prematurity and many congenital imperfections is not fully understood, scientific explanations of these events often cannot be given. Even when scientific explanations are available, they do little to remove the personal sense of failure these mothers often feel.

Guilt causes people to feel uncomfortable. When a mother feels guilty about her baby's imperfections, she may reject it outright or may spend the rest of her life punishing herself for failing to give her child a perfect body. This punishment may take the form of slavishly serving the child in an attempt to make up in every possible way for the child's poor start in life. This reaction is one of the disguised forms that rejection may take.

As in many other situations, the nurse cannot alter the reality of the difficult situation but can encourage the mother to talk about her feelings. If the mother can be helped to discuss some of these feelings, she may come to feel less guilty and may be able to clear away some of the emotion about the problem so that constructive steps can be taken and solutions can be planned.

Some women who have set high achievement goals for themselves find it particularly difficult to accept an imperfect baby. The following clinical report demonstrates this point.

> An English professor from a large midwestern university found that she was pregnant for the first time at the age of 40. She and her husband were moderately happy about this new development in their lives. However, they were sorry to have to give up their plans for a sabbatical leave and a trip abroad. When the baby boy was born, he had a bilateral harelip and a cleft palate. When the nurse brought the baby to the mother, she looked at him and said, "That can't possibly be my child." The nurse assured the mother that it was her little boy. She said to the nurse, "Don't bring that baby in here again. I won't have a baby that looks like that!" In 5 days the mother left the hospital without asking to see her baby again. The father arranged for a nurse to help him take his son to a distant city where he had an appointment with a famous surgeon who specialized in repairing harelips. Within a few weeks, the mother began to experience overwhelming feelings of anxiety and guilt for which she saw no cause. These feelings became so intense that she sought professional help. Through psychotherapy this mother eventually was able to understand the highly personalized meaning that the birth of her imperfect baby had for her.

EMOTIONAL REACTIONS PRECIPITATED BY AN ABORTION

There are few situations in a woman's life that have such a potential for producing a variety of emotional responses as does abortion. The response on the part of the woman involved is a highly individual one dependent on many factors. Some of these factors include her religious beliefs and cultural background. Some religious groups are explicit in their teaching against abortion, whereas others are more inclined to leave such a decision to the woman and her physician. Some cultures emphasize the relationship between a woman's intrinsic value to society and her ability to produce children; others place more importance on the quality of life that can be provided for the mother and child. Another factor is the woman's relationship with the father. If the relationship is a stable one and the man agrees that abortion is a wise decision, the reaction of the woman may be less emotionally distressing than if he wishes her to maintain the pregnancy. If the pregnancy is unwanted because of the circumstances surrounding conception (such as rape) or if by genetic counseling techniques the fetus has been identified as being seriously defective, the opportunity for abortion may be greeted with relief.

Some individuals may be convinced that they have discarded the early religious instructions that they received and the attitudes taught within the family about such controversial questions as abortion. However, these attitudes are difficult to discard and may greatly influence the woman's emotional response even though they are not recognized consciously.

Many women are able to accept an abortion without experiencing any untoward emotional reactions. However, it is not uncommon for selected individuals to express feelings of serious personal loss, deep regret, shame, guilt, a loss of self-esteem, and sadness. Such individuals may have difficulty in sleeping, experience a loss of appetite, exhibit a lack of interest in their home and work, express resentment toward the man involved, and cry frequently.

Unless the nurse visits in the home or works with women in a clinic situation, there is little opportunity to be helpful to these individuals, since abortion is usually a procedure that is completed within an 8- or 10-hour period and usually does not require overnight hospitalization.

If opportunities are available, it is helpful to encourage the woman to discuss her feelings and how she perceives the situation. In selected individuals an abortion may precipitate a crisis. In this case the person should be treated as any other individual who is overwhelmed by a problem of daily living.

Women who are anticipating an abortion should have an opportunity to think the situation through with the help of a nurse therapist. Since abortion is irreversible, alternatives should be thoroughly explored before a choice is made.

EMOTIONAL ASPECTS OF DEATH AND DYING

No discussion of the emotional needs of the physically ill would be complete without addressing the needs of the individual who is dying. With the development of complex medical technology the ability to prolong life has increased. This ability has raised questions about the quality of life and in the opinion of some has contributed to the unconsciously held belief that death occurs only as a result of the failure of the individual or the health care team to "try hard enough."

It is important for all health care personnel to understand that death is an inevitability and that dying persons have a right to be treated in a humane manner. The specter of a dying person surrounded by machines and technicians so that the family cannot even reach him is frightening. The opposite often occurs as well, namely, that the person who is terminally ill is figuratively abandoned. Individuals in this situation are often relegated to rooms furthest away from the nurse's station, receive only cursory attention from medical and nursing staff, and may have few visitors.

The nurse must be concerned about remedying both of these extreme situations. Nursing, more than any other health care profession, has the opportunity and the obligation to assist the dying person and his family to achieve a satisfactory resolution of this last phase of life. To fulfill this responsibility the nurse needs to develop an understanding of the emotional needs of the terminally ill person.

Dr. Elisabeth Kübler-Ross, a pioneer in thanatology, has studied the responses of hundreds of terminally ill persons. Her subjects included persons of all ages, socioeconomic levels, and cultural backgrounds. These persons also represented a wide variety of illnesses and injuries, both acute and chronic. Regardless of their differences, Dr. Kübler-Ross found that all dying persons progress through a similar process of emotional response. Her formulation, which is probably familiar to most nurses, delineates five stages of dying.

Denial is the initial response caused by the person not being able to deal emotionally with the reality of his impending death. To deal with the intense anxiety that this news engenders, the person uses the ego defense of denial. As a result, persons in this stage often express the belief that a mistake has been made in laboratory reports or that the physician is incompetent. As with any person who is using the defense of denial, the nurse will be most helpful if she understands that this defense is operative because the individual has sustained a massive emotional assault with which he cannot deal directly without endangering the integrity of his personality. Consequently, the wise nurse intervenes in a manner that allows the individual to maintain this defense while simultaneously not avoiding the reality of the situation. For example, the nurse would not encourage a person who is in this stage of the dying process to make plans for his funeral, but she would encourage him to take his medications as they were prescribed. Because the reality of the situation is such that the individual soon becomes sicker, the length of this stage is relatively short in individuals who are mentally healthy. It should be noted that illnesses that initially do not have symptoms that cause incapacitation, such as chronic lymphocytic leukemia, may enable even mentally healthy persons to cling to the denial of the fact that they are dying.

Anger characterizes the second stage of the dying process. During this stage individuals often feel as if they are victims of fate, circumstances, medical incompetence, or a vengeful God. Their thoughts and verbalizations center around the question of, "Why me?" They fear the dependency their illness creates and often resent their family and the health care workers who try to be of help. Since feeling and expressing anger are not acceptable to many people, some dying persons may express their anger in covert, rather than overt ways. Most nurses recognize the anger and underlying anxiety in terminally ill individuals who complain about everything and everyone. Only the sensitive, insightful nurse recognizes the same dynamics in the individual who expresses his anger in passive ways, such as "forgetting" to take his medication and then asking the nurse what he should do.

Bargaining is the third stage of the dying process characterized by the individual attempting to gain more time by trading off "good" behavior. Most commonly, the dying individual bargains with supernatural powers—God, fate, or whatever higher Being he believes can effect a change in his condition. Bargaining takes the form of, "If you (let me live until Christmas) then I (will bequeath half of my money to the church)." The behavior that the person "trades off" is highly individualized and is probably related to earlier unresolved conflicts. The bargaining stage is helpful to the dying person in that it temporarily eases his anxiety and enables him to deal with the pain and dependence that may accompany his illness.

The *depression* stage follows bargaining. Depression begins when the reality of the situation can no longer be ignored and the uselessness of denial, anger, and bargaining is apparent. The depression that the individual feels is a response to an overwhelming sense of anticipated loss—the loss of his entire world. At this stage the dying person looks and acts depressed and often has no need to talk with others about how he feels. He must use his energy to confront the fact that what is done is done, and what is undone will remain so. Because he is depressed, the person in this stage of dying makes few demands. Consequently, his behavior is often misinterpreted as "cooperative."

Acceptance is the final stage of the dying process when the individual has come to peace with himself about the fact that his death is imminent. Acceptance is characterized by an affective void; the person is not happy, nor is he depressed. His interests, even in his own care, narrow. During this time only those persons who are most significant to him are able to elicit a positive response. The presence of others is merely tolerated. This does not mean, however, that the dying person cannot receive comfort from the nursing interventions of a warm, caring nurse. It does mean that the most effective interventions are likely to be nonverbal in the form of physical comfort measures delivered in a competent, compassionate way.

Understanding the emotional needs of the dying person is of value to the nurse only if she is able to combine this knowledge with self-understanding. Since death and dying is not viewed by our culture as a natural phenomenon, nurses, like most people, have been taught since early childhood to avoid the subject of death. This cultural attitude may be compounded by the developmental stage of the nurse herself. The developmental stages of adulthood and middle age are the stages most nurses are in and may prove to be particularly problematic in regard to the issue of death and dying. The stage of adulthood, especially early adulthood, is a time when people view all things as being possible. As a result, the nurse in this stage may be prone to view the terminally ill person as representative of the failure of the health care team. The nurse who is dealing with the developmental tasks of middle age may be actively dealing with the awareness of her own mortality reinforced by the declining health of her parents. The terminally ill person may represent the nurse's vulnerability to the prospect of her own death.

In either instance, the nurse may feel anxious and guilt ridden and avoid dealing with her feelings by avoiding the patient. During those times when the nurse cannot avoid the person, she avoids the reality of the situation by assuming a false air of cheerfulness, by changing the subject when the person or his family start to talk about death, or by not answering the client's questions. Other nurses may respond angrily to the dying person, as if his dying were his fault. This counterproductive response seems especially justifiable to the nurse when the dying person's poor health habits, such as smoking, have obviously contributed to his terminal illness. Only if the nurse can be helped to explore and confront her own feelings about the dying process will she be able to give the skilled, compassionate care the dying person deserves.

SELF-HELP GROUPS

The nurse should make an effort to become aware of the increasing number of community-based organizations designed to provide information and support to individuals and their families who have experienced certain medical or surgical procedures or the death of a family member. For example, there are Ostomy Clubs throughout the country whose members are people who have had ileostomies or colostomies and who meet regularly to discuss with each other the ways in which they have solved the problems they encounter. In some parts of the country, similar groups are available for persons who have undergone mastectomies, laryngectomies, abortions, or myocardial infarcts. By being aware of the availability of these organizations in the community, the nurse will be in a position to inform others of them. Although these clubs are not designed to substitute for medical supervision, the value of the support and understanding that can be gained from persons who have had similar experiences is inestimable in helping individuals and families to regain or attain a state of positive mental health.

CONCLUDING STATEMENTS

1. The large majority of complaints made by individuals concerning their hospital care have to do with the failure of professional nurses to establish satisfying interpersonal relationships with them.
2. The understanding and emotional support that physically ill people deserve and are demanding is omitted more often because the nurse does not understand the character of the emotional needs of the individuals and how to cope with them, rather than because time is not available to give this type of help.
3. Any physical illness for which hospitalization is necessary forces the individual to assume a dependent role that may be disturbing and may cause him to react with what is sometimes called uncooperative behavior.
4. People who are newly admitted to general hospitals may feel frightened and may develop a sense of having lost their identity.
5. Individuals who must rely on mechanical devices, such as dialysis machines and pacemakers, often feel that they have lost control of their bodies and of their destinies.
6. Providing an organ for an individual from the body of another can be an emotionally disturbing experience, both for the person donating the organ and for the recipient. There are few situations in which an individual is placed under so much tension as when he undergoes an organ transplant.
7. Every individual has a mental picture of his body, which is called the body image and which may be realistic or part of the individual's wish-fulfilling fantasy about himself.
8. Surgical removal of a breast or the uterus is among the most emotionally disturbing surgical procedures that women may be called on to accept.

9. Although people respond in highly individual and unique ways to the same surgical procedures, almost all women unconsciously feel they have been mutilated by amputation of a breast or the removal of the uterus.
10. All individuals who submit to disfiguring surgery of any type have a variety of fears that focus on their concern about being acceptable to other people, especially their sexual partners.
11. In this culture the emphasis placed on cleanliness and fastidiousness in personal hygiene creates a serious emotional conflict for individuals who find it medically necessary to resort to a colostomy.
12. The nurse is being therapeutic when she helps individuals to talk about the way they feel regarding the surgical procedure that they have experienced.
13. Mothers of imperfectly formed or premature babies may be distressed by doubts concerning their own adequacy as women and are guilt ridden concerning their own responsibility for the existence of the problem.
14. As in many other situations, the nurse cannot alter the reality of the difficult situation for the new mother with an imperfect baby but can encourage her to talk about her feelings and help to lessen her guilt. This may make it possible for the new mother to view the problem realistically and to plan solutions.
15. It is important for all health care personnel to understand that death is an inevitability and that dying persons have a right to be treated in a humane manner.
16. Dr. Elisabeth Kübler-Ross has deliniated five stages in the dying process: denial, anger, bargaining, depression, and acceptance.
17. Understanding the emotional needs of the dying person is of value to the nurse only if she is able to combine this knowledge with self-understanding.
18. The value of the support and understanding that can be gained from participation in self-help groups is inestimable in helping individuals and families regain or attain a state of positive mental health.

Suggested sources of additional information

CLASSICAL

Craytor, Josephine K.: Talking with persons who have cancer, Am. J. Nurs. **69**:744-748, 1969.

Francis, Gloria M.: Cancer: the emotional component, Am. J. Nurs. **69**:1677-1681, 1969.

Ingals, Thelma: Do patients feel lost in a general hospital? Am. J. Nurs. **60**:648-651, 1960.

Kübler-Ross, Elisabeth: On death and dying, New York, 1969, Macmillan Publishing Co., Inc.

Larsen, Virginia A.: What hospitalization means to patients, Am. J. Nurs. **61**:44-47, May, 1961.

Martin, Harry W., and Prange, Arthur J.: The stages of illness—psychosocial approach, Nurs. Outlook **4**:168-171, March, 1962.

Mead, Margaret: Understanding cultural patterns, Nurs. Outlook **4**:260-262, May, 1956.

Quint, Jeanne C.: The impact of mastectomy, Am. J. Nurs. **63**:89-92, Nov., 1963.

Van Bree, Nancee S.: Sexuality, nursing practice, and the person with cardiac disease, Nurs. Forum **14**:397-411, 1975.

Velazquez, Janet M.: Alienation, Am. J. Nurs. **69**:301-304, 1969.

Wesseling, Elizabeth: The adolescent facing amputation, Am. J. Nurs. **65**:90-94, Jan., 1965.

CONTEMPORARY

Brolin, Rose Homan, and Auld, Margaret E.: Hodgkin's disease, Am. J. Nurs. **74**:1982-1986, 1974.

Bowlby, John: Loss, New York, 1980, Basic Books, Inc., Publishers.

Boyle, Mary A., and Cinca, Rudy L. Amyotrophic lateral sclerosis, Am. J. Nurs. **76**:66-68, 1976.

Bragg, T.L.: Psychological response to myocardial infarction, Nurs. Forum, **14**:383-395, 1975.

Breu, Christine, and Dracup, Kathleen: Helping the spouses of critically ill patients, Am. J. Nurs. **78**:50-53, Jan., 1978.

Burgess, Helen A., et al.: When a patient on lithium is pregnant, Am. J. Nurs. **79**:1989-1990, Nov., 1979.

Cantor, Robert C.: And a time to live, New York, 1980, Harper & Row, Publishers.

Copp, Laurel Archer: The spectrum of suffering, Am. J. Nurs. **74**:491-495, 1974.

Covelli Pat: Borrowing time, Philadelphia, 1980, J.P. Lippincott Co.

Cressy, Mary K.: Psychiatric nursing intervention with a colostomy patient, Perspect. Psychiatr. Care **10**:69-71, April-June, 1972.

Dafflitti, Judith Gregorie, and Swanson, Donna: Group sessions for the wives of home-hemodialysis patients, Am. J. Nurs. **75**:633-635, 1975.

Davidson, Shirlee, and Noyes, Russell: Psychiatric nursing consultation on a burn unit, Am. J. Nurs. **73**:1715-1718, 1973.

Davis, Marcella Z.: Socioemotional component of coronary care, Am. J. Nurs. **72**:705-709, 1972.

Doyle, Phyllis B., et al.: Helping the severely handicapped child, New York, 1980, Lippincott and Crowell.

Ellis, Rosemary: Unusual sensory and thought disturbances after cardiac surgery, Am. J. Nurs. **72:**2021-2025, 1972.

Fagerhaugh, Shizuko Yoshimura: Mental illness and the tuberculosis patient, Nurs. Outlook **18:**38-41, Aug., 1970.

Featherstone, Helen: A difference in the family, New York, 1980, Basic Books, Inc., Publishers.

Foster, Sue, and Andreoli, Kathleen: Behavior following acute myocardial infarction Am. J. Nurs. **70:**2344-2348, 1970.

Francone, Carol A.: My battle against Wilson's disease, Am. J. Nurs. **76:**247-249, 1976.

Fultz, John M., et al.: When a narcotic addict is hospitalized, Am. J. Nurs. **80:**478-482, March, 1980.

Garfield, Charles A.: Stress and survival: the emotional realities of life-threatening illness, St. Louis, 1979, The C.V. Mosby Co.

Grace, Mary Jo: The psychiatric nurse specialist and medical surgical patients, Am. J. Nurs. **74:**481-483, 1974.

Hagin, Joan M.: Infant death: nursing interaction and intervention with grieving families, Nurs. Forum **13:**371-385, 1974.

Harrell, Helen C.: To lose a breast, Am. J. Nurs. **72:**676-677, 1972.

Heusinkveld, Karen Billars: Cues to communication with the terminal cancer patient, Nurs. Forum **11:**103-113, 1972.

Jansson, Diane P.: Student consultation: a liaison psychiatric experience for nursing students, Perspect. Psychiatr. Care **17:**77-82, March-April, 1979.

Jontz, Donna Lynn: Presceiption for living with M.S., Am. J. Nurs. **73:**817-818, 1973.

Kleinman, Carol S.: Psychological processes during pregnancy, Perspect. Psychiatr. Care **15:**175-178, 1977.

Kübler-Ross, Elisabeth: Questions and answers on death and dying, New York, 1974, Macmillan Publishing Co., Inc.

Lambert, Vickie A., and Lambert, Clinton E.: The impact of physical illness and related mental health concepts, Englewood Cliffs, N.J., 1979, Prentice-Hall, Inc.

Lerner, Gerda: A death of one's own, New York, 1980, Harper & Row, Publishers.

Loxley, Alice Keating: The emotional toll of crippling deformity, Am. J. Nurs. **75:**1839-1840, 1972.

McLachlan, Eileen: Recognizing pain, Am. J. Nurs. **74:**496-497, 1974.

Maxwell, Sister Marie Bernadette: A terminally ill adolescent and her family, Am. J. Nurs. **72:**925-927, 1972.

Neu, Carlos: Coping with newly diagnosed blindness, Am. J. Nurs. **75:**2161-2163, 1975.

Noble, Mary Ann: Communication in the ICU: therapeutic or disturbing, Nurs. Outlook **27:**195-198, March, 1979.

Perron, Denise M.: Deprived of sound, Am. J. Nurs. **74:**1057-1059, 1974.

Pisarcik, Gail, et al.: Psychiatric nurses in the emergency room, Am. J. Nurs. **79:**1264-1266, July, 1979.

Reix, Laura: Managing a life with chronic disease, Am. J. Nurs. **73:**261-264, 1973.

Santopietro, Mary-Charles S.: Meeting the emotional needs of hemodialysis patients and their spouses, Am. J. Nurs. **75**:629-632, 1975.

Schneidman, Edwin: Voices of death, New York, 1980, Harper & Row, Publishers.

Severin, Nelda K., and Becker, Robert E.: Nurses as psychiatric consultants in a general hospital emergency room, Community Ment. Health J. **10**:261-267, Fall, 1974.

Seward, Elizabeth M.: Preventing postpartum psychosis, Am. J. Nurs. **75**:520-523, 1972.

Shufer, Shirley: Communication with young children: teaching via the play-discussion group. I., Am. J. Nurs. **77**:1960-1962, Dec., 1977.

Simenon, Georges: The bells of bicetre, New York, 1965, The New American Library Inc.

Tatelbaum, Judy: The courage to grieve, New York, 1980, Lippincott and Crowell.

Tiedt, Eileen: The psychodynamic process of the oncological experience, Nurs. Forum **14**:265-277, 1975.

Weinstein, Leslie J., Chapman, Mary M., and Stallings, Mary A.: Organizing approaches to psychiatric nursing consultation, Perspect. Psychiatr. Care **17**:66-71, March-April, 1979.

Whitman, Helen M., and Lukes, Shelby J.: Behavior modification for terminally ill patients, Am. J. Nurs. **75**:98-101, 1975.

Williams, Margaret A.: Cultural patterning of the feminine role—a factor in the response to hysterectomy, Nurs. Forum **12**:379-387, 1973.

Wittkower, Eric D., and Warnes, Hector: Psychosomatic medicine: its clinical applications, New York, 1977, Harper & Row, Publishers.

Zahourek, Rothyln, and Jensen, Joseph S.: Grieving and loss of the newborn, Am. J. Nurs. **73**:838-839, 1973

Zahourek, Rothlyn, and Tower, Margene: Therapeutic abortion: the psychiatric nurse as therapist, liaison, and consultant, Perspect. Psychiatr. Care **9**:64-71, March-April, 1971.

OF PARTICULAR INTEREST

Kübler-Ross, Elisabeth: Questions and answers on death and dying, New York, 1974, MacMillan Publishing Co., Inc.

This is a classic book about the process of death and dying. It contains the author's formulation of the stages of the dying process. It is essential reading for all students of nursing.

Simenon, Georges: The bells of bicetre, New York, 1965, The New American Library Inc.

This book is recommended for every student and every member of the therapeutic team. It is concerned with the experiences and reactions of a patient hospitalized after a cerebrovascular accident.

SECTION SEVEN

Altering maladaptive behavioral patterns through the use of treatment modalities and settings

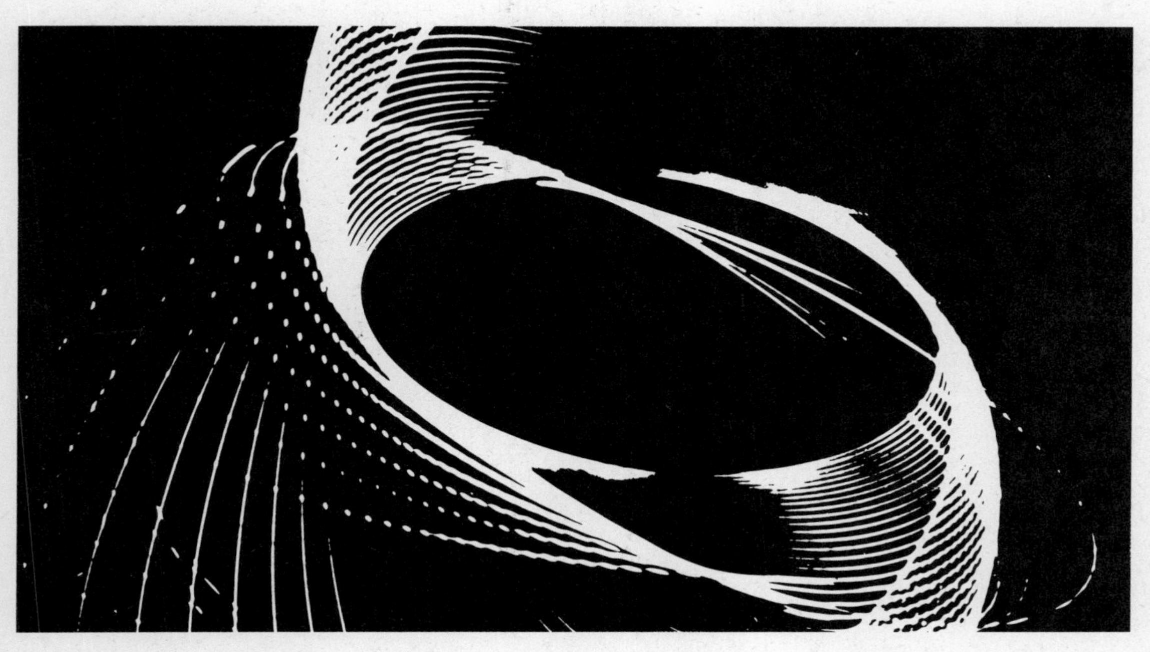

Section Seven presents a discussion of treatment modalities and settings that have general relevance to the care of the mentally ill. In addition, the roles and functions of other mental health workers are presented so that the nurse can use this knowledge to facilitate interdisciplinary collaboration in the care of the mentally ill.

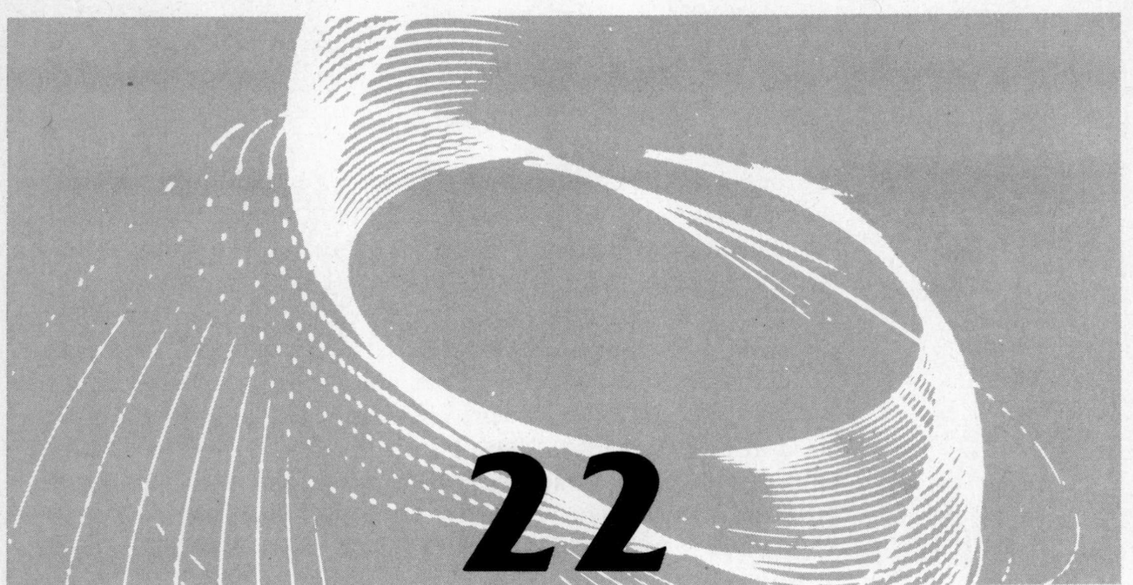

22

Somatic therapies

- Psychotropic drugs
- Insulin shock therapy
- Electroconvulsive therapy
- Psychosurgery
- Other somatic therapies

Through the ages the human race has searched for treatments with which to solve the problem of mental illness, a problem that has been present among a few members of the human family since the beginning of time. Treatment has ranged from trephining the skull, which was used by prehistoric man, to soft music and beautiful surroundings, which were used by the ancient Greeks. Floggings, purgings, and starvation were used in more recent times. A variety of primitive shock treatments have been used in past centuries. These have included throwing individuals into a pit filled with snakes and ducking them in ice-cold water. Benjamin Rush, who was America's first psychiatrist, lived between the years of 1745 and 1813. He worked at Pennsylvania Hospital in Philadelphia and devised an instrument, the gyrator, for the treatment of mental illness. It employed a system of centrifugal action to whirl the person about to increase the flow of blood to his brain. About 1792 Dr. Rush invented the "tranquilizer," a type of restraint, and the ducking stool.

Many of these strenuous attempts to restore a person's normal behavior were based on the belief that the person had lost his senses as a result of an emotional crisis and that restoration would be achieved when he experienced another equally disturbing event. Tranquility for emotionally disturbed individuals has always been one of the goals of treatment and remains one of the goals today.

In more modern times the cold, wet sheet pack and the continuous tub bath were used in attempts to help individuals achieve more tranquil emotional states. The individual reactions to these measures varied widely.

One of the first drugs to be used for its tranquilizing effect was reserpine, which is the purified alkaloid of *Rauwolfia serpentina*. Although reserpine is somewhat effective in relaxing and quieting overactive individuals, this drug has a delayed action, tends to intensify depression, and is associated with gastrointestinal hemorrhage. It has been largely replaced by the newer psychopharmacological agents that were introduced in the United States in 1953 on a research basis. Use of these drugs in the treatment of mental illness has had a dramatic effect on the care of emotionally ill people and on the national attitude toward all aspects of mental illness.

Although much is still to be learned about the psychological effect of the psychotropic drugs, they appear to modify certain aspects of mental and emotional illness without having a stupefying effect. Many of these drugs have the advantage of producing normalization of thinking and behavior rather than tranquilization. Although these drugs can be effective in a wide range of mental illnesses, it appears that the more acute the symptoms, the more dramatic the individual's response to the drug will be.

PSYCHOTROPIC DRUGS

The psychotropic drugs have been widely prescribed and remarkably effective in their own right. Because of them, other treatment modalities, such as psychotherapy and the various group therapies, have been made available to large numbers of individuals. Although the psychotropic drugs do not cure mental illness, they do normalize behavior. Thus many people are able, for the first time, to participate therapeutically with others in a variety of group activities. Mental health centers are able to focus more attention on providing therapeutic experiences instead of expending most of the available manpower in controlling behavior and in keeping individuals fed, clothed, and bathed.

One of the most dramatic results of the use of psychotropic drugs is the ability of many severely disturbed persons to return to their community after the administration of antipsychotic drugs. Some are able to reestablish their roles in the family, and others return to their jobs. These drugs have made possible the movement of thousands of individuals out of large public psychiatric hospitals into community treatment centers. Thus the care and treatment of mentally ill people has been dramatically altered by the introduction of the psychotropic drugs.

The term *psychotropic drugs* refers to any drug that has the effect of altering the mind. Drugs that have an antipsychotic effect, such as the phenothiazine derivatives, and drugs that have an antianxiety effect, such as the benzodiazepine derivatives, are commonly referred to as major and minor tranquilizers. Many authorities believe that these terms are misnomers in that the main effect of these drugs is not tranquilization, but rather clearing of the sensorium in the case of the antipsychotic drugs, and lowering of anxiety in the case of the antianxiety drugs. To be sure, "tranquilization" often occurs with the administration of these drugs, but it is thought to be a result of the individual's increased ability to test and deal with reality. At the very least, the designation of these drugs as major or minor is misleading in that all these drugs are potent chemical agents that have a major effect on the body chemistry. The false belief that the antianxiety drugs are "minor tranquilizers" may have contributed to their being inappropriately prescribed for individuals who are not mentally ill but who are experiencing the anxiety associated with crisis states. In many instances these drugs are abused by individuals who seek relief from anxiety. This practice is dangerous because these drugs not only create a physiological disequilibrium, but they may also create a false sense of well-being, decreasing the person's motivation to address and solve those problems from which the anxiety stems.

In addition to the antipsychotic and antianxiety drugs, there are two other categories of commonly used psychotropic drugs: the antidepressants and lithium carbonate. The psychiatric nurse must be knowledgeable about the actions, side effects, and untoward effects of the drugs in each of these four categories, since their use is so prevalent and since the nurse is most often in the position of administering them and monitoring their effects.

Antipsychotic drugs

In 1956 the most useful of the new drugs, chlorpromazine, was introduced. It was marketed under the name of Thorazine and is only one of several examples of the family of drugs known as the *phenothiazine derivatives.* All the drugs in this group have essentially the same action. They are especially helpful to individuals who demonstrate psychotic symptoms related to schizophrenia. For this reason they are referred to as antipsychotic drugs because they seem to reduce psychotic symptoms. Thus excited, overactive individuals are calmed by these drugs; withdrawn, inactive individuals become normally active; and hallucinated, de-

Table 5 *Antipsychotic psychotropic drugs*

Generic name	Trade name	Range of daily oral dosage (mg)	Comments
Phenothiazine derivatives: dimethylamine subgroup			
Chlorpromazine	Thorazine	100-1500	
Triflupromazine	Vesprin	20-200	
Phenothiazine derivatives: piperidine subgroup			
Thioridazine	Mellaril	100-800	
Piperacetazine	Quide	20-160	
Mesoridazine	Serentil	30-400	Schizophrenia, organic mental disorders, and alcoholism are often treated with Serentil.
Phenothiazine derivatives: piperazine subgroup			
Acetophenazine	Tindal	40-80	
Fluphenazine	Prolixin	1-5	Often given intramuscularly at a dosage two to three times *less* than orally.
Perphenazine	Trilafon	6-64	
Trifluoperazine	Stelazine	2-40	
Prochlorperazine	Compazine	30-150	Specific for controlling severe nausea and vomiting.
Butyrophenone derivatives			
Haloperidol	Haldol	2-100	Optimum dosage highly variable.
Thioxanthene derivatives			
Chlorprothixene	Taractan	100-600	Specific for moderate to severe agitation, anxiety, and tension related to schizophrenia.
Thiothixene	Navane	10-60	
Dihydroindolone derivatives			
Molindone	Moban	15-225	Specific for use in schizophrenia.
Dibenzoxazepine derivatives			
Loxapine succinate	Loxitane	20-200	

lusional people become less psychotic. Some authorities state that from 65% to 75% of the schizophrenic individuals who receive adequate doses of one of the phenothiazine derivatives are helped.

Because chlorpromazine (Thorazine) proved to be so effective for psychotic individuals, scientists began searching for even more beneficial combinations of the essential chemicals used in the formula. As a result, there are now many phenothiazine derivatives, each with slight variations in its formula. In addition, other antipsychotic drugs with an entirely different chemical for-

Table 6 *Possible untoward effects from antipsychotic drugs*

Untoward effect	Comment
Hypotension	Drug should be given with great caution if cardiovascular disease is present. Individual should be warned about possible occurrence of hypotensive reactions.
Skin reactions	Urticarial, maculopapular, edematous, or petechial responses may occur 1 to 5 weeks after initiation of treatment.
Photosensitivity	Redness and itching of skin occur most frequently with chlorpromazine.
Abnormal skin pigmentation	Gray-blue discoloration of areas exposed to sun develops in some individuals after receiving prolonged high doses.
Jaundice	Develops in about 4% of the clients and is a dangerous complication; drug should be discontinued.
Agranulocytosis and leukopenia	Chlorpromazine depresses production of leukocytes. Initial symptoms of sore throat, high temperature, and lesions in mouth indicate that drug should be stopped immediately. Outcome may be lethal, but this is rare.
Endocrine changes	Weight gain, edema, lactation, and menstrual irregularities may take place.
Ocular changes	Corneal and lenticular changes and pigmentary retinopathy may occur with high dosages over long periods of time. Periodic ocular examinations are recommended.
Convulsions	Antipsychotic agents lower seizure threshold, making seizure-prone persons more likely to have seizures. Persons with a history of seizures or organic conditions associated with seizures require an increased dosage of anticonvulsant medication if antipsychotics are used.
Extrapyramidal reactions	Dose and duration related. Managed by adjusting dose of drug or adding antiparkinsonism drug.
Pseudoparkinsonism	Typical shuffling gait, masklike facies, tremor, muscular ridigity, slowing of movements, and so on occur.
Akathisia	Continuous restlessness, fidgeting, and pacing occur.
Dystonia	Spasm of neck muscles, extensor rigidity of back muscles, carpopedal spasm, eyes rolled back, swallowing difficulties occur. There is acute onset, but is reversible with appropriate medication. Reassurance should be provided until symptoms subside.
Tardive dyskinesia	Insidious onset of fine vermicular movements of tongue occurs, which is reversible if drug is discontinued at this time. Can progress to rhythmical involuntary movements of the tongue, face, mouth, or jaw with protrusion of tongue, puffing of cheeks, chewing movements. No known treatment; often irreversible. Prevention is imperative. Females over 50 years on prolonged high doses are particularly at risk.

mula have been developed. With so many antipsychotic drugs available, the situation becomes confusing. In the hope of clarifying the facts about these drugs, Table 5 was prepared. The majority of the antipsychotic drugs are listed with their generic name, trade name, and range of daily oral dosage in milligrams.

Antipsychotic drugs are all considered useful in the management of the manifestations of psychotic disorders, although they are usually *not* indicated for psychotic depressions. Drug manufacturers often make claims that a drug is specifically useful in alleviating a particular symptom, implying that there are major differences between drugs within a given chemical group. Clinicians, on the other hand, more commonly report that the effect of the drug seems to be idiosyncratic to the individual and that if a drug in one chemical group is not successful in alleviating the symptomotology without untoward effects, success can often be achieved by the administration of an antipsychotic drug from another chemical group. Because of this observation, Table 5 presents the antipsychotic drugs according to chemical group.

Table 6 describes some of the untoward effects that can be brought on by the use of some of these drugs with selected individuals. The nurse is often the first health care professional to notice the occurrence of untoward effects and therefore must be aware of their danger to differentiate them from unpleasant but benign side effects and initiate the institution of appropriate nursing and medical measures. These measures vary from reassuring the client in instances when side effects occur, to withholding the drug and contacting the physician immediately when untoward effects occur.

Antianxiety drugs

In addition to the antipsychotic drugs, which are called the major tranquilizers by some, there is a group of widely used drugs referred to as antianxiety drugs. These drugs may be called minor tranquilizers. They do not have an antipsychotic quality and therefore do not help schizophrenics. These drugs are best used to (1) treat individuals suffering from delirium tremens, (2) relieve anxiety in individuals experiencing moderate situational stress (e.g., preoperatively), (3) potentiate anticonvulsant drugs,

Table 7 *Antianxiety psychotropic drugs*

Generic name	Trade name	Range of daily oral dosage (mg)	Comments
Benzodiazepine group			
Chlordiazepoxide	Librium	10-100	
Diazepam	Valium	4-40	Useful for relief of skeletal muscle spasm.
Oxazepam	Serax	30-120	Particularly useful in older persons.
Doxepin	Sinequan	75-300	Has an antidepressant effect in addition to antianxiety effect.
Flurazepam	Dalmane	15-30 h.s.	Effective hypnotic agent for temporary use.
Clorazepate dipotassium	Tranxene	7.5-60.0	
Glycerol derivatives			
Meprobamate	Miltown, Equanil	400-1600	Useful as a muscle relaxant.
Tybamate	Solacen, Tybatran	250-2000	

(4) relieve muscle spasm, and (5) reduce high to moderate levels of endogenous anxiety to a moderate or mild level, rendering the client able to benefit from psychotherapy.

Although the antianxiety drugs have a limited number of side effects, they all have the potential for creating physical and emotional dependence. Sedation occurs when large doses are given, and the client needs to be warned not to engage in activities that require complete mental alertness. Ataxia is occasionally observed.

Table 7 provides the generic name, trade name, range of daily oral dosage in milligrams, and comments about the specific uses for some of the most commonly used antianxiety drugs. It should be noted that the glycerol derivatives are less often used than the benzodiazepines because overdoses can be treated successfully only with hemodialysis, and intentional overdoses are therefore more likely to result in death.

Antidepressant drugs

The third major category of psychotropic drugs is made up of the antidepressants, which are extremely useful in the treatment of

Table 8 *Antidepressant psychotropic drugs*

Generic name	Trade name	Range of daily oral dosage (mg)	Comments
Tricyclic antidepressants			
Imipramine	Tofranil	75-300	More effective when used for retarded depressive reactions of manic-depressive psychosis than for any other condition. Helpful in severe anxiety attacks and enuresis in children.
Amitriptyline	Elavil	75-300	Hypnotic effect useful when depressed individuals have severe sleep disturbance.
Desipramine	Pertofrane, Norpramin	75-200	More quickly effective therapeutically than imipramine or amitriptyline.
Nortriptyline	Aventyl	40-150	
Monoamine oxidase inhibitors			
Isocarboxazid	Marplan	20-60	Monoamine oxidase inhibitors potentiate effects of many other drugs, including sedative, hypnotic actions of alcohol and barbiturates. When cautiously administered with appropriate dietary restrictions and careful observation of blood pressure, their therapeutic effect may outweigh their danger in individuals who have not responded to an adequate trial of tricyclic antidepressants.
Phenelzine	Nardil	40-60	
Nialamide	Niamid	75-450	
Tranylcypromine	Parnate	20-60	

individuals who are depressed. In fact, statistics show that about 70% of the depressed individuals treated with these drugs improve markedly. Unfortunately, when drugs from this category are given, there is a delay of several weeks in the therapeutic effect. This fact suggests that suicidal individuals are best hospitalized during this period, not only for their protection, but also to allow the professional staff to assess the onset of the drug's effect, which clients often do not report because of their depression.

The antidepressants fall into two main chemical structures: the tricyclic antidepressants and the monoamine oxidase inhibitors. Table 8 gives the generic name, trade name, range of daily oral dosage in milligrams, and comments about the specific uses for some of the most commonly used antidepressant drugs.

Untoward side effects of antidepressant drugs. Dryness of the mouth is experienced by all who take any one of the tricyclic antidepressants. Other side effects that may be experienced by many who take one of the tricyclic antidepressants include palpitation, difficulties in accommodation, perspiration about the head and neck, dizziness, tachycardia, and postural hypotension that often leads to injuries. A mild degree of urinary retention or constipation may also occur. These drugs aggravate glaucoma. In addition, they may also produce a variety of minor symptoms of the central nervous system that may include tremor of the upper extremities, convulsions, twitching, and ataxia. If such symptoms appear, they can be easily controlled by decreasing the dosage.

Monoamine oxidase inhibitors potentiate epinephrine, so over-the-counter cold remedies are prohibited. In addition, persons receiving the monoamine oxidase inhibitors should be warned to avoid cheese, wines, yeast products (including beer), yogurt, fava beans, chicken livers, and pickled herring. As a result of eating any of these foods, a *hypertensive crisis* may occur. It occurs most frequently in individuals who are taking tranylcypromine (Parnate) and who ingest one of the prohibited foods. This reaction is called the *Parnate-cheese reaction* and is caused by a substance in the foods called *tyramine.* Its pressor effect is markedly enhanced by the monoamine oxidase inhibitors. These dietary restrictions should be maintained for at least 2 weeks after the drug is discontinued to allow for the complete resynthesis of the drug.

These drugs share common side effects that include hypotension, dizziness, vertigo, and fainting. Monoamine oxidase inhibitors should not be administered with the tricyclic antidepressants and, because of their side effects, are often used only after an adequate trial of the tricyclic antidepressant has failed. If a client's medication is changed from one category of antidepressant to another, a lag period of at least 2 weeks should elapse to avoid an untoward synergistic effect.

Lithium carbonate

The fourth category of psychotropic drugs is lithium carbonate. This drug is now recognized as effective in the treatment of manic attacks and in preventing the recurrence of manic-depressive episodes when given on a maintenance basis. About three fourths of the individuals who have a definitive diagnosis of bipolar manic-depression improve remarkably when treatment with lithium is properly carried out. Lithium does not impair intellectual activity, consciousness, or range or quality of emotional life. However, the toxic levels of lithium are close to the therapeutic levels. Lithium toxicity is closely related to serum lithium levels, and facilities for prompt and accurate serium lithium determinations should be readily available. Toxicity is indicated by nausea, abdominal cramps, vomiting, diarrhea, thirst, and polyuria. These symptoms can occur at lithium levels below 2 mEq/L. If the drug is not reduced at the first sign of toxicity, serious symptoms of the central nervous system and cardiovascular system may ensue. Recent studies have shown that prolonged use of lithium even without symptoms of toxicity may lead to renal tubule damage, cardiac toxicity, and thyroid damage. Therefore, despite its effectiveness, lithium is being prescribed cautiously and is unlikely to fulfill its promise of curing manic-depressive psychosis.

The nurse and use of psychopharmacological agents

The widespread use of the psychopharmacological agents in the treatment of mental illness has greatly influenced the role of the nurse in psychiatric settings. Because of the large number of medications to be given, many nurses find themselves fulfilling only one aspect of the many-faceted role of the nurse. It is not unusual for a nurse to spend the largest part of her time pouring and dispensing drugs. This is especially discouraging in view of current thinking regarding the effectiveness of the drugs. Most authorities agree that these drugs do not cure mental illness or solve basic emotional problems. Instead, the drugs relieve tension and provide varying degrees of symptomatic relief from the disabilities of mental illness. Because the acute symptoms are alleviated, many physicians, nurses, and families are encouraged to believe that the individual is basically changed when his improvement may be temporary and superficial.

Mentally ill individuals may be too ill to be left with the responsibility of remembering to take their medications or of accurately reporting the amount taken. This should be a responsibility of the nurse, in most cases.

The nurse's responsibilities and opportunities have increased with the advent of new drugs. It is necessary to know the therapeutic dosage and action of each drug and the specific untoward reactions that may be encountered.

The safety of the individual requires that he be observed closely and his response to the medication be recorded accurately. His physical well-being depends on the nurse's being vigilant in observing him in relation to untoward reactions to the drug. The nurse's records guide the physician in making decisions about dosage and change in medication.

The nurse must do far more than administer drugs and observe the individual's response if the needs of the mentally ill person are to be met. The attitude and approach used by the nurse as medications are dispensed are thought to be almost as significant in the individual's therapy as the actual drugs themselves (Fig. 22-1). When drugs are administered to a crowd without in-

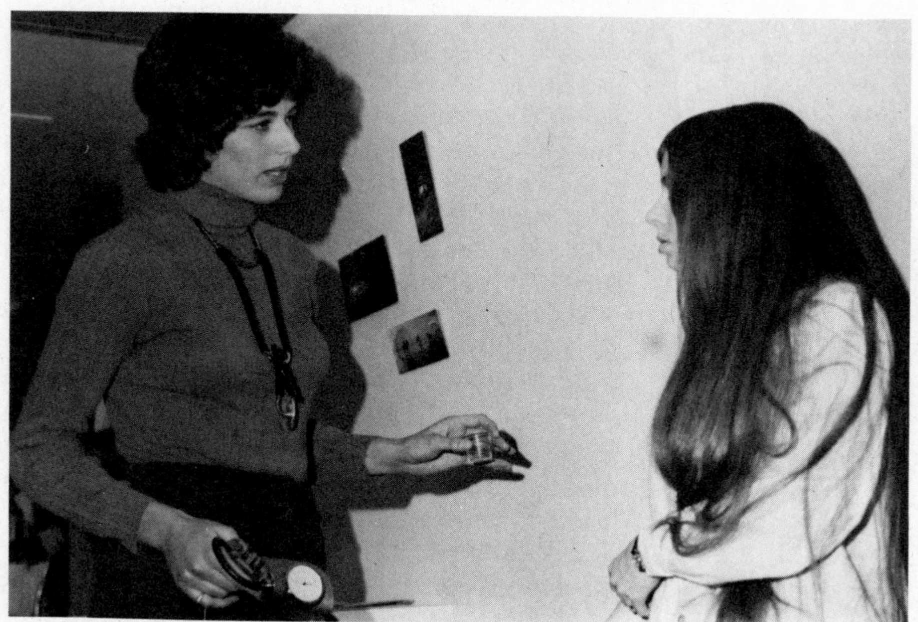

Fig. 22-1 *The attitude and approach used by the nurse as she dispenses medications are almost as significant as the actions of the drugs themselves.*

dividualizing the approach to each individual, much of the possible therapeutic effect of the drug may be lost.

Because of the effectiveness of the drugs, nursing staffs in psychiatric hospitals have been relieved of much of the problem of coping with destructive, uncontrolled behavior that once took so much of their time. Today the usual individual who is receiving one of the psychotropic drugs is able to assume much of the responsibility for his own physical care. This provides the nurse with an opportunity to use skills in communicating, listening, giving emotional support, and helping the individual become involved in the social and recreational activities provided in the hospital. More recently, large numbers of individuals have been treated by community mental health centers and live at home or in halfway houses. They are given the responsibility for administering their own medications.

INSULIN SHOCK THERAPY

Insulin shock therapy is a procedure where a series of hypoglycemic shocks are induced by injections of insulin. Although its use has declined markedly, insulin shock therapy has been used longer than any of the other somatic therapies that are still employed. Insulin shock therapy was first reported by Manfred Sakel in 1933 while he was working in the Psychiatric Clinic at the University of Vienna. In 1935 Dr. Sakel and Dr. Theo Dussick published a report of their experiences in treating 200 cases of schizophrenia with insulin shock.

Even today some authorities believe that insulin is the most effective treatment for schizophrenic individuals, especially those who are under 25 years of age, who have been ill for less than a year, and who have had well-integrated prepsychotic personalities. Persons who are delusional and hallucinatory respond better than do those who show the deteriorated symptoms of hebephrenia. Unfortunately, there is a high rate of recurrence among schizophrenic individuals who are treated with insulin therapy.

Like electroconvulsive therapy, the reason for the therapeutic effects of insulin shock is not understood. Some authorities believe that they are related to the glucose deprivation that the brain experiences during hypoglycemia. Other authorities believe that the therapeutic effects may be related to the nursing care and individual attention provided for these individuals during the period of hypoglycemia that they experience.

The decline in the use of insulin shock therapy results from the effectiveness and widespread use of the psychotropic drugs as well as other treatment modalities such as psychotherapy and group, family, occupational, and recreational therapies. These therapies are employed to a greater extent because individuals on drug therapy are able to participate in and benefit from them. In addition, insulin shock therapy has lost its appeal because it is dangerous. Persons undergoing this treatment require constant attention from skilled physicians and nurses. This professional vigilance is necessary to avoid some of the unfortunate problems that may arise from prolonged hypoglycemia.

Only individuals in good physical health should be given this treatment. Those suffering from diseases of the heart, blood vessels, kidneys, or liver are not good candidates for insulin shock therapy. Individuals with active pulmonary tuberculosis and hypertension do not tolerate insulin shock therapy well.

More recently, some treatment centers have been using small doses of insulin. This appears to be effective and much less dangerous.

ELECTROCONVULSIVE THERAPY

Electroconvulsive therapy is one of the most convenient and practical forms of somatic therapy. It was introduced in 1938 by two Italian clinicians, Ugo Cerletti and Bini, who had done ample experimentation on dogs before they applied this treatment to human beings. Although its use has been replaced to a great extent by psychopharmacological therapy, it is still used with excellent results by some physicians in the treatment of individuals suffering from agitated or retarded depression and to a lesser degree in the treatment of overactivity.

Electroconvulsive therapy is a relatively safe procedure in that it has few contraindications. It can be given to most elderly individuals with greater safety than many other somatic therapies.

Hypertensive cardiorenal disease, active tuberculosis, acute infections, and severe debility are contraindications to its use.

Electroconvulsive therapy is a fairly simple procedure to administer. It consists of producing a typical grand mal convulsion by applying controlled electric current. The current enters the individual's frontal lobes through electrodes placed on his temples. Each week 2 or 3 treatments are given until approximately 20 have been given. Breakfast is not served to the patient until after the treatment is over. Continuation of treatments depends to some extent on the individual's response to the therapy. This treatment can be successfully used for individuals who remain in the community.

Preparation of the individual

When electroconvulsive therapy is to be initiated, it is the responsibility of the physician to discuss the treatment plans with the individual, to order the routine x-ray examinations and laboratory work before the treatment is begun, and to obtain the signed treatment permit. The nurse is also involved in preparing the individual for the procedure. Sometimes the person has not understood the physician's explanation when the treatment was discussed and does not understand why breakfast is withheld. The nurse may discover that he is frightened at the thought of receiving treatment. She is then confronted with the responsibility of reassuring the person and helping him to accept treatment.

Nurses should avoid using the words *electric shock* when talking about this therapy. It is much better to refer to it simply as *the treatment* when discussing it with people who are to receive it, because electric shock may be frightening to a confused person and may suggest electrocution.

When reassuring the individual and encouraging him to cooperate with treatment plans, the nurse can say honestly that there will be no pain connected with the treatment and that the individual will remember nothing except the desire to sleep. It may be helpful to promise to accompany the person and to stay with him throughout the experience. If this promise is made, the nurse must actually carry it out. It may also be reassuring to the individual to learn that there will be a physician and other nurses with him during the actual treatment.

Sometimes the nurse is not able to reassure or convince the individual to accept the treatment. At this point the physician should be called. If the physician is unsuccessful in convincing the individual and still believes that treatment is essential, enough help should be summoned to make it possible to transport the client safely to the therapy room. After the first few electroconvulsive treatments, many individuals accept the treatment without question. However, because this treatment disturbs the memory, individuals do not remember having had the experience and usually require encouragement before each time it is given.

Before the therapy is given, the individual should be toileted. If this is not done, the person is inevitably incontinent during the treatment. Temperature, pulse, respirations, and blood pressure should be checked before the individual is allowed to go to the therapy room. If any of these findings are unusual, the physician should be notified. The treatment is usually canceled for individuals who exhibit signs of physical illness.

Because some individuals do not react to electroconvulsive therapy with a convulsion after having received sedatives, most physicians request that sedatives be withheld for 24 hours before treatment.

An airway is placed in the individual's mouth and one of the muscle-relaxing drugs is usually injected before the treatment is started. Emergency equipment is kept on hand in case the individual experiences respiratory difficulty after the treatment has been given. During and following the treatment the care of the individual is the same as that provided for any unconscious person who has just had a convulsive seizure.

Untoward reactions

Respiratory arrest is one of the untoward reactions to electroshock. Artificial respiration given immediately after the electroconvulsive therapy will stimulate respiration and will reduce the period of apnea. The head should be moved from side to side while the jaws are held in a fixed position.

Dislocation of the jaw is another problem that may follow this treatment. The jaw can be reduced by downward pressure on the molars and upward pressure on the chin.

Occasionally, electroconvulsive therapy is followed by a period of extreme excitement. An intravenous injection of 2 to 3 grains of amobarbital sodium will promote a restful period of sleep after the treatment.

After five or six treatments, patients frequently complain of confusion and loss of memory, particularly for recent events. This situation puzzles and perplexes the individual. He may fear that his memory will not return. Relatives are likely to express concern about this development unless the treatment has been carefully explained to them before it was undertaken. They should be prepared to expect such unusual developments and to understand that the symptoms will clear up completely after the series of treatments has been concluded. They should be reassured that there will be no permanent untoward aftereffects from the treatments.

Therapeutic effect

In the treatment of depressions, particularly midlife depression, improvement begins early and is usually noted after the first 2 or 3 treatments. Recovery usually occurs after a series of 6 to 10 convulsive treatments. Electroconvulsive therapy is discontinued when the individual attains a feeling of well-being, is no longer preoccupied with morbid thoughts, and is free of agitation. If symptoms reappear, a second series of treatments is given. As with any other form of somatic treatment, when the individual's emotional tone improves, an excellent opportunity is provided for the nurse as well as for the physician to establish a therapeutic relationship with the individual and to help him solve emotional problems that contributed to the mental illness.

Nurse's responsibility

Although very little is known about how electroconvulsive therapy achieves its results, it seems to break through the psychotic process and releases the individual to become more accessible to other people. Thus, after he has received a series of treatments, it is frequently possible for the nurse to develop a relationship with him and to begin to help him become an active participant in group activities.

Immediately following the treatment the individual should not be left alone until the nurse is positive that the respirations and pulse are within normal limits and that he is sleeping. Because some individuals become very confused and overactive following electroconvulsive therapy, it is wise to use a recovery room in which several people can remain under the watchful eye of one member of the nursing staff until they are awake and have fully regained contact with the environment. As an additional precaution, many treatment centers have added side rails to the beds.

Some authorities believe that one of the chief values of electroconvulsive therapy is that individuals become more accessible to psychotherapy following its use, and thus they may be helped to begin socializing with others and taking part in other therapeutic activities.

Some psychiatrists segregate individuals who are receiving electroconvulsive therapy and concentrate on helping them to develop relationships with other people and to involve themselves with their environment. This is done with the cooperative planning of the occupational therapist, the recreational therapist, the nurses, and other workers involved in the individual's care. Such plans usually include filling the days and evenings with a variety of interesting activities designed to help individuals to express themselves, to gain personal satisfaction, and to function as members of a group.

PSYCHOSURGERY

The prefrontal lobotomy is a surgical procedure during which the association fibers between the frontal lobes and the thalamus are severed. The theoretical explanation for surgical intervention in this particular portion of the brain is that severing these fibers will reduce the emotional component attached to the psychotic ideation that renders the individual incapable of living productively in society. Since the thalamus is thought to be the center of emotional energy, it has been reasoned that severing it from the center of thought, the frontal lobes, will result in improvement in social behavior. In other words, the individual may continue to have psychotic ideation but not the will or emotional energy to act on it.

The surgical procedure was developed by Egas Moniz, a Portuguese neurologist. His co-worker, Almeida Lima, a neurosurgeon, performed the first prefrontal lobotomy in 1935. In 1936 the procedure was introduced in the United States by Dr. Walter Freeman and Dr. James Watts.

From the time the operation was introduced until the mid-1950s, a good many individuals received this treatment. Because of its irreversibility, it was usually regarded as a drastic procedure to be used only after all other therapies had failed to produce favorable results. Consequently, it was performed on many who suffered from a chronic mental illness. Unfortunately, the major complication proved to be convulsive seizures that did not always appear immediately after surgery.

As physicians had an opportunity to study this procedure and its long-term results, it became evident that the frequency of postoperative complications, including convulsions, made the procedure a controversial one. In fact, it is said by some authorities to be one of the most controversial procedures in modern medicine.

Recently the usefulness of prefrontal lobotomy has been reconsidered by both the medical and legal professions. As a result, this procedure is now available only with a court order. However, since people who have undergone a prefrontal lobotomy may be among the individuals for whom the nurse will provide care, this care is discussed here.

Nursing care

As soon as the individual is physically able, an active system of retraining and reeducation should be established. The individual should be required to get out of bed, to toilet himself, to shower, to dress, and to feed himself using the proper tableware. From the earliest possible moment after surgery, activities that will interest him should be introduced even though this may require toys and games that might usually be chosen for children. Many of these individuals behave in childlike ways and enjoy activities that a child would enjoy.

After a prefrontal lobotomy, most individuals regress, with some developing more severely regressed behavior than others. The major nursing task is to help them become resocialized through a regimen of habit training. This is sometimes difficult and trying, since lobotomized individuals procrastinate and seem to lack any understanding of the concept of time.

Operant conditioning is a method of modifying an individual's response to the environment. This method may be employed profitably with lobotomized individuals. The modification of the behavior is achieved by reinforcing desirable patterns of behavior through rewards and extinguishing undesirable patterns of behavior by withholding the rewards. Among the rewards that have been used successfully are praise, candies, or tokens that may be exchanged for desired objects or for privileges. The positive changes in behavior that the use of a token economy has achieved with some types of individuals are remarkable.

At best, the individual who has had a prefrontal lobotomy can become an acceptable member of society and may return to his former occupation but cannot be expected to enter into new ventures, make sound judgments on complicated matters, or maintain the emotional calm required in conducting any activity requiring concerted, concentrated effort. In general, previous emotional conflicts remain, but the intensity of the emotional charge is reduced.

OTHER SOMATIC THERAPIES

Continuing research on the cause of mental illness indicates that it is likely that a major contributing factor to mental illness is physiological in nature. Therefore it is understandable that there is much current interest in somatic therapies. In addition to those previously discussed, the literature documents remarkable improvement in a few psychotic persons who have been treated with hemodialysis and in others who have been systematically treated with one form or another of nutritional therapy. The reader would be wise to maintain an open mind to these developments, particularly since the holistic view of individuals as stated in Chapter 1 of this text directs that mental health or mental illness results from the interrelationship of both physical and emotional factors.

CONCLUDING STATEMENTS

1. The use of psychotropic drugs that help to normalize behavior has had a dramatic effect on the care of mentally ill individuals in this country and on the national attitude toward all aspects of mental illness.
2. The psychotropic drugs include antipsychotic drugs, antianxiety drugs, antidepressant drugs, and lithium carbonate.
3. Authorities agree that the psychopharmacological agents do not cure mental illness or solve basic emotional problems but relieve tension and provide varying degrees of symptomatic relief.
4. The attitude and approach used by the nurse in dispensing medications are thought to be almost as significant in the individual's therapy as the actual drug received.
5. Because of the effectiveness of the psychopharmacological agents, nursing staffs in psychiatric treatment centers have been relieved to a large extent of coping with destructive, uncontrolled behavior, which once took a great deal of time. The nurse is now able to use psychiatric nursing skills in relating to individuals and in helping them become involved in the social and recreational activities provided.
6. The decline in the use of insulin shock therapy results from the effectiveness of other treatment modalities, from the fact that it is a treatment that can be dangerous, and from the fact that individuals undergoing such a treatment require constant skilled professional attention.
7. Electroconvulsive therapy has been replaced to a large extent by psychopharmacological therapy, but it is still used by some physicians with excellent results in the treatment of individuals suffering from agitated or retarded depression and to a lesser degree in the treatment of overactivity.
8. Although very little is known about how electroconvulsive therapy achieves its result, it seems to break through the psy-

chotic process and to allow the individual to become more accessible to other people. This provides the nurse with an opportunity to develop a therapeutic relationship with the individual.

9. Prefrontal lobotomy, a surgical procedure that severs the association fibers between the frontal lobes and the thalamus, is no longer being used as a viable treatment for mental illness.
10. Other forms of somatic therapies, such as hemodialysis and nutritional therapy, have been used with remarkable success with a few psychotic individuals. The reader would be wise to maintain an open mind to reports of the development of new types of somatic therapies for mental illness.

Suggested sources of additional information

CLASSICAL

Maloney, Elizabeth M., and Johannesen, Lucile: How the tranquilizers affect nursing practice, Am. J. Nurs. **57**:1144-1146, 1957.

Miller, Edgar: Psychological theories of ECT: a review, Int. J. Psychiat. **5**:154-165, Feb., 1968.

CONTEMPORARY

Bassuk, Ellen L., and Schoonover, Stephen C.: The practitioner's guide to psychoactive drugs, New York, 1977, Plenum Publishing Corp.

Distasio, Carol, and Nawrot, Marcia: Methaqualone, Am. J. Nurs. **73**:1922-1925, 1973.

Goodman, Lois S., and Gillman, Alfred, editors: The pharmacological basis of therapeutics, ed. 5, New York, 1975. Macmillan Publishing Co., Inc.

Hitchens, Emily A.: Helping psychiatric outpatients accept drug therapy, Am. J. Nurs. **77**:464-466, March, 1977.

Kalinowski, Lothar B.: Electric and other convulsive treatments. In Arieti, Silvano, editor: American handbook of psychiatry, vol. 5, ed. 2, New York, 1974, Basic Books, Inc., Publishers, pp. 531-547.

Laquer, H. Peter: Insulin coma therapy. In Arieti, Silvano, editor: American handbook of psychiatry, vol. 5, ed. 2, New York, 1974, Basic Books, Inc., Publishers, pp. 525-529.

Lehman, H.E.: Physical therapies of schizophrenia. In Arieti, Silvano, and Brody, Eugene B., editors: American handbook of psychiatry, vol. 3, ed. 2, New York, 1974, Basic Books, Inc., Publishers.

Lipkin, Gladys B., and Cohen, Roberta G.: Effective approaches to patients' behavior, New York, 1980, The Springer Publishing Co.

Livingston, Kenneth E.: Surgical contributions to psychiatric treatment. In Arieti, Silvano, editor: American handbook of psychiatry, vol. 5, ed. 2, New York, 1974, Basic Books, Inc., Publishers, pp. 548-563.

Morgan, Arthur James: Minor tranquilizers, hypnotics, and sedatives, Am. J. Nurs. **73:**1220-1222, 1973.

Pilette, Wilfrid L.: What is an adequate therapeutic trial of psychotropic medication? Perspect. Psychiatr. Care **15**(4):170-174, Oct.-Dec., 1977.

Wendt, Roselyn L.: Good morning, world. I'm glad to be back, Am. J. Nurs. **79:**949, May, 1979.

OF PARTICULAR INTEREST

Hitchens, E.A.: Helping psychiatric outpatients accept drug therapy, Am. J. Nurs. **77:**464-466, March, 1977.

This is an excellent article on the various issues related to the use of psychotropic medications for discharged psychiatric clients.

Kline, N.I., and Davis, J.M.: Psychotropic drugs, Am. J. Nurs. **73:**54, 1973.

This article presents a comprehensive discussion of the psychotropic medications. It is essential reading for all nurses working in the clinical area.

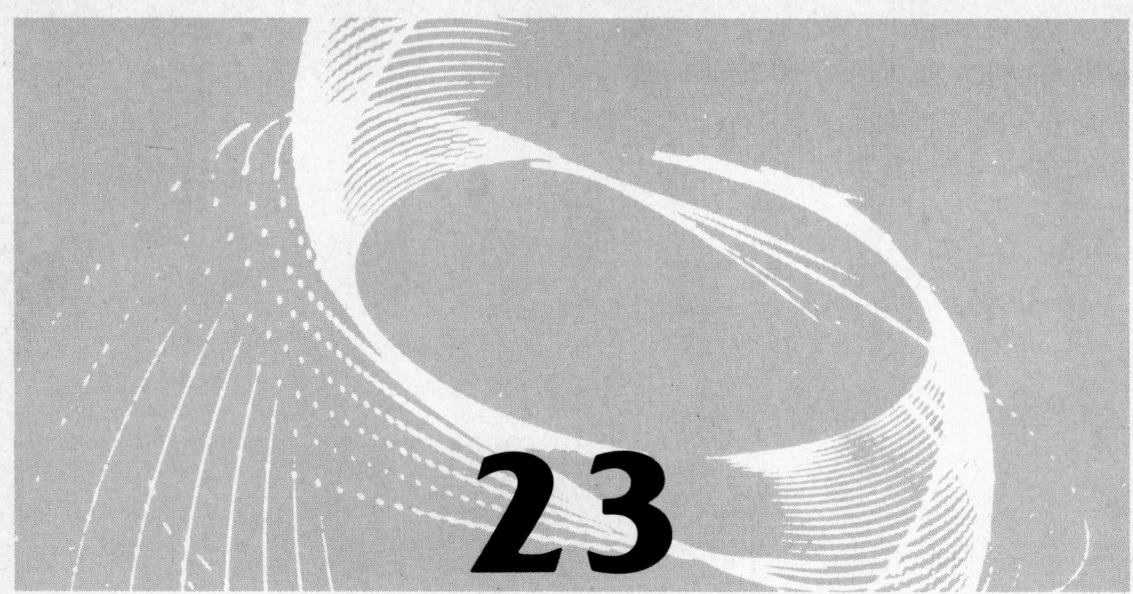

23

Interpersonally based treatment modalities

- Roles and functions of mental health professionals
- Psychotherapy
- Psychoanalysis
- Psychodrama
- Transactional analysis
- Gestalt therapy
- Hypnotherapy

In addition to the interpersonally based treatment modalities (e.g., group therapy, the nurse-client relationship) with which the nurse is most often involved, there are a number of other such therapies the principles of which nurses need to understand if they are to be knowledgeable participants in the treatment plan.

The implementation of interpersonally based treatment modalities is not limited to professionals of any one discipline, although the discipline of the therapist often influences the style and emphasis of treatment employed. Because of this, a brief description of the educational preparation and functions of the major mental health professionals follows.

ROLES AND FUNCTIONS OF MENTAL HEALTH PROFESSIONALS

Although any physician may call himself a *psychiatrist,* the vast majority of practicing psychiatrists not only hold an M.D. degree but also have had several years of supervised residency training in psychiatry. The law does not require licensing beyond that necessary for any physician, but the medical profession makes available a voluntary examination in this clinical specialty. Physicians who successfully complete this examination are "Board Certified" and identify themselves as such. This designation helps to ensure the lay public of the services of a physician who has advanced knowledge and experience in psychiatry. Psychiatrists function in private practice as well as treating hospitalized clients. In the latter instance the psychiatrist is frequently the leader of the treatment team, although there is a trend toward the treatment team leader being the person who is most knowledgeable about the client, regardless of professional discipline. The psychiatrist's unique function is the prescribing of medications and the administration of other somatic treatments such as insulin and electroconvulsive therapies. In addition, he is the only professional equipped to make a medical diagnosis and is particularly skilled in identifying and treating persons whose problems have highly interrelated emotional and physiological components.

Psychologists are professionals who have advanced education in the study of mental processes and the treatment of mental disorders. They are not physicians but rather hold M.A. or Ph.D. degrees. As is true in the field of medicine, psychology has become such a broad discipline that most psychologists specialize. Those who are most directly involved in the diagnosis of mental illness and in the treatment of the emotionally ill are called *clinical psychologists.* Those clinical psychologists concerned with the diagnosis of mental illness have developed expertise in the use of inferential tools that are designed to assist in the diagnostic process and assessment of treatment effects. Such tools are projective techniques best exemplified by the Rorschach test, personality inventories such as the Minnesota Multiphasic Personality Inventory, and intelligence tests. Only clinical psychologists are trained in the use and interpretation of these highly complex instruments. Other clinical psychologists have chosen to develop expertise in the treatment of the emotionally ill. Since the entire education of these psychologists has been geared to the study of human behavior, they are particularly effective when the problems of the individual or the family are clearly psychogenic in origin and manifestation. Most clinical psychologists work in close collaboration with a psychiatrist who assists in the treatment program if somatic therapies seem indicated. Some states make legal certification mandatory for practice as a clinical psychologist.

Social workers are health professionals many of whom have educational preparation at the master's degree level. Although social workers are prepared to work with individuals and families who have a wide variety of physical, emotional, and social problems, some specialize in psychiatric social work. Psychiatric social workers are particularly skilled in assessing familial, environmental, and social factors that contribute to the maladaptive behavior of the individual and the family. They also are major contributors to the planning and implementation of follow-up care.

Nurses are professionals whose initial educational preparation is through either diploma, associate degree, or baccalaureate degree programs. After this preparation the nurse becomes licensed as a registered nurse through successful completion of state board examinations. Without additional educational or experiential preparation, this nurse is prepared to function as a generalist in any setting. An increasing number of nurses with baccalaureate degrees have continued their education to attain a master's degree in a particular clinical specialty. Nurses prepared at the graduate level in psychiatric–mental health nursing have advanced preparation in promoting the mental health of individuals, groups, families, and communities, as well as in assisting these persons in increasing the effectiveness of their adaptations. The nursing profession has recently developed an examination process whereby these expert nurses can be certified, although there is no legal mandate requiring this. Psychiatric nurses are increasingly assuming more responsibility for psychotherapeutic interventions.

It should be noted that anyone may legally call himself a *psychotherapist* or *psychoanalyst,* and these designations do not guarantee a level of expertise. All reputable therapists and analysts, however, have years of advanced education and supervised clinical training in their particular discipline.

The following interpersonally based treatment modalities can be implemented by any prepared professional mental health worker, and as the number of persons requiring treatment increases and the preparation of mental health workers becomes more extensive, there is a concomitant increase in role blurring.

PSYCHOTHERAPY

Any procedure that promotes the development of courage, inner security, and self-confidence can be called psychotherapy. However, the traditional use of this term is limited to sustained interpersonal interactions between the psychotherapist and client where the goal is to help the client to develop behaviors that are more functional. Psychotherapy is not a fixed technique; it is more an art than a science, and its methods must be adapted and modified to fit the individual situation. In plain language, it is a form of mental exploration. It is universally acknowledged that one cannot standardize psychotherapy, that it must be individualized, and that it will vary from client to client.

Psychotherapy falls into two general types: supportive psychotherapy and "uncovering" or "insight" psychotherapy. *Supportive psychotherapy* helps the individual cope with his problems and includes such techniques as diagnosis, advice, education, guidance, counseling, assurance, and medication. *Uncovering* or *insight psychotherapy* involves exploring and bringing to consciousness the source of repressed and suppressed conflicts and experiences that operate at unconscious levels to cause anxiety. Uncovering psychotherapy gives meaning to abnormal or irrational feelings and maladaptations in normal-to-usual life situations.

The type of psychotherapy used is dependent on the therapist's assessment of the interrelationship of a number of variables. Chief among these variables are the extent and severity of the client's maladaptation, the client's goals, his intellectual ability, and his personal and interpersonal resources. Generally the more mentally ill the client is, the fewer resources he has, and the less intellectually capable he is, the more he will be a candidate for supportive psychotherapy. Supportive psychotherapy requires the psychotherapist to assume a direct role by offering direction and guidance. The client may not develop an understanding of the dynamics underlying his behavior, but he can learn behaviors that are more functional.

Clients who give evidence of available ego strength, a viable support system, and at least average intelligence can often benefit from uncovering or insight psychotherapy. During this type of psychotherapy, the client is encouraged to talk about his life experiences. He is encouraged to talk freely about anything that comes to his mind, as long as he relates his own ideas and concerns. This random talk allows the client to follow freely the associations that come into his mind and is accurately described as *mental ventilation.* The therapist will note that there are certain occasions and events that the client dismisses quickly or avoids mentioning except in a superficial way. These sensitive areas are then explored more fully. The client is encouraged to talk about them more freely until they no longer cause excess emotion, a process known as *desensitization.*

The client is guided to an understanding of how his repressed feelings are related to his behavior. This is done in a simple, clear style, thereby helping the client to gain insight into the exact nature of his problem. Thus begins the process of reeducation.

It should be noted that a client who initially requires supportive psychotherapy may be able to increase his self-esteem to the point where uncovering or insight psychotherapy is indicated. A skilled psychotherapist has the ability to make this assessment and to respond accordingly.

Prerequisite to any form of psychotherapy is the identification of the chain of events and situations that caused or contributed to the emotional illness. No period in the client's history should be overlooked. Information should be gathered concerning family background and experiences of early life, as well as current or recent happenings and conditions at home and at work.

Regardless of the type of psychotherapy employed, the client is encouraged to face his distressing problems; he is urged to think of them instead of running away from them, to become familiar with them rather than to "forget" them, and to approach their solution in a candid, open manner. He is encouraged to take an active part in his own therapy. If all goes well, he should take more and more constructive steps in the management of his own treatment. He can then answer some of his own questions and make his own decisions. The therapist measures therapeutic success by the degree to which she makes herself less and less necessary.

The most important element in any psychotherapeutic process is the relationship between the therapist and the client. The client must have confidence in the therapist and some respect for the therapist's knowledge and experience. A word of assurance alone may be the deciding factor in relieving many anxious clients of their fears. Such a relationship is dependent on a positive rapport between the therapist and the client.

A very important aspect of the therapist-client relationship is the unconscious attitude of the client toward his therapist. The therapist is cast into a variety of roles, including that of a parent. The client's attitude may be competitive or even erotic. This shifting toward the therapist of desires, feelings, and relations originally experienced by the client with regard to his own parents, siblings, and other persons is known as *transference*. Hence every nuance of feeling, ranging from trustful dependence to open hostility, may be directed toward the therapist. When the client's attitude toward the therapist appears to be favorable, the transference is regarded as being positive. Resistant or antagonistic attitudes of the client toward the therapist imply a negative transference. The client's transference reaction to the therapist may elicit an unconscious counterresponse by the therapist. This attitude of the therapist toward the client is called *countertransference.*

The development of a transference reaction between the client and the psychotherapist is often viewed as a positive sign, for it indicates that the therapist has become significant to the client, thereby establishing the potential for the client to benefit from a corrective emotional experience. For example, if the client responds to the psychotherapist in the clinging, dependent manner that he learned in early life was necessary to maintain his mother's love, the psychotherapist can subtly but consistently encourage the client to make his own decisions while still conveying approval. Through this process the client can learn that it is possible for him to take steps toward independence without jeopardizing the highly valued relationship with the psychotherapist. The client may or may not be helped to become aware of his transference reaction and the process engaged in by the therapist to use the transference therapeutically.

A countertransference reaction is rarely, if ever, seen as having therapeutic potential except insofar as it provides the therapist with an understanding of the psychodynamics underlying the client's behavior. In other words, by becoming aware of her own reaction to the client, the therapist can better understand the unconscious purpose of the client's behavioral patterns. An example of a nontherapeutic countertransference is when the client behaves toward the psychotherapist as if the therapist were his parent (transference), and the psychotherapist unconsciously responds by treating the client as if he were a child for whom all decisions need to be made (countertransference). Since both transference and countertransference occur on a unconscious level, and since countertransference is not desirable, many teachers of psychotherapy require their students to undergo psychotherapy themselves as a means of discovering their own emotional vulnerabilities and increasing their own overall level of self-awareness. Whether or not a psychotherapist has undergone personal psychotherapy, supervision of psychotherapy by a skilled colleague is necessary to identify and prevent countertransference. The occurence of the transference and countertransference phenomena is a testimony to the fundamentally human nature of the psychotherapeutic process.

In summary, the success of the psychotherapeutic process depends to a large extent on the quality of the interpersonal experience between the client and the therapist. The therapy can be a success only if the therapist succeeds in motivating the client toward promoting his own well-being on his own behalf rather than to please another person. The relationship between the two must remain at a professional level and never at a social one.

PSYCHOANALYSIS

Psychoanalysis is more than assisting the client to recall some childhood experience, such as being locked in a dark room, or to recall some long-concealed hate of a sibling. Such exhuming of old memories by suggestion, narcosis, or hypnosis may relieve the symptoms of a deep-seated emotional problem, but it rarely dissolves the basic difficulty.

The analyst by a long and often tedious process looks for clues to the fundamental disturbance—in free association, in the content of dreams, in the nature of the client's transference, and in those matters the client appears to avoid because of resistance to their open recognition. The analyst leads the client back to forgotten events and emotional crises, to his childhood fears, frustrations, and other residuals that operate at unconscious levels and cause the individual to be an insecure and unhappy person. As one exponent phrased it, "The patient acquires a more conscious knowledge of his inner conflicts and gains freedom from the tyranny of the unconscious."

Because of the intensive intrapsychic exploration required by the psychoanalytic process, only persons with a relatively intact ego can benefit from this relationship.

PSYCHODRAMA

Another type of therapeutic experience that is sometimes provided for a group of clients is called psychodrama. This technique was developed by J. L. Moreno, a psychiatrist who began working with emotionally disturbed individuals in a theater in Vienna as early as 1941. Psychodrama is usually conducted by a leader who has been especially prepared to direct this type of activity. Although a variety of methods may be used, one of the more frequent techniques places the leader on a stage in front of an audience of clients and staff members. The leader identifies a situation in which interpersonal conflict is involved. He invites members of the audience to come to the stage for the purpose of acting out this human relations problem.

When members of the audience agree to accept parts in the drama, they are told the essential facts about the roles they are to play. The chosen situation frequently focuses on a conversation with the significant members of a family. In the role of an actor, the individual is given a specially selected part that affords him an opportunity to give free expression to his inner conflicts as a situation is acted out with other performers who symbolize or represent persons who are the real objects of his love or hate. For example, a son who normally represses his hostility toward his father may freely express it as an actor and may even reveal the cause. On the other hand, if he is induced to take the father role, he may, after doing so, tolerate his own father's point of view in a more objective and understanding manner. It is surprising how effectively individuals fill the roles to which they are assigned and how realistically feelings are expressed. The leader stops the action when he believes the enactment has progressed far enough to provide the audience with a basis for a fruitful discussion.

Another method that has been used productively in psychodrama is for the leader to request a volunteer from among the audience to come forward and set up a situation that he wishes to portray. He is also asked to select individuals from the audience to play the parts required and to provide the role players with the necessary data about the roles they will enact. This technique focuses specifically on some personal concern of the individual who volunteered to develop the psychodramatic situation. With either of these methods individuals from the audience may be asked to come forward to play the role of alter ego for the major characters in the psychodrama.

After the role playing is completed, the people in the audience are given an opportunity to participate in a discussion of the situation they have witnessed and experienced vicariously. The participants from the audience may focus attention on various aspects of the situation and frequently present similar life experiences.

Psychodrama provides individuals with an opportunity to express feelings and concerns that relate to a personal human relations situation that is like, but not identical to, a personal problem of their own. Thus psychodrama has somewhat the same therapeutic effect as *abreaction,* the lessening of emotional trauma by reenacting the situation. It also furnishes individuals with an opportunity for *catharsis,* an opportunity to freely express feelings. As in other group therapy situations, the individual is helped by the group to express feelings and consider them objectively.

The nurse is frequently involved in psychodrama as a role player or as a discussant. Skill and understanding of psychodrama are developed through continued participation in this treatment modality. Eventually the nurse may accept the role of the leader of the psychodrama sessions.

TRANSACTIONAL ANALYSIS

Transactional analysis is both a theoretical framework and a treatment method developed by Eric Berne. Its popularity and usability is attested to by the amount of literature available to lay persons on the subject. Transactional analysis, as a theory, postulates that each person has three elements of his personality that are in greater or lesser operation at any given point in time. These elements are (1) the immature, need-gratifying aspect, referred to as the Child, (2) the moralistic, rigid standard-setting aspect, referred to as the Parent, (3) and the mature reality-based aspect, referred to as the Adult. The student will notice the similarity between this theoretical formulation and Freud's conception of the id, superego, and ego, respectively. Unlike Freudian theory, however, Berne's construct does not imply a judgment about the existence of these personality elements. Rather, he states that problems arise only when there is an incongruency between the elements that are operating when people relate with each other. This belief is the foundation for his use of the term *transactional.* The emphasis on dysfunctional interpersonal relationships as the crux of emotional problems is reminiscent of Sullivan's theories. Consequently, Berne's theory of transactional analysis is seen by many as effectively combining the salient intrapsychic features of Freudian theory and the aspects of Sullivanian theory that provide direction for therapeutic intervention.

When persons communicate and the adult elements of their personalities are operative, it is likely that they will be effective in hearing and responding to each other. In addition, the nonverbal aspects of the process will be congruent with the verbal content, and no hidden messages will be perceived by either person. Each will reality test on the basis of feedback received, and each is likely to feel that the interaction has been satisfying. This is not to imply that no differences of opinion will arise during such an interaction, but the individuals will probably feel that any differences are based on content issues, rather than on covert attempts to dominate, control, or otherwise minimize the value of the other person. Adult-Adult interactions are effective and therefore desirable interactional processes when the participants are engaged in problem-solving or task-oriented activities.

Another effective and desirable interactional process occurs when two or more chronological adults simultaneously have the child element of their personalities in preeminence. It is at these times they have fun "playing." Many adults have had the experience of spontaneously engaging in what appear to be foolish or childlike activities with another adult, such as frolicking through a park on a beautiful autumn day instead of attending a scheduled meeting. As long as this behavior does not have major irreversible consequences and does not become a persistent pattern, it can serve to enhance feelings of well-being of the individual and strengthen the relationship.

Problems arise, however, when two persons characteristically relate to each other through divergent elements of their personalities. For example, a husband who relates to his wife through the parent element of his personality is going to feel continuously dissatisfied with their interactions unless she responds with the child element of her personality. If she does respond in this way, there may be little initial conflict, since both their needs are being met superficially. However, it should be noted that neither is engaged in reality-testing behaviors and neither can change interactional elements without open conflict emerging. Therefore this pattern is growth-stifling for both partners.

The previous situation is presented merely as one example of a common interactional problem. The reader can speculate as to the large variety of interactional problems that can occur when two or more people interact from the basis of incongruent personality elements. For more detailed explanations of transactional analysis, the student is referred to the many excellent books on the subject.

Transactional analysis as a method of treatment is most effective as a form of family therapy. When this is not possible, it can be effectively implemented as a method of group therapy, in which the group members consciously and unconsciously assume characteristic familial roles. In either the family or group setting the participants have the immediate opportunity to analyze their reactions and subsequent behavior in light of the Child-Parent-Adult framework and experience how they affect others and are affected by them. They also have the opportunity to experiment with using other elements of their personality and can receive immediate feedback.

Transactional analysis is also used as a form of individual treatment. The effectiveness of this form of treatment modality is limited, however, since the client has only one other person with whom to interact, and feedback about behavioral changes in life situations is delayed. Nevertheless, many therapists are successfully adopting some of the concepts of transactional analysis in their treatment of individuals because these concepts are seen by many clients as easy to understand and relevant to their life situations.

Regardless of setting, the primary role of the transactional therapist is to observe and tactfully comment on the discrepancies between the personality elements of those engaged in the interactional process. The therapist often suggests and supports role playing with another personality element so that the person can experience its effects. The dynamics that underlie the person's use of one personality element as opposed to the other two are not always explored. If they are discussed, it is usually done in the context of the present rather than in terms of childhood experiences.

GESTALT THERAPY

Gestalt therapy is as much a philosophy as it is an intervention technique. Its developer is Frederic S. Perls, who has trained many others in its use. The emphasis in gestalt therapy is on treatment of the person as a holistic being, placing as much importance on somatic responses as on emotional responses. Proponents of gestalt therapy believe that the problems of many persons emanate from the fact that individuals have lost touch with their feelings, both physical and emotional. If one is unaware of what one is feeling, the likelihood of being able to express these feelings is greatly diminished and therefore one is unlikely to have one's needs met. Therefore treatment consists primarily of helping the individual increase sensory awareness of his present state. Once the individual begins the process of getting in touch with himself, his current relationships with others and with his environment are explored. The configuration of the holistic being in interaction with others and with the environment is referred to as the *gestalt* and is heavily based on systems theory. Although it is acknowledged that there are multiple causative factors that produced the individual's current responses, the understanding of these factors is not believed to alleviate the present problems and they are therefore not explored.

As with transactional analysis, the principles of gestalt therapy can be used in a one-to-one psychotherapeutic relationship but are most commonly practiced as a form of group therapy. Eight to ten participants are seen as an ideal number for a gestalt group. The environment in which the group meets is viewed as instrumental in facilitating self-awareness. Therefore factors such as comfortable chairs, a pleasing decor, and adequate space are seen as essential. Techniques such as role playing and ventilation are used frequently. The ultimate goal of gestalt therapy is to assist the client to fulfill his potential, and therefore it is appropriately used with individuals interested in self-growth as well as with persons who are emotionally disturbed.

HYPNOTHERAPY

Hypnotherapy is a method by which the client is induced into a relative state of disassociation through such techniques as gazing at a fixed spot, concentrating on a consistent movement, or listening to a monotonous sound. Of more importance than the induction technique is the previously established relationship of trust between the client and the hypnotist. By allowing himself to be hypnotized, the client is in fact relinquishing some degree of ego control to the therapist. The hypnotist is thus enabled to give the client instructions concerning therapeutic behavioral alterations, which will be acted on after the hypnotic trance when precipitated by a posthypnotic suggestion. For example, a compulsive overeater can avoid eating binges by reproducing the posthypnotic suggestion, which in turn precipitates the avoidance of food.

Another use of hypnotherapy is to gain direct access quickly to information and feelings that are stored in the client's unconscious and that seem to be particularly relevant to the therapeutic issues being currently explored. However, most authorities agree that nothing can be achieved through hypnotherapy that cannot ultimately be achieved through other forms of psychotherapy. There are instances, however, when it is in the client's interest to achieve speedy behavioral change or information, and it is in these instances when hypnotherapy is likely to be employed.

CONCLUDING STATEMENTS

1. The implementation of interpersonally based treatment modalities is not limited to professionals of any one discipline, although the discipline of the therapist often influences the style and treatment employed.
2. Psychotherapy is a sustained interpersonal interaction between the therapist and client where the goal is to help the client develop behaviors that are more functional. The two types of psychotherapy are supportive psychotherapy and uncovering or insight psychotherapy.

3. Psychoanalysis is a long and tedious process that requires the client to have a moderate degree of ego strength. The analyst assists the client to discover the underlying basis of his problems through such techniques as free association and dream analysis.
4. Psychodrama is a form of group therapy that allows individuals to role play problem situations by alternating various roles and to receive feedback from observers in the audience.
5. Transactional analysis uses the Child-Parent-Adult framework to analyze and improve interactional patterns.
6. Gestalt therapy focuses on helping persons fulfill their potential through increased sensory awareness of themselves and their relationships with others and with the environment within the context of the present.
7. Hypnotherapy is used to achieve relatively rapid alterations in behavior or access to unconscious material.

Suggested sources of additional information

CLASSICAL

Glasser, William: Reality therapy, a new approach to psychiatry, New York, 1975, Harper & Row, Publishers.

Skinner, B.F.: Science and behavior, New York, 1965, The Free Press.

CONTEMPORARY

Bales, Robert: Interaction process analysis: a method for the study of small groups, Reading, Mass., 1950, Addison-Wesley Publishing Co., Inc.

Balgopal, Pallassana, R., and Vassil, Thomas V.: The group psychotherapist: a new breed, Perspect. Psychiatr. Care **17:**132-135, May-June, 1979.

Geach, Barbara, and White, James C.: Empathic resonance: a counter transference phenomenon, Am. J. Nurs. **74:**1282-1285, 1974.

Hediger, Karen H.: The place of the dream in therapy, Perspect. Psychiatr. Care **17:**223-227, Sept.-Oct., 1979.

Huber, Cathee J., and Hanson, Shirley: Sensitivity training: a step toward involvement with patients, Nurs. Forum **14:**175-187, 1975.

Jones, Maxwell: Beyond the therapeutic community, New Haven, Conn., 1968, Yale University Press.

Kerr, Norine: Neurosis and primal therapy, Nurs. Forum **15:**34-46, 1976.

Kohnke, Mary, and Lego, Suzanne: Point/counterpoint: a psychotherapist is a psychotherapist . . . , Perspect. Psychiatr. Care **18:**26-27, Jan.-Feb., 1980.

Krizinofski, Marian: Evolution of the communication model of therapy. In Kneisl, Carol Ren, and Wilson, Holly Skodol, editors: Current perspectives in psychiatric nursing: issues and trends, vol. 2, St. Louis, 1978, The C.V. Mosby Co.

Nelson, Priscilla: Involvement with Betty: an experience in reality therapy, Am. J. Nurs. **74:**1440-1441, 1974.

Ruffin, Janice E.: The relevence of racism to the goals of psychotherapy, Perspect. Psychiatr. Care **14:**160-164, 1976.

Shaw, Dale, et al.: Multiple impact therapy, Am. J. Nurs. **77:**246-248, 1977.

Singer, Erwin: Key concepts in psychotherapy, ed. 2, New York, 1970, Basic Books, Inc., Publishers.

White, Eleanor M.: Principles and practice of gestalt therapy. In Kneisl, Carol Ren, and Wilson, Holly Skodol, editors: Current perspectives in psychiatric nursing: issues and trends, vol. 2, St. Louis, 1978, The C.V. Mosby Co.

OF PARTICULAR INTEREST

Ehrenwald, J.: The history of psychotherapy, New York, 1976, Jason Aronson, Inc.
This book is an excellent resource for the various models of psychotherapy. It is interesting and informative.

Skinner, B.F.: Science and behavior, New York, 1965, The Free Press.
This is a classic text on behavior therapy that created heated discussion on its original publication. It is interesting reading for all students interested in behavioral alterations.

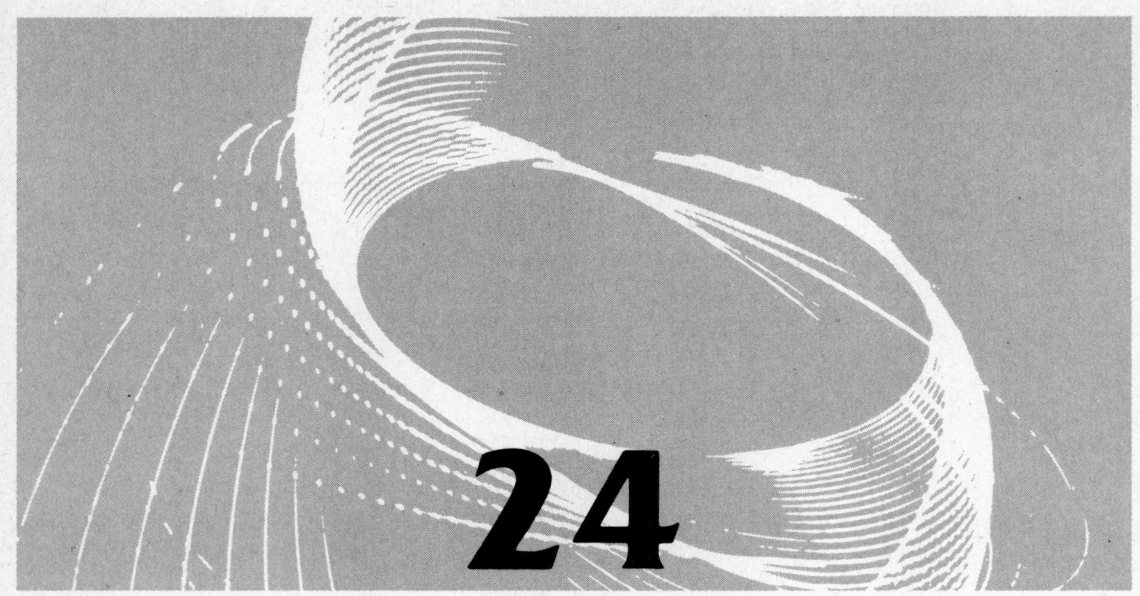

24 Activity therapies

- History of activity therapies
- Goals of activity therapies
- Specific activity therapies
- Implications of activity therapies for nursing practice

The disciplines that make up the activity therapies include occupational therapy, recreational therapy, music therapy, vocational or industrial therapy, educational therapy, and patient library services (bibliotherapy). Within these specialties other services may be provided, such as dance therapy, drama therapy, art therapy, horticulture therapy, and manual arts therapy.

Activity therapies are most commonly provided in hospital settings, but their value is such that they are increasingly being found in community-based mental health facilities. Another common pattern is when the client who is being treated in the community attends activity therapies at the local hospital. This pattern is often used for reasons of economy of resources and personnel, but it is less therapeutically desirable than the provision of activities within a community setting. A community-based treatment center that provides little more than supervision of medications and interpersonally based interventions misses an important opportunity to assist clients in ways that are relevant to their daily lives.

The activity therapies are briefly discussed in this chapter because close coordination must be maintained between the nursing staff and the activity therapists if the client is to receive optimum benefit from these auxiliary services. This is especially true if the client's program of activity centers around activities of daily living, since the nurse is in a position to supervise and reinforce the use of those skills learned in activity therapy.

HISTORY OF ACTIVITY THERAPIES

In the care of emotionally disturbed persons the activity therapies have, until recently, been considered to be less important in the treatment of emotional disturbances than interpersonally based psychotherapeutic measures. This has been the case despite the fact that ancient Greek and Egyptian civilizations have left evidence of their use of music, games, and dancing as forms of treatment for the mentally ill.

By the turn of the twentieth century two kinds of occupational therapy had developed and were categorized by their purpose. The first kind was designed to provide diversionary activities, primarily through the use of arts and crafts. Hospitalized persons were taught to make simple objects such as ashtrays, leather slippers, and wallets. Other activities such as painting and sculpturing were also available. Some patients were quite talented in these areas and created objects that were not only aesthetically pleasing but that also could be sold for profit. Many persons, however, used these activities merely as a means of whiling away the hours in an effort to combat the tedium of long-term hospitalization.

The second type of occupational therapy at that time involved the functional usefulness of the activity. Large state mental hospitals, in particular, carried on the centuries-old tradition of isolating the mentally ill in rural settings that were designed to be as self-sufficient as possible. This meant that the hospital often included a machine shop, heating plant, farm, kitchen, and laundry. These departments were major enterprises, since they had to meet the living needs of thousands of patients as well as many of the staff who lived on the hospital's grounds. Clients who were able to work were assigned tasks that included farming, meal preparation and serving, cleaning, sewing, machine maintenance and repair, and grounds maintenance. Although there is no doubt that many clients learned valuable skills as a result of these activities, economic factors played a larger part in their use than did therapeutic factors. Clients who worked in the hospital were not paid even a token salary; in fact, it was seen as a privilege to be given a work assignment. Therefore the hospital did not have to employ outside workers. Contributing to the overall welfare of the institution and its inmates must certainly have created a sense of belonging and worthiness in some clients, but these benefits were offset by the simultaneous development of a sense of dependency on the hospital, thereby increasing the syndrome of institutionalization.

Aside from these activities, the field of activity therapies was still very limited, since many authorities believed that the best treatment for emotional illnesses was a strict regimen of rest and inactivity. This belief resulted in many persons spending their days sitting side by side on uncomfortable ward benches, not having sufficient ego strength to interact with each other or to structure their time in a meaningful way. The trained nurses who worked in such settings must be given credit for seeing the lack of therapeutic effects of idleness and for attempting to engage clients in diversionary or functional activities. In fact, the first book written on the subject of occupational therapy was written by a nurse, Susan E. Tracy. This book, *Studies in Invalid Occupation,* was published in 1910. Miss Tracy also gave the first course of instruction on the subject in 1906 at the Adams Nervine in Boston. As such, nurses were the first occupational therapists, although that term was not used until 1921.

Some physicians also saw the potential therapeutic benefit of a planned activities program. As early as 1892 Dr. E.N. Brush wrote of his belief that even the most simple and routine tasks keep the mind occupied, awaken new trains of thought and interest, and divert the client from the delusions or hallucinations that harass and annoy him. Dr. Brush particularly advocated the use of outdoor activities in the belief that physical exertion had a beneficial effect on the emotional health of the client. Since the nursing staff was still seen as being responsible for initiating and supervising all client activities, a book titled *Occupation Therapy, A Manual for Nurses* was published in 1915. The author was Dr. William Rush Dunton, one of the earliest leaders in the field of occupational therapy. Dr. Dunton advised that the nurse "provide herself with an armamentarium which should consist at least of the following: playing cards, dominoes or card dominoes, cribbage board, scrap book with puzzles and catches, and one or more picture puzzles. . . . She is also urged to cultivate a particular craft in order that she may herself have a hobby and also that she may have special ability in instructing her client."*

Activity programs for mentally ill clients were formerly called *workcures* and *moral treatment.* These terms provide insight into both the ways in which mental illness was conceptualized at that time as well as the dominance of the work ethic in the American culture at large. The work ethic dictated that there was inherent value in activity, regardless of its purpose or outcome. It was not until 1921 that the term *occupational therapy* was coined and de-

*Dunton, William Rush: Occupation therapy, a manual for nurses, Philadelphia, 1915, W.B. Saunders Co., p.8.

fined. After that time, activity programs for the mentally ill increased, but their primary purpose was to keep clients busy, with scant attention paid to the therapeutic benefits that could be achieved. In recent decades, with the advent of a greater number of professionally trained activity therapists, there has been increased recognition of the positive role the discipline can play in the diagnosis and treatment of emotional disturbances.

GOALS OF ACTIVITY THERAPIES

Although each form of activity therapy has a specific focus, they all share in common the principle that it is helpful to the emotionally disturbed person to be engaged in an activity that focuses on objects outside himself. The concept of *object relations* is a fundamental one in activity therapies. This concept includes not only the materials used in the therapy but also the setting, the therapist, and the other participants. These objects all have symbolic value, and through their use the individual expresses feelings, needs, and impulses. In this sense, all activity therapies are creative and therefore can be used in varying ways and for varied purposes. They are developed into a program based on psychodynamic insights but are highly individualized to meet the needs of the person for whom they are designed. The nurse therefore may work in a mental health setting where most of the clients attend occupational therapy, but it must not be assumed that all are engaged in the same activity.

The following four goals are common to all activity therapies in a mental health setting:

1. To provide opportunities for structured normal activities of daily living. Activities are designed to help the clients deal with their basic problems. In addition, the activities permit the maintenance as well as reinforcement of the healthy aspects of the client's personality.
2. To assist in diagnostic and personality evaluation. Activity therapists, as trained members of the health care team, can assist with diagnostic and personality evaluations through their observations of clients while they are participating in the activities. In addition, the process of participation, such as the type of activity chosen and the interaction that takes

place between the client and the therapist and between the client and other participants, gives the therapist much valuable information about the personality structure of the client.

3. To enhance psychotherapy and other psychotherapeutic measures. The activity prescribed for the client often provides a nonverbal means for the client to express and resolve the feelings that are being discussed verbally in other settings. In addition, the interpersonal relationship established between the client and the therapist provides another vehicle for the provision of corrective emotional experiences.
4. To assist the client in making the transition from the sick role to becoming a contributing member of society. Some activities provide opportunity for work experience, often with the use of community resources. Through these activities the client is able to learn a skill that may be marketable. Other activities in this category focus on the development of the client's talents and interests so that he might learn to use his time in ways that are satisfying to him.

All activity therapies have in common the fact that they are purposefully designed to achieve a specified goal, and the role of the therapist is to observe, direct, and guide the client in the activity. The therapist continuously assesses the client's reactions to the activity both as a means of providing information to other members of the treatment team and as a basis on which to alter the activity as the needs of the client change.

SPECIFIC ACTIVITY THERAPIES

Occupational therapy

Occupational therapy is defined by the American Occupational Therapy Association as the art and science of directing man's response to selected activity to promote and maintain health, to prevent disability, to evaluate behavior, and to treat or train clients with physical or psychosocial dysfunction. This broad definition encompasses many activities, and thus the occupational therapy department is usually the largest of the activity therapy departments found in mental health settings. Although all occupational therapists have an educational and experiential background in the use of a wide variety of activities for many purposes, most develop particular expertise in the use of a few activities for a specified purpose. For example, occupational therapists who work with the mentally ill have more skill in the use of objects that help people identify, express, and resolve their feelings than they do in the use of objects that are designed to aid the physically handicapped in carrying out the activities of daily living.

Although occupational therapy can be carried out in almost any setting, most mental health centers have an occupational therapy department to which clients go. This setting may be one or more large, brightly decorated rooms that contain many types of equipment, which is organized into different sections of the room. For example, all the artist supplies may be on one side of the room and the weaving and sewing equipment on another. The advantage of this arrangement is more than organizational in that clients who are engaged in similar kinds of activities will be working in physical proximity to one another, which promotes social interaction. Often persons who lack the social skills required to converse spontaneously with others will be able to do so if they can focus their conversation on an object in which all are interested. An individual's self-esteem can be increased by the positive regard shown by others for a painting or other project on which he is working.

It is not unusual for individuals who are emotionally disturbed to have difficulty in verbally expressing or even identifying the emotions they are currently feeling. Through the use of various objects, the occupational therapist can help the individual discover and express these feelings. For example, the client who is very angry but who has directed his anger inwardly and therefore feels depressed, may not be able to develop insight into these dynamics merely through talking with a psychotherapist, no matter how skilled the psychotherapist may be. The astute occupational therapist, however, will take advantage of her observation that the client enjoys the hammering associated with building a bookcase and will suggest other activities that require aggressive movement. The client is able to engage in these activities because they provide a constructive, indirect outlet for his anger, in contrast to the destructive, direct impulses he unconsciously harbors and fears. Whether or not the client and the occupational therapist verbally discuss his feelings is highly dependent on the treatment goals and the client's ability to tolerate such an interpretation.

Although many examples could be given, it should be obvious that to achieve the optimum benefit of occupational therapy, the individualized attention of the therapist is required. It is rarely possible to provide one-to-one situations, but the group of clients participating in occupational therapy at any one time is usually kept small. To achieve this, appointments are made with clients, and the nursing staff frequently has the responsibility of ensuring that other activities of the unit do not interfere with these appointments. If the members of the nursing staff are unaware of the purpose and value of occupational therapy, they might view these sessions as unimportant and therefore feel free to schedule conflicting activities. It is not sufficient to make sure that there are no conflicting activities scheduled; it is also the responsibility of the nursing staff to encourage the client to attend the occupational therapy sessions. Nurses can be helpful to clients in this regard by inquiring about their projects and otherwise expressing interest in their activities.

Recreational therapy

Recreational therapy is described as the use of recreational activities, including, but not limited to, games, sports, crafts, discussion groups, and local community functions, for the purposes of aiding the client's recovery from illness or injury and assisting him in his adjustment to hospitalization. The latter purpose of recreational therapy has been widely known and used in the past through the use of diversionary activities. It has not been until recently, however, that the therapeutic effects of recreational activities have been recognized. A dramatic example occurs when a group of schizophrenic individuals who have probably never achieved the developmental task of learning how to compete and compromise are successful in engaging in a team sport such as baseball or football. Card games such as bridge that require cooperation between two players against a team of two other players can accomplish the same objective in a less dramatic but equally effective manner.

As mental health centers have been gradually relocating in the communities whose populations they serve, recreational therapists have been taking increasing advantage of community functions as therapeutic activities for groups of clients. Activities such as concerts, plays, and lectures simultaneously provide clients with an enjoyable activity as well as a focus for subsequent group discussion. For the client who has been hospitalized for a period of time, attendance at community-sponsored events is a relatively painless means of reentering community life. Despite enlightened treatment of persons with mental illness and the trend to return them to the community as soon as possible, there is still a sizeable number of persons who have been hospitalized for such a long period of time that they need to learn how to purchase a ticket to an event or how to dress appropriately. Therefore recreational therapists often aid and encourage clients to make their own arrangements when they wish to attend a community-sponsored event.

One of the many values of recreational therapy is to help the client develop skill in a diversionary activity that he finds enjoyable and can engage in by himself. Some emotionally disturbed individuals become immobilized when left by themselves with nothing to do. This can result in a marked increase in anxiety, causing the individual to retreat into a fantasy world or to use other unhealthy defenses. The person who is helped to develop his interest in such activities as stamp or coin collecting will be helped to develop a socially constructive and emotionally healthy means of coping with unstructured time. This goal is particularly appropriate for persons whose depression has been precipitated by such events as retirement from an active career or the youngest child's leaving home.

Recreational therapy, as all other activity therapies, attempts to build on existent interests and skills of the client as well as to help the client develop new ones. The nurse can be particularly helpful as she works in close collaboration with the recreational therapist if she is alert to the client's expression of interest in certain activities and conveys this information to the recreational therapist.

Music therapy

For reasons that are not clearly known, many emotionally disturbed persons derive a great deal of enjoyment from music. In fact, it is not unusual for a severely emotionally disturbed person who seems unresponsive to everything else to respond to music. Music therapy is described simply as the purposeful use of music as a participative or listening experience in the treatment of clients to improve their health. Mental health centers with sufficient financial resources provide a music library for their clients. Clients are encouraged to select records to play in soundproof rooms. The person's selection is often an indication of his emotional state at the time; persons who feel sad tend to select music that expresses sadness and the client may even cry while listening. This emotional response is sometimes misinterpreted by the staff as meaning that the client should be directed toward music that is more cheerful, rather than being recognized as a therapeutic emotional release. Changes in the nature of the person's selection of music over time provide some indication as to the progress he is making in treatment.

Group activities structured around music are also a commonly used therapeutic endeavor. Clients discuss not only the history of the musical selection and its composer but also can be helped to discuss the feelings the music elicited in them. In this way the individual not only expresses his own feelings but also learns that others may share these feelings, thereby decreasing his sense of aloneness.

Vocational therapy

Vocational therapy is also sometimes termed *industrial therapy.* This form of activity therapy deals with the development and provision of therapeutic work opportunities for clients under medical care, especially for those who are emotionally disturbed.

Many such persons have never developed an occupational skill or find themselves unable to engage in the occupation for which they were trained. Vocational therapy recognizes that in American society the ability to earn a living is a major factor in enhancing a person's self-concept and thereby his mental health. Vocational therapists are often skilled in the administration and interpretation of vocational interest and aptitude tests, and the therapy often begins with the client's taking a battery of such tests. After the results have been interpreted by the therapist, she and the client engage in one or more discussions about the results and mutually evolve a plan whereby the client can improve an existent skill or develop a new one. Whenever possible, the client is helped to develop these skills in an on-the-job setting where he is paid as he learns.

The purpose of vocational therapy is not merely to find something for the client to do to pass the time or to use his abilities to meet the needs of an institution but rather to place the client in a situation where he will be able to develop skills that will be relevant and applicable in the future. Therefore it is important that the client's needs and the needs of the work situation be closely matched. This sometimes means that the client will work in the mental health setting itself doing such jobs as typing or mechanical repair. Increasingly often, however, clients are taking apprentice-type jobs in the community, since the community needs are wider in scope than are the needs of the institution, thereby providing a larger variety of appropriate work opportunities. Positive relationships between the community and the mental health center are therefore becoming increasingly important. Although many employers in the community have little, if any, understanding of the dynamics of mental illness, most have been found to be very cooperative when the vocational therapist takes the time to elicit their help.

Some clients who are still hospitalized may progress to the point that they are working in the community full-time through the vocational therapy department of the hospital and return to the hospital only in the evening. In these instances the most qualified nursing staff should be available during those times when the client is present rather than automatically working during the day, as is usually the case. Halfway houses provide the best setting for such a client, but these are not always available.

It should be noted that vocational therapy not only provides the client with the opportunity to learn and practice a marketable skill but also with the opportunity to interact with peers in a work situation. Some clients quickly become skilled at the assigned task but have difficulty in relating to their co-workers. The sensitive vocational therapist will recognize these problems and either help the client deal with them or suggest that these interpersonal difficulties be discussed in psychotherapeutically oriented sessions.

Educational therapy

Educational therapy is closely related to vocational therapy but has as its specific focus the gathering of information and the providing of credentials for the client, rather than the development of skills. Some clients have never completed high school or may have begun but not completed their college education because of their emotional disturbance. This is not to say that all these persons are intellectually incompetent but rather that their emotional problems have interfered with their intellectual achievement. In American society, having the proper credentials is seen as a prerequisite to many types of employment, and one of the goals of the educational therapist is to assist such an individual to complete his education, usually through nontraditional routes such as the High School Equivalency Program or external degree programs. The establishment of programs of this type in many states has inadvertently provided the emotionally disturbed individual with an opportunity to obtain credentials without further lowering his self-esteem by forcing him to attend classes with persons who are much younger than he.

Educational therapy is also used in instances when the client has problems that result from a great deal of misinformation. Although his problems may be emotional, they may partially stem from years of reinforcement of inaccurate information. The educational therapist is in a position to provide the client with readings and learning experiences that can do a great deal to eliminate this misinformation and resultant anxiety. The emotional conflict that this precipitates is usually explored in psychotherapeutic sessions but is sometimes dealt with by the skilled educational therapist.

Patient library services (bibliotherapy)

The patient library services are also referred to as *bibliotherapy*, which is described as the prescription of reading materials that will help to develop emotional maturity and nourish and sustain mental health. Some emotionally disturbed individuals are able to relate therapeutically to the experiences of others when they read about them rather than experiencing them directly. In other words, sufficient distance between the individual and the situation is achieved by reading about the situation so that the person's anxiety level is not increased, and he therefore can potentially benefit from learning about the experiences of others. This benefit is usually achieved through the use of novels and biographies.

Another benefit of bibliotherapy is the increase in the individual's fund of general information. Regardless of what is read, the person is likely to pick up new ideas that can be used later in conversation with others, thereby enhancing the person's feelings of self-esteem. Some clients benefit greatly from the reading of the daily newspaper, which helps them to become reoriented to the world around them in a variety of ways. Not only are they helped to become aware of local, national, and world events, but they can gain a practical base of information that will enable them to function more effectively within the community. For example, the mere perusal of grocery store advertisements gives the reader a knowledge of food prices, which is necessary to plan a budget and shop efficiently. Clients who have expressed interest in a particular subject are encouraged to become familiar with the literature in that area. Not only can this form of reading activity be enjoyable, since it is about a subject in which the client is interested, but it can also help him gain expertise in the area.

Reading itself is usually a solitary activity. However, it is therapeutically desirable for small groups to be formed to discuss a particular book or subject. The discussion is focused around the content that was read, but the therapeutic benefit occurs as a result of the social interaction required for the discussion.

IMPLICATIONS OF ACTIVITY THERAPIES FOR NURSING PRACTICE

The nurse has an important role in enhancing the therapeutic effects of activity therapies. The activity in which the client is engaged is likely to elicit a variety of feelings in him, which he will express to the activity therapist and to the nurse. Therefore it is important for the nurse to be aware of the specific activities prescribed for each client.

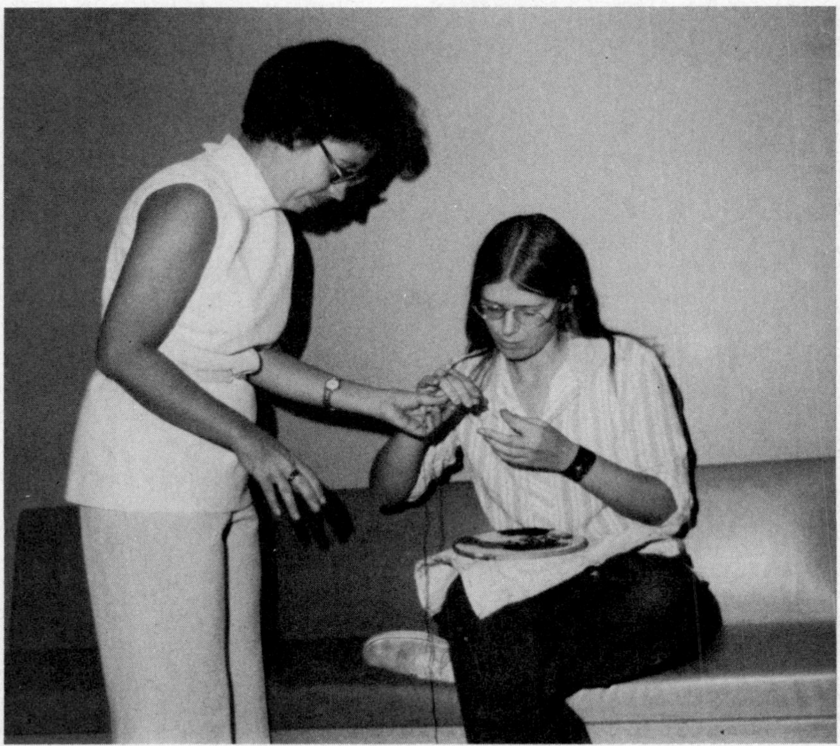

Fig. 24-1 *The nurse's interest in the client's project enhances the therapeutic effects of activity therapies.*

Close coordination between the nursing staff and the activity therapy departments is essential. The activity therapists usually take the initiative in establishing and maintaining this coordination, but nursing staff members should be receptive to these conferences, thereby acknowledging the therapeutic value of activity therapies in the total treatment program.

The nurse's interest in the client's project enhances the therapeutic effects of the activity therapies (Fig 24-1). This is particularly true if the client's program of activity centers around activities of daily living, because the nurse is in a position to supervise and reinforce the use of those skills learned in an activity therapy. It is also the nurse who often has the opportunity to gather clients together in small informal groups. The projects being worked on in the activity therapies program provide an excellent topic for discussion.

Nursing staff members sometimes participate in the activities planned as part of the recreational therapy program. Such activities include dances, sports activities, and parties. By engaging in these activities, the nurse not only has an opportunity to support the therapeutic efforts of the recreational therapist but also has an invaluable opportunity to observe the client in a setting that is not only different from the one in which she usually sees him but is more like settings usually encountered in daily living. Through her observations of the client's behavior during these activities, the nurse will gain valuable information that she can subsequently use to therapeutic advantage in the working phase of the nurse-client relationship.

CONCLUDING STATEMENTS

1. The disciplines that make up the activity therapies include occupational therapy, recreational therapy, music therapy, vocational or industrial therapy, educational therapy, and patient library services (bibliotherapy).
2. Activity therapies have been used since ancient times but until recently have been considered to be less important in the treatment of emotional disturbances than interpersonally based psychotherapeutic measures.
3. The first book on the subject of occupational therapy, pub-

lished in 1910, was written by a nurse, Susan E. Tracy, and was titled *Studies in Invalid Occupation.*

4. It was not until 1921 that the term *occupational therapy* was coined and defined. After that time, activity programs for the mentally ill increased, but their primary purpose was to keep clients busy, with scant attention paid to the therapeutic benefits that could be achieved.
5. Recently there has been increased recognition of the positive role that activity therapies can play in the diagnosis and treatment of emotional disturbances.
6. The concept of object relations is fundamental to activity therapy. Objects have symbolic value, and through their use the individual expresses feelings, needs, and impulses.
7. All activity therapies have four goals in common:
   a. To provide opportunities for structured normal activities of daily living.
   b. To assist in diagnostic and personality evaluation.
   c. To enhance psychotherapy and other psychotherapeutic measures.
   d. To assist the client in making the transition from the sick role to becoming a contributing member of society.
8. Occupational therapy is the art and science of directing man's response to selected activity to promote and maintain health, to prevent disability, to evaluate behavior, and to treat or train clients with physical or psychosocial dysfunction.
9. Recreational therapy is described as the use of recreational activities, including, but not limited to, games, sports, crafts, discussion groups, and local community functions, for the purposes of aiding the client's recovery from illness or injury and assisting him in his adjustment to the hospital.
10. Music therapy is the purposeful use of music as a participative or listening experience in the treatment of clients to improve their health.
11. Vocational therapy is sometimes termed *industrial therapy* and deals with the development and provision of therapeutic work opportunities for clients under medical care, especially for those who are emotionally disturbed.

12. Educational therapy has as its specific focus the gathering of information and the providing of credentials for the client.
13. Patient library services are also referred to as bibliotherapy, which is described as the prescription of reading materials that will help to develop emotional maturity and nourish and sustain mental health.
14. The nurse has an important role in enhancing the therapeutic effects of activity therapies. This role is implemented through close coordination with the activity therapist and support of the goals of activity therapy with clients on an individual and small group basis.

Suggested sources of additional information

CLASSICAL

Dunton, William Rush, and Licht, Sidney: Occupational therapy, principles and practice, ed. 2, Springfield, Ill., 1957, Blackwell Scientific Publications.

Irwin, B.: Play therapy for a regressed schizophrenic patient, J. Psychiatr. Nurs. **9**:30-32, Sept.-Oct., 1971.

CONTEMPORARY

Burch, J.W., and Meredith, J.L.: Nurses as the core of the psychiatric team, Am. J. Nurs. **74**:2037-2038, 1974.

Gerace, Laina, and Rosenberg, Lisa: The use of art prints in group therapy with aftercare patients, Perspect. Psychiatr. Care **17**(2):83-86, March-April, 1979.

Kasiman, C.M.: Issues between professional and paraprofessional nursing staff in community mental health, J. Psychiatr. Nurs. **12**(5):31-35, 1974.

Kyes, Joan, and Hofling, Charles K.: Basic psychiatric concepts in nursing, ed. 4, Philadelphia, 1980, J.B. Lippincott Co., pp. 478-493.

Labarca, Judith R.: Communication through art therapy, Perspect. Psychiatr. Care **17**:118-124, May-June, 1979.

McMorrow, Martin J., Cullinan, Douglas, and Epstein, Michael H.: The use of the premack principle to motivate patient activity attendance, Perspect. Psychiatr. Care **16**:14-17, Jan.-Feb., 1978.

Smith, Marie M.: The use of the premack principle to motivate patient activity attendance, Perspect. Psychiatr. Care **16**:14-18, Jan. Feb., 1978.

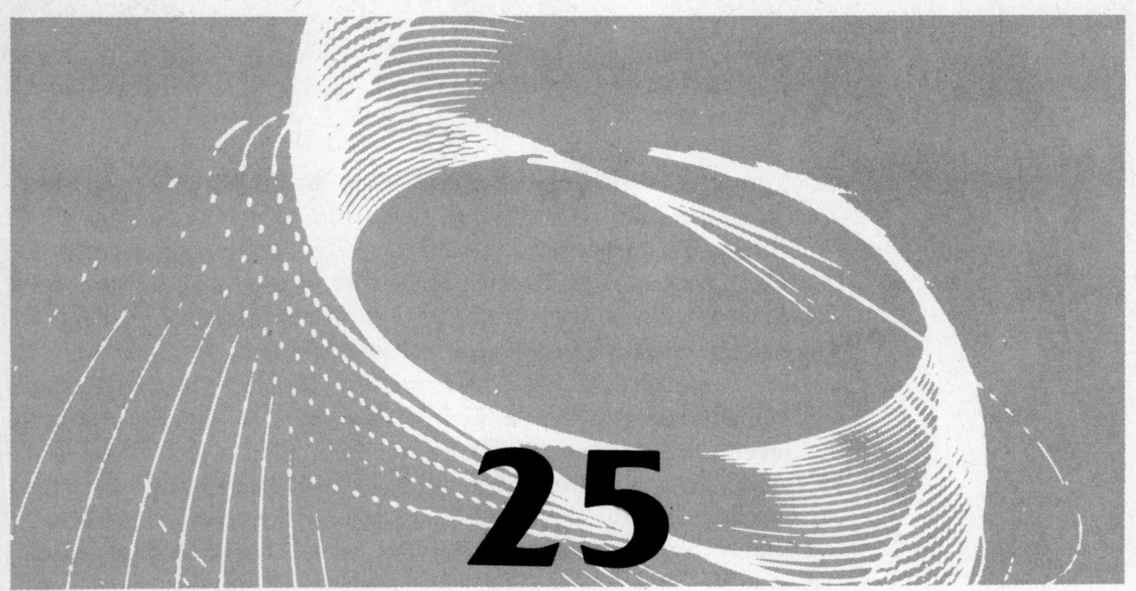

25

Community mental health: a treatment philosophy

- Philosophical assumptions underlying the concept of community mental health
- Development of the community mental health movement
- Characteristics of a comprehensive community mental health center
- Role of the nurse in comprehensive community mental health centers
- Accomplishments of the Community Mental Health Centers Act

Community mental health, as a treatment philosophy, was mandated by the Community Mental Health Centers Act of 1963 and was introduced to revolutionize the care of the mentally ill. In 1963 it was a relatively new and expanding concept. The basic principles underlying this concept were put into practical use in centers called *comprehensive community mental health centers.*

Community mental health is said to be the fourth revolutionary development in the field of psychiatry. The first of these was achieved by Pinel in 1793 when he struck off the chains of mentally ill patients who were confined in Bicêtre outside of Paris. The second was the development in the psychoanalytic method of treatment by Freud about 100 years later. The third was the development in the early 1950s of the antipsychotic drugs.

The concept of community mental health is new in that it requires a total realignment of the roles of professional mental health workers and a change in their philosophical approach to the prevention of mental illness and the treatment of people in need of emotional and psychological help.

PHILOSOPHICAL ASSUMPTIONS UNDERLYING THE CONCEPT OF COMMUNITY MENTAL HEALTH

The basic assumption underlying the community mental health movement is that behavior is a function of two sets of variables: the person and the situation. That is, behavior is related both to the characteristics of the individual and to the nature of his environment. Thus the term *community mental health* has come to represent all mental health activities carried out in a community, and this theoretical formulation has evolved as an alternative to the medical model.

The medical model successfully used by physicians to identify and treat physically ill individuals was employed for many years by psychiatrists because they were trained as physicians, often as neurologists. In dealing with a mentally ill individual, the psychiatrist frequently removed him from the community and prescribed a treatment program designed to correct the sickness that presumably lay within the individual's personality. Even the treatment technique known as psychoanalysis was developed out of Freud's experiences, some of which he had as a neurologist. Psychoanalysis seeks to help the individual to identify his own interpersonal or intrapsychic problems and to make appropriate changes through developing self-understanding and insight.

As social science research has developed and grown in importance, it has become increasingly evident that mental health problems are intimately related to the environment and that there are many environmental factors that contribute to the mental health or mental illness of an individual. Thus there has been a growing dissatisfaction with the medical model or the idea that mental illness is inherent within the personality of the individual. As dissatisfactions grew, attempts have been made to develop a theoretical model to replace the medical model that has been in use so long.

Thus the theoretical formulations underlying the current movement in community mental health have been developed. They deal with the belief that much deviant behavior is learned behavior and develops in response to a negative environmental situation that reinforces and encourages the development of deviance. It follows that if a type of behavior is learned, it can be unlearned or a more socially acceptable type of behavior can be substituted. It also follows that if deviant behavior develops in relation to environmental influences, as much social science research has demonstrated, the environment should be the focus of the attention of professional workers who seek to alter the situation in a positive direction. Social scientists have come to recognize that inadequate, overcrowded housing, poor or nonexistent community recreation facilities, unemployment, poverty, broken homes, and poor schools are all factors that contribute to high rates of deviant behavior or mental illness among the population in some communities. One approach to preventing mental illness in individuals living in a community is to improve the conditions existing in the community. Thus community mental health not only focuses on helping the individual and his family but also on altering the environment in the community itself.

Another philosophical assumption underlying the community mental health movement is that removing the mentally ill person from his family and community for treatment encourages chronicity rather than a return to a productive life. Thus the current trend is to treat the individual immediately in the community, no matter how disturbed his behavior may be. In this way it is hoped that the development of chronic symptomatology and the rupturing of familial and community ties through institutionalization can be avoided. When hospitalization is necessary, the staff members of the comprehensive community mental health center expect the period of institutionalization to be for a relatively short period. The individual will be treated as an outpatient or in a day-care center as soon as possible and will be encouraged to resume a reasonable number of his former responsibilities, including a return to work. Thus the depersonalization effect of a large institution will be avoided.

DEVELOPMENT OF THE COMMUNITY MENTAL HEALTH MOVEMENT

Knowledge of the historical background of the community mental health movement helps us to understand and appreciate it. Some authorities place its earliest beginnings in 1908 when Clifford Beers, a psychiatric patient who was hospitalized several times during an otherwise productive life, published a book entitled *A Mind That Found Itself*. This book about his experiences as a mentally ill patient provided the impetus for the beginning of the mental health movement in the United States. Child guidance clinics developed and flourished from the early 1920s through the 1930s. A heritage from this era is the staffing pattern of the traditional clinic team, which included a psychiatrist, a psychologist, and a social worker. The nurse was omitted. This oversight probably grew out of the belief that the expertise of the nurse lay solely in caring for the physically ill. Since most children who required help from child guidance clinics were not physically ill, the usefulness of the nurse in such clinics was thought to be limited or nonexistent.

Schools of nursing did not traditionally include mental health or psychiatric nursing in the curriculum until the late 1930s. Thus most physicians and social workers thought of the nurse's work as dealing almost entirely with physical illness. Unfortunately, this attitude continues today among many professional people who represent the three professions that traditionally staffed the child guidance clinics.

One of the most forward-looking actions the nation has ever

taken in relation to mental illness was the passage of the National Mental Health Act in 1946. Among other accomplishments was the establishment of the National Institute of Mental Health within the Public Health Service of the Department of Health, Education, and Welfare. A similar act was passed about the same time in Canada, and it has had a similar effect in moving Canada into the forefront in the field of mental health. Both these acts provided for the financing of research and training programs. Through their enactment the governments expressed their belief that it was necessary to acquire more knowledge concerning the cause, prevention, and treatment of mental illness and that more professionally trained workers were needed to improve the care and treatment of the mentally ill. Financial support for the education of psychologists, psychiatric social workers, psychiatrists, and psychiatric nurses was provided in the United States for many years through the National Mental Health Act.

The National Mental Health Act grew out of the experiences the nation had during World War II when more men in the Armed Forces were disabled by mental illness than by all the other problems related to actual military action. The many soldiers who were incapacitated by acute and chronic mental illness alerted the nation to the need for many more trained professional workers in the field, for greater knowledge about the cause and prevention of mental illness, and for greatly improved treatment techniques.

During World War II the psychiatrists in the medical corps, led by Dr. William Menninger, learned the importance of early recognition of psychiatric problems and the significance of initiating treatment rapidly and close to the place where the difficulty occurred. They developed a method of crisis-oriented treatment, which promoted adaptation and an early return to duty. To individuals in decision-making positions, they demonstrated the usefulness of consultation when issues that affected the mental well-being of soldiers were concerned. This knowledge and skill, which was developed pragmatically in the Armed Forces, has been incorporated today into the principles of the community mental health movement.

The psychotropic drugs, particularly the antipsychotic agents, played a large role in the development of community mental health. They were first used experimentally in 1953. By 1956 the populations of the state mental hospitals were reported to have fallen slightly, instead of increasing as they had done for decades. This development was largely a result of the fact that, with the help of the drugs, persons could control their behavior and thus could spend time outside the hospital in the community. Had it not been for these drugs, many individuals would never have been able to control their unusual behavior sufficiently to remain at home and thus be available for help on an outpatient basis.

In the late 1940s and the early 1950s the large public institutions for the care of the mentally ill began to change significantly through the development of new methods for approaching and understanding human problems. Some of these new methods included family diagnosis, the introduction of short- and long-term treatment programs, and the advent of crisis-oriented therapy. At about the same time, several new ideas were introduced into public psychiatric hospitals. Such developments as the therapeutic community concept, which attempted to alter certain sections of larger psychiatric institutions to provide clients with an opportunity for achieving a more constructive social adjustment, the concept described as milieu therapy, and the approach known as the open-door hospital were introduced and refined. Some of these ideas, especially the open-door hospital and the therapeutic community, came to the United States directly from experimentation carried on in England.

In 1955 the Congress of the United States passed the Mental Health Study Act. This act provided money for a 5-year study of the problem of mental illness in the United States. As a result of the act, the Joint Commission on Mental Illness was established. On December 31, 1960, this commission submitted its final report to the Congress, to the Surgeon General of the Public Health Service, and to the governors of the 50 states. The published report was entitled *Action for Mental Health* and was available to the public in 1961. It was widely read and provided an impetus for developing more effective services for people in need of psychiatric help and was the basis for additional legislation. Because of its statements concerning the need to develop and use the potential therapeutic abilities of all other professional workers in psychiatric settings, in addition to psychiatrists, it added strength to the position that had already been taken by professional nurses who were working in psychiatric situations. Many of these nurses had maintained for years that the nurse had a legitimate and specific role in providing therapy for the mentally ill.

A milestone in the nation's developing awareness of the need for an improved approach to the problems of mental health and illness was reached on February 5, 1963, when President John F. Kennedy delivered his special message to the Congress on mental illness and mental retardation. In this speech he mentioned a few goals: "Central to a new mental health program is comprehensive community care. . . . The mentally ill can achieve . . . a constructive social adjustment. . . . The centers will focus on community resources. . . . Prevention as well as treatment will be a major activity." In that same year, 1963, the Community Mental Health Centers Act was passed, followed in 1965 by the Staffing Act for the Community Mental Health Centers. These acts made money available to build and staff the centers and were the impetus for the rapid development of many centers in a relatively short period of time. The first federally funded centers began operation in 1966.

In 1975 the Congress of the United States enacted the Community Mental Health Centers Amendments of 1975. This law provided for the continuation of federal funds to community mental health centers but also designated specific guidelines for services that must be provided. Specified in these guidelines is a full range of inpatient, outpatient, and emergency services. Certain population groups such as children and the elderly were targeted as particularly requiring services. Individuals suffering from drug and alcohol abuse and addiction and those persons being discharged from mental institutions also were included in the population groups given priority for services.

In 1977 President Jimmy Carter called for the development of a President's Commission on Mental Health, which was charged with identifying "the mental health needs of the nation." Nursing was represented on such a commission for the first time by Martha Mitchell, a nurse educator and clinical specialist in psychiatric–mental health nursing. The report of the 1977 Commission recommended the development of a new federal grant program designed to strengthen existent community efforts and to develop new initiatives to address the mental health needs of communities. Special emphasis was placed on meeting the needs of underserved and high-risk populations such as the elderly, children, the chronically mentally ill, cultural minorities, rural communities, and inner-city neighborhoods. The very timely issue of the economics of mental health care was addressed by a recommendation that mental health coverage be included in all health insurance and that this coverage not be limited to hospitalization. The Commission also recommended that evaluation of federally funded community mental health centers be centralized.

In October of 1980 Congress passed the Mental Health Systems Act of 1980. This legislation grew out of the Commission's recommendations, and it addresses, among other topics, research and training priorities and patients' rights. It is too soon to postulate about the impact of this latest legislation. However, there is no doubt that the mental health needs of the nation are of great concern to its citizenry.

CHARACTERISTICS OF A COMPREHENSIVE COMMUNITY MENTAL HEALTH CENTER

The comprehensive community mental health center is organized around a demographic unit with a population small enough to permit the development of comprehensive mental health services. It seeks to serve the people who reside in a specific geographic area of a city or a locality that is referred to as a *catchment area.* The workers in the center attempt to assist the community to improve its level of mental health and to help individuals and families who have developed emotional problems to maintain their ties with the community and, when hospitalization is necessary, to return to community living as soon as possible. To achieve these goals, it becomes essential that all helping agencies share information freely and cooperate effectively.

Specific requirements for a fully developed comprehensive community mental health center were identified in the law that made government funding available. When fully developed, a comprehensive community mental health center includes inpatient services, outpatient services, day and night hospital units, crisis intervention centers, halfway houses, family therapy centers, rehabilitation centers, transitional facilities where individuals may receive board and care, and suicide prevention centers. In addition, the community mental health center is expected to offer services to the community that include consultation to community agencies and professional personnel, diagnostic services, and rehabilitative services including vocational and educational programs. Finally, the community mental health center is expected to provide training for professional and paraprofessional workers, to conduct research into the prevention, cause and treatment of mental illness, and to evaluate the effectiveness of the program being carried forward.

Although inpatient services, outpatient services, and partial hospitalization were required, the government expected individual communities to identify those services that would be developed first, those services that would be emphasized most, and what the specific focus of the outreach centers would be.

The need for suicide prevention and crisis clinics was identified early in the development of some mental health services in some communities, whereas other communities concentrated on the development of day-care and night-care centers. Thus each comprehensive community mental health center developed somewhat differently, depending on the needs of the community it served, the philosophy of the professionals involved in the development of the services, and the relationship the community had with the center.

In spite of many differences, there are some significant similarities in comprehensive community mental health centers. There are also departures from the more traditional approach to the treatment of psychiatric problems, including the following:

1. The treatment modality is focused on helping the individual through the use of groups of which he is a member rather than by relying entirely on the use of the individual one-to-one relationship. Thus the treatment focus may be on family therapy, group therapy, the therapeutic community, or crisis intervention. The development of knowledge and skill in the use of the group process and in intervening

therapeutically in crisis situations is essential for all professional workers who hope to be involved with comprehensive community mental health centers.

2. The services of individuals who are already working with the larger population of the catchment area are used. These individuals may include welfare workers, police, clergy, teachers, public health nurses, and other community leaders. Some community mental health centers have involved individuals identified as indigenous workers. These are people who may lack formal education but who have lived in the community and understand the unofficial community organization. They are aware of the real hopes, interests, and concerns of the people. In addition, they speak and understand the language commonly used by the people being served. With professional guidance the indigenous workers have been surprisingly successful in some community mental health centers because of their ability to relate in a meaningful way with the people seeking help and to offer it to them on a level that is acceptable and useful.
3. Role definitions are becoming blurred as the various representatives of the professional disciplines work in the interdisciplinary climate of the comprehensive community mental health centers. All disciplines share treatment responsibilities in these centers. The leadership of the team may be held by any one of its members, depending on the background, experience, interests, and abilities of the individual team members. Group or family therapy may be carried on by the nurse as a therapist or as a cotherapist with some other member of the professional team. Thus the nurse who looks forward to working in a comprehensive community mental health center needs to think in terms of seeking preparation in individual and group therapy before undertaking such responsibility.
4. Prevention is a major focus in community mental health centers. Thus consultation and educational activities become as important in the centers as treatment. Many of the professional workers spend more time in the consultation

and educational aspects of their work than in the treatment aspects. They seek to help mothers of children, schoolteachers, public health nurses, workers in the juvenile courts, and individuals employed in social agencies to understand the concepts of mental health and the contribution they can make in the areas of prevention of mental illness and the promotion of mental health among the groups with whom they deal.

5. Planned social change is another focus of comprehensive community mental health centers. Professional workers are concerned not only with the individuals who seek help but also with the community itself, which is the incubator, in a sense of the word, of the mental health problems from which the population suffers. Thus the professional staff of the community mental health center works to improve the social systems that serve the population within the community, that is, the family, the churches, the schools, the hospitals, recreational facilities, the court system, housing, local government, industry, and so on.
6. Comprehensive and continuous service to the individual is emphasized in community mental health centers. The individual is seen immediately when he presents himself for help. No longer are individuals asked to wait for weeks or months for an appointment. Some clinics function as crisis clinics. Others are referred to as *coping clinics* to emphasize the fact that they are available to anyone who feels that he is in some kind of urgent difficulty or trouble and needs help in coping with the situation. Still others are called *walk-in clinics* to emphasize the fact that they are available to anyone who wishes to walk in. Many of these clinics have a psychiatrist available around the clock. Cooperation among agencies is basic if these centers are to offer a comprehensive program that can deal with the range of mental problems that arise in any community.
7. Research into the cause and treatment of mental illness is a part of every well-developed community mental health center.

ROLE OF THE NURSE IN COMPREHENSIVE COMMUNITY MENTAL HEALTH CENTERS

As has been stated, the role definitions of the professional workers in community mental health centers are becoming blurred, since the workers are free to use the knowledge and skill that they bring to the situation or that they have developed in the course of their experience at the center.

Many nurses who work in community mental health centers are involved in carrying on a variety of therapeutic activities that focus on group and family therapy, crisis intervention, and mental health education and consultation.

An initial visit to the family after the individual has been referred to the community mental health center has been one of the contributions made by the nurse. Through this visit the nurse is able to evaluate the situation, relay this information to the treatment team, and initiate whatever therapeutic intervention is indicated in relation to the social situation.

The community mental health center provides the professionally prepared nurse with an unusual opportunity to fill an expanding therapeutic role. In no other clinical situation does the nurse have so many opportunities to use her professional potential to achieve the maximum therapeutic benefit for the individual, his family, and the community.

In some communities where community mental health centers are not prepared to offer a full complement of services, the public health nurse is called on to supervise individuals in their homes who have been discharged from treatment centers. Since the introduction of the psychotropic drugs, hundreds of individuals who continue to require professional supervision are discharged to their homes. The public health nurse is frequently the key professional person who helps the family develop an understanding and acceptance of the individual so that the period after his discharge will be a constructive part of his return to the community. Families may be afraid to accept the hospitalized member back in the home because they remember how difficult his sick behavior was for them to handle. They may feel guilty and ashamed because they placed the individual in the hospital. Some families have used the individual's living space for another person and may require help in finding enough room for him. The public health nurse can be of inestimable assistance to a family group in preparing for the return of a discharged member. The nurse can assist the family to make realistic plans for the future. After the individual resumes his place in the home, the nurse's visits can provide an opportunity for the family to ventilate their concerns about new problems that the individual's behavior may precipitate and new needs they have identified.

During the visits to the family, the public health nurse is able to evaluate the adjustment the client is making and will report the findings to the appropriate individual at the clinic. The nurse can encourage the client to continue taking the medication prescribed by the physician and to keep his clinic appointments. The nurse can also offer valuable assistance in supporting the family members and helping them to recognize the progress the returning member is making. If the individual is having a difficult time in adjusting, the public health nurse can help make the decision that he should reenter the hospital if such a step is indicated. Today, public health nurses need to be as skilled in meeting the needs of the emotionally ill individual and his family as they are in meeting the needs of other individuals who require assistance with health problems.

The public health nurse is usually aware of the agencies in the community that offer help to families and can assist them in contacting appropriate agencies when additional services are required.

ACCOMPLISHMENTS OF THE COMMUNITY MENTAL HEALTH CENTERS ACT

The Community Mental Health Centers Act sought to revolutionize the provision of mental health care by emphasizing prevention and decentralized, local "community treatment" as opposed to "institutional care" for even those persons who manifest severe psychiatric difficulties. There is much debate as to whether these goals are even beginning to be achieved.

It is a fact that the number of actual public mental hospitals has not significantly decreased, although the patient population has become markedly smaller. This phenomenon is thought to be the result of political and economic issues that were not clearly envisioned when the Community Mental Health Centers Act was passed. Because of their size, public mental hospitals are major employers of residents of the community in which they are located. Attempts to close these hospitals have been met by cries of outrage from citizens who would lose their means of livelihood if these institutions were closed. Furthermore, because these mental hospitals are publically supported, their future is in the hands of elected officials who strongly consider the desires of their constituency. Another factor mitigating against the closure of these institutions is the continuing resistance of most neighborhood groups against having small treatment centers in their midst. Newspapers and television news reports give almost weekly accounts of neighborhoods organizing to prevent the establishment of day treatment facilities, halfway houses, or residential centers for the emotionally ill or the mentally retarded.

Despite the decrease in patient population in public mental institutions, the number of admissions to public mental hospitals has increased every year since 1955. This fact becomes somewhat alarming when one realizes that it includes a large number of readmissions. The current early discharge and rapid readmission phenomenon in public mental hospitals is referred to as the *revolving door syndrome.* Although more individuals are now out of the institution and in the community than 20 years ago, there has been considerable public and professional concern regarding the quality of life experienced by many of these individuals. Critics have even suggested that individuals have simply been moved from the "back wards" of the hospital to the "back alleys" of the community.*

The decrease in the size of the population of public mental hospitals may not be due entirely to the community mental health movement. The psychotropic drugs have been widely used since the mid-1950s and have made it possible for many individuals to return to life in the community because of their ability to control behavior with the assistance of the drugs. The growth of nursing homes has occurred over about the same period of time.

---

*Test, Mary Ann, and Stein, Leonard: Practical guidelines for the community treatment of markedly impaired patients, Community Ment. Health J. **12**:73-74, Fall, 1976.

These facilities have offered an alternative to hospitalization in the public mental hospitals for a large number of aged individuals. In addition, psychiatric units in general hospitals have been developed in many parts of the country. This alternate care facility, where hospitalization benefits are as applicable as for physical illness, has played a part in lowering the rate of admissions to public mental hospitals. Thus it is difficult to evaluate the effect on the public mental hospitals of the community mental health movement. However, the majority of individuals now in the community and being treated through the activities of day-care centers and working in sheltered workshops would probably be hospitalized in public mental institutions if treatment facilities were not available in the community.

Underlying the treatment philosophy of most community mental health centers is the belief that the disturbed behavior of mentally ill individuals responds positively when the person is maintained in the community because, as with all people, the environmental demands are powerful determinants of his behavior. Thus every effort is made to achieve early discharge for mentally ill individuals from short-term treatment centers or day-care facilities. As a result, however, many communities are distressed by the presence of individuals who appear to require 24-hour care.

It seems reasonable to believe that there will continue to be a need for long-term treatment situations for some clients for many years to come. Undoubtedly there will continue to be some chronically disturbed individuals who require close supervision and a rigidly structured environment. To recover, selected individuals need to be removed from their normal surroundings including family, friends, and work. When this need is not acknowledged and these individuals are hospitalized only for short periods, damage is done to the individual, the community, and the community mental health movement.

To date, the community mental health movement has had limited success in treating those mentally ill individuals who are markedly impaired. According to some authorities, community treatment of such individuals should focus primarily on the teaching of basic coping skills necessary to live as autonomously as possible. These learning needs include (1) daily living skills, (2) vocational skills, (3) leisure time skills, and (4) social and interpersonal skills. In some situations treatment has been most effective when "taken to the patient" in the individual's natural environment. It is also thought by some that a nonsheltered facility may be more therapeutic than a sheltered arrangement because greater expectations for appropriate, responsible behavior encourage socially acceptable responses.*

Thus far, many individuals in this country who are poor and members of minority groups are relatively untouched by the programs provided by community mental health centers. Programs must be developed to meet the needs of these groups, who may not respond positively to therapeutic methods that focus primarily on the sharing of feelings. Instead, these clients often require treatment techniques that emphasize actions rather than words, that deal directly with the problems of living rather than with fantasies, and that provide immediate assistance in coping with emergencies when they arise. These clients respond to therapeutic intervention that assists them to find a job, make friends, improve their domestic relations, improve their physical well-being, and get along better with relatives.†

As time has passed, this nation has become increasingly concerned about human rights. The court system has become an advocate for the client. The individual who is in need of treatment of mental illness now has a legal right to adequate treatment that adheres to minimum professional standards and that is designed appropriately to assist him in solving his problems. Among other legal rights is the right to the least restrictive setting necessary to achieve the treatment he requires and a right to an understandable explanation of the treatment planned for him. The community mental health approach has been successful in altering the detrimental effects of long-term treatment in public hospitals, in clarifying the legal rights of the mentally ill, and in promoting an enlightened community response to the problems of the mentally

---

*Test, Mary Ann, and Stein, Leonard: Practical guidelines for the community treatment of markedly impaired patients, Community Ment. Health J. **12:**73-74, Fall, 1976.

†Levy, Rona: Behavior therapy techniques as a fulfillment of community mental health ideology, Community Ment. Health J. **12:**417-418, Winter, 1976.

ill. Therefore this approach has revolutionized the delivery of mental health services and is here to stay. However, much more needs to be done to develop new treatment methods that will effectively serve clients in relieving psychological distress and in intervening in social stress. The preparation and supervision of the workers in many centers must be upgraded. The professional and paraprofessional workers need to work toward solving the conflicts that arise when treatment responsibilities are shared. A more systematic approach to treatment and research is necessary. The requirements of the original act for significant programs in primary prevention, consultation, public education, community planning, and development are all essential factors that need more attention if the goals in the 1963 Community Mental Health Centers Act are to be brought into reality. More effective techniques for achieving these goals must be developed.

In summary, the community mental health approach required a reorientation of the treatment philosophy traditionally held by most of the treatment team, especially the psychiatrists. The desired change was from the "medical model," which decreed that the individual's problem is a reflection of something inherently wrong within the person to a focus on the problems of living that have their origin within the system in which the client functions. The fact that this change has not yet been fully achieved is not surprising, since the change is a fundamental one and there has been insufficient time to feel the impact of mental health professionals who have been trained since the passage of the Community Mental Health Centers Act.

CONCLUDING STATEMENTS

1. The basic principles underlying the concept of community mental health are being used in comprehensive community mental health settings.
2. Community mental health requires a total realignment of the roles of the professional workers who are involved and a change in their philosophical approach to the prevention of mental illness and the treatment of mentally ill people.
3. The term *community mental health* has come to represent all mental health activities carried on in a community, and the

theoretical formulation basic to their functioning has evolved as an alternative to the medical model of treatment.

4. It has become increasingly evident that mental health problems are intimately related to the environment and that many environmental factors contribute to the individual's mental health or illness.
5. The theoretical formulations underlying community mental health deal with the belief that much deviant behavior is learned behavior in response to a negative environmental situation.
6. One approach to preventing mental illness and improving the mental health of individuals in a community is to improve the social conditions that exist in the community.
7. The comprehensive community mental health center attempts to treat mentally ill individuals while helping them to maintain their ties with their families and the community.
8. The National Mental Health Act was passed by the U.S. Congress in 1946 and made it possible for the nation to begin its attack on the problem of mental illness through the financing of research and training programs.
9. The psychotropic drugs, first used experimentally in 1953, played a large role in the development of community mental health care by helping mentally disturbed individuals to control their behavior and thus to remain in the community.
10. The final published report of the Joint Commission on Mental Illness was entitled *Action for Mental Health* and was issued in 1961. This report provided the basis for the legislation known as the Community Mental Health Centers Act.
11. Federal legislation in 1975 and 1980 has continued to address the mental health needs of the nation with a community approach.
12. When fully developed, a comprehensive community mental health center includes inpatient services, outpatient services, crisis intervention and suicide prevention centers, facilities for partial hospitalization, consultation and education services, diagnostic services, rehabilitation services, training for professional and paraprofessional workers, and a research program.

13. Each comprehensive community mental health center has developed differently, depending on the needs of the community it serves, the philosophy of the professional workers involved, and the relationship of the community to the center.
14. The treatment modality in the comprehensive community mental health center is focused on helping the individual through the use of a variety of group techniques.
15. Role definitions are becoming blurred as representatives of several professional disciplines work together in an interdisciplinary climate.
16. The major foci of the comprehensive community mental health centers include (a) prevention, (b) planned social change, (c) comprehensive and continuous service to the client, (d) research into the cause and treatment of mental illness, and (e) consultation and community education.
17. The fact that the goals embodied in the 1963 Community Mental Health Centers Act have not yet been fully achieved is not surprising, since the desired changes are fundamental ones, and there has been insufficient time to feel the impact of mental health professionals who have been trained since the passage of the act.
18. Public mental hospitals have not disappeared, but their patient population has grown markedly smaller. Unfortunately, a tremendous number of admissions are readmissions, leading to the description of this phenomenon as the "revolving door syndrome."
19. It seems reasonable to believe that for many years to come there will continue to be a need for long-term treatment situations for selected clients.
20. More effective treatment programs must be developed to provide the assistance required by the poor and by the members of minority groups, who respond best to action-oriented techniques.

Suggested sources of additional information

CLASSICAL

Blackman, Sheldon, and Goldstein, Kenneth M. Some aspects of a theory of community mental health, Community Ment. Health J. **4**:85-90, 1968.

Bulbuylan, Ann, Davidites, Rose Marie, and Williams, Florence: Nurses in a community mental health center, Am. J. Nurs. **69**:328-331, 1969.

Caplan, Gerald: An approach to community mental health, New York, 1966, Grune & Stratton, Inc.

Carty, Rita Cardillo, and Breault, Gretchen Clemento: Gheel: a comprehensive community mental health program, Perspect. Psychiatr. Care **5**:281-285, Nov.-Dec., 1967.

Elwell, Richard: Community mental health centers, and community mental health nursing, Am. J. Nurs. **70**:1014-1021, 1970.

Fagin, Claire M., editor: Readings in child and adolescent psychiatric nursing, St. Louis, 1974, The C.V. Mosby Co.

Freed, Harvey M., et al.: Community mental health-second class treatment? Ment. Hyg. **56**:26-29, Summer, 1972.

Gorman, Mike: Community mental health: the search for identity. Community Ment. Health J. **6**:347-355, Oct., 1970.

Joint Commission on Mental Illness and Health: Action for mental health, New York, 1961, Basic Books, Inc., Publishers.

Jones, Maxwell: Beyond the therapeutic community, New Haven, Conn., 1968, Yale University Press.

Leininger, Madeleine M.: Community psychiatric nursing: trends, issues, and problems, Perspect. Psychiatr. Care **7**:10-20, Jan.-Feb., 1969.

Lief, Victor F., and Brotman, Richard: The psychiatrist and community mental health practice, Community Ment. Health J. **4**:134-143, April, 1968.

McGee, Richard K.: Community mental health concepts as demonstrated by suicide prevention programs in Florida. Community Ment. Health J. **4**:144-152, April, 1968.

Margolin, Reuben J.: A concept of mental illness: a new look at some old assumptions, Community Ment. Health J. **4**:417-424, Oct., 1968.

Mereness, Dorothy: The potential significant role of the nurse in community mental health services, Perspect. Psychiatr. Care **1**:34-39, May-July, 1963.

Mistr, Virginia R.: Community nursing service for psychiatric patients, Perspect. Psychiatr. Care**6**:36-41, Jan.-Feb., 1968.

Ozarin, Lucy D.: The community mental health center: concept and commitment, Ment. Hyg. **52**:76-80, 1968.

Richards, Hilda: The role of the nurse in therapy of lower socioeconomic psychiatric patients. Perspect. Psychiatr. Care **5**:82-91, March-April, 1967.

Rosenblum, Gershen, and Hassol, Leonard: Training for new mental health roles, Ment. Hyg. **52**:81-85, 1968.

Sheldon, Alan, and Hope, Penelope: The developing role of the nurse in a community mental health program, Perspect. Psychiatr. Care **5**:272-279, Nov.-Dec., 1967.

Stretch, John J.: Community mental health: the evolution of a concept in social policy, Community Ment. Health J. **3**:5-12, Spring, 1967.

Ujhely, Gertrud B.: The nurse in community psychiatry, Am. J. Nurs. **69**:1001-1005, 1969.

Zahourek, Rothlyn: Nurses in a community mental health center, Nurs. Outlook **19**:592-595, 1971.

CONTEMPORARY

Adler, Peter T.: The community as a mental health system, Ment. Hyg. **56:**29-32, Fall, 1972.

Bayer, Mary: Easing mental patients' return to their communities, Am. J. Nurs. **76:**406-608, 1976.

Bellak, Leopold, and Barten, Harvey H., editors: Progress in community mental health, vol. 3, New York, 1975, Brunner/Mazel, Inc.

Brown, Frances Gold: Social linkability, Am. J. Nurs. **71:**516-520, 1971.

Buckwald, Susan: Families of the mentally ill-are we meeting their needs? Ment. Hyg. **56:**48-51, Spring, 1972.

Bushnell, Marilyn E.: Alice in mental healthland, Perspect. Psychiatr. Care **15:**11-14, 1977.

Carruth, Beatrice F.: Modifying behavior through social learning, Am. J. Nurs. **76:**1804-1806, Nov., 1976.

Carter, A.B.: Rural emergency psychiatric services, Am. J. Nurs. **73:**868-869, 1973.

Coghlan, Albon, J., Pixley Lawrence, and Zimmerman, Roger S.: Community mental health concepts and methadone maintenance: are they compatible? Community Ment. Health J. **10:**426-433, Winter, 1974.

Geller, Joseph J.: The relationship between psychoanalysis and the Community Mental Health Program, Perspect. Psychiatr. Care **13:**113-118, July-Sept., 1975.

Gibbs, Margaret S., and Lachenmeyer, Juliana R.: Community psychology; theoretical and empirical approaches. Sigal, Janet, editor: New York, 1979, Halsted Press.

Gorman, Mike: Community absorption of the mentally ill: the new challenge, Community Ment. Health J. **12:**119-127, Summer, 1976.

Greaves, George: An evolution of a 24-hour crisis intervention clinic, Can. Ment. Health **21:**13-15, May-Aug., 1973.

Henschen, Rita Sue: Learning impulse control through day care, Perspect. Psychiatr. Care **9:**219-224, Sept.-Oct., 1971.

Hitchcock, Janice E.: Community mental health nursing: an innovative use of the nurse's evolving role, Community Ment. Health J. **7:**3-12, March, 1971.

Johns, Marion Meaux: What has been done about the mental health of minorities? Ment. Hyg. **60:**21-30, Spring, 1976.

Kaplan, Howard M., and Bohr, Ronald H.: Change in the mental health field, Community Ment. Health J. **12:**244-251, Fall, 1976.

Kasiman, C.M.: Issues between professional and paraprofessional nursing staff in community mental health, J. Psychiatr. Nurs **12**(5):31-35, 1974.

Knight, Jeane Harris: Applying nursing process in the community, Nurs. Outlook **76:**708-711, 1974.

Krauss, Judith B.: The chronic psychiatric patient in the community—a model of care, Nurs. Outlook **28:**308-314, May, 1980.

Lego, Suzanne: The community mental health system: is it an improvement over the old system? Perspect. Psychiatr. Care **13:**105-112, July-Sept., 1975.

Levy, Rona L.: Behavior therapy techniques as a fulfillment of community mental health ideology, Community Ment. Health J. **12:**415-421, Winter, 1976.

Lowery, Barbara J., and Janulis, Diane: Community mental health and the unanswered questions, Perspect. Psychiatr. Care **11:**26-28, Jan., 1973.

Lyon, Glee G., and Hitchins Emily A.: Ways of intervening with the psychotic individual in the community, Am. J. Nurs. **79:**490-493, March, 1979.

Mirelowitz, Seymour: Alienation and bureaucratization of mental health organizations, Ment. Hyg. **56:**6-21, Winter, 1972.

Moran, Janet C.: An alternative to constant observation: the behavioral checklist, Perspect. Psychiatr. Care **17:**114-117, May-June, 1979.

Murray, Jacquelyn E.: Failure of the community mental health movement, Am. J. Nurs. **75:**2034-2036, 1975.

President's Commission on Mental Health: Report to the President, vol. 1, Washington, D.C., 1978.

Ruiz, Pedro, and Langrod, John: The role of folk healers in community mental health services, Community Ment. Health J. **12:**392-398, Winter, 1976.

Silverman, Wade H., and Val, Eduardo: Day hospital in the context of a community mental health program, Community Ment. Health J. **11:**82-90, Spring, 1975.

Stein, Edna, and Sorenson, Karl Dan: A cooperative apartment for transitional patients, Ment. Hygiene **56:**68-74. Winter, 1972.

Test, Mary Ann, and Stein, Leonard I.: Practical guidelines for the community treatment of markedly impaired patients, Community Ment. Health J. **12:**72-82, Spring, 1976.

OF PARTICULAR INTEREST

Jansson, D.P.: Return to society: problematic features of the re-entry process, Perspect. Psychiatr. Care **13:**136, 1975.

Some of the realities of the "re-entry process" are discussed here with recommendations for interventions to accomplish the process effectively.

Schulberg, H., Becker, A., and McGrath, M.: Planning the phasedown of mental hospitals, Community Ment. Health J. **12:**3, Spring, 1976.

This article addresses some of the challenges to the accomplishment of continuity of care in the community mental health model.

Institutional care as a treatment modality

- The newly admitted client
- Clinical situations encountered in the hospital setting
- Creating a therapeutic environment
- The therapeutic community

Until recently, the care of the mentally ill in the United States has taken place almost entirely in large, publicly supported hospitals devoted solely to this purpose. However, over the past several decades, most general hospitals have established units for inpatient treatment of emotionally disturbed persons. These units tend to be relatively small compared to the other units within the hospital. Most recently, there is a trend toward treating mentally ill individuals through outpatient services based in the client's community. Proponents of this community-based model make every effort to avoid hospitalizing clients or, if hospitalization is necessary, to limit the client's stay to only the length of time that is absolutely necessary. This trend is a result of much evidence that prolonged hospitalization produces a syndrome called *institutionalization,* wherein the individual adapts well to the hospital community, making it increasingly difficult, if not impossible, for him to function effectively within the society at large. Consequently, prolonged hospitalization for psychiatric reasons is viewed as a major factor in increasing the amount and degree of chronicity among emotionally disturbed persons.

Despite the trend toward a community-based outpatient treatment approach, authorities agree that there is still a need to provide inpatient treatment services for some individuals whose needs are best met in the controlled environment a hospital can offer. Persons in this category are usually those who are actively self-destructive or dangerous to others. In addition, there are some emotionally ill persons who have so few social resources and so little initiative that a period of hospitalization may be the only means to provide them with structured therapeutic interactions with other human beings. Hospitalization for a short period is also used as a planned part of the treatment program for some persons who are experiencing a major life crisis and who can benefit from temporary placement in a neutral environment.

THE NEWLY ADMITTED CLIENT

For many reasons, the nurse who has the responsibility for admitting mentally ill individuals to a psychiatric facility should be skilled in the use of tact and reassurance. Initial admission to any hospital may be an upsetting and frightening experience. Mentally ill persons frequently fear other people and what other people may do to them. They, like all human beings, cherish freedom and the ability to come and go at will. When they realize that they must remain at the hospital, they may develop a feeling of resentment. Sometimes these persons are extremely upset by separation from family members. For these and many other reasons, the nurse who admits a mentally ill person to a psychiatric unit needs to be kind, tactful, reassuring, persuasive, and patient.

The admission procedure, like all other experiences in the hospital, should be designed to strengthen the client's self-esteem, to help him feel safe, and to build his feeling of confidence in the hospital personnel. Unfortunately, not all admission procedures achieve these results, and some psychiatric facilities have developed admission procedures that do little or nothing to reassure fearful patients.

It is usually wise to postpone for 1 or 2 hours the activities involved in officially admitting the client. This will give the nurse an opportunity to welcome him, to introduce him to other clients, to show him the physical arrangement of the unit, and to talk with him in an informal and friendly way so that he can begin to feel safe in his new environment. After the nurse has begun the process of gaining the new client's confidence and has answered his questions, he will probably be better able to accept the admission procedure without suspicion or fear.

Some hospital authorities may believe that assigning a nurse to spend a few hours with a newly admitted client is too great an expenditure of time. Staying with a new client does take time, but the positive results are worth the effort expended. If clients are helped empathically and tactfully to get acquainted with the hospital setting, they will be able to accept the hospital routine without becoming unduly anxious or fearful.

There are some persons who are so confused and upset on the first day of admission that it is not practical to attempt to introduce them to the setting or the other persons. With extremely upset clients it is also very important to wait for an hour or so before trying to carry out the admission procedure. This lapse of time gives the individual an opportunity to regain some emotional control and a chance for his fear to subside. It also gives the nurse time to reassure this person and to begin to get acquainted with him. Any newly admitted client who is waiting to have the admission procedure completed should be accompanied by a member of the nursing staff.

The hospital is to be the client's home for a period of time. If he is to benefit from this experience in living, it seems reasonable to believe that a congenial and pleasant atmosphere should be developed. It also seems important for the environment to be free from anxiety-producing experiences. Opportunities should be provided for the client to participate in occupational and resocialization activities from the first day of hospital admission. It is therapeutically important for mentally ill persons to be allowed to wear their own clothing in the hospital, beginning with the first day of admission. Practices such as requiring that pajamas be worn during the first few weeks of hospitalization, even though the client is physically well, make it almost impossible to provide a variety of therapeutic experiences. The all too frequent plan of eliminating newly admitted persons from many hospital activities as a safety measure seems indefensible. The need to become self-destructive and to strike out against the environment will greatly diminish if clients are provided with challenging activities, if they are helped to feel secure and safe, and if the hospital personnel provide meaningful interpersonal relationships for them.

Of course, it is necessary to exercise reasonable precautions to protect and safeguard both the clients and hospital personnel. Probably the most significant aspect of any combination of safety measures is an adequately prepared and interested staff large enough to ensure individual attention and a variety of therapeutic activities for all clients. Mentally ill persons, like all human beings, require individualized treatment if they are to recover and be able to resume a role in the community as contributing members of society.

A serious mistake that has been made in the past in the care of the mentally ill is the failure to realize that all persons need to be recognized as unique and important human beings. Because individualized care is so significant in the client's total therapy, hospitals that have routinized the care of the mentally ill have defeated their own purposes.

CLINICAL SITUATIONS ENCOUNTERED IN THE HOSPITAL SETTING

The following discussion gives examples of clinical situations that are frequently encountered and are best dealt with in hospital settings.

Feeding problems. Ensuring adequate food intake for mentally ill persons is a major nursing responsibility when they refuse to eat. Responses to hallucinations, delusions, and illusions are frequent reasons for the refusal of food by some mentally ill persons. The voices may tell them not to eat because someone is poisoning or contaminating the food in some shocking manner. The person appears to be terrified at the thought of eating. Such suspicious individuals may eat if they are allowed to have foods that are not easily contaminated. A list of such foods might include hard-cooked unshelled eggs, baked potatoes, unpeeled fruits, and bread from an unopened package. It is discouraging to hear some clients comment that poison could have been instilled in these foods if a hypodermic needle were used. Tasting the food in the presence of a suspicious person who believes that the food is poisoned is another well-known suggestion. In this way the nurse may demonstrate that she does not believe that the food is contaminated. Dietary problems that arise from illusions may be controlled by avoiding the offending food altogether. Some of the common illusionary problems involving foods include seeing tomato juice as blood, tapioca as living animal eyes, small whole potatoes as toes, and macaroni as worms. When refusal of food is related to psychotic symptoms, the administration of antipsychotic drugs often has a dramatic effect in altering the symptoms, thereby enabling the client to eat.

All but a few of the most acutely ill individuals hospitalized in a psychiatric facility begin to eat soon after being admitted to the neutral, relatively anxiety-free environment of the hospital. It is helpful for these persons to be required to go to meals at regular, stated intervals even though they may not actually eat. Appetites frequently return when clients are encouraged to retire and rise at regular hours. Restoration of some semblance of an eating and sleeping schedule in the lives of mentally ill persons frequently does much to encourage food intake.

It is not a good plan to coax or threaten a client in relation to his food intake. It is more therapeutic to invite him to come to the dining room or to serve the tray without comment. If he refuses to eat, it is wise to accept his refusal without comment. It is usually not therapeutically helpful to use any coercion, even persuasion, until the client has spent 2 or 3 days without food. When the nurse first realizes that the client is refusing food, it is a good plan to discuss the problem with the professional person in charge of the client's treatment. If the refusal of food becomes an actual health problem, tube-feeding may be indicated, although this procedure should be avoided if at all possible.

Clients sometimes respond positively to spoon-feeding. This is especially true if the person is disoriented, confused, or tremulous.

It is probably never wise to force-feed a person. Force-feeding rarely accomplishes anything positive, and it may be interpreted as an attack. When a client persists in refusing food for days because of an irrational fear of eating or deep-seated self-destructive tendencies, it is futile to hope that anything can be accomplished by force-feeding. In an incident after a client had received a meal by force, the client induced an emesis. The client said, "No one can make me eat." It would be helpful for nurses to remember that persons cannot be made to retain food even if they are forced to swallow it.

Because the first experiences human beings have in receiving love from the mothering person are associated with feeding, food is unconsciously associated with mothering and with receiving love and acceptance. It is important for the nurse who is developing a therapeutic environment for mentally ill persons to create and maintain a happy, friendly atmosphere during mealtime. There is probably never a time in the care of an emotionally ill person when it is therapeutic for anyone to become aggressive toward the client concerning food. The mere physical acceptance of food is only part of the therapeutic significance of feeding a client. Unless the feeding experience also provides a friendly, warm, accepting atmosphere, it loses much of its potential value.

Mentally ill persons, like all people, deserve attractively prepared meals served in pleasant, homelike surroundings that contribute to a therapeutic environment.

Toileting problems. Extremely regressed clients may be careless with regard to excreta. This means that the client is so much out of touch with the demands of reality that he does not go to the toilet when he needs to void or defecate. This behavior is part of the regression to infantile reaction patterns resorted to by some psychotic persons. Initiating a toileting routine is one way of coping with this problem.

Some catatonic persons withhold urine and bowel content, a condition that can result in a seriously distended bladder or in fecal impaction. Hence it is important to record daily bowel movements and to report to the physician when a client has had no defecation for 2 or 3 days. Enemas should be avoided, since clients frequently misinterpret the enema procedure as a sexual assault. Most clients establish regular bowel habits in the hospital after receiving a balanced diet over a period of time. Women may suffer a concomitant loss of menstrual function when suffering from a severe emotional illness. The menstrual cycle is usually reestablished after a period of experiencing the hospital routine.

Suicidal individuals. Actively suicidal individuals are almost always hospitalized, even if for only a short time. Almost all actively suicidal persons are suffering from severe feelings of worthlessness, guilt, and depression. Therapeutic efforts must be directed at alleviating these feelings. Information about the underlying dynamics and manifestations of depression as well as suggestions for therapeutic intervention is found in Chapter 13.

When a person is hospitalized because he is actively suicidal, it is important that he be protected against his self-destructive impulses. Sometimes an attempt is made to ensure the client's safety by removing from his environment all the equipment with which he might injure himself. This is extremely difficult because every piece of clothing, all eating utensils, cigarettes, furniture, bathroom equipment—literally everything an individual needs in the process of daily living—could be used if the individual wished to injure or destroy himself. One client strangled herself by using a toothbrush to fashion a tourniquet from her long braided hair; another client dived headlong into the toilet and suffered a serious head wound; a third client destroyed herself by using the armholes of her knitted underwear as a noose; and a fourth client injured herself seriously by setting fire to her dress with a cigarette. If the philosophy of making the environment safe were carried to its logical conclusion, the client would be placed in an absolutely barren room with a pallet on which to lie. To make self-destruction even more unlikely, hospitals have frequently followed the plan of placing the client under constant observation so that he is observed by a hospital worker during every minute of the day and night. Variations of this procedure have been developed for clients who are thought to have less drive to injure or destroy themselves. At best, this procedure of environmental control and constant observation is only a preventive measure.

Depriving clients of freedom to move about and placing them under constant observation may increase their self-destructive tendencies. These steps may convince them that their worst fears are true and that they are worthless and unworthy or that they have committed an unforgivable crime and are being justly punished. An illustration of such an occurrence is an incident in which the nurse was playing cards with a young man who was actively suicidal and confined to an empty seclusion room, dressed only in trousers. As both sat cross-legged on the floor, the client over a period of hours dealt the cards a few inches to the right and the nurse unconsciously shifted her position to accommodate to the cards. This client eventually succeeded in shifting the nurse's position so that he had free access to the door through which he fled and proceeded to fling himself through a window. This incident illustrates that even with all precautions, prevention of suicide is not always possible, and its occurrence may be increased by establishing an environment that serves as a constant reminder to the client of his destructive wishes. Although there is no question that the actively suicidal client should be closely supervised, the hospital staff would be wise to emphasize the client's participation in safe activities with others rather than the environmental modifications so often unsuccessfully employed.

CREATING A THERAPEUTIC ENVIRONMENT

For many years the professional staffs of most hospitals encouraged the belief that any actual improvement in hospitalized clients was achieved through the efforts of the physician. As a result of this attitude, nurses demonstrated a reluctance to accept responsibility for developing therapeutic relationships with clients or to accept credit for positive changes in client behavior. Today it is believed that a variety of people can provide therapeutic help for mentally ill persons. The time has come when the nursing staff must assume its share of the responsibility for providing the therapeutic experiences in living that are necessary for persons who need to achieve more mature patterns of behavior. It is interesting to note that the idea of a hospital environment having therapeutic potential is not new.

Historical background

The historical archives of American psychiatry include records of early, successful attempts to develop a homelike atmosphere for mentally ill persons with provision for social and recreational activities. Physicians and their families joined other staff members in initiating and directing some of these activities. Early in the ninteenth century, emphasis on a homelike environment, recreational activities, and a sympathetic approach to clients was referred to as *moral treatment*. In 1842 Boston State Hospital was reported to have placed emphasis on moral treatment for mentally ill individuals. At about the same time a similar approach was being carried out in Worcester, Massachusetts, at the public psychiatric hospital there. The superintendent of one psychiatric hospital in Massachusetts is reported to have invited patients to his home for Sunday dinner. Intimate discussions of the patient's personal problems and difficulties were part of the therapy offered in those institutions at that time.

Some authorities believe that the era of moral treatment for the mentally ill ceased to exist as a direct result of the large numbers of immigrants who arrived in the United States after the Civil War. Many of these people could not cope with the problems of adjustment presented by the radically different environment they found in this country. Some could not accept the loss of the close family ties that existed in the European villages from which they came. Many immigrants reacted to these social and personal deprivations with such unusual behavior that institutionalization was necessary. When the client population in mental institutions began to increase rapidly, the clients were no longer culturally homogeneous. Many of them did not speak English. Developing a homelike environment for people from such different backgrounds was difficult. The nation became preoccupied with the task of national growth and expansion. For reasons that are not entirely clear, the era of moral treatment for mentally ill persons passed. By 1940 large public hospitals were filled to overflowing. Few patients recovered sufficiently to return to the community. Because of the ever-increasing patient population the task of the hospital personnel was staggering. They were able to do little more than keep the patients bathed, dressed, and fed.

When the nation had time to evaluate national needs after World War II, attention became focused on improving the care of mentally ill persons. Since 1945 many new approaches to care and treatment have been proposed. Among these was the old, partially forgotten idea that the hospital environment could provide therapeutic experiences for clients.

Influence of physical environment on the therapeutic climate

A therapeutic climate for mentally ill persons depends on the attitude of the staff toward mental illness and the needs of the clients and does not develop as the result of any fixed type of hospital architecture. It can be developed in any type of hospital if the staff focuses on meeting the needs of clients. However, it is helpful if certain structural features are present. The needs of individuals can be met more effectively if provisions for privacy, socialization, and planned activities are available. If such facilities are not already present in the unit where clients live, innovations must be introduced if a therapeutic environment is to be achieved. The goals of a therapeutic environment are to help the individual develop a sense of self-esteem and personal worth, to improve his ability to relate to others, to help him learn to trust others, and to return him to the community better prepared to resume his role in living and working.

If a person's self-esteem is to be elevated, it is essential to provide an opportunity for privacy and a place where his personal belongings can be kept. In most situations a substitute has been found for the barrack-like dormitories and public showers with which many large psychiatric hospitals were once equipped. The mass approach to the care of human beings destroys self-esteem and the sense of individual worth. The key to a therapeutic environment is provision for the unique needs of individuals rather than dealing with clients as members of a crowd. The idea that nothing should be arranged for one client unless it could be arranged for the group has led many hospital staffs in the past away from treating people as individuals. This attitude sometimes increased the client's difficulties rather than providing opportunities for him to solve problems.

If clients are to receive individualized care, and if the environment is to be therapeutic, living quarters must be attractive and inviting. In most instances no more than two or three persons should share the same room. If possible, single rooms should be provided for individuals who have strong feelings about sharing a room with another person. Clothes closets and dressers or satisfactory substitutes for this equipment must be available. It is important for mentally ill persons to bring personal clothing and other equipment to the hospital so that they can be attractively and appropriately groomed. The use of hospital clothing may be necessary in rare instances, but in the past this dress contributed to depersonalization of the patient population and reduced them to a group of human beings with a universal attitude of hopelessness. Because it is therapeutic for clients to assume responsibility for their personal cleanliness, laundry facilities should be available.

Dining room facilities are important in developing a therapeutic environment. Mealtime should be a leisurely experience and a time for sharing ideas and reinforcing friendly relationships. It is not merely a time for the intake of food. The nurses can profitably assume a therapeutic role by serving as hostesses at small tables that seat groups of four to six clients. The role of hostess is more effective if the nurse shares the meal with the clients. This plan has been used successfully in some hospitals. As a hostess the nurse can encourage conversation and can help make mealtime a happy, relaxed, and rewarding group experience. Such mealtime experiences cannot be initiated unless there is a dining room attached to the unit itself. Serving meals in large, noisy dining rooms where hundreds of people are fed achieves the purpose of getting food to clients but negates the accomplishment of other therapeutic goals.

Bathrooms should provide privacy. Although locks on doors may not be advisable for safety reasons, it is possible to provide toilet doors that close and shower rooms that are equipped with screens. The old practice of showering 10 or 15 persons at a time contributed to reducing the individual to a member of a crowd and negated other attempts to help him feel like a respected human being. The therapeutic environment can develop most effectively when the physical surroundings lend themselves to helping clients feel that they are respected and that their personal preferences are recognized, appreciated, and considered.

Emotional climate essential to a therapeutic environment

The physical environment of the hospital is vitally important in developing a situation in which the individual can feel comfortable and safe and in which he can develop more effective ways of coping with stress. Even more important, however, in helping clients achieve the goal of improved emotional health is the interpersonal climate present in the unit where the individual is to live during his hospital stay. This climate is largely the responsibility of the nursing staff members who are assigned to the unit.

Like all people who embark on a new experience, clients need to be helped to become familiar with the hospital situation and to learn what the staff expects of them.

Since a new environment is likely to be frightening to emotionally ill persons, a sensitive nursing staff will strive to develop a climate that encourages the clients to feel that the hospital is a safe place in which they are protected from the dangers in the outside world. Some clients want and need reassurance that the staff will protect them from their own impulses to injure themselves or others.

Providing safety for a client includes safeguarding him against making significant decisions when he is not well enough to do so. Thus the nursing staff may find it necessary to help him avoid making legal decisions about a pending divorce or separation, about the sale of property or other financial matters, or about the choice of a school for his children.

The therapeutic emotional climate in a hospital is established by a nursing staff who is friendly, sensitive, and concerned about the welfare of the clients. Such staff members are aware of the client's individual rights and needs. They respect him as a worthwhile, important human being, even though his behavior may sometimes be socially unacceptable.

A nursing staff striving to develop a therapeutic environment establishes as few rules and regulations as possible for client behavior and restricts activity only when necessary. Opportunities for freedom of choice are provided. As the client demonstrates his ability to accept more responsibility for his behavior, opportunities for making choices are increased.

It is expected that as the client's emotional health improves, he will experiment with new mechanisms of adjustment and develop new ways of responding to others and of coping with stress. Some of these new methods of dealing with problems may not be appropriate. He will require encouragement to continue testing new patterns of behavior until he has achieved a more mature way of relating to other people.

The nursing staff fulfills a key role in providing the warmth, friendliness, acceptance, and optimism essential to the development of a therapeutic emotional climate.

The following characteristics of a therapeutic environment are adapted from Brown and Fowler*:

1. The client is familiar with the situation and what is expected of him.

---

*Brown, Martha M., and Fowler, Grace R.: Psychodynamic nursing—a biosocial orientation, ed. 3, Philadelphia, 1972, W.B. Saunders Co.

2. The client feels comfortable in the situation and is free from a fear of danger.
3. Provision is made to meet the client's immediate physical needs.
4. Provision is made for the client to have clean surroundings and to be cared for with clean equipment.
5. The environment provides the client with optimum safety from injury to his person from his own impulses or from the impulses of others, from anxieties related to his former environment, and from decisions beyond his current level of responsibility.
6. The personnel in the environment respect him as an individual, recognize his rights, needs, and opinions, and accept his behavior as an expression of his needs.
7. The environment provides for a limited number of restrictions and for opportunities for freedom of choice.
8. The environment provides a testing ground for the establishment of new patterns of behavior.

Setting limits

Words such as *acceptance* and *permissiveness* confuse some inexperienced professional workers and may encourage them to function in a psychiatric setting as if any type of behavior is allowed. Nothing could be further from the truth, and such an attitude is actually detrimental to clients who by their sick behavior may be asking for controls. Acceptance means that the hospital staff members assume an emotionally neutral attitude toward individual behavior and refrain from placing a judgmental label on it. It further means that the behavior is recognized as an expression of the person's needs. Permissiveness refers to the prevailing attitude in psychiatric settings that allows a client to behave as he needs to behave within limits of safety. It also allows a client to experiment with new ways of behaving as he progresses toward more successful and satisfying behavioral patterns. The staff cannot allow a client to injure himself or others or to engage in behavior that will be legally or morally detrimental to himself or others. When a client's behavior cannot be permitted, the nurse should frankly tell him that the behavior cannot be allowed and should give him a logical reason for this decision.

Setting limits frequently becomes the responsibility of the nurse, although the psychiatric team usually makes the initial decision concerning the limit to be established. Certainly the nurse would be wise to seek an opportunity to discuss the setting of limits with other professional colleagues when such responsibility is entirely up to her. She will want to be certain that she is not imposing her own personal standards on clients. If a form of client government is operating, much of the limit setting can be established by this group.

An example of a limit frequently established in psychiatric settings is the requirement that all clients attend breakfast fully dressed and ready for the activities of the day. Usually this requirement is made because some mentally ill persons seem to prefer to stay up most of the night and remain in bed most of the day. This habit can help the client avoid participating in most activities of the day and relieve him of the need to relate to people. If the client is required to be up and dressed for breakfast, he is then available to participate in group activities. This rule also requires the client to establish some kind of living pattern that involves getting to bed at a reasonable hour in the evening. Some authorities argue that many well persons enjoy sleeping until noon and that they often skip breakfast. It seems reasonable to allow some clients to decide when they will retire and arise and what morning activities they will become involved in, including breakfast. It is apparent that before any rule that regulates client activity is established, all aspects of the result of such action should be considered, including the problem of enforcing the rule once it is established. Consideration should be given to the way in which a rule assists or impedes the growth of mature attitudes on the part of clients.

The populations of modern psychiatric units are likely to include both men and women. This calls for some limit setting concerning the relationship between men and women. Since sexual behavior is often a problem area for many mentally ill persons, they may feel much more comfortable if fairly specific limits are established for their coming and going on the unit where they are to live. The question essentially involves the limits that would be most helpful to men and women who are fearful of each other but who should be helped to establish more mature behavioral patterns in relation to the opposite sex.

The nurse can easily confuse limit setting with control of behavior. She may rationalize that many of the unnecessary controls that may have been imposed are limits placed on the situation for safety and security of clients. Sometimes unnecessary controls are placed on behavior because of one unfortunate incident. For instance, one psychiatric hospital refused to allow clients to go outdoors for a walk because several years earlier one male client attacked a nurse with whom he was walking. The responsibility for setting limits should not be assumed by one individual until the proposed action has been discussed with other people and all possible alternatives have been explored.

Nurse's role

It is not possible to develop a therapeutic environment without the strong, intelligent leadership of a nurse. When many of the traditional rules and regulations of the psychiatric unit are discarded and it becomes a place that focuses on meeting the needs of the individual and the group, the nurse is forced to accept a more active therapeutic role with clients. She finds it necessary to assign the clerical work, which formerly kept her confined to the nurse's station, to a ward secretary to free herself to give leadership to the personnel as they participate with clients in all the planned activities. Mentally ill persons require mature help and guidance in initiating and carrying out social activities.

When clients begin to experiment with new ways of behaving, they will make use of the nurse as an understanding person with whom they can discuss daily problems and emotional stresses. The nurse needs to be more alert than ever to changes in behavior. In a therapeutic environment many of the traditional safeguards are removed, and therefore safety of clients depends more than ever on an alert nursing staff. Thus it becomes the responsibility of the nurse to recognize changes in mood and behavior of clients and to intervene at appropriate times.

Skill in understanding group behavior and in directing groups is essential in the therapeutic environment. The nurse needs to work actively with patient government to solve many unit problems. Finally, active, functioning channels of communication are essential. The nurse's relationships as the leader of the nursing staff will be reflected in the total effectiveness of the psychiatric team and ultimately in the therapeutic climate of the psychiatric unit. To a large extent the effectiveness of the client's total hospital experience will depend on the level of professional leadership provided by the nurse.

THE THERAPEUTIC COMMUNITY

Historical background

In 1953 a small book by Dr. Maxwell Jones entitled *Social Psychiatry* was published in England. It has been one of the motivating forces in the movement in the United States to use the hospital environment therapeutically in the treatment regimen of mentally ill persons. When Dr. Jones's book was published in this country, the title was changed to *The Therapeutic Community*. It is essentially a report of efforts at Belmont Hospital in England during and after World War II to rehabilitate neurotic patients through the use of group methods. That experience in group living at Belmont Hospital came to be known as the therapeutic community, and thus this name was applied to the report. Particular attention was paid to the development of the social structure of the hospital and to communication between patients and the hospital staff. Dr. Jones dedicated his book to "The Nursing Staff who have formed a framework around which our therapeutic communities have been built." Although the nurses to whom he referred were not registered nurses, they were intelligent, capable, mature women who used the interpersonal skill and understanding required in psychiatric nursing. The dedication is appropriate. Without a nursing staff with insight, understanding, personal warmth, and skill in directing groups, the concept of a therapeutic community could not have developed into a reality.

Theoretical considerations

The therapeutic community is a contemporary approach to the care of mentally ill persons through group activity. It is an attempt to introduce democracy into the hospital setting. The therapeutic community strives to involve the client in his own therapy, to restore self-confidence by providing an opportunity for decision making, and to focus his attention and concern away from self and toward the needs of others. It has been organized in various ways in different settings. Sometimes the principles of the therapeutic community are used throughout the hospital, and in other situations they may be limited to one or two units where the clients are almost ready to be discharged.

One important aspect of a democratic situation is that the people who are to be influenced by a decision are involved in making the decision. Until recently, administrators and professional staffs of hospitals have taken the position that persons who require hospital care are incapable of making wise judgments and therefore must have all decisions made for them. Clients in most hospitals where this philosophy has been implemented have been reduced to a dependent state. Recently there has been a growing realization that forcing an adult person into such a dependent role is not usually necessary and is not therapeutic. Of course, there are some completely dependent persons for whom all decisions must be made. This is obviously true of acutely ill or unconscious patients. However, in spite of the reason for hospitalization, a majority of adults are able to make valid decisions about many things involving their welfare. Forcing the dependent role on some mentally ill persons may be particularly unfortunate. Some of them have spent a lifetime struggling against an unconscious desire to accept a dependent role. When hospitalization forces this role on such an individual, he may never be able to relinquish it.

Today there is a growing belief that a therapeutic environment for mentally ill persons should provide an opportunity for them to participate in the formulation of hospital rules and regulations that affect their personal liberties. Following through with such a plan means that clients would be involved in formulating policies that regulate smoking, bedtime, late night privileges, weekend passes, social activities, control of the radio, television, and piano, check-in time when returning to the hospital from a weekend, reporting for meals, and the many other aspects of personal life that are influenced by rules in the usual psychiatric setting. Also, it is thought to be therapeutic to involve clients in making decisions about behavior and relationships among the ward population. Thus clients in a therapeutic community might be given responsibility for rendering a judgment about the infringement of ward rules, settling arguments between clients, judging the appropriateness of granting weekend privileges for certain members of the group, and many other decisions regarding the regulation of life on the unit.

Careful preparation of both the hospital staff and the clients should be assured before a therapeutic community is initiated. The hospital staff may have a good deal of difficulty accepting the activities and responsibilities granted to clients. Before a therapeutic community is initiated, a thorough exploration of the implications of such an undertaking should be carried on through group discussions. All levels of hospital workers from physicians to attendants, kitchen helpers, and cleaning people should be involved in these group discussions because all will be affected by this new activity. All members of the staff need to have a thorough understanding of the goals and limitations of the undertaking. Clients in the units where the new philosophy is to be initiated should also have an opportunity to explore its implications through group discussions. These discussions should be directed by the physicians and nurses who will be directly involved in the future activities of the new organization. Both clients and hospital staff need to understand what responsibilities they can and cannot assume.

Active administrative sanction, acceptance, and interest are essential if the therapeutic community is to be successful. Involving clients in decision making represents a drastic change in the entire administrative philosophy of many hospitals. The therapeutic community cannot be expected to function smoothly at all times, and problems will undoubtedly arise. Decisions made by clients will not always be reality based. Unless the entire hospital staff believes that involving clients in decision making is therapeutically valuable and worth the struggle, dissenting forces may destroy the undertaking.

Meetings of the therapeutic community should be held regularly and at specific times if they are to be effective. Meetings should not be allowed to deteriorate into complaint sessions or to focus entirely on what the hospital should do for clients. This can be avoided if the group has some real responsibility for solving problems relating to clients' needs.

In one instance the members of a therapeutic community in a small unit of a large New York psychiatric hospital held a meeting to consider the problem of three suicide attempts made in 1 week by a young woman on the unit. Their decision was to institute a buddy system so that she would be accompanied at all times by one of a group of clients, each of whom would be assigned to spend a specific amount of time with her daily. Several weeks after this decision was made, the system was working well, and the woman had made no further suicide attempts. At this same meeting other problems considered were the problem of a client who did not return on time from a weekend holiday, a fight between two clients, and the request by a new client for a weekend pass.

It is far easier for the hospital staff to make all decisions for clients, but there is little that is therapeutic in this procedure. When clients have the opportunity to make decisions about their own and other people's behavior, they are presented with a realistic learning experience.

Significant aspects of a therapeutic community

1. The emphasis in a therapeutic community is placed on social and group interaction, with both individual clients and staff being important members of the community.
2. The goal of the therapeutic community is to provide a favorable climate in which clients can gain an awareness of their feelings, thoughts, impulses, and behavior, try new interpersonal skills in a relatively safe environment, increase personal self-esteem, and realistically appraise the potentially helpful and destructive aspects of their behavior.
3. The work of the therapeutic community and the maintenance of an open network of communication are achieved through a daily meeting attended by all staff members and all clients who work and live on the specific unit.

4. A successful therapeutic community requires that both staff and individual clients become fully aware of their roles, limitations, responsibilities, and authority.
5. Staff members in a therapeutic community make information openly available to clients with whom they share treatment responsibilities.
6. The treatment arena in the therapeutic community includes all relationships among the members of the community, with special attention being given to the network of communication between members.

CONCLUDING STATEMENTS

1. There is still a need for hospitalization for some emotionally ill persons, especially those who are actively self-destructive or dangerous to others.
2. The procedures for admitting a client to a hospital should be designed to strengthen the client's self-esteem, to help him feel safe, and to build his feeling of confidence in the hospital personnel.
3. Ensuring adequate food intake for clients is a major nursing responsibility.
4. Initiating a toileting regimen is one way of coping with the careless elimination habits of extremely regressed clients.
5. Actively suicidal clients need to be protected from their self-destructive impulses, but this is best achieved by focusing on their participation in safe activities with others rather than on environmental control.
6. The nursing staff members who work on psychiatric units need to assume their share of the responsibility for providing therapeutic experiences in living for clients.
7. A therapeutic climate for mentally ill persons is dependent on the attitude of the staff toward mental illness and toward the needs of the clients and does not develop as the result of any fixed type of hospital architecture. However, it is helpful if certain structural features are present.
8. The goals of a therapeutic environment are to help the client develop a sense of self-esteem and personal worth, to improve his ability to relate to others, to help him learn to trust oth-

ers, and to return him to the community better prepared to resume his role in living and working.

9. The key to a therapeutic environment is to provide for the unique needs of individual clients rather than to deal with them as members of a crowd.
10. In spite of the reason for hospitalization, the majority of adults are able to make valid decisions about many things concerning their welfare and should be provided with opportunities to do so.
11. Limit setting frequently becomes the responsibility of the nurse, although decisions about what limits need to be established are usually made by the entire psychiatric team.
12. It is not possible to develop a therapeutic environment without the strong, intelligent leadership of a nurse.
13. In a therapeutic environment the nurse will find it necessary to be free from clerical work to give leadership to the ward personnel as they participate with clients in planned activities.
14. *The Therapeutic Community* by Dr. Maxwell Jones, published in England in 1953, has been a motivating force in the United States in focusing attention on the contribution that a therapeutic hospital environment can make to the care and treatment of mentally ill persons.
15. The therapeutic community is a contemporary approach to the care of the mentally ill through the sharing of treatment responsibility by clients and staff.
16. One important aspect of a therapeutic community is a democratic situation in which the people who are to be influenced by a decision are involved in making the decision.
17. Both clients and members of the hospital staff need to understand what responsibilities are involved in initiating a therapeutic community.
18. Active administrative sanction, acceptance, and interest are essential to achieving a successful therapeutic community.
19. The work of the therapeutic community and the maintenance of an open network of communication are achieved in a daily community meeting attended by all staff and all clients who live and work on the specific unit.

Suggested sources of additional information

CLASSICAL

Abrams, G.M.: Defining milieu therapy, Arch. Gen. Psychiatry **21**:553-560, 1969.

Bennet, Leland R.: A therapeutic community, Nurs. Outlook **9**:423-425, 1961.

Berliner, Arthur K.: The two milieus in milieu therapy, Perspect. Psychiatr. Care **5**:266-271, Nov.-Dec., 1967.

Briggs, Dennie Lynn: Social psychiatry in Great Britain, Am. J. Nurs. **59**:215-221, 1959.

Greenblatt, M., York, R.H. and Brown, I.L.: From custodial to therapeutic patient care in mental hospitals, New York, 1979, Arno Press, Inc.

Holmes, Marguerite J., and Werner, Jean A.: Psychiatric nursing in a therapeutic community, New York, 1966, Macmillan Publishing Co., Inc.

Huey, Florence: In a therapeutic community, Am. J. Nurs. **71**:926-933, 1971.

Irvine, LaVerne F., and Deery, S. Joel: An investigation of problem areas relating to the therapeutic community concept, Ment. Hyg. **45**:367-373, 1961.

Jones, Maxwell: The therapeutic community: a new treatment method in psychiatry, New York, 1953, Basic Books, Inc., Publishers.

Loomis, Maxine E.: Nursing management of acting out behavior. Perspect. Psychiatr. Care **8**:168-173, 1970.

Peplau, Hildegarde E.: Interpersonal relations in nursing, New York, 1952, G.P. Putnam's Sons.

Schwartz, Morris S., and Shockley, Emmy L.: The nurse and the mental patient, New York, 1956, John Wiley & Sons, Inc.

Siegel, Nathaniel H.: What is a therapeutic community? Nurs. Outlook **12**:49-51, May, 1964.

Simpson, George, and Kline, Nathan S.: A new type psychiatric ward, Am. J. Psychiatry **119**:511-514, 1962.

Stainbrook, E.: The hospital as a therapeutic community. In Freedman, A.M., and Kaplan H.I.: Comprehensive textbook of psychiatry, Baltimore, 1975, The Williams & Wilkins Co.

Stanton, A., and Schwartz, M.: The mental hospital. A study of institutional participation in psychiatric illness and treatment, New York, 1954, Basic Books, Inc., Publishers.

Stevens, Leonard F.: What makes a ward climate therapeutic? Am. J. Nurs **61**:95-96, 1961.

Von Mering, Otto, and King, Stanley H.: Remotivating the mental patient, New York, 1957, Russell Sage Foundation.

CONTEMPORARY

Adelson, Pearl Yaruss: The backward dilemma, Am. J. Nurs. **80**:422-426, March, 1980.

Brooks, Rath E.: Behind the heavy metal door, Am. J. Nurs. **79**:1547-1550, Sept., 1979.

Calnen, Terrence: Whose agent? A re-evaluation of the role of the psychiatric nurse in the therapeutic community, Perspect. Psychiatr. Care **10**:210-219, Dec., 1972.

Carson, Verna: Meeting the spiritual needs of hospitalized psychiatric patients, Perspect. Psychiatr. Care **18**:17-20, Jan.-Feb., 1980.

Cavens, Annie, and Williams, Robert L.: The budget plann: (behavior modification of long-term patients), Perspect. Psychiatr. Care **9:** 13-16, Jan.-Feb., 1971.

Clark, Carolyn C.: A social systems approach to short-term psychiatric care, Perspect. Psychiatr. Care **10:**178-182, Oct.-Nov., 1972.

Closurdo, Janette S.: Behavior modication and the nursing process, Perspect. Psychiatr. Care **13:**25-36, Jan.-Mar., 1975.

Craig, Anne E., and Hyatt, Barbara A.: Chronicity in mental illness: a theory on the role of change, Perspect. Psychiatr. Care, **16:**139-144, May-June, 1978.

Dall, William: Home is not sweet anymore, Ment. Hyg. **75:**22-24, Winter, 1975.

Fanning, V.: Patient involvement in planning own care: staff and patient attitudes, J.Psychiatr. Nurs. **10:**5-8, Jan.-Feb., 1972.

Fitzgerald, Roy C., and Long, Imelda: Seclusion and the treatment and management of severely disturbed manic-depressed patients, Perspect. Psychiatr. Care **11**(2):59-64, 1973.

Gardner, Kathyrn: Patient groups in a therapeutic community, Am. J. Nurs. **71:**528-531, 1971.

Jones, Maxwell: Nurses can change the social systems of hospitals, Am. J. Nurs. **78:**1012-1014, June, 1978.

Kiev, Ari: The courage to live, New York, 1980, Lippincott & Crowell.

McDonagh, Mary Jo, et al.: Nurse-therapists in a state psychiatric hospital, Am. J. Nurs. **80:**102-105, Jan., 1980.

Penningrath, Philip E.: Control of violence in a mental health setting, Am. J. Nurs. **75:**606-609, 1975.

Reuell, Virginia M.: Nurse-managed care for psychiatric patients, Am. J. Nurs. **75:**1156-1157, 1975.

Schmieding, Norma Jean: Institutionalization: a conceptual approach, Perspect. Psychiatr. Care **6:**205-212, Sept.-Oct., 1968.

Stewart, David W.: The future of the state mental hospital, Perspect. Psychiatr. Care **13**(3):120-122, 1975.

OF PARTICULAR INTEREST

Jones, J.: Social psychiatry in practice, Harmondsworth, England, 1968, Penguin Books, Ltd.

The author's elaboration on the concept of the therapeutic community is especially relevant for the nurse in considering the impact of institutionally based nursing care.

Will, G.T.: A sociopsychiatric nursing approach to intervention in a problem of mutual withdrawal on a mental hospital ward, Psychiatry: J. Stud. Interpers. Proc. **15:**193, 1952.

This classic article is essential reading for any student of psychiatric nursing. It describes the phenomenon of mutual withdrawal on a psychiatric unit and describes therapeutic interventions to address the problem.

Wolf, M.S.: A review of literature on milieu therapy, J. Psychiatr. Nurs., **15:**26-33, May, 1977.

This comprehensive overview of milieu therapy is especially relevant for the nurse in considering the ramifications of providing psychiatric nursing care within an institution.

SECTION EIGHT

Psychiatric nursing: its past, present, and future

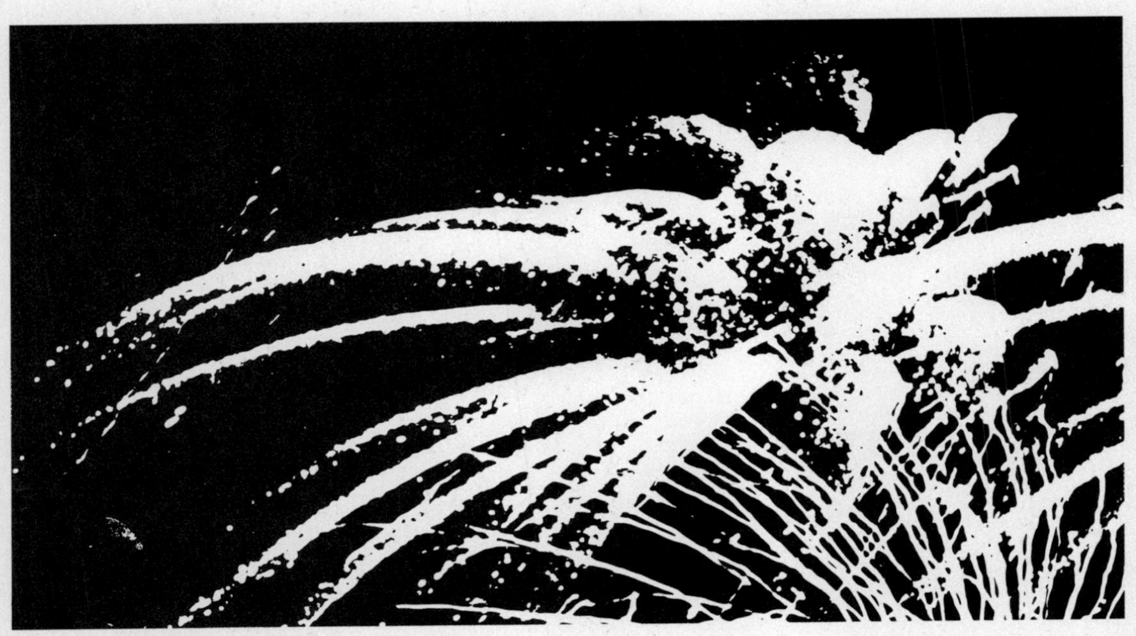

Section Eight provides an overview of the past, present, and possible future of the field of psychiatric nursing. An understanding of this material helps the reader to place the practice of psychiatric nursing as discussed in previous sections in perspective. As such, this section could appropriately serve as an introduction to the study of psychiatric nursing.

27

Historical development of psychiatric nursing

- Historical background of the treatment of the mentally ill
- Development of psychiatric nursing

HISTORICAL BACKGROUND OF THE TREATMENT OF THE MENTALLY ILL

Although the development of modern psychiatric nursing did not begin until 1882, the history of the development of psychiatry has significance for nursing.

In his slow development through the ages, primitive man gradually acquired a sense of compassion for his fellow creatures; he then began to recognize mental disorders and to make attempts at treating them. In the light of modern knowledge these attempts were undeniably crude and meaningless.

From the study of contemporary primitive peoples and their attitude toward mentally ill individuals, it can be safely inferred that after certain tribal rites had failed to effect a cure, the victim of mental illness in the dim past was disposed of by the simple expedient of being abandoned to die quickly of starvation in a barren waste or to be devoured by animals in the wilderness. That some prehistoric peoples had, however, developed a high degree of knowledge about the brain and its functions is the conclusion of anthropologists who have studied the remains of several civilizations in both the New and the Old Worlds. Excavations have revealed skeletons that clearly bear evidences of such successful trephining of the skull that the subjects survived for several years. It is assumed that such operations were done to relieve headache and probably mental derangement and that even some knowledge of asepsis may have existed in those remote days.

In recorded ancient history, such as that of the Eastern Mediterranean civilizations, there are references to mental disorders. Thus an Egyptian papyrus of 1500 BC contains a discourse on old age and says of it that "the heart grows heavy and remembers not yesterday." In later Egyptian civilization, particularly during the Alexandrian era, medicine developed a high status; sanatoriums known as the temples of Saturn were operated for the care of those who were mentally afflicted. The Old Testament records authentic cases of mental illness, of which King Saul offers a famous example.

The Golden Age of Greece was noted for its humane regard for the sick. The Greek physicians were poor anatomists because they deified the human body and dared not dissect it, but they were astute observers and excellent clinicians. Hippocrates (460-375?

BC), the greatest of the old Greek physicians, knew well the symptoms of melancholia and regarded epilepsy not as the "sacred disease" but insisted that "it has a natural cause from which it originates like other afflictions." The Greeks used as hospitals temples that had an abundance of fresh air, pure water, and sunshine. These temples of Aesculapius "as often as they had patients, such as were unhinged, did make use of nothing so much for the cure of them as symphony and sweet harmony of voices." Theatricals, riding, walking, and listening to the sound of a waterfall were all recommended as methods to divert the melancholic. With this amazingly humane attitude, there were, however, instances when the treatment was not always free of its vicious aspects; even in the best of the Greek temples, starving, chains, and flogging were advocated "because with these it was believed that when those who refused food began to eat, frequently the memory was also refreshed thereby."

There is a surprising paucity of data about the Roman era in reference to mental illness. Galen, a Greek who practiced in Rome, based his treatment on the teachings of his Greek predecessors. Other physicians of the Roman era treated mental illness by bleeding, purging, and sulfur baths.

With the collapse of Greek and Roman civilization, medicine, along with other cultural developments, suffered an almost complete eclipse. The treatment of mental illness was left to priests, and every sort of superstitious belief flourished. The insane were flogged, fettered, scourged, and starved in the belief that the devils that possessed them could be driven out by these means.

A few bright spots in this tragic picture were some monasteries or shrines where this technique of "exorcising" the evil spirit was performed by the gentle laying on of hands instead of the whip. Members of the nobility, self-appointed ascetics, and holy men of varying degrees of sincerity practiced this art, which at least was not physically cruel.

Out of this tradition and belief in the "holy" or "royal touch" arose several great shrines, of which the one at Gheel in Belgium is most famous. The legend behind the beginnings of this colony is worth telling. Sometime in the dim past there lived a king in Ireland who was married to a beautiful woman and who became the father of an equally beautiful daughter. The good queen developed a fatal illness, and at her deathbed the daughter dedicated herself to a life of purity and service to the poor and the mentally bereft. The widowed king was beside himself with grief and announced to his subjects that he must at once be assuaged of sorrow by marrying the woman in his kingdom who most resembled the dead queen. No such paragon was found. But the devil came and whispered to the king that there was such a woman—his own daughter. The devil spurred the king to propose marriage to the girl, but she was appropriately outraged and fled across the English Channel to Belgium. There the king overtook her and, with Satan at his elbow, slew the girl and her faithful attendants. In the night an angel came, recapitated the body, and concealed it in the forest near the village of Gheel. Years later five lunatics chained together spent the night with their keepers at a small wayside shrine near this Belgian village. According to the legend, all the victims recovered overnight. Here indeed must be the place where the dead girl, reincarnated as St. Dymphna, was buried, and here was the sacred spot where her cures of the insane were effected. In the fifteenth century, pilgrimages to Gheel from every part of the civilized world were organized for the mentally sick. Many of the pilgrims remained in Gheel to live with the inhabitants of the locality, and in the passing years it became the natural thing to accept them into the homes, and thus the first colony for the mentally ill, and for that matter the only one that has been consistently successful, was formed. In 1851 the Belgian government took charge of this colony of mentally ill persons. It continues to exist to the present day. Some 1500 certified mentally ill individuals live in private homes, work with the inhabitants, and suffer no particular restriction of freedom, except to refrain from visiting public places and from the use of alcohol and to report regularly to the supervising psychiatrist. In spite of the success of the Gheel colony and its great humanizing value, most attempts at duplicating it elsewhere have been complete or partial failures. The community mental health movement in the United States is, in a sense, an attempt to capture some of the values of community involvement demonstrated in Gheel.

Although the treatment of the mentally ill in the Middle Ages had little to recommend it, the period that followed was in some respects a great deal worse. When the church and the monastery gave up the care of the insane, it was gradually taken over by the so-called almshouse, the contract house, and the secular asylum. The more violent persons were placed in jails and dungeons. In the sixteenth century Henry VIII officially dedicated Bethlehem Hospital in London as a lunatic asylum. It soon became the notorious "Bedlam" whose hideous practices were immortalized by Hogarth, the famous cartoonist. There, keepers were allowed to exhibit the most boisterous of the patients for 2 pence a look, and the more harmless inmates were forced to seek charity on the streets of London as the "Bedlam beggars" of Shakespear's *King Lear.*

In those dark days of psychiatry, society was interested in its own self-security, not in the welfare of the insane. The almshouses were a combination of jail and asylum, and within their walls petty criminals and the insane were herded indiscriminately. In the seventeenth and eighteenth centuries the dungeons of Paris were the only places where the violently insane could be committed. Drastic purgings and bleedings were the favorite therapeutic procedures of the day, and "madshirts" and the whip were applied religiously by the cell keepers.

Superstition about mental disease took a horrible turn in the seventeenth century. God and Satan were still thought to be engaged in a ceaseless battle for possession of one's soul. The year after the *Mayflower* sailed into Plymouth Harbor, Burton published his classic work *Anatomy of Melancholy,* wherein he stated that "witches and magicians can cure and cause most diseases." To seek out and execute witches became a sacred religious duty. At least 20,000 persons were said to have been burned in Scotland alone during the seventeenth century. Small wonder that Cotton Mather precipitated the witch mania in Salem, since he was merely subscribing to the dogma of the day.

The political and social reformations in France toward the end of the eighteenth century influenced the hospitals and jails of Paris. In 1792 Philippe Pinel (1745-1826), a young physician who was medical director of the Bicêtre asylum outside of Paris, was given permission by the Revolutionary Commune to liberate the miserable inmates of two of the largest hospitals, some of whom had been in chains for 20 years. Had his experiment proved a failure, he might well have lost his head by the guillotine. Fortunately, he was right, since by his act he proved conclusively the fallacy of inhuman treatment of the insane. The reforms instituted by Pinel were continued by his pupil Esquirol, who founded no less than 10 asylums and was the first regular teacher of psychiatry. The Quakers, under the Brothers Tuke, had at this time established the York Retreat and effected the same epoch-making reforms in England.

In America, under the guidance of Benjamin Franklin, the Pennsylvania Hospital was completed in 1756. There the insane were still relegated to the cellar but at least they were assured clean bedding and warm rooms. Benjamin Rush (1745-1813), a prime humanitarian and the "father of American psychiatry," began his duties at the Pennsylvania Hospital in 1783. Subscribing in part to the lunar theory of insanity and inventing an inhuman restraining device called the "tranquilizer" but at the same time insisting on more humane treatment of the mentally afflicted, he stands as a prominent transitional figure between the old era and the new.

Most of the states were still without special institutions for mentally ill persons in the first quarter of the nineteenth century. The poorhouse or almshouse was still popular, but it invariably became a catchall for all types of offenders, and the mentally ill received the brunt of its manifold evils. Most shocking to people of today was the placing of the poor and the mildly demented on the auction block, where those with the strongest backs and the weakest minds were sold to the highest bidder, the returns from the sale being assigned to the township treasury.

About 1830 a vigorous movement for the erection of suitable state hospitals spread simultaneously through several states. The excellent results obtained by private institutions such as the Hartford Retreat, founded in 1818, probably served as an object lesson. Horace Mann took an enthusiastic interest in the plight of the mentally ill, and the advantages of a state hospital system were publicized to promote construction of such institutions. The first public psychiatric hospital in America was built in Williamsburg, Virginia, in 1773. Today it is known as the Eastern Psychiatric Hospital.

However, it remained for an asthenic, 40-year-old schoolteacher to expose the sins of the poorhouse. From that day in 1841 when Dorothea Lynde Dix (1802-1887) described the hoarfrost on the walls of the cells of the East Somerville jail in Massachusetts to the day when she retreated into one of the very hospitals she was instrumental in creating, she effected reforms that shook the world. She so aroused the public conscience that millions of dollars were raised to build suitable hospitals, and 20 states responded directly to her appeals. She played an important part in the founding of St. Elizabeth's Hospital in Washington, D.C., directed the opening of two large institutions in the maritime provinces of Canada, completely reformed the asylum system in Scotland and in several other foreign countries, and rounded out a most amazing career by organizing the nursing forces of the northern armies during the Civil War. A resolution presented by the U.S. Congress in 1901 characterized her as "among the noblest examples of humanity in all history."

By the middle of the nineteenth century the asylum, "the big house on the hill" surrounded by its landscaped park and topped by high turrets and senseless cupolas, became a familiar landmark in every state capital. In it mentally afflicted men and women lived and enjoyed a modicum of comfort and freedom from abuse. But to the general public it had a fortresslike appearance, and its occupants were a strange and foreboding lot. From this smug isolation the psychiatrist made no attempt to teach the public anything to ease their fear and horror of mental illness. As a matter of fact, the psychiatrist could not impart much information because he had little to give. Although such matters as management, housing, and feeding of mental patients were slowly attaining decent humanitarian standards, as late as 1840 there was no clear classfication of mental disorders, and a German teacher, Dr. Heinroth, was still advancing the theory that insanity and sin were identical. Not until 1845 when Griesinger published the first authentic textbook on mental disease was the position of psychiatry in relation to other medical sciences clearly defined.

Formal research into the cause and nature of nervous and mental disease gained impetus under the inspiration of Jean Charcot (1825-1893), the great French neurologist whose clinics attracted students from every country in the world. Toward the end of the nineteenth century much new knowledge was derived from the microscopic study of the brain and the introduction of laboratory methods. The development of outpatient departments for psychiatric care dates back to 1885, when persons suffering with incipient mental disease were treated at the Pennsylvania Hospital and, a few months later, at Warren in the same state.

In 1883 Emil Kraepelin (1856-1926), a professor of psychiatry in Germany, published the first edition of *Psychiatrie,* which in English translation changed the whole view of classifications of mental disorders in America. He classified human behavior on the basis of symptomatology and offered a description of dementia praecox. Eugene Bleuler (1857-1939), a psychiatrist from Zurich, elaborated the concept of dementia praecox and expanded it into schizophrenia in 1911.

The emphasis on prevention and recognition of early stages of mental illness was not made until the turn of the present century, when Clifford Beers entered on the scene. Having spent several years in various mental institutions as a patient, he emerged in 1907 to write his famous book *A Mind That Found Itself*. Being of a vivid, colorful temperament, he had unlimited enthusiasm, which he directed in founding the National Committee for Mental Hygiene. Under the momentum of his aggressive leadership the movement became worldwide and now has ramifications in the form of child guidance, prison psychiatry, vocational guidance, and other practical activities that are important to all concerned people.

Simultaneously with the mental hygiene program came the astounding contributions of Sigmund Freud (1856-1939), which revolutionized the orthodox concepts of the mind, proposed a new technique for exploring it, and brought psychiatry as a living subject to the attention of every intelligent man and woman. Psychiatry at last left its flying buttresses and ramparts and participated in everyday human activity.

Freud's formulations dealing with the dynamics of the unconscious mind have resulted in a deeper understanding of human behavior and a better approach to the treatment of personality problems and psychoneurotic disorders. Psychotherapy in all its many phases continues to be the core of many methods of treatment, and its techniques are being refined and improved with each succeeding year. Recently psychoanalysis has come under severe attack. Among other criticisms, it is viewed by some as being sexist in that the female is given the role accorded women in Vienna in the late 1800s. It also focuses entirely on the concept of the medical model in explaining mental illness.

Along with psychotherapy, successful attacks on mental disorders have been made by means of special physical remedies, testifying to the fact that present-day psychiatry is willing to use any measure that offers a promise to control or to relieve physical and psychological problems.

Outstanding was the introduction of malaria and other types of fever therapy in 1917 by Wagner-Jauregg (1857-1940), a psychiatrist in Vienna. This work was indispensable in the treatment of neurosyphilis before the advent of the antibiotics. This was followed by the discovery and isolation of the various vitamin principles and their remarkable effects on delirium and deficiency states such as alcoholism, pellagra, and polyneuritis.

During the third decade of the twentieth century came the unique shock method of treating schizophrenia with insulin, as introduced by Sakel. This was followed shortly by Meduna's treatment of mental depressions by the convulsion-producing drug pentylenetetrazol (Metrazol) and in 1938 by electroconvulsive therapy introduced by Cerletti and Bini. Finally, surgery entered the psychiatric field and boldly cut into brain substance, particularly in the region of the frontal lobe, to help allay some of the worst features of otherwise hopeless agitation and deterioration. This operation is called prefrontal lobotomy. The procedure has been almost totally rejected since a longitudinal study of recipients of this surgery disclosed the fact that the negative outcomes, including seizures, greatly outweighed the positive outcomes such as less socially destructive behavior.

The period during and after World War II brought outstanding developments that virtually made it a golden age for psychiatry.

Modern technologies brought countless conveniences, leisure, sanitation, immunity to infectious diseases, and freedom from heavy toil, but the challenging problems that remained were mental illness and the degenerative diseases. Hence there was a great resurgence of interest in mental disease. The gospel of mental health was communicated nationally through all media, including radio, television, magazines, newspapers, sermons, and lectures.

In 1946 the first National Mental Health Act became law. The enactment of this law greatly changed the care of the mentally ill in the United States. It supported the first broad-based national approach to the long neglected problems of mental illness and the promotion of mental health.

In 1956 the first of the many psychotropic drugs, chlorpromazine, was adopted for use in the care of the mentally ill. The effect these psychotropic drugs have had falls just short of miraculous. Under the influence of these drugs, particularly the antipsychotic agents, the atmosphere of disturbed wards changed from bedlam to an environment conducive to therapeutic interventions. Consequently, the morale and interest of all mental health workers greatly increased.

Action for Mental Health, the Report of the Joint Commission on Mental Illness and Health, was published in 1961. It was a study of the needs of the nation in relation to preventing and treating mental illness. Among other things, it stressed the need to use the therapeutic potential of all the health workers involved with mentally ill persons, especially nurses. The momentum created by this report eventually resulted in the passage of the Community Mental Health Centers Act in 1963 and the implementation of recommendations for community-based care. The focus of community-based care was not solely on the individual, but it was also on the creation of a community that promotes mental health. Despite the fact that 2 decades have elapsed since the passage of this act, most authorities believe it is too soon to accurately evaluate the efficiency and effectiveness of the community mental health movement.

Despite federal legislation in 1975 and the 1977 President's

Commission on Mental Health, most authorities believe that the change in national priorities in the seventh decade of the twentieth century resulted in little of substance being achieved in the care of the mentally ill. The period between 1946 and 1971 is seen to be the time when the best of American psychiatry developed. During those years the care of the mentally ill was brought into the mainstream of the health care in this nation. Much of the stigma and isolation that the mentally ill had suffered was reduced, innovative patterns of community-based mental health care emerged, and sophisticated research programs were mounted.

Despite the current pessimism, it is good for psychiatry to take pride in pointing to a fine record wherein a mere century has carried it out of the ignorance and mysticism of the days when the mentally ill were whipped regularly at the full of the moon to the present era of humane treatment in modern treatment centers where every facility for diagnosis and treatment is provided. In developing the therapeutic aspects of psychiatry, an all-important step forward was achieved with the introduction of professional nurses in all psychiatric hospitals and the placing of professional nurses at the head of the nursing staffs. This system, first introduced by Dr. Samuel Hitch in 1841 at Gloucester Asylum in England, has been instrumental in improving the care of the mentally ill, has engendered a better public attitude toward psychiatric treatment centers, and has done more than anything else to soften the atmosphere of tension and mystery that still lingers about the mentally ill individual.

DEVELOPMENT OF PSYCHIATRIC NURSING

The first school of nursing in a psychiatric setting was established at McLean Hospital in Boston in 1882, which was 9 years after the first schools of nursing in the United States had been founded. Up to this time poorly trained, nonprofessional workers had dominated the care of patients in psychiatric institutions. After McLean Hospital opened a school of nursing, many other hospitals that specialized in the care of the mentally ill followed its example. By 1917 41 mental institutions were operating training schools for nurses. Unfortunately, the standards for admission and graduation established by most of these schools were much lower than those of schools of nursing in general hospitals.

Beginning in 1906 nurse educators began to work toward establishing affiliations in psychiatric situations for students enrolled in schools of nursing in general hospitals. Today all programs that prepare registered nurses include some experience with individuals who are being treated in psychiatric treatment centers. Schools of nursing in psychiatric hospitals no longer exist. The clinical learning opportunities in psychiatric hospitals are now used for students of nursing enrolled in schools in general hospitals and in colleges. As a result of the preparation of nurses interested in the care of psychiatric patients, a struggle began with traditional caretakers for control of the nursing care in mental hospitals.

The practice of psychiatric nursing was initially limited to the application of medical-surgical principles to the care of the mentally ill. Little organized thought was given to the psychosocial aspects of the nursing care, although undoubtedly there were numerous mature, intelligent nurses who became aware of the fact that their interactions with clients had a therapeutic effect. The title of the first psychiatric nursing textbook, *Nursing Mental Diseases,* by Harriet Bailey* indicates that the focus of the nursing care was on the illness, not on the person. As long as physical care remained the focus, psychiatric nurses had little more to offer the physically well, but mentally ill, person than did the nonprofessional caretaker. On the other hand, in instances where the cause of the mental illness was physiologically based or where the treatment was somatic, the quality of care rendered by psychiatric nurses was generally superior to that given by the unprepared hospital attendant.

An event significant to the development of psychiatric nursing was the establishment in 1949 of the National Institute of Mental Health. The Institute was empowered to make grants-in-aid to the states, to fund training programs and demonstration projects,

---

*Bailey, Harriet: Nusing mental diseases, New York, 1920, Macmillan Publishing Co., Inc.

and to provide support for basic and applied research. The Mental Health Act of 1949 identified the need for training four groups of key mental health workers: psychiatrists, psychologists, psychiatric social workers, and psychiatric nurses. Graduate programs to prepare clinical specialists in psychiatric nursing were first funded in the mid-1940s by appropriations made possible by the Mental Health Act. This funding stimulated advanced education and research among psychiatric nurses so that many of today's nurse leaders in education were prepared through this mechanism. By 1980 over 60 graduate programs in psychiatric nursing had been established. Unfortunately, this funding was seriously reduced by the reorientation of the national government concerning the support of education for nurses that took place after the presidential election of 1972.

In 1947 McGraw-Hill Book Company published *Nurse Patient Relationships in Psychiatry* by Helena Willis Render. She was the first author to introduce the idea that the relationship the nurse establishes with the client has a significant therapeutic potential. This book stimulated much attention on the part of nurses concerning the potential therapeutic possibilities inherent in their work role in psychiatric settings. In 1952 G.P. Putnam's Sons published the book *Interpersonal Relations in Nursing* by Dr. Hildegard E. Peplau, an active nurse clinician and educator. This book in many ways revolutionized the teaching and practice of psychiatric nursing in this country. Dr. Peplau's theoretical framework provided a basis for the development of the therapeutic roles that nurses play in helping clients with emotional problems. The year following the publication of Dr. Peplau's book, a small book by Dr. Maxwell Jones, *The Therapeutic Community,* was released in the United States. Peplau's text focused on the therapeutic potential of the one-to-one-relationship; Jones's book emphasized the therapeutic potential of groups. It was not, however, until the widespread use of the psychotropic drugs rendered clients amenable to interpersonally based treatment modalities that psychiatric nursing began to take the form it has today, making use of the concepts originally proposed by Peplau and Jones.

In 1963 two new journals, *Perpectives in Psychiatric Care* and the *Journal of Psychiatric Nursing and Mental Health Services,* were published. These journals continue to provide a forum for the communication and discussion of issues specific to the current practice of psychiatric nursing. Thus they serve to advance the quality of psychiatric nursing practice while simultaneously supporting the development of a theory base through the republication of articles of timeless value written by pioneer psychiatric nurses.

By 1963 psychiatric nursing had truly come of age. It had moved into the mainstream of the nursing profession, instead of being adjunctive to the field of psychiatry. All schools of nursing were required to provide their students with learning experiences in the care of mentally ill persons; the practice of psychiatric nursing had moved away from managing the daily lives of mentally ill individuals to providing highly skilled therapy for individuals, families, and groups; and the body of knowledge foundational to the practice of psychiatric nursing was growing in geometric proportions.

The passage of the Community Mental Health Centers Act in 1963 has had a profound effect on the practice of psychiatric nursing. Because of the philosophy of the community mental health movement, the psychiatric nurse is no longer able to limit her interventions to the traditional individual and group modalities. She must also play a significant role in prevention through education and consultation for community groups, including mothers, teachers of young children, and other providers of care for children. First and foremost, the nurse must become skilled in community assessment, diagnosis, intervention, and evaluation. How well psychiatric nursing is going to be able to develop this expertise while still maintaining its professional identity is thought by some to be the challenge of the 1980s.

CONCLUDING STATEMENTS

1. Although the development of modern psychiatric nursing did not begin until 1882, the history of the development of psychiatry has significance for nursing.
2. With the collapse of the Greek and Roman civilizations the humane treatment of mental illness deteriorated markedly, and patients were flogged, fettered, scorged, and starved in

the belief that the devils that possessed them could be driven out by these means.

3. In the Middle Ages a technique developed that involved "exorcising" the evil spirit that was causing the patient to behave in a strange way. This was performed by a laying on of hands.
4. In England during the sixteenth century, keepers of the lunatic asylums, as they were called, were allowed to exhibit boisterous patients to the public for a small fee, and more harmless patients were forced to beg on the streets of London.
5. In Paris in the seventeenth and eighteenth centuries the insane were kept in dungeons.
6. In 1792 Philippe Pinel (1745-1826), director of the Bicêtre asylum outside of Paris, liberated miserable inmates of two of the largest hospitals for the insane, some of whom had been in chains for 20 years. This was the beginning of many reforms in the care of the mentally ill.
7. In 1756, in Philadelphia, the Pennsylvania Hospital was completed. It provided good custodial care for insane patients.
8. Benjamin Rush (1745-1813), who is known as the father of American psychiatry, began work at the Pennsylvania Hospital in 1783.
9. About 1830 a movement to erect suitable hospitals for the mentally ill swept the United States.
10. The first public psychiatric hospital in America was built in Williamsburg, Virginia, in 1773 and is still being used today under the name of the Eastern Psychiatric Hospital.
11. Dorothea Lynde Dix (1802-1887) was instrumental in effecting tremendous reforms in the care of the mentally ill in the United States. She played an important role in founding St. Elizabeth's Hospital in Washington, D.C.
12. Emil Kraepelin (1856-1926), a German psychiatrist, published the first edition of *Psychiatrie,* which in English translation changed the whole view of classifications of mental disorders.
13. Eugene Bleuler (1857-1939), a psychiatrist from Zurich, elaborated the concept of dementia praecox and expanded it into schizophrenia in 1911.

14. In 1907, Clifford Beers, a former mental patient, wrote *A Mind That Found Itself,* which revolutionized thinking about prevention and early recognition of mental illness.
15. Clifford Beers founded the National Committee for Mental Hygiene, which spearheaded the mental hygiene movement and initiated child guidance, prison psychiatry, and vocational guidance.
16. Although his theories are now under attack by some authorities, Sigmund Freud (1856-1939) revolutionized thinking about the mind and proposed a new treatment technique called *psychoanalysis.*
17. Electroconvulsive therapy was introduced in 1938 by Cerletti and Bini.
18. The National Mental Health Act of 1946 supported the first broad-based national approach to the long neglected problems of mental illness and the promotion of mental health.
19. In 1956 the first of the many psychotropic drugs, chlorpromazine, was adopted for use in the care of the mentally ill. Under the influence of psychotropic drugs the atmosphere of disturbed wards changed dramatically.
20. *Action for Mental Health,* published in 1961, stressed the need to use the therapeutic potential of all health workers involved with the mentally ill, especially nurses.
21. The Community Mental Health Centers Act of 1963 shifted the focus of mental health care from large publicly supported institutions to community-based centers.
22. In 1882 the first school of nursing in a psychiatric setting was established at McLean Hospital outside of Boston in recognition of the need for nursing care of the mentally ill. The practice of psychiatric nursing was initially limited to the application of medical-surgical principles to the care of the mentally ill.
23. The first textbook on psychiatric nursing was published in 1920 and was entitled *Nursing Mental Diseases* by Harriet Bailey.
24. The Mental Health Act of 1949 funded training programs for all members of the psychiatric treatment team. As a result,

advanced education and research among psychiatric nurses were greatly stimulated.

25. In 1952 the book *Interpersonal Relations in Nursing* by Hildegard E. Peplau was published, which revolutionized the teaching and practice of psychiatric nursing and provided the theoretical framework for the development of the therapeutic roles being practiced today.
26. In 1963 two journals devoted to the communication and discussion of issues specific to psychiatric nursing were first published.
27. The passage of the Community Mental Health Centers Act in 1963 has had a profound effect on the practice of psychiatric nursing.
28. The psychiatric nurse's role can no longer be limited to the use of traditional treatment modalities. Her role must also include a focus on prevention and community assessment, diagnosis, intervention, and evaluation.

Suggested sources of additional information

CLASSICAL

Angrist, Shirley S.: The mental hospital; its history and destiny, Perspect. Psychiatr. Care **1**:20-26, Dec., 1963.

Beers, Clifford: A mind that found itself, New York, 1948, Doubleday & Co., Inc.

Bockhoven, J.S.: Moral treatment in American psychiatry, New York, 1963, Springer Publishing Co., Inc.

Carty, Rita Cardillo, and Breault, Gretchen Clemento: Gheel: a comprehensive community mental health program, Perspect. Psychiatr. Care **5**:281-285, Nov.-Dec., 1967.

Deutsch Albert: The shame of the states, New York, 1948, Harcourt, Brace & World, Inc.

Grinker, Roy R.: Mid-century psychiatry, Springfield, Ill., 1953, Charles C Thomas, Publisher.

Leininger, Madeleine M.: Trends, issues and problems, Perspect. Psychiatr. Care **10**:11-20, Jan.-Feb., 1969.

Marshall, Helen E.: Dorothea Dix, forgotten samaritan, New York, 1967, Russell Sage Foundation.

Mereness, Dorothy: Problems and issues in contemporary psychiatric nursing, Perspect. Psychiatr. Care **2**(1):14-16, 1964.

Peplau, Hildegarde E.: Historical development of statement of some facts and trends, presented at the Working Conference on Graduate Education in Psychiatric Nursing, Williamsburg, Va., 1956 (mimeographed).

Thompson, Clara: Psychoanalysis; evolution and development, New York, 1950, Hermitage House.

CONTEMPORARY

Donaldson, Ken: Looking back, Ment. Hyg. **60**:5-9, Spring, 1976.

Goshen, Charles E.: The background of today's social psychiatry, Ment. Hyg. **55**:5-9, Oct., 1971.

Gregg, Dorothy E.: Hildegard Peplau: her contributions, Perspect. Psychiatr. Care **16**:118-121, May-June, 1978.

Lewis, Nolan D.C.: American psychiatry from its beginnings to World War II. In Arieti, Silvano, editor: The American handbook of psychiatry, vol. 1, ed. 2, New York, 1974, Basic Books, Inc., Publishers, pp. 28-42.

Liston, Mary F.: Educational issues confronting mental health nursing. In Leininger, Madeleine M., editor: Contemporary issues in mental health nursing, Boston, 1973, Little, Brown and Co., pp. 137-154.

Ramshorn, Mary T.: The major thrust in American psychiatry: past, present, and future, Perspect. Psychiatr. Care **9**:145-153, July-Aug., 1971.

Sills, Grayce M.: Historical developments and issues in psychiatric mental health nursing. In Leininger, Madeleine M., editor: Contemporary issues in mental health nursing, Boston, 1973, Little, Brown and Co., pp. 125-136.

Sills, Grayce M.: Hildegard Peplau: leader, practitioner, academician, scholar, and theorist, Perspect. Psychiatr. Care **16**:122-128, May-June, 1978.

Two hundred years of mental health care in America: Hosp. Community Psychiatry (entire issue), July, 1976.

Woloshin, Arthur A., and Dennis, Everette E.: The romance and rodomontade of comprehensive community mental health, Ment. Hyg. **54**:280-287, April, 1970.

OF PARTICULAR INTEREST

Leininger, Madeleine M., editor: Contemporary issues in mental health nursing, Boston, 1973, Little, Brown and Co.

This excellent book is a compilation of articles from nursing leaders on the topic of psychiatric nursing as it relates to the various social sciences.

Ujhely, G.: The nurse as psychotherapist: what are the issues? Perspect. Psychiatr. Care **11**(4):155-160, 1973.

In this article the author focuses on several important aspects of the role of the nurse as psychotherapist.

28

Impact of the law on the current practice of psychiatric nursing

- Methods of psychiatric admission
- Clients' rights
- Professional accountability
- Community accountability

Psychiatric nursing and the law both are primarily concerned with the behavior of human beings. Psychiatric nursing is concerned with assisting individuals, families, and community groups to achieve satisfying and productive patterns of living. The law provides rules for behavioral conduct to facilitate orderly social functioning while simultaneously protecting the rights of the individual. Thus psychiatric nursing and the law impact greatly on one another. The psychiatric nurse can practice effectively only if she is knowledgeable about the rudimentary principles of the law that concern the mentally ill, since she is accountable for providing care that is not only clinically sound but also protects both the society and the client. Many authorities believe that the psychiatric nurse can best fulfill this responsibility by assuming the role of client advocate. Thorner* states that the primary responsibility of the client advocate is to assist the client to learn about his rights and to protect and assert those rights within the health care context.

This chapter addresses those legal issues that are most likely to be encountered in the practice of psychiatric nursing in the hope that the psychiatric nurse can satisfactorily fulfill the client advocate role.

METHODS OF PSYCHIATRIC ADMISSION

The detention of persons considered to be mentally ill is permitted by law; however, laws differ from state to state. Wilhelm† emphasizes that the state is authorized to segregate and isolate those persons who psychiatrists find to be committable because of mental illness.

In 1953 the U.S. Public Health Service published the Draft Act Governing Hospitalization of the Mentally Ill on which states could model their commitment laws. The following distinctions were suggested:

1. Voluntary admission is to be characterized by the individual's admission and discharge via his own signature.

---

*Thorner, Nancy: Nurses violate their patients' rights, J. Psychiatr. Nurs. **14**(1):7-12, Jan., 1976.

†Wilhelm, Yvonne M.: A look at psychiatric commitment, Perspect. Psychiatr. Care **10**:49-86, March-April, 1971.

2. Involuntary admission is undertaken by someone other than the client.

The least restrictive manner of obtaining treatment for mental illness is voluntary admission. Since many mentally ill individuals lack insight concerning their behavior and will not seek hospitalization of their own will, voluntary hospitalization is not always possible. The psychiatric nurse must remember that it is a combination of overt behaviors and legal status, not a diagnostic category, that determines whether an individual can be treated voluntarily or involuntarily. Suicidal, violent, acute psychotic, and antisocial behaviors in persons unwilling to be treated commonly indicate the need for the person to be involuntarily admitted to a psychiatric treatment center.

There are two types of involuntary admissions that result in commitment. One is an *emergency commitment* for observation. The length of this hospitalization is limited, usually for 10 to 60 days. The other type of commitment is called *indefinite* or *regular commitment* and extends for an unspecified period of time, usually subject to periodic judicial review. When persons charged with crimes awaiting trial and defendants acquitted by reason of insanity are hospitalized against their will, this is a form of indefinite commitment called *criminal commitment.*

Generally only state facilities and some private psychiatric institutions admit persons on an involuntary status. Psychiatric units in general hospitals usually accept only persons who voluntarily choose to be treated. These units have often excluded individuals who have such poor impulse control that attempts to treat them on an unlocked unit would be dangerous for them and others. Such an admission policy permits treatment to be adapted to the needs of a select client population, defined largely on behavioral grounds and on the basis of willingness to accept treatment and hospitalization. There is no uniformity of commitment methods among the states, but no one can be deprived of his liberty without due process of law.

In general, the commitment proceedings consist of (1) application, (2) examination, (3) determination, and (4) detention if indicated. The action is initiated generally by relatives or friends, although any legally appointed officer of the law, members of charitable organizations, a public health official, or any private citizen may make the application, which will bring the matter to the attention of the proper court. In most states the court that settles matters of psychiatric commitment is the common pleas court or the probate court. Here the application is submitted, statements by interested parties are heard under oath, and all available information about the individual and his behavior is recorded.

Frequently the application must be accompanied by the certificates of one or more physicians. The judge may, however, appoint one or two physicians to conduct a psychiatric examination. Some states require that at least one physician must be a psychiatrist. The testimony of lay witnesses and of the examining physicians must be sufficient to convince a judge or jury that the person in question is potentially dangerous to himself or others and needs to be restrained and treated. If the court finds that the need exists for hospitalization, the individual is generally committed to a publicly supported psychiatric treatment center.

The issue of commitment is more than simply a legal and psychiatric question. Ideally, it is an issue of freedom of choice. Each nurse must decide whether to take a stand for or against commitment. It is imperative that psychiatric nurses know and understand the commitment procedures in the states in which they practice. Furthermore, they must work for the necessary legislative amendments that would facilitate appropriate reforms so as to fulfill the dictum *primum nil nocere*—we must minimize harm.

CLIENTS' RIGHTS

A right is the enjoyment of a privilege that is secured by law to a person. Mentally ill persons who are hospitalized may experience a double limitation on their rights—one created by the organization of the hospital system and the other created by their illness. While the individual's illness may limit him to some extent, the prejudging of his competency by the staff may be a greater obstacle. This may mean that a simple request, such as the right to make a telephone call to his home, is subject to interpretation, evaluation, and possible rejection if it is not deemed to be in the best interest of both the client and the hospital organization.

Thus a tension exists in all psychiatric institutions between the client's need to exercise his civil rights and the hospital's need to provide care in an effective and efficient manner. When the hospital's organizational needs take precedence over the client's treatment needs or his civil rights, dehumanization, frustration, resignation, and despair occur.

To protect the individual's rights and property, a guardian may be appointed by the court or by state authorities if it is proved that the individual is incapable of conducting his affairs. If the amount of property warrants the expense of guardianship or if necessary business involving such property is transacted, the guardian's responsibilities are not tivial. In some states this property guardian is called a conservator. A guardian is one who has direct responsibility for the individual's personal welfare. He is generally a near relative. He cannot confine the individual in an institution without permission or approval of the court but can dictate, within certain limits, the nature of the treatment, and he can sign a permit for a major operation. He may also have custody of the minor children of the individual if there is no relative who is capable of accepting this responsibility.

The wife or husband of a client, rather than the parents, is regarded as the natural guardian. Every guardian must give bond for the proper performance of his duties. At regular intervals the guardian is required to make an accounting of expenses and income. His first consideration must be the comfort of the client. The guardian is required to guard the client's welfare judiciously.

The law has defined certain rules for the control of human conduct, including protection from injury-producing situations. These rules have been developed from rights that pertain to each individual and may not be violated without legal repercussion, unless the individual consents to their invasion. The first 10 amendments to the U.S. Constitution, adopted in 1791, deal with human rights. Some of the rights included in these amendments are the freedom of speech, the right of protection from unreasonable search and seizure, the right to a speedy trial, and the right to due process of law before being denied life, liberty, or property.

A serious loss of civil rights was often the consequence of involuntary psychiatric commitment. As a result, in many states the committed person was not able to make valid contracts, vote, marry, or divorce. However, in almost all legal jurisdictions, legally committed individuals presently retain their constitutional and human rights, particularly those pertaining to their person, property, and civil liberties. Various rights have been listed in recent legislation, such as the following:

1. The right to keep clothing and personal effects
2. The right to communicate by telephone, to correspond, and to visit with persons outside the institution
3. The right to vote
4. The right to religious freedom
5. The right to enter contractual relationships
6. The right to make purchases
7. The right to make wills
8. The right to education
9. The right to habeas corpus
10. The right to be employed
11. The right to independent psychiatric examinations
12. The right to civil service status
13. The right to marry
14. The right to sue and to be sued
15. The right to retain licenses or permits established by law
16. The right not to be subjected to unnecessary mechanical restraint

Rubin states that

> When a person's freedom is abrogated or his civil liberties are denied him, this power should be exercised for compelling reasons, at the most propitious moment and for a minimum period of time. It should be clear that such power is exercised only if the person is mentally ill and *a danger to others or himself.* To compel another person for less than those reasons—as, for example to help them to do "good," or to tyrannize them because their behavior offends—is unsupportable.*

In 1973 the American Hospital Association published a Patient's Bill of Rights (see Appendix D). The rights of clients are only as secure as the dedication of nurses and physicians who have the authority to protect them. These professionals must re-

*Rubin, Bernard: Psychiatry and the law. In Arieti, Silvano, editor: American handbook of psychiatry, vol. 5, New York, 1974, Basic Books, Inc., Publishers.

alize that most judges believe that personal freedom takes priority over endeavors to promote mental health that limit this freedom.

In 1976 the American Nurses' Association (ANA) developed a Code for Nurses (see Appendix C). The code deals with issues of ethical nursing conduct. In developing the code, the ANA recognized that the recipients of health care have basic rights that must not be intruded on by those who provide service. It is the responsibility of the nurse to recognize and respect the client's dignity as a human being by protecting his rights.

In 1977 the President's Commission on Mental Health recommended that each state have a bill of rights for all mentally ill individuals. A copy of these rights must be displayed in all psychiatric settings, be given to each client using the facilities, and be explained in an easily understandable manner.

Ennis* states that clients are not always right, but disagreement between the client and professional raises the possibility that the professional is acting as an agent of the profession or state, rather than as an agent of the client. Each psychiatric nurse must examine her motivation in regard to her actions with clients.

Statements regarding clients' rights have evolved because of judicial disillusionment with the basic assumptions underlying the way mental health professionals have traditionally dealt with mentally ill individuals. It is imperative that judges and legislators continually reexamine the fundamental assumptions that have gone unchallenged throughout the years. Swan and Dipert† believe that the simple enactment of legislation about clients' rights is inadequate. Facilities with no internal structure to enforce rights are in a vulnerable position, because clients may be forced to go outside institutions, possibly to court, to see that their rights are protected. Nurses seeking employment in psychi-

*Ennis, Bruce J.: Emerging legal rights of the mentally handicapped. In Issac Ray Symposium: Human rights, the law and psychiatric treatment, Pittsburgh, 1974, University of Pittsburgh School of Law.

†Swan, Marlene, and Dipert, Dennis: A survey of the impact of a patients' rights law on state facilities in Indiana, Hosp. Community Psychiatry **30**(4):234, 237, April, 1979.

atric institutions must be certain that these facilities have the proper internal structure to protect the clients' rights.

Following is a discussion of some client rights that have particular applicability to the practice of psychiatric nursing.

The right to habeas corpus. The object of the right to habeas corpus is to ensure the speedy release of any individual who claims that he is being deprived of his liberty and being detained illegally. This fundamental right has not always been respected. Kenneth Donaldson, a client in a civil commitment case decided by the Supreme Court, was refused writs of habeas corpus 18 times during his 15 years of hospitalization before he finally won his chance to have a court hear his case.

The right to treatment. In 1960 Morton Birnbaum advocated the enforcement and recognition of the legal right of a mentally ill individual hospitalized in a public psychiatric institution to adequate medical treatment for psychiatric illness. Adequate treatment for the institutionalized mentally ill and mentally retarded is a constitutional right. The U.S. Second Federal Appeals Court and the Alabama Federal District Court have elaborated the following legal doctrines: (1) persons in custody for mental illness have a right to treatment, (2) they may not be held without treatment, and (3) treatment can be legally defined.

In 1971 the guardians of civily committed patients and some employees of Bryce State Mental Hospital filed a class action suit against the Commissioner of Mental Health, members of the Alabama Mental Health Board, and others *(Wyatt vs Stickney)*. The defendants were charged with providing inadequate treatment to approximately 5000 mentally ill persons. The court based its decision on the constitutional guarantee of a right to treatment. In 1972 the court issued an order that detailed criteria for adequate treatment: (1) a humane psychological and physical environment, (2) qualified staff in sufficient numbers to administer adequate treatment, and (3) individualized treatment plans.

The right to informed consent. If clients consent to treatment, their consent must be informed by staff explanation. It is important to understand what consent means. For a consent to be valid it must be based on adequate knowledge and information and must be given by a person who has the legal capacity to consent. Furthermore, it must be voluntarily given. A rapidly growing mental health doctrine requires that the clients be given specific and adequate information about the proposed treatment procedure. This is to include the administration of the treatment, its probability of success or failure, its risks and side effects, alternative treatment procedures, and the probable consequences of not receiving treatment.

It is the duty of the mental health professional to provide the necessary information whether or not the client requests it. The precise information given will depend on the nature, severity, and consequences of the proposed treatment. Szasz* believes that the risks of psychiatric treatment should be emphasized. The mental health professional misleads the client when the beneficial effects of a treatment are exaggerated, while the dangers of the treatment are minimized or withheld. If the client is injured, the mental health professional could be held responsible via malpractice or negligence claims.

The right to confidentiality-privacy. Confidentiality and privacy of information about the client must be respected. Hemelt and Mackert† state that the exchange of information about the client between health care centers does not reduce any of the requirements of the law to protect his privacy. The individual revealing information about the client's condition without authorization could be subject to legal difficulties. A lawsuit for invasion of privacy, liability, or slander is possible, depending on the facts of the situation and the type of information revealed.

Statutes that pertain to the confidentiality of psychiatric hospital records vary greatly among the states. Some statutes only prohibit disclosure of information about the client's diagnosis and treatment, while others prohibit disclosure of the fact of hospitalization. Most statutes permit disclosure to private physicians, welfare officials, police, and insurance companies. Some

---

*Szasz, Thomas: Law, liberty, and psychiatry, New York, 1968, Collier Books.

†Hemelt, Mary Dolores, and Mackert, Mary Ellen: A Nursing '79 handbook: your legal guide to nursing practice. II. Nurs. '79 **9**(11):57-64, Nov., 1979.

may permit disclosure to prospective employers. Other statutes prohibit disclosure to almost everyone, unless the person consents to disclosure.

The client should be told of the need to share information with other persons and agencies. He should be asked to sign the appropriate consent form.

Some states consider mental health professional-client communication, including nurse-client communication, as privileged. Four criteria are accepted for judging the appropriateness of privileged information:

1. The communication was given with confidence in its non-disclosure.
2. Confidentiality must be essential to the maintenance of the relationship.
3. The relationship must be one that, in the opinion of the community, ought to be zealously fostered.
4. The injury that would result to the relationship by disclosure of the communication must be greater than the benefit gained in winning litigation.

The unnecessary disclosure of confidential information is considered improper by law. A breach of confidence is considered to be the discussion of the client's confidential information with a third party. This type of unlawful disclosure may provide the client with a cause of action against the party revealing such information.

The right to independent psychiatric examination. Ennis and Emery* believe that arguments can be made in support of the client's right to have an independent psychiatric examination by a physician of his choice. Fairness or due process requires an independent judgment because the judgments made by mental health professionals in commitment proceedings may not be very reliable. If the state is allowed to use such testimony, the client should have the same right. Furthermore, the constitutional right to present witnesses may also necessitate that clients be allowed to chose expert witnesses. Ennis and Emery also believe that each

---

*Ennis, Bruce J., and Emery, Richard D.: The rights of mental patients, New York, 1978, Avon Books.

state should provide the client with sufficient funds to retain at least one expert witness.

The right to refuse treatment. An important basis of the right to refuse treatment is the constitutional right to privacy and personal autonomy. As long as the public health, safety, or morals remain unharmed, the courts will respect a client's decision to refuse treatment. Ford* states that "The constitutional origins of the right to refuse medication stem from a long-standing recognition by the courts that each person has a strong interest in being free from nonconsensual invasion of his bodily integrity. . . ."

In 1976 the Third Circuit Court of Appeals found at least three constitutional deprivations that may accompany the involuntary administration of medication *(Scott vs Plante).* The first involves the involuntary administration of psychotropic drugs, which affect mental processes and which may interfere with a person's First Amendment rights to freedom of speech and association. In the second, the person, even though committable, may retain the ability to consent to medical treatment. In the third, the court considered that the administration of involuntary medication may raise an Eighth Amendment issue concerning cruel and unusual punishment. The psychiatric nurse must be knowledgeable about these issues before forcefully administering medication that the client refuses. The consequence of such an action on the nurse's part could result in a charge of assault.

The right from unnecessary treatment or the right to least restrictive treatment. During his hospital stay, the client may become violent. Robitscher† states that the hospital is obliged to control him so that he does not harm others or himself. If a delirious postoperative patient were left unattended by an open window and jumped from it, the hospital would be considered negligent.

However, the right to restrain a client is a right limited only to the duration of real necessity. While no one would dispute

---

*Ford, Maurice D.: The psychiatrist's double bind: the right to refuse medication, Am. J. Psychiatry **137**(3): 332-339, March, 1980.

†Robitscher, Jonas B.: Pursuit of argument: psychiatry and the law, Philadelphia, 1966, J.B. Lippincott Co.

the right of hospital personnel to prevent a delirious individual from pulling out a catheter, in most situations the hospital personnel cannot interfere with the actions of a client. If, for example, he shouts obscenities but is not a threat to himself or others, hospital personnel cannot tie him down or lock him up. To commit such an act invites the risk of a suit for false imprisonment.

Some state laws have specified the type of physical restraints that may be used, including the consistency of the actual material from which the restraint is made. Psychiatric nurses must be mindful of such regulations. The restraint need not be physical; threats of force are sufficient cause for legal action. One who is physically restrained may have an action for battery. Alternatives for restraining clients must be considered. One such alternative is the provision of constant observation by nursing personnel. Nurses must also be aware that the issue of understaffing is not a suitable justification for the use of chemical or physical restraints. The issue of safety is the primary concern.

PROFESSIONAL ACCOUNTABILITY

Creighton* defines negligence as the omission to do something that a reasonable person, guided by ordinary considerations that regulate human affairs, would do, and the commission of an act as doing something that a wise and reasonable person would not do. Nursing malpractice has been defined by a California court as the neglect of the nurse to apply a degree of learning and skill in treating and caring for a client, which is customarily practiced in caring for and treating the sick. This definition also includes taking actions out of the realm of authorized nursing practice.

A *tort* is a legal wrong, injury, or damage committed on a person or property independent of a contract. A *contract* is an agreement between two or more parties. Not every agreement is a contract. In general, moral agreements, agreements of conscience, or

---

*Creighton, Helen: Law every nurse should know, Philadelphia, 1975, W.B. Saunders Co.

agreements involving social obligations are not classified as contracts.

When an individual becomes a psychiatric patient, he automatically contracts with licensed health care personnel, including the psychiatric nurse, for treatment. In such a contract both parties agree that the nurse will provide reasonable and prudent care for the client.

If this contract is violated, the client may initiate action to obtain a remedy for an injury to his rights. In this instance the client is referred to as the *plaintiff*. The psychiatric nurse, or *defendant,* is then required to answer and defend her action or be judged by default. A psychiatric nurse may be a defendant in a negligent tort. Under the law of negligent tort, the plaintiff must prove the following:

1. A legal duty of care existed.
2. The nurse performed her duty negligently.
3. Damages were suffered by him as a result.
4. The damages were substantial.

The majority of lawsuits in psychiatric nursing involve negligence in the observation of suicidal precautions, assistance in the administration of electroconvulsive therapy, and the reporting of information or lack of such reporting in regard to medications.

COMMUNITY ACCOUNTABILITY

By providing rules of behavioral conduct to facilitate orderly social functioning, the law not only protects the individual from society, but also society from the individual. Forensic psychiatry, which is a branch of psychiatry, is involved in the criminal justice system. Forensic psychiatrists are concerned with determinations of dangerousness, mental incompetency, and insanity.

Dangerousness

The body of law dealing with various crimes and their legal penalties, the Model Penal Code, has been promoting extended sentences for the dangerous. Numerous legal definitions of dangerousness have been used for the care and treatment of dangerous offenders. Rubin* believes that if fear of bodily harm from violent behavior could be reduced by being able to define, predict, and modify such behavior, the quality of life in the United States would be greatly improved.

The abnormal offender is defined in the Model Penal Code by having the psychiatrist demonstrate that the offender

1. Possesses a gravely abnormal mental illness
2. Has engaged in criminal conduct that has been characterized by a pattern of repetitive behavior or by persistent aggressive behavior with indifference to consequences
3. Is a serious danger to others as a result of the two above conditions

Special dangerous offenders are provided for in the Proposed Federal Criminal Code. Sentences of up to 25 years may be imposed on a number of special categories of persons, including the dangerous, mentally ill offender. This category requires the following:

1. The offender possesses a mental illness.
2. Such a mental condition makes the offender a serious danger to others' safety.
3. The offender committed a major crime such as murder, treason, a felony, or other crime as an instance of aggressive behavior without heed to the consequences.

It is evident that it is difficult to define and predict dangerousness. The psychiatrist is often in a dilemma by assisting in the determination of dangerousness. The process of making such a determination is often contrary to the physician-client relationship.

The doctrine of mental incompetency

Mental incompetency exists when the defendant, because of mental illness or other reasons, does not understand the object and nature of the proceedings against him. It may also mean that the defendant cannot comprehend his own condition in relation to

*Rubin, Bernard: Psychiatry and the law. In Arieti, Silvano, editor: American handbook of psychiatry, vol. 5, New York, 1974, Basic Books, Inc., Publishers.

the proceedings or for some other reason is unable to assist his lawyer in his own defense. If the defendant is deemed incompetent, all criminal proceedings are suspended and the state is denied the power to proceed against him. To prosecute an incompetent is to deny his right to due process of law. Psychiatrists are often given the responsibility for making decisions regarding competency.

The defense of insanity

In the seventeenth century, Sir Matthew Hale, Chief Justice of the Court of King's Bench, wrote, "Human beings are naturally endowed with these two great faculties, understanding and liberty of will. . . . The consent of the will is that which renders human actions commendable or culpable. . . . "* Hale elaborated that the choice of will or liberty presupposes an act of understanding to the knowledge of a thing or an action chosen by the will. Where there is a total defect in understanding, there is no free act of will. As a result, judges began to charge juries that a defendant was not to be held responsible for his actions unless he had the capacity to distinguish evil from good.

In May 1800, believing that he was commanded by God to sacrifice himself for the world's salvation, Manes Hatfield fired a shot at George III. Hatfield's counsel argued that although the defendant was not mentally ill, his delusion was truly characteristic of mental illness. The trial was stopped and the jury returned a verdict of not guilty by reason of insanity. In 1843 Daniel M'Naghten shot Daniel Drummond, Secretary to Prime Minister Robert Peel. The M'Naghten rule, a test of right and wrong, was developed as a result of the arguments and testimony.

Most American jurisdictions accepted the M'Naghten rule and began to supplement it with the "irresistible impulse test." This test states that the defendant must have had a mental disease that kept him from controlling his behavior. In 1962 the Ameri-

*Rubin, Bernard: Psychiatry and the law. In Arieti, Silvano, editor: American handbook of psychiatry, vol. 5, New York, 1974, Basic Books, Inc., Publishers, p. 872.

can Law Institute developed a Model Penal Code, which stated that "a person is not responsible for criminal conduct if at the time of such conduct, as a result of disease or defect, he lacked substantial capacity either to appreciate the wrongfulness of his conduct or to conform his conduct to the requirements of law."* This modification in the M'Naghten rule is accepted in most jurisdictions. The American Psychiatric Association favors the American Law Institute test because it allows psychiatric testimony to clearly describe the history, adaptation, development, and function of patients' behavioral processes and the results of other medical tests to evaluate the clinical symptoms of mental illness in relation to alleged criminal acts.

CONCLUDING STATEMENTS

1. The psychiatric nurse can practice effectively only if she is knowledgeable about the rudimentary principles of law that concern the mentally ill.
2. As a client advocate, the psychiatric nurse's primary responsibility is to assist the client to learn about his rights and to protect and assert those rights within the health care context.
3. It is a combination of overt behaviors and legal status, not a diagnostic category, that determines whether an individual can be treated voluntarily or involuntarily.
4. There is no uniformity of commitment methods among the states, but no one can be deprived of his liberty without due process of law.
5. Psychiatric nurses must work for the necessary legislative amendments that would facilitate appropriate reforms so as to fulfill the dictum *primum nil nocere*—we must minimize harm.
6. A right is the enjoyment of a privilege that is secured by law to a person.
7. Mentally ill persons who are hospitalized may experience a double limitation on their rights—one created by the orga-

*Rubin, Bernard: Psychiatry and the law. In Arieti, Silvano, editor: American handbook of psychiatry, vol. 5, New York, 1974, Basic Books, Inc., Publishers, p. 873.

nization of the hospital system and the other created by their illness.

8. The psychiatric nurse must be knowledgeable about a Patient's Bill of Rights published by the American Hospital Association in 1973.
9. The Code for Nurses developed in 1976 by the American Nurses' Association (ANA) deals with issues of ethical nursing conduct.
10. Psychiatric nurses seeking employment in psychiatric institutions must be certain that these facilities have the proper internal structure to protect clients' rights.
11. The following client rights have particular applicability in the practice of psychiatric nursing:
    a. The right to habeas corpus
    b. The right to treatment
    c. The right to informed consent
    d. The right to confidentiality-privacy
    e. The right to independent psychiatric examination
    f. The right to refuse treatment
    g. The right from unnecessary treatment or the right to least restrictive treatment
12. A tort is a legal wrong, injury, or damage committed on a person or property independent of a contract.
13. By virtue of the psychiatric client being in need of nursing care, the client and the psychiatric nurse have a contract in which both parties agree that the nurse will provide reasonable and prudent care to the client.
14. The law not only protects the individual from society, but also society from the individual.
15. Forensic psychiatry is concerned with determinations of dangerousness, mental incompetency, and insanity to promote orderly social functioning.

Suggested sources of additional information

CLASSICAL

Ginsberg, Leon H.: Civil rights of the mentally ill—a review of the issues, Community Ment. Health J. **4**:244-250, June, 1968.

Szasz, Thomas: Law, liberty, and psychiatry, New York, 1968, Collier Books.

Zilboorg, Gregory: The psychology of the criminal act and punishment, Westport, Conn., 1968, Greenwood Press, Inc.

CONTEMPORARY

Applebaum, Paul S., and Gutheil, Thomas G.: Drug refusal: a study of psychiatric inpatients, Am. J. Psychiatry **137**(3):340-346, March, 1980.

Cohen, R.J.: Malpractice: a guide for mental health professionals, New York, 1979, The Free Press.

Creighton, Helen: Law every nurse should know, Philadelphia, 1975, W.B. Saunders Co.

Crowder, John E., and Klatte, Ernest W.: Involuntary admission to general hospitals: legal status is not the same issue, Hosp. Community Psychiatry **31**(5):325-327, May, 1980.

Ennis, Bruce J.: Emerging legal rights of the mentally handicapped. In Issac Ray Symposium: Human rights, the law and psychiatric treatment, Pittsburgh, 1974, University of Pittsburgh School of Law.

Ennis, Bruce J., and Emery, Richard D.: The rights of mental patients, New York, 1978, Avon Books.

Ennis, Bruce J., and Friedman, Paul R., editors: Legal rights of the mentally handicapped, vol 1, Pittsburgh, 1973, Practicing Law Institute, The Mental Health Law Project-University of Pittsburgh School of Law.

Ford, Maurice D.: The psychiatrist's double bind: the right to refuse medication, Am. J. Psychiatry **137**(3):332-339, March, 1980.

Gonzalez, H: The consumer movement: the implications for psychiatric care, Perspect. Psychiatr. Care **14:**186, Oct.-Dec., 1976.

Greenblatt, Milton: Class action and the right to treatment, Hosp. Community Psychiatry **25:**449-452, 1974.

Gutheil, Thomas, Shapiro, Robert, and St. Clair, R. Lawrence: Legal guardianship in drug refusal: an illusory solution, Am. J. Psychiatry **137**(3):347-352, March, 1980.

Hemelt, Mary Dolores, and Mackert, Mary Ellen: A Nursing '79 handbook: your legal guide to nursing practice. II. Nurs. '79 **9**(11):57-64, Nov., 1979.

Hemelt, Mary Dolores, and Mackert, Mary Ellen: A Nursing '79 handbook: your legal guide to nursing practice. III. Nurs. '79 **9**(12):49-56, Dec., 1979.

Johnston, Robert, and Fraser, Margaret: Right to treatment, Ment. Hyg **56:**13-19, Summer, 1972.

Kaimowitz vs Michigan Department of Mental Health Civil Action, 73-19434-AW (Mich Cir Ct, July 10, 1973).

Knecht vs Gillman, 4882d 1136 (8th Cir 1973).

Kumasaka, Yorihiko: The lawyer's role in involuntary commitment-New York's experience, Ment. Hyg. **56:**21-29, April, 1972.

Leeman, Cavin: Involuntary admissions to general hospitals: progress or threat? Hosp. Community Psychiatry **31**(5):315-317, May, 1980.

Leeman, Cavin, and Berger, Howard S.: The Massachusetts psychiatric society's position paper on voluntary psychiatric admissions to general hospitals, Hosp. Community Psychiatry **31**(5):318-324, May, 1980.

Mackey vs Procunier, 477F2d 877 (9th Cir 1973).

Mancini, Marguerite: Nursing, minors and the law, Am. J. Nurs. **78:**124, Jan., 1978.

National Association of Mental Health Position Statement: Civil rights of mental patients, Ment. Hyg. **56:**67-69, Spring, 1972.

Nations, Wanda C.: Nurse-lawyer is patient advocate, Am. J. Nurs. **73:**1039-1041, 1973.

O'Connor vs Donaldson, 422 U.S. 563 (1975).

Padberg, Joan: Nursing and forensic psychiatry, Perspect. Psychiatr. Care **10:**163-167, Nov., 1972.

President's Commission on Mental Health: report to the president, vol. 1, Washington, D.C., 1978.

Reiser, Stanely J.: Refusing treatment for mental illness: historical ethical dimensions, Am. J. Psychiatry **137**(3):329-331, March, 1980.

Report of the task panel on legal and ethical issues: task panel reports submitted to the President's Commission on Mental Health, vol. 4, Washington, D.C., 1978, U.S. Government Printing Office.

Robitscher, Jonas B.: Pursuit of argument: psychiatry and the law, Philadelphia, 1966, J.B. Lippincott Co.

Robitscher, Jonas B.: Medical, moral and legal issues in mental health care, Hosp. Community Psychiatry **25:**446-448, 1974.

Robitscher, Jonas B.: The powers of psychiatry, Boston, 1980, Houghton Mifflin Co.

Rosner, S. Steven: The rights of mental patients—the new Massachusetts law, Ment. Hyg. **56:**117-119, Winter, 1972.

Rubin, Bernard: Psychiatry and the law. In Arieti, Silvano, editor: American handbook of psychiatry, vol. 5, New York, 1974, Basic Books, Inc., Publishers.

Scott vs Plante, 532F2d 939, 946 (3rd Cir 1976).

Stone, A.A.: Informed consent: special problems for psychiatry, Hosp. Community Psychiatry **30:**321-327, May, 1978.

Swan, Marlene, and Dipert, Dennis: A survey of the impact of a patients' rights law on state facilities in Indiana, Hosp. Community Psychiatry **30**(4):234-237, April, 1979.

Tancredi, Laurence R., Lieb, Julian, and Slaby, Andrew E.: Legal issues in psychiatric care, New York, 1975, Harper & Row, Publishers.

Thorner, Nancy: Nurses violate their patients' rights, J. Psychiatr. Nurs. **14**(1):7-12, Jan., 1976.

Weihofen, Henry, and Usdin, Gene L.: Who is competent to make a will? Ment. Hyg. **54:**37-43, Jan., 1970.

Wilhelm, Yvonne M.: A look at psychiatric commitment, Perspect. Psychiatr. Care **10:**49-86, March-April, 1971.

OF PARTICULAR INTEREST

Nations, Wanda C.: Nurse-lawyer is patient advocate, Am. J. Nurs. **73:**1039-1041, 1973.

This is an excellent article depicting the innovative role of nurse-lawyer. It is relevant for the beginning nurse in outlining pertinent legal issues in nursing and providing direction toward patient advocacy.

Stachyra, M.: Nurses, psychotherapy, and the law, Perspect. Psychiatr. Care **2:**200, Sept.-Oct., 1969.

This article addresses specific issues related to nurses practicing psychotherapy. It discusses various practice acts and suggests direction for changes in existing laws.

Issues influencing the future of psychiatric nursing

- Economic issues
- Social issues
- Identity issues
- Clinical issues
- Delivery system issues
- Educational issues

The last 20 years of the twentieth century will be a time of challenge for psychiatric nursing. The very existence of this health care specialty is in question, while simultaneously the potential for it to make a valuable and unique contribution to the welfare of society has never been so great.

This chapter is designed to highlight some of the major issues that confront psychiatric nursing. The nature of any issue is that solutions are not readily discernible. If they were, issues would not be present. Another characteristic of issues is the multiplicity of factors that interrelate to create an issue. However, whenever a discussion of issues is attempted, it becomes necessary to artificially separate each factor to facilitate discussion. Consequently, this chapter presents my view of those issues facing psychiatric nursing and does not purport to supply solutions. It is hoped that the reader's awareness of these issues will be increased whether or not the reader agrees with my analysis of them. As a result of an increased awareness, it is further hoped that the reader will be motivated to formulate her own concerns and develop a plan to address them.

ECONOMIC ISSUES

Not since the Great Depression of the 1930s has the U.S. economy been as influential a factor in shaping daily events as it is today. Unlike the depression when there was too little money available, we are currently living in a period of inflation where, in a sense, there is too much money available. The tragedy of inflation, however, is that despite the abundance of money, most persons are unable to attain or maintain the standard of living they desire because the cost of goods and services is also very high. Consequently, many individuals and families find themselves in a position where they have more income than ever before, but their expenses are also higher than ever before.

The economic issue of inflation is all pervasive. It is a direct or indirect factor that influences all other issues in psychiatric nursing. For example, the consumer who is faced with expenses equal to or greater than his income must establish priorities for the expenditure of the available funds. Often health care takes a low priority, particularly health care designed to promote health and prevent illness. Furthermore, health care providers are being called to ever greater accountability for the expenditure of their time. Unfortunately, it is not usually possible to prove that time spent in crisis intervention with an individual or family has prevented costly mental illness. At least, this expenditure of time cannot be compared to the administration of a parenteral diuretic, the results of which are quickly visible in the improved cardiopulmonary function of the recipient.

Psychiatric nurses, by the very virtue of their function, are highly vulnerable to the economic issue. As the reader is well aware, the crux of psychiatric nursing is believed to be the provision of corrective emotional experiences for clients. This process often manifests itself by the nurse's and client's engaging in such activities as walking or talking together, playing cards, or sitting silently with each other. It is understandable that the casual observer of these activities would raise questions as to their value. Psychiatric nurses must assume the initiative and responsibility for engaging in research that documents the efficacy of such approaches.

Economic constraints that result in demands for increased accountability also inevitably result in increased paperwork. Unfortunately, the persons required to do this paperwork are often those who least wish to do so—people prepared to function as clinicians. In addition, events that can be quantified, that is, reduced to numbers, are more easily accounted for than events that are not quantifiable. Take, for example, the difference between health counseling, which may take 30 minutes, and changing a Foley catheter, which may take 15 minutes. The latter intervention can be easily documented as to need, action taken, and results achieved, while the former may prove difficult to justify in terms of these criteria. Therefore the necessity for accountability has increased the value of activities that can be quantified and has devalued activities that cannot be easily translated into numerical values.

SOCIAL ISSUES

A major social trend that has had a direct impact on psychiatric nursing is the continued, organized effort of women to achieve social and economic equality. Since nursing is primarily a women's profession, changes in the status of women are closely intertwined with changes in the profession. No longer are women content to be dependent on men; no longer are nurses willing to be handmaidens to physicians. Women are demanding more education; nurses are becoming increasingly better educated. Women are demanding financial remuneration commensurate with their preparation and responsibilities; nurses are organizing and striking to receive salaries more closely reflective of their preparation and responsibilities.

An unfortunate but, it is hoped, temporary result of the women's movement is the tendency of young women to choose careers other than those traditionally associated with women, namely, teaching and nursing. While it is certainly desirable for all young people, both men and women, to have the opportunity to pursue careers for which they are best suited, it is unfortunate that many young women are dismissing nursing as a career merely because it has been historically associated with women.

A social phenomenon that is unprecedented is the self-help phenomenon. Consumers no longer believe that professionals necessarily know best. Popular magazines regularly feature articles about health issues, ranging from diet to human behavior. Self-help books are readily available on a wide range of subjects, and some that deal with human emotions have been best-sellers. The result of this phenomenon is a citizenry that is well educated about health matters and that consequently demands quality care at reasonable cost. The field of psychiatry, which less than a century ago was scorned, has now become demystified. The implication of this trend is that all mental health care professionals, including psychiatric nurses, are increasingly held accountable by consumers and cannot hide behind professional jargon and unexplained actions.

IDENTITY ISSUES

A major issue is the question of whether the psychiatric nurse is really a nurse like any other or whether by virtue of her specialty she has forfeited her identity as a nurse. This issue affects medicine as well as nursing and stems from two factors.

One factor underlying this issue is that, despite knowledge and verbalizations to the contrary, health care professionals still practice in a manner that perpetuates a dichotomy between the mind and body. In addition, knowledge and care of the body seem to be more valued by lay persons and professionals alike than knowledge and care of the mind. Perhaps this is the case because physiological functioning is better understood and more predictable than psychological functioning. Whatever the reason, the result is that when nurses or physicians choose to specialize in the care of the mentally ill, they run the risk of divorcing themselves from the mainstream of health care delivery. Some persons* have gone so far as to state that mental illness, as currently defined, is not an illness at all but rather a reflection of societal problems. Therefore preparation for the care of these persons should not be within the health care disciplines. When this issue is exacerbated by economic constraints, it is logical for the system to attempt to replace the psychiatric nurse with less expensive attendants or aides who can be trained in a short period of time to focus only on behavior and engage in many of the activities performed by a psychiatric nurse.

Research continues to document the fact that humans are holistic beings, that the the whole of the person is greater than the sum of his parts. Therefore health care that is directed only to the body or only to the mind is bound to be ultimately ineffective and at worst harmful. All health care professionals must have an in-depth knowledge of both the biophysical and the psychosocial sciences to practice effectively. Consequently, it is necessary for psychiatric nurses to remain knowledgeable about physiological as well as psychological precesses and to document the difference that this knowledge makes in the nursing care they give.

Another factor underlying the identity issue facing psychiatric nursing is role blurring. Before the advent of the phenothiazine derivatives, the roles of mental health care workers were more clearly defined. The nurse was primarily concerned with the

---

*See, for example, Szasz, Thomas: Myth of mental illness, New York, 1974, Harper & Row, Publishers.

client's activities of daily living, the psychiatrist focused on diagnosing and prescribing, the psychologist focused on testing and research, and the social worker had the client's family as her domain. Very little treatment occurred. When psychotropic drugs made clients more accessible to therapeutic interventions, all mental health disciplines began to claim these interventions as being within their scope of practice. The result was role blurring where members of all disciplines engage in individual, family, and group therapy. The question then arises as to what, if anything, differentiates the nurse from the physician, the psychologist, or the social worker? Psychiatric nursing must convincingly answer this question or run the risk of extinction.

CLINICAL ISSUES

The incidence of mental illness in our society is clearly on the increase. Factors such as economic pressures, changing moral values, and an increase in violent crimes all result from and contribute to a stress-laden life-style to which individuals and families must adapt. Intervention measures designed to promote mental health and to prevent mental illness are needed in addition to measures designed to treat those who are already mentally ill. Meeting the mental health needs of the citizenry constitutes an enormous challenge to society.

Most authorities acknowledge that the most cost-effective and best way to meet these needs is through programs geared to prevention. These programs are designed to alter the environment in a way that is conducive to better mental health or to helping individuals, families, and communities to increase and diversify their coping mechanisms. An example of the former is efforts directed toward decreasing violence on the streets; examples of the latter are Head Start programs, victim assistance programs, and self-help groups such as Recovery, Inc.

Although there is almost universal agreement that prevention of mental illness and promotion of mental health is the best route in terms of long-term goals, it is exceedingly difficult to document the effects of such programs in the short term. With a scarcity of resources, government and private agencies are less likely to allocate funds to such programs, feeling a need to concentrate limited resources on short-term, obvious problems, namely, the treatment of those already mentally ill.

Most major forms of mental illness are now viewed as chronic in the sense that the individual will always need a greater or lesser degree of supervision and care. With the advent of community mental health centers there was concomitantly great hope that the bulk of those persons requiring mental health care could be maintained in and benefit from care in the community. This hope was short-lived, however, as the "revolving door" syndrome developed. This syndrome is a phenomenon whereby persons receive intensive care through hospitalization, are discharged to the community where they may or may not continue to receive care, and shortly require hospitalization again wherein the cycle is again repeated. The response to the revolving door syndrome was initially a sense of failure on the part of mental health care workers and the system. That attitude has gradually shifted from a sense of failure to an acceptance of the chronicity of mental illness.

Whichever view turns out to be correct, it is obvious that major changes need to take place in the mental health care delivery system. Because of the enormity and severity of the problem, there is a need for the development of treatment modalities and intervention techniques that address large population groups. Traditional one-to-one, family, and even group interpersonally based treatment modalities are no longer viable as the main forms of intervention. These techniques have proved to be costly and, at worst, not necessarily therapeutically effective. In addition, these modalities clearly benefit only those who value feelings and thoughts, are verbally fluent, have financial resources, are highly motivated, and have the intelligence necessary to deal with the abstractions inherent in these treatment modalities. Obviously these criteria rule out large numbers of individuals as well as certain population groups such as cultural minorities, children, the elderly, and the poor. It is these groups in which there is the greatest incidence of mental illness and for whom we have the least understanding of its cause and the fewest effective means of treatment. While the need for change is well accepted by most mental health disciplines, there seems to be a paucity of ideas as to what changes can and should occur. Consequently, mental health workers are still being educationally and experientially prepared in the traditional modes of treatment while being told that in most instances their developing skills will be to no avail in solving the larger issues of the day.

What then is required? First and foremost, research must be instituted if reliable answers to these problems are to be found. Research needs to focus on the cause, prevention, and treatment of mental illness. This is easier said than done. Research regarding human behavior is substantively different from pure laboratory research in a variety of ways. First, there is a multiplicity of variables that are difficult if not impossible to control. In a laboratory, chemical elements can be isolated and then systematically combined with other elements one by one and the effects clearly observed. When dealing with human beings it is impossible to isolate a subject's personality from his intelligence or from his culture. Second, many laboratory experiments yield results in a relatively short period of time, at least within the lifetime of the researcher. In contrast, much behavioral science research is longitudinal in nature, requiring the observation and study of the subjects over a generation or two. In addition to the time and money involved, longitudinal research also runs the risk of incurring environmental changes that may affect the outcome, for example, a war.

A prime concern in behavioral research, perhaps the seminal issue, is the necessity felt in a democratic society to protect the rights of each individual. Therefore procedures involved in research as well as treatment are subjected to vigorous scrutiny and are not approved if there is any potential for harm to the persons involved. It is clearly unethical, for example, to create situations that are believed to produce schizophrenia in an effort to determine the cause of this tragic illness. Consequently, the best that behavioral research can show is a relationship between and among variables after the fact. Despite these obstacles, however, it is mandatory that society continue to support behavioral science research that is directed toward understanding the cause of mental illness and developing effective treatment modalities.

DELIVERY SYSTEM ISSUES

The philosophical basis of the community mental health movement was and still is seen as desirable. Not only is it more humane, but also it is more cost effective to maintain persons outside of institutions. While the society and the health care professions endorse the end result, it appears that little thought has been given to the changes that this would require in treatment methods and, therefore, in educational preparation of health care workers. Unfortunately, in too many instances the community mental health movement has meant little more than a change of setting: the same treatment philosophy and modalities have been moved from the institution to a decentralized center in the community.

Rather than solving any problems, this short-sighted approach has in many instances compounded existent problems and created new ones. Chief among these are the revolving door syndrome, the community disorganization resulting from scores of mentally ill persons with few or no resources being thrust into the streets, and the inadequate treatment received by the mentally ill. Another irony or paradox of the community mental health movement is the fact that the best prepared health care workers, including nurses, are slowly but steadily moving into the community as a result, in part, of a powerful attitudinal shift elevating the status of those working in the community and denigrating those who choose to work in institutions. Consequently, some authorities fear that the care of institutionalized, chronically and acutely ill persons will be left to the least well-prepared health care workers. This situation, it is feared, will result in such terrible treatment that the "back wards" of the late nineteenth and early twentieth centuries will be seen as model treatment settings in comparison. This view may be an overstatement of the reality, but there is no doubt that the potential for this situation to occur is great enough to warrant grave concern.

Another major delivery system issue is the geographical maldistribution of mental health care workers and treatment centers that tend to be clustered together in large urban areas, particularly on the East and West coasts of the United States. It is in these areas that professionals can receive not only appropriate financial remuneration, but also the intellectual, cultural, and social stimulation they desire. As a result, there are large groups of consumers who do not have geographical access to continuous mental health care.

As previously stated, mental health professionals continue to be educationally prepared in the traditional treatment modalities, so it is understandable that they choose to work with those clients who can benefit from these measures. Therefore, in addition to geographical maldistribution, there is also a disproportionately small number of mental health care workers who choose to work with the poor, including the inner-city poor, the educationally and culturally disadvantaged, minority groups, children, and the elderly. Since these groups represent the largest number of mentally ill, it should be clear that the mental health needs of this country are not being met. This situation is so serious that the U.S. Congress has directed the National Institute of Mental Health to fund only those training programs that address one or more of these target populations.

EDUCATIONAL ISSUES

The cost of higher education in this country is skyrocketing daily and therefore placing postsecondary education out of the reach of more and more people at a time when scientific and technological advances require increasingly more educational preparation for those who wish to make a societal contribution. This situation is particularly true for women and members of cultural minorities who are attempting to achieve equality, in part, through education. Consequently, a smaller proportion of black and Hispanic people and women are able to afford the cost of higher education, which in turn results in fewer health care workers from those populations that require the most health care.

Of great concern is the fact that there are fewer and fewer nurses who are choosing to work in psychiatric settings or to pursue a graduate education in this field. It is believed that the reasons for this are multiple and complex. Many psychiatric nurse educators, however, believe that a major contributing factor is the trend in undergraduate nursing programs to integrate content. This trend is a result of nursing's attempt to teach in a way that helps the student view the client holistically and to move away from the medical model that tends to segment clients according to the disease or illness from which they are suffering. While these goals are commendable, one unanticipated effect has been that some students of nursing do not have a specific learning experience with the mentally ill. Consequently, it becomes understandable that graduates of these programs are unlikely to choose psychiatric nursing as a field in which to work, and therefore the pool of persons who are interested in and qualified to pursue graduate education in psychiatric nursing is lessened. As with all other issues, the cyclical nature of this problem is evident in the fact that as fewer nurses become prepared at the graduate level there ultimately will be fewer psychiatric nurses prepared to teach, which in turn results in poorer preparation of beginning practitioners in psychiatric nursing, ending with fewer choosing to work in the area. Thus the cycle is complete and is set to repeat itself. Unless efforts are made to recruit qualified persons into psychiatric nursing, this health care specialty will die a natural death and need not fear extinction from external forces.

CONCLUDING STATEMENTS

1. The last 20 years of the twentieth century will be a time of challenge for psychiatric nursing.
2. The economic issue of inflation directly or indirectly affects all other issues in psychiatric nursing.
3. Psychiatric nurses must assume the initiative and responsibility for engaging in research that documents the efficacy of nurse-client activities that are designed to provide corrective emotional experiences for clients.
4. Economic constraints lead to demands for increased accountability, which leads to increased paperwork, which in turn leads to a valuing of activities that are quantifiable in nature. Therefore psychiatric nurses, by the very virtue of their function, are vulnerable to the economic issue.
5. The women's movement and the self-help movement are social issues that have direct relevance for psychiatric nursing.
6. Identity issues that affect psychiatric nursing include the psy-

chiatric nurse's identity as a nurse like all others and the role blurring among mental health professionals.

7. The incidence of mental illness in our society is clearly on the increase, and meeting the mental health needs of the citizenry constitutes an enormous challenge to society.
8. Major changes need to take place in the mental health care delivery system so that the treatment needs of large population groups can be met.
9. Despite the difficulties involved in behavioral research, it is mandatory that society continue to support behavioral science research that is directed toward understanding the cause of mental illness and developing effective treatment modalities.
10. Delivery system issues include the need for changes in treatment methods and in the educational preparation of health care workers. In addition, the trend toward the best prepared health care workers leaving the care of a hospitalized person to less well-prepared workers raises grave concern.
11. Geographical maldistribution of mental health care workers and treatment centers results in large groups of consumers who do not have geographical access to continuous mental health care.
12. Fewer and fewer nurses are choosing to work in psychiatric settings or to pursue graduate education in this field.
13. Efforts must be made to recruit qualified persons into psychiatric nursing.

APPENDIX

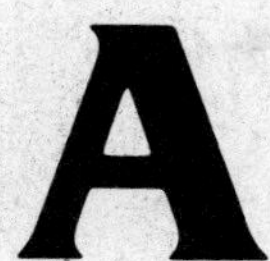

DSM-III Multiaxial Evaluation*

AXIS I: Clinical syndromes
Conditions not attributable to a mental disorder that are a focus of attention or treatment
Additional codes
AXIS II: Personality disorders
Specific developmental disorders

All official DSM-III codes and terms are included in ICD-9-CM. However, in order to differentiate those DSM-III categories that use the same ICD-9-CM codes, unofficial non-ICD-9-CM codes are provided in parentheses for use when greater specificity is necessary. The long dashes indicate the need for a fifth-digit subtype or other qualifying term.

*From American Psychiatric Association: Diagnostic and statistical manual of mental disorders, ed. 3, Washington, D.C., 1980, pp. 15-19, 27, 29-30. Reprinted with permission from the American Psychiatric Association.

DISORDERS USUALLY FIRST EVIDENT IN INFANCY, CHILDHOOD OR ADOLESCENCE

Mental retardation

(Code in fifth digit: 1 = with other behavioral symptoms [requiring attention or treatment and that are not part of another disorder], 0 = without other behavioral symptoms.)

317.0(×) Mild mental retardation, ______
318.0(×) Moderate mental retardation, ______
318.1(×) Severe mental retardation, ______
318.2(×) Profound mental retardation, ______
319.0(×) Unspecified mental retardation, ______

Attention deficit disorder

314.01 with hyperactivity
314.00 without hyperactivity
314.80 residual type

Conduct disorder

312.00 undersocialized, aggressive
312.10 undersocialized, nonaggressive
312.23 socialized, aggressive
312.21 socialized, nonaggressive
312.90 atypical

Anxiety disorders of childhood or adolescence

309.21 Separation anxiety disorder
313.21 Avoidant disorder of childhood or adolescence
313.00 Overanxious disorder

Other disorders of infancy, childhood or adolescence

313.89 Reactive attachment disorder of infancy
313.22 Schizoid disorder of childhood or adolescence
313.23 Elective mutism
313.81 Oppositional disorder
313.82 Identity disorder

Eating disorders

307.10	Anorexia nervosa
307.51	Bulimia
307.52	Pica
307.53	Rumination disorder of infancy
307.50	Atypical eating disorder

Stereotyped movement disorders

307.21	Transient tic disorder
307.22	Chronic motor tic disorder
307.23	Tourette's disorder
307.20	Atypical tic disorder
307.30	Atypical stereotyped movement disorder

Other disorders with physical manifestations

307.00	Stuttering
307.60	Functional enuresis
307.70	Functional encopresis
307.46	Sleepwalking disorder
307.46	Sleep terror disorder (307.49)

Pervasive developmental disorders

Code in fifth digit: 0 = full syndrome present, 1 = residual state.

299.0×	Infantile autism, ______
299.9×	Childhood onset pervasive developmental disorder, ______
299.8×	Atypical, ______

Specific developmental disorders
Note: These are coded on Axis II.

315.00	Developmental reading disorder
315.10	Developmental arithmetic disorder
315.31	Developmental language disorder
315.39	Developmental articulation disorder
315.50	Mixed specific developmental disorder
315.90	Atypical specific developmental disorder

ORGANIC MENTAL DISORDERS
Section 1

ORGANIC MENTAL DISORDERS WHOSE ETIOLOGY OR PATHOPHYSIOLOGICAL PROCESS IS LISTED BELOW (TAKEN FROM THE MENTAL DISORDERS SECTION OF ICD-9-CM).

Dementias arising in the senium and presenium

Primary degenerative dementia, senile onset,

290.30 with delirium
290.20 with delusions
290.21 with depression
290.00 uncomplicated

Code in fifth digit:
1 = with delirium, 2 = with delusions, 3 = with depression, 0 = uncomplicated.

290.1× Primary degenerative dementia, presenile onset, ______

290.4× Multi-infarct dementia, ______

Substance-induced
Alcohol

303.00 intoxication
291.40 idiosyncratic intoxication
291.80 withdrawal
291.00 withdrawal delirium
291.30 hallucinosis
291.10 amnestic disorder

Code severity of dementia in fifth digit: 1 = mild, 2= moderate, 3 = severe, 0 = unspecified.

291.2× Dementia associated with alcoholism, ______

Barbiturate or similarly acting sedative or hypnotic

305.40 intoxication (327.00)
292.00 withdrawal (327.01)
292.00 withdrawal delirium (327.02)
292.83 amnestic disorder (327.04)

Opioid

305.50	intoxication (327.10)
292.00	withdrawal (327.11)

Cocaine

305.60	intoxication (327.20)

Amphetamine or similarly acting sympathomimetic

305.70	intoxication (327.30)
292.81	delirium (327.32)
292.11	delusional disorder (327.35)
292.00	withdrawal (327.31)

Phencyclidine (PCP) or similarly acting arylcyclohexylamine

305.90	intoxication (327.40)
292.81	delirium (327.42)
292.90	mixed organic mental disorder (327.49)

Hallucinogen

305.30	hallucinosis (327.56)
292.11	delusional disorder (327.55)
292.84	affective disorder (327.57)

Cannabis

305.20	intoxication (327.60)
292.11	delusional disorder (327.65)

Tobacco

292.00	withdrawal (327.71)

Caffeine

305.90	intoxication (327.80)

Other or unspecified substance

305.90	intoxication (327.90)
292.00	withdrawal (327.91)
292.81	delirium (327.92)
292.82	dementia (327.93)

292.83	amnestic disorder (327.94)
292.11	delusional disorder (327.95)
292.12	hallucinosis (327.96)
292.84	affective disorder (327.97)
292.89	personality disorder (327.98)
292.90	atypical or mixed organic mental disorder (327.99)

Section 2

ORGANIC BRAIN SYNDROMES WHOSE ETIOLOGY OR PATHOPHYSIOLOGICAL PROCESS IS EITHER NOTED AS AN ADDITIONAL DIAGNOSIS FROM OUTSIDE THE MENTAL DISORDERS SECTION OF ICD-9-CM OR IS UNKNOWN.

293.00	Delirium
294.10	Dementia
294.00	Amnestic syndrome
293.81	Organic delusional syndrome
293.82	Organic hallucinosis
293.83	Organic affective syndrome
310.10	Organic personality syndrome
294.80	Atypical or mixed organic brain syndrome

SUBSTANCE USE DISORDERS

Code in fifth digit: 1 = continuous, 2 = episodic, 3 = in remission, 0 = unspecified.

305.0×	Alcohol abuse, ______
303.9×	Alcohol dependence (Alcoholism), ______
305.4×	Barbiturate or similarly acting sedative or hypnotic abuse,
304.1×	Barbiturate or similarly acting sedative or hypnotic dependence, ______
305.5×	Opioid abuse, ______
304.0×	Opioid dependence, ______
305.6×	Cocaine abuse, ______
305.7×	Amphetamine or similarly acting sympathomimetic abuse, ______
304.4×	Amphetamine or similarly acting sympathomimetic dependence, ______

	305.9×	Phencyclidine (PCP) or similarly acting arylcyclohexylamine abuse, _______ (328.4×)
	305.3×	Hallucinogen abuse, _______
	305.2×	Cannabis abuse, _______
	304.3×	Cannabis dependence, _______
	305.1×	Tobacco dependence, _______
	305.9×	Other, mixed or unspecified substance abuse, _______
	304.6×	Other specified substance dependence, _______
	304.9×	Unspecified substance dependence, _______
	304.7×	Dependence on combination of opioid and other nonalcoholic substance, _______
	304.8×	Dependence on combination of substances, excluding opioids and alcohol, _______

SCHIZOPHRENIC DISORDERS

Code in fifth digit: 1 = subchronic, 2 = chronic, 3 = subchronic with acute exacerbation, 4 = chronic with acute exacerbation, 5 = in remission, 0 = unspecified.

Schizophrenia

295.1×	disorganized, _______
295.2×	catatonic, _______
295.3×	paranoid, _______
295.9×	undifferentiated, _______
295.6×	residual, _______

PARANOID DISORDERS	297.10	Paranoia
	297.30	Shared paranoid disorder
	298.30	Acute paranoid disorder
	297.90	Atypical paranoid disorder

PSYCHOTIC DISORDERS NOT ELSEWHERE CLASSIFIED	295.40	Schizophreniform disorder
	298.80	Brief reactive psychosis
	295.70	Schizoaffective disorder
	298.90	Atypical psychosis

NEUROTIC DISORDERS

These are included in Affective, Anxiety, Somatoform, Dissociative, and Psychosexual Disorders. In order to facilitate the identification of the categories that in DSM-II were grouped together in the class of Neuroses, the DSM-II terms are included separately in parentheses after the corresponding categories. These DSM-II terms are included in ICD-9-CM and therefore are acceptable as alternatives to the recommended DSM-III terms that precede them.

AFFECTIVE DISORDERS

Major affective disorders

Code major depressive episode in fifth digit: 6 = in remission, 4 = with psychotic features (the unofficial non-ICD-9-CM fifth digit 7 may be used instead to indicate that the psychotic features are mood-incongruent), 3 = with melancholia, 2 = without melancholia, 0 = unspecified.

Code manic episode in fifth digit: 6 = in remission, 4 = with psychotic features (the unofficial non-ICD-9-CM fifth digit 7 may be used instead to indicate that the psychotic features are mood-incongruent), 2 = without psychotic features, 0 = unspecified.

Bipolar disorder

296.6× mixed, ______
296.4× manic, ______
296.5× depressed, ______

Major depression

296.2× single episode, ______
296.3× recurrent, ______

Other specific affective disorders

301.13 Cyclothymic disorder
300.40 Dysthymic disorder (or Depressive neurosis)

	Atypical affective disorders	
	296.70	Atypical bipolar disorder
	296.82	Atypical depression
ANXIETY DISORDERS	**Phobic disorders (or Phobic neuroses)**	
	300.21	Agoraphobia with panic attacks
	300.22	Agoraphobia without panic attacks
	300.23	Social phobia
	300.29	Simple phobia
	Anxiety states (or Anxiety neuroses)	
	300.01	Panic disorder
	300.02	Generalized anxiety disorder
	300.30	Obsessive compulsive disorder (or Obsessive compulsive neurosis)
	Post-traumatic stress disorder	
	308.30	acute
	309.81	chronic or delayed
	300.00	Atypical anxiety disorder
SOMATOFORM DISORDERS	300.81	Somatization disorder
	300.11	Conversion disorder (or Hysterical neurosis, conversion type)
	307.80	Psychogenic pain disorder
	300.70	Hypochondriasis (or Hypochondriacal neurosis)
	300.70	Atypical somatoform disorder (300.71)
DISSOCIATIVE DISORDERS (OR HYSTERICAL NEUROSES, DISSOCIATIVE TYPE)	300.12	Psychogenic amnesia
	300.13	Psychogenic fugue
	300.14	Multiple personality
	300.60	Depersonalization disorder (or Depersonalization neurosis)
	300.15	Atypical dissociative disorder

PSYCHOSEXUAL DISORDERS

Gender identity disorders

Indicate sexual history in the fifth digit of Transsexualism code: 1 = asexual, 2 = homosexual, 3 = heterosexual, 0 = unspecified.

302.5×	Transsexualism, ______
302.60	Gender identity disorder of childhood
302.85	Atypical gender identity disorder

Paraphilias

302.81	Fetishism
302.30	Transvestism
302.10	Zoophilia
302.20	Pedophilia
302.40	Exhibitionism
302.82	Voyeurism
302.83	Sexual masochism
302.84	Sexual sadism
302.90	Atypical paraphilia

Psychosexual dysfunctions

302.71	Inhibited sexual desire
302.72	Inhibited sexual excitement
302.73	Inhibited female orgasm
302.74	Inhibited male orgasm
302.75	Premature ejaculation
302.76	Functional dyspareunia
306.51	Functional vaginismus
302.70	Atypical psychosexual dysfunction

Other psychosexual disorders

302.00	Ego-dystonic homosexuality
302.89	Psychosexual disorder not elsewhere classified

FACTITIOUS DISORDERS	300.16	Factitious disorder with psychological symptoms
	301.51	Chronic factitious disorder with physical symptoms
	300.19	Atypical factitious disorder with physical symptoms

DISORDERS OF IMPULSE CONTROL NOT ELSEWHERE CLASSIFIED	312.31	Pathological gambling
	312.32	Kleptomania
	312.33	Pyromania
	312.34	Intermittent explosive disorder
	312.35	Isolated explosive disorder
	312.39	Atypical impulse control disorder

ADJUSTMENT DISORDER	309.00	with depressed mood
	309.24	with anxious mood
	309.28	with mixed emotional features
	309.30	with disturbance of conduct
	309.40	with mixed disturbance of emotions and conduct
	309.23	with work (or academic) inhibition
	309.83	with withdrawal
	309.90	with atypical features

PSYCHOLOGICAL FACTORS AFFECTING PHYSICAL CONDITION

Specify physical condition on Axis III.

316.00 Psychological factors affecting physical condition

PERSONALITY DISORDERS

Note: These are coded on Axis II.

301.00	Paranoid	301.82	Avoidant
301.20	Schizoid	301.60	Dependent
301.22	Schizotypal	301.40	Compulsive
301.50	Histrionic	301.84	Passive-Aggressive
301.81	Narcissistic	301.89	Atypical, mixed or other personality disorder
301.70	Antisocial		
301.83	Borderline		

V CODES FOR CONDITIONS NOT ATTRIBUTABLE TO A MENTAL DISORDER THAT ARE A FOCUS OF ATTENTION OR TREATMENT	V65.20	Malingering
	V62.89	Borderline intellectual functioning (V62.88)
	V71.01	Adult antisocial behavior
	V71.02	Childhood or adolescent antisocial behavior
	V62.30	Academic problem
	V62.20	Occupational problem
	V62.82	Uncomplicated bereavement
	V15.81	Noncompliance with medical treatment
	V62.89	Phase of life problem or other life circumstance problem
	V61.10	Marital problem
	V61.20	Parent-child problem
	V61.80	Other specified family circumstances
	V62.81	Other interpersonal problem

ADDITIONAL CODES	300.90	Unspecified mental disorder (nonpsychotic)
	V71.09	No diagnosis or condition on Axis I
	799.90	Diagnosis or condition deferred on Axis I

V71.09	No diagnosis on Axis II
799.90	Diagnosis deferred on Axis II

AXIS III: Physical disorders and conditions

AXIS IV: Severity of psychosocial stressors

Code	Term	Adult examples	Child or adolescent examples
1	None	No apparent psychosocial stressor	No apparent psychosocial stressor
2	Minimal	Minor violation of the law, small bank loan	Vacation with family
3	Mild	Argument with neighbor; change in work hours	Change in schoolteacher; new school year
4	Moderate	New career; death of close friend; pregnancy	Chronic parental fighting; change to new school; illness of close relative; birth of sibling.
5	Severe	Serious illness in self or family; major financial loss; marital separation; birth of child	Death of peer; divorce of parents; arrest; hospitalization; persistent and harsh parental-discipline
6	Extreme	Death of close relative; divorce	Death of parent or sibling; repeated physical or sexual abuse
7	Catastrophic	Concentration camp experience; devastating natural disaster	Multiple family deaths
0	Unspecified	No information, or not applicable	No information; or not applicable

AXIS V: Highest level of adaptive functioning during the past year

Levels	Adult examples	Child or adolescent examples
1 *SUPERIOR*—Unusually effective functioning in social relations, occupational functioning and use of leisure time.	Single parent living in deteriorating neighborhood takes excellent care of children and home, has warm relations with friends, and finds time for pursuit of hobby.	A 12-year-old girl gets superior grades in school, is extremely popular among her peers, and excels in many sports. She does all of this with apparent ease and comfort.
2 *VERY GOOD*—Better than average functioning in social relations, occupational functioning, and use of leisure time.	A 65-year-old retired widower does some volunteer work, often sees old friends, and pursues hobbies.	An adolescent boy gets excellent grades, works part time, has several close friends, and plays banjo in a jazz band. He admits to some distress in "keeping up with everything."
3 *GOOD*—No more than slight impairment in either social or occupational functioning.	A woman with many friends functions extremely well at a difficult job, but says "the strain is too much."	An 8-year-old boy does well in school, has several friends, but bullies younger children.
4 *FAIR*—Moderate impairment in either social relations or occupational functioning, or some impairment in both.	A lawyer has trouble carrying through assignments; has several acquaintances, but hardly any close friends.	A 10-year-old girl does poorly in school, but has adequate peer and family relations.
5 *POOR*—Marked impairment in either social relations or occupational functioning, or moderate impairment in both.	A man with one or two friends has trouble keeping a job for more than a few weeks.	A 14-year-old boy almost fails in school and has trouble getting along with his peers.
6 *VERY POOR*—Marked impairment in both social relations and occupational functioning.	A woman is unable to do any of her housework and has violent outbursts toward family and neighbors.	A 6-year-old girl needs special help in all subjects and has virtually no peer relationships.
7 *GROSSLY IMPAIRED*—Gross impairment in virtually all areas of functioning.	An elderly man needs supervision to maintain minimal personal hygiene and is usually incoherent.	A 4-year-old boy needs constant restraint to avoid hurting himself and is almost totally lacking in skills.
0 *UNSPECIFIED*	No information.	No information.

APPENDIX

B

ANA Standards of Psychiatric–Mental Health Nursing Practices*

STANDARD I Data are collected through pertinent clinical observations based on knowledge of the arts and sciences, with particular emphasis upon psychosocial and biophysical sciences.

STANDARD II Clients are involved in the assessment, planning, implementation and evaluation of their nursing care program to the fullest extent of their capabilities.

STANDARD III The problem solving approach is utilized in developing nursing care plans.

*From American Nurses' Association: *Standards of psychiatric–mental health nursing practice*, Kansas City, Mo., 1973, A.N.A. Reprinted with permission of the American Nurses' Association. The ANA booklet also contains the rationale and assessment factors for each standard.

STANDARD IV Individuals, families and community groups are assisted to achieve satisfying and productive patterns of living through health teaching.

STANDARD V The activities of daily living are utilized in a goal directed way in work with clients.

STANDARD VI Knowledge of somatic therapies and related clinical skills are utilized in working with clients.

STANDARD VII The environment is structured to establish and maintain a therapeutic milieu.

STANDARD VIII Nursing participates with interdisciplinary teams in assessing, planning, implementing and evaluating programs and other mental health activities.

STANDARD IX Psychotherapeutic interventions are used to assist clients to achieve their maximum development.

STANDARD X The practice of individual, group or family psychotherapy requires appropriate preparation and recognition of accountability for the practice.

STANDARD XI Nursing participates with other members of the community in planning and implementing mental health services that include the broad continuum of promotion of mental health, prevention of mental illness, treatment and rehabilitation.

STANDARD XII Learning experiences are provided for other nursing care personnel through leadership, supervision and teaching.

STANDARD XIII Responsibility is assumed for continuing educational and professional development and contributions are made to the professional growth of others.

STANDARD XIV Contributions to nursing and the mental health field are made through innovations in theory and practice and participation in research.

APPENDIX

C

The Code for Nurses (with interpretive statements)*

1. The nurse provides services with respect for human dignity and the uniqueness of the client unrestricted by considerations of social or economic status, personal attributes, or the nature of health problems.
2. The nurse safeguards the client's right to privacy by judiciously protecting information of a confidential nature.
3. The nurse acts to safeguard the client and the public when health care and safety are affected by the incompetent, unethical, or illegal practice of any person.

---

*From American Nurses' Association: Code for nurses (with interpretive statements), Kansas City, Mo., 1976. Reprinted with permission from the American Nurses' Association.

4. The nurse assumes responsibility and accountability for individual nursing judgments and actions.
5. The nurse maintains competence in nursing.
6. The nurse exercises informed judgment and uses individual competence and qualifications as criteria in seeking consultation, accepting responsibilities, and delegating nursing activities to others.
7. The nurse participates in activities that contribute to the ongoing development of the profession's body of knowledge.
8. The nurse participates in the profession's efforts to implement and improve standards of nursing.
9. The nurse participates in the profession's efforts to establish and maintain conditions of employment conducive to high quality nursing care.
10. The nurse participates in the profession's effort to protect the public from misinformation and misrepresentation and to maintain the integrity of nursing.
11. The nurse collaborates with members of the health professions and other citizens in promoting community and national efforts to meet the health needs of the public.

APPENDIX

D

A Patient's Bill of Rights*

1. The patient has the right to considerate and respectful care.
2. The patient has the right to obtain from his physician complete current information concerning his diagnosis, treatment, and prognosis in terms the patient can be reasonably expected to understand. When it is not medically advisable to give such information to the patient, the information should be made available to an appropriate person in his behalf. He has the right to know, by name, the physician responsible for coordinating his care.
3. The patient has the right to receive from his physician information necessary to give informed consent prior to the start of any procedure and/or treatment. Except in emergencies, such information for informed consent should include but not

*Reprinted with the permission of the American Hospital Association, copyright 1972.

necessarily be limited to the specific procedure and/or treatment, the medically significant risks involved, and the probable duration of incapacitation. Where medically significant alternatives for care or treatment exist, or when the patient requests information concerning medical alternatives, the patient has the right to such information. The patient also has the right to know the name of the person responsible for the procedures and/or treatment.

4. The patient has the right to refuse treatment to the extent permitted by law and to be informed of the medical consequences of his action.
5. The patient has the right to every consideration of his privacy concerning his own medical care program. Case discussion, consultation, examination, and treatment are confidential and should be conducted discreetly. Those not directly involved in his care must have the permission of the patient to be present.
6. The patient has the right to expect that all communications and records pertaining to his care should be treated as confidential.
7. The patient has the right to expect that within its capacity a hospital must make reasonable response to the request of a patient for services. The hospital must provide evaluation, service, and/or referral as indicated by the urgency of the case. When medically permissible, a patient may be transferred to another facility only after he has received complete information and explanation concerning the needs for and alternatives to such a transfer. The institution to which the patient is to be transferred must first have accepted the patient for transfer.
8. The patient has the right to obtain information as to any relationship of his hospital to other health care and educational institutions insofar as his care is concerned. The patient has the right to obtain information as to the existence of any professional relationships among individuals, by name, who are treating him.
9. The patient has the right to be advised if the hospital pro-

poses to engage in or perform human experimentation affecting his care or treatment. The patient has the right to refuse to participate in such research projects.

10. The patient has the right to expect reasonable continuity of care. He has the right to know in advance what appointment times and physicians are available and where. The patient has the right to expect that the hospital will provide a mechanism whereby he is informed by his physician or a delegate of the physician of the patient's continuing health care requirements following discharge.
11. The patient has the right to examine and receive an explanation of his bill regardless of source of payment.
12. The patient has the right to know what hospital rules and regulations apply to his conduct as a patient.

Glossary

The following words are frequently used by the psychiatric nurse. Many of the definitions were taken from *A Psychiatric Glossary.** A larger and equally useful book is the *Psychiatric Dictionary.*†

acting out Expression of unconscious emotional conflicts or feelings of hostility or love in actions that the protagonist does not consciously know are related to such conflicts or feelings.

addiction Strong emotional and physiological dependence on alcohol or a drug that has progressed beyond voluntary control.

affect A person's emotional feeling tone; affect and emotional response are commonly used interchangeably.

affective psychosis A psychotic reaction in which the predominant feature is a severe disorder of mood or emotional feelings.

aggression In psychiatry, a forceful attacking action (physical, verbal, or symbolic).

agitation State of chronic restlessness; psychomotor expression of emotional tension.

agoraphobia Fear of open spaces.

ambivalence Coexistence of two opposing drives, desires, feelings, or emotions toward the same person, object, or goal; may be conscious or partially conscious.

anxiety Apprehension, tension, or uneasiness that stems from the anticipation of danger, the source of which is largely unknown or unrecognized; primarily of intrapsychic origin, in distinction to fear, which is the emotional response to a consciously recognized and usually external threat or danger.

autism (autistic thinking) Form of thinking that attempts to gratify unfulfilled desires without due regard for reality; objective facts are distorted, obscured, or excluded in varying degrees.

autoeroticism Securing or attempting to secure sensual gratification from oneself as in masturbation; a characteristic of an early stage of emotional development.

blocking Difficulty in recollection or interruption of a train of thought or speech due to emotional factors usually unconscious.

brain syndrome A group of symptoms resulting from impaired function of the brain; may be acute (reversible) or chronic (irreversible).

*American Psychiatric Association, Diagnostic and Statistical Manual of Mental Disorders, Third Edition, Washington, D.C., APA, 1980.

†Campbell, Robert J.: Psychiatric dictionary, ed. 5, New York, 1981, Oxford University Press, Inc.

catatonia Type of schizophrenia characterized by immobility with muscular rigidity or inflexibility; alternating periods of physical hyperactivity and excitability may occur; generally there is marked inaccessibility to ordinary methods of communication.

cathexis Investment of an object or idea with special significance or value to the individual.

cerea flexibilitas The "waxy flexibility" often present in catatonic schizophrenia in which the person's arm or leg remains passively in the position in which it is placed.

cognitive Refers to mental processes of comprehension, judgment, memory, and reasoning.

compensation (1) Mental mechanism, operating unconsciously, by which the individual attempts to make up for real or fancied deficiencies; (2) conscious process by which the individual strives to make up for real or imagined defects in such areas as physique, performance, skills, or psychological attributes—the two types frequently merge.

complex A group of associated ideas that have a common strong emotional tone; these may be in part unconscious and may significantly influence attitudes and associations.

compulsion An insistent, repetitive, intrusive, and unwanted urge to perform an act that is contrary to the person's ordinary conscious wishes or standards; a defensive substitute for hidden and still more unacceptable ideas and wishes (anxiety results from failure to perform the compulsive act).

concept Mental image.

condensation Psychological process often present in dreams in which two or more concepts are fused so that a single symbol represents the multiple components.

confabulation Unconscious, defensive "filling in" of actual memory gaps by imaginary or fantastic experiences, often complex, that are recounted in a detailed and plausible way as though they were factual.

conflict Clash, conscious or unconscious, between two opposing emotional forces; if unconscious, an internal (instinctual) wish or striving is opposed by another internal and contradictory wish.

confusion Disturbed orientation in respect to time, place, or person; sometimes accompanied by disturbances of consciousness.

consciousness Clear awareness of self and the environment.

conversion Mental mechanism, operating unconsciously, by which intrapsychic conflicts, which would otherwise give rise to anxiety, are instead given symbolic external expression; the repressed ideas or impulses plus the psychological defenses against them are converted into a variety of somatic symptoms.

countertransference The therapist's conscious or unconscious emotional reaction to her client.

delirium Disturbance in thinking with disorientation and confusion; illusions, delusions, or hallucinations may be present.

delusion False belief out of keeping with the individual's level of knowledge and his cultural group; the belief is maintained against logical argument and despite objective contradictory evidence.

delusions of grandeur Exaggerated, unrealistic ideas of one's importance or identity.

delusions of persecution Unrealistic ideas that one has been singled out for persecution.

delusions of reference Incorrect assumption that certain casual or unrelated remarks or the behavior of others applies to oneself.

dementia Old term denoting madness or insanity; now used entirely to denote organic loss of intellectual function.

dementia praecox Obsolescent descriptive term for schizophrenia.

denial Mental mechanism, operating unconsciously, used to resolve emotional conflict and to allay consequent anxiety by denying some of the important elements; the feelings denied may be thoughts, wishes, needs, or external reality factors; what is consciously intolerable is simply disowned by the protectively automatic and unconscious denial of its existence.

dependency needs Vital infantile needs for mothering, love, affection, shelter, protection, security, food, and warmth; these needs may continue beyond infancy in overt or hidden forms or be increased in the adult as a regressive manifestation.

depersonalization Feelings of unreality or strangeness concerning either the environment or the self.

depression In the psychiatric sense, a morbid sadness, dejection, or melancholy; may vary in depth from neurosis to psychosis; to be differentiated from grief that is realistic and proportionate to what has been lost.

dereistic Describes mental activity that is not in accordance with reality, logic, or experience; similar to autistic.

disorientation Loss of awareness of the position of self in relation to space, time, or persons.

displacement A mental mechanism, operating unconsciously, by which an emotion is transferred or "displaced" from its original object to a more acceptable substitute object.

dissociation Psychological separation or splitting off; an intrapsychic defensive process, which operates automatically and unconsciously, through which emotional significance and affect are separated and detached from an idea, situation, or object.

dynamic psychiatry Psychiatry stressing the existence of mental forces that energetically demand expression; dynamic psychiatry implies the study of the active, energy-laden, and changing factors in human behavior, as opposed to the older, more static, and descriptive study of clinical patterns, symptoms, and classification.

dysarthria Impaired, difficult speech, usually due to organic disorders of the nervous system; sometimes applied to emotional speech difficulties such as stammering and stuttering.

ego Refers to the conscious self, the "I"; in Freudian theory, the central part of the personality that deals with reality and is influenced by social forces; the ego modifies behavior by largely unconscious compromise between the primitive instinctual drives (the id) and the conscience (the superego).

ego ideal That part of the personality which comprises the aims and goals of the self; usually refers to the conscious or unconscious emulation of significant persons with whom it has identified.

emotion Subjective feeling such as fear, anger, grief, joy, or love.

empathy Objective and insightful awareness of the feelings, emotions, and behavior or another person and their meaning and significance; to be distinguished from sympathy, which is nonobjective and usually noncritical.

euphoria Exaggerated feeling of physical and emotional well-being not consonant with apparent stimuli or events; usually of psychological origin, but also seen in organic brain disorders and toxic states.

exhibitionism Commonly, showing off; psychiatrically, body exposure, usually of the male genitals to females; sexual stimulation or gratification usually accompanies the act.

extroversion State in which attention and energies are largely directed outward from the self, as opposed to interest primarily directed toward the self as in introversion.

fabrication Relating imaginary events as true, not in the sense of lying but to cover up gaps in memory.

fixation Arrest of psychosexual maturation at an immature level; depending on degree, may be either normal or pathological.

flight of ideas Verbal skipping from one idea to another before the preceding one has been concluded; the ideas appear to be continuous but are fragmentary and determined by chance associations.

free association In psychoanalytic therapy, unselected verbalization by the person of whatever comes to mind.

free-floating anxiety Pervasive anxiety that the individual cannot explain to his own satisfaction.

functional mental illness Illness of emotional origin in which organic or structural changes are either absent or are developed secondarily to prolonged emotional stress.

general paresis A psychosis associated with organic disease of the central nervous system resulting from chronic syphilitic infection.

globus hystericus Sensation of having a ball in the throat; a hysterical spasm of the esophagus.

grandiose In psychiatry, refers to delusions of great wealth, power, and fame.

hallucination False sensory perception in the absence of an actual external stimulus; may be of emotional or chemical (drugs, alcohol, etc.) origin and may occur in any of the five senses.

homosexual panic Acute and severe attack of anxiety based on unconscious conflicts involving homosexuality.

homosexuality Sexual attraction or relationship between members of the same sex; active homosexuality is marked by overt activity, whereas latent homosexuality is marked by unconscious homosexual desires or conscious desires consistently denied expression.

hypnosis Altered state of conscious awareness induced in a suggestible subject; under hypnosis a person manifests increased receptivity to suggestion and direction.

hysteria Illness resulting from emotional conflict and generally characterized by immaturity, impulsiveness, attention seeking, dependency, and use of the mental mechanisms of conversion and dissociation.

id In Freudian theory, that part of the personality structure which harbors the unconscious instinctive desires and strivings of the individual.

ideas of reference Incorrect interpretation of casual incidents and external events as having direct reference to oneself; may reach sufficient intensity to constitute delusions.

identification Mental mechanism, operating unconsciously, by which an individual endeavors to pattern himself after another; plays a major role in the development of one's personality and specifically of one's superego (conscience).

idiopathic Term applied to diseases of unknown cause, for example, idiopathic epilepsy.

illusion Misinterpretation of a real external sensory experience.

incorporation Primitive mental mechanism, operating unconsciously, by which a person or parts of another person are symbolically ingested and assimilated; for example, infantile fantasy that the mother's breast has been ingested and is a part of oneself.

infantilism Applied to adults who are childish or mentally or physically immature.

inhibition Unconscious interference with or restriction of instinctual drives.

insight Self-understanding; a major goal of psychotherapy; the extent of the individual's understanding of the origin, nature, and mechanisms of his attitudes and behavior.

instinct Inborn drive; human instincts include those of self-preservation, sexuality, and (according to some authorities) the ego instincts and the herd or social instincts.

integration Useful organization of both new and old data, experience, and emotional capacities incorporated into the personality; also refers to the organization and amalgamation of functions at various levels of psychosexual development.

introjection Mental mechanism, operating unconsciously, whereby loved or hated external objects are taken within oneself symbolically; the converse of projection; may serve as a defense against conscious recognition of intolerable hostile impulses; for example, in severe depression the individual may unconsciously direct unacceptable hatred or aggression toward himself, that is, toward the introjected object within himself; related to the more primitive mechanisms of incorporation.

introversion Preoccupation with oneself, with accompanying reduction of interest in the outside world; roughly the reverse of extroversion.

involutional psychosis Psychotic reaction taking place during the involutional period, climacteric or menopause, characterized most commonly by depression and occasionally by paranoid thinking; the course tends to be prolonged, and the condition may be manifested by feelings of guilt, anxiety, agitation, delusional ideas, insomnia, and somatic preoccupation.

kleptomania Compulsive stealing, largely without any apparent material need for the stolen objects.

Korsakoff's psychosis (Korsakoff's syndrome) Disorder marked by disturbance of attention and memory, as evidenced by confabulation and by involvement of the peripheral nerves; may be due to alcohol, certain poisons, or infections.

labile Rapidly shifting emotions.

latency period In psychoanalysis, a phase between the phallic (or oedipal) and adolescent periods of psychosexual development; characterized by a marked decrease of sexual behavior and interest in sex.

libido Psychic drive or energy usually associated with the sexual instinct (sexual is used here in the broad sense to include pleasure and love-object seeking); also used broadly to connote the psychic energy associated with instincts in general.

lucid interval Period during which there is a remission of symptoms in a psychosis.

malingerer Conscious simulation of illness used to avoid a personally unpleasant or intolerable alternative.

manic-depressive psychosis Major emotional illness marked by severe mood swings alternating from elation to depression and a tendency toward remission and recurrence; depressed type is characterized by depression of mood with retardation and inhibition of thinking and physical activity; manic type is characterized by elation, overtalkativeness, extremely rapid ideation, and increased motor activity.

megalomania Syndrome marked by delusions of great self-importance, wealth, or power.

melancholia Pathological dejection, usually of psychotic depth.

mental mechanisms Also called defense mechanisms and mental dynamisms; specific intrapsychic defensive processes, operating unconsciously, that are employed to seek resolution of emotional conflict and freedom from anxiety; conscious efforts are frequently made for the same reasons, but true mental mechanisms are out of awareness (unconscious).

milieu The environment; the people and objects with which the individual deals.

mysophobia Morbid fear of dirt, germs, or contamination.

narcissism Self-love; in a broader sense indicates a degree of self-interest normal in early childhood but pathological when seen in similar degree in adulthood.

narcolepsy Condition in which the individual is overcome by short irresistible periods of sleep.

negative feelings As used in psychiatry, refers to hostile, unfriendly feelings.

negativism Perverse opposition and resistance to suggestions or advice; often observed in people who subjectively feel "pushed around."

neologism In psychiatry, new word or condensed combination of several words coined by a client to express a highly complex meaning related to his conflicts; not readily understood by others; common in schizophrenia.

nihilism In psychiatry, refers to the delusion of nonexistence of the self or part of self.

obsession Persistent, unwanted idea or impulse that cannot be eliminated by usual logic or reasoning.

oral erotism Pleasurable sensation obtained from the mouth; first experienced in suckling at the breast; later modified and sublimated but still persisting, as in kissing.

oral stage Includes both the oral-erotic and oral-sadistic phases of infantile psychosexual development, lasting from birth to 12 months or longer; oral-erotic phase is the initial pleasurable experience of nursing; oral-sadistic phase is the subsequent aggressive (biting) phase; both erotism and sadism normally continue in later life in disguised and sublimated forms.

orientation Awareness of oneself in relation to time, place, and person.

orthopsychiatry Psychiatry concerned with the study of children; emphasis is placed on preventive techniques to promote normal, healthy emotional growth and development.

overcompensation Conscious or unconscious process by which a real or fancied physical or psychological deficit inspires exaggerated correction.

panic In psychiatry, refers to an attack of acute, intense, and overwhelming anxiety, accompanied by a considerable degree of personality disorganization.

paranoia Psychotic disorder that develops slowly and becomes chronic; characterized by an intricate and internally logical system of persecutory or grandiose delusions, or both; stands by itself and does not interfere with the remainder of the personality, which continues essentially normal and apparently intact; to be distinguished from paranoid schizophrenic reactions and paranoid states.

penis envy Literally, envy by the female of the penis of the male; more generally, the female's wish for male attributes, position, or advantages; believed by many to be a significant factor in female character development.

perversion Substitution of another aim for the usual aim in any activity; usually related to sexual activity when a component of sex or an earlier stage of sexual development is substituted for normal coitus.

phallic stage Period of psychosexual development from the age of about $2^1/_2$ to 6 years during which sexual interest, curiosity, and pleasurable experience center about the penis and, in girls, to a lesser extent, the clitoris.

phobia Obsessive, persistent, unrealistic fear of an external object or situation such as heights, open spaces, dirt, and animals; fear believed to arise through a process of displacing an internal (unconscious) conflict to an external object symbolically related to the conflict.

pleasure principle Basic psychoanalytic concept that humans instinctually seek to avoid pain and discomfort and strive for gratification and pleasure; in personality development theories, the pleasure principle antedates and subsequently comes in conflict with the reality principle.

preconscious Referring to thoughts that are not in immediate awareness but that can be recalled by conscious effort.

projection Mental mechanism, operating unconsciously, whereby that which is emotionally unacceptable in the self is unconsciously rejected and attributed (projected) to others.

psyche The mind, in distinction to the soma, or body.

psychodynamics The systematized knowledge and theory of human behavior and its motivation, the study of which depends largely on the functional significance of emotion; psychodynamics recognizes the role of unconscious motivation in human behavior; a predictive science, based on the assumption that a person's total makeup and probable reactions at any given moment are the product of past interactions between his specific genetic endowment and the environment in which he has lived from conception onward.

psychogenesis Production or causation of a symptom or illness by mental or psychic factors as opposed to organic ones.

psychosexual development The changes and stages that characterize the development of the psychological aspect of sexuality during the period from birth to adult life.

pyromania Morbid compulsion to set fires.

rapport Confidential relationships between the client and the professional person who is in a helping relationship with him.

rationalization Mental mechanism, operating unconsciously, by which the individual attempts to justify or make consciously tolerable by plausible means those feelings, behaviors, and motives that would otherwise be intolerable (not to be confused with conscious evasion or dissimulation).

reaction formation Mental mechanism, operating unconsciously, wherein attitudes and behavior are adopted that are the opposite of impulses the individual disowns either consciously or unconsciously—for example, excessive moral zeal may be the product of strong but repressed antisocial impulses.

reality principle In Freudian theory, the concept that the pleasure principle in personality development in infancy is normally modified by the inescapable demands and requirements of external reality; the process by which this compromise is effected is technically known as reality testing, both in normal growth and in psychiatric treatment.

regression Partial or symbolic return to more infantile ways of gratification; most clearly seen in severe psychoses.

repression Mental mechanism, operating unconsciously; the common denominator and unconscious precursor of all mental mechanisms in which there is involuntary relegation of unbearable ideas and impulses into the unconscious from whence they are not ordinarily subject to voluntary recall but may emerge in disguised form through use of one of the various mental mechanisms; particularly operative in early years.

resistance In psychiatry, an individual's massive psychological defense against bringing repressed (unconscious) thoughts or impulses into awareness, thus avoiding anxiety.

Rorschach test Psychological test developed by the Swiss psychiatrist Hermann Rorschach (1884-1922), which seeks to disclose conscious and unconscious personality traits and emotional conflicts through eliciting the person's associations to a standard set of inkblots.

sadism Pleasure derived from inflicting physical or psychological pain on others; the sexual significance of sadistic wishes or behavior may be conscious or unconscious; the reverse of masochism.

schizoid Adjective describing traits of shyness, introspection, and introversion.

schizophrenia Severe emotional disorder of psychotic depth characteristically marked by a retreat from reality with the formation of delusions, hallucinations, emotional disharmony, and regressive behavior; formerly called dementia praecox.

sensorium Roughly approximates consciousness; includes the special sensory perceptive powers and their central correlation and integration in the brain; a clear sensorium conveys the presence of a reasonably accurate memory together with a correct orientation for time, place, and person.

soma The body; the physical aspect of a human as distinguished from the psyche.

somatic Bodily; having reference to the body or its organs.

stereotypy Persistent, mechanical repetition of an activity; common in schizophrenia.

subconscious Psychiatrically obsolescent; refers in general to both that which is not subject to recall and to that which may, with independent effort, be recalled.

sublimation Mental mechanisms, operating unconsciously, through which consciously unacceptable instinctual drives are diverted into personally and socially acceptable channels.

substitution Mental mechanism, operating unconsciously, by which an unattainable or unacceptable goal, emotion, or object is replaced by one that is more attainable or acceptable.

suggestibility Referring to a person's susceptibility to having his ideas or actions changed by the influence of others.

superego In Freudian theory, that part of the mind which has unconsciously identified itself with important and esteemed persons from early life, particularly parents; the supposed or actual wishes of these significant persons are taken over as part of one's own personal standards to help form the "conscience."

suppression Conscious effort to overcome unacceptable thoughts or desires by forcing them out of the conscious mind.

symbolization Mental mechanism, operating unconsciously, in which a person forms an abstract representation of a particular object, idea, or constellation. The symbol carries, in more or less disguised form, the emotional feelings vested in the initial object or ideas.

tardive dyskinesia A serious side effect of antipsychotic medication characterized by grimacing, choreiform, or athetoid movements of the arms, fingers, ankles, and toes, and tonic contractions of the neck and back muscles. At the present time it is irreversible.

toxic psychosis Psychosis resulting from the toxic effect of chemicals and drugs, including those produced in the body.

transference Unconscious attachment to others of feelings and attitudes that were originally associated with important figures (parents, siblings, etc.) in one's early life. The transference relationship follows roughly the pattern of its prototype; the therapist uses the phenomenon as a therapeutic tool to help the client understand his emotional problems and their origin; in the client-therapist relationship the transference may be negative (hostile) or positive (affectionate).

transvestism Sexual pleasure derived from dressing or masquerading in the clothing of the opposite sex; the sexual origins of transvestism may be unconscious.

unconscious In Freudian theory, that part of the mind or mental functioning the content of which is only rarely subject to awareness; a repository for data that have never been conscious (primary repression) or that may have become conscious briefly and were then repressed (secondary repression).

undoing Primitive defense mechanism, operating unconsciously, by which something unacceptable and already done is symbolically acted out in reverse, usually repetitiously, in the hope of "undoing" it and thus relieving anxiety.

verbigeration Stereotyped and seemingly meaningless verbal responses without relevance to the attempt of another to converse.

volition The will.

word salad Voluble speech in which words and phrases have no logical connection or meaning.

zones, erotic Regions such as the lips, breasts, and genitoanal area, stimulation of which causes erotic excitement.

Index